Modern System of Ophthalmology (MSO) Series

Disorders of
Uvea and Sclera

Modern System of Ophthalmology (MSO) Series

Disorders of
Uvea and Sclera

Editor-in-Chief

AK Khurana MS, FAICO, CTO (London)
Fellow, Moorfields Eye Hospital, London
Senior Professor and Head-II
Regional Institute of Ophthalmology
Pt BD Sharma Postgraduate Institute of Medical Sciences
Rohtak, Haryana

Editors

Jyotirmay Biswas MS, FMRF, FNAMS, FIC Path., FAICO
Director
Department of Uveitis and Ocular Pathology
Sankara Nethralaya
Chennai

Parthopratim Dutta Majumder
Consultant
Department of Uveitis and Intraocular Inflammation
Sankara Nethralaya
Chennai

Padmamalini Mahendradas MD
Head of Department of Uveitis and Ocular Immunology
Narayana Nethralaya
Bengaluru

Aruj K Khurana DNB, FICO
Fellow, Vitreo-Retina Services
Narayana Nethralaya
Bengaluru

Vishali Gupta MD
Advanced Eye Centre
Postgraduate Institute of Medical Education and
Research, Chandigarh

Bhawna Khurana MS, DNB, FICO
Fellow, Orbit, Oculoplasty and Oncology
Narayana Nethralaya
Bengaluru

Foreword by
Bhujang K Shetty

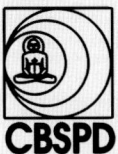

CBSPD

CBS Publishers & Distributors Pvt Ltd

New Delhi • Bengaluru • Chennai • Kochi • Kolkata • Lucknow • Mumbai
Hyderabad • Jharkhand • Nagpur • Patna • Pune • Uttarakhand

Modern System of Ophthalmology (MSO) Series

Disorders of
Uvea and Sclera

ISBN: 978-93-85915-24-6

Copyright © AK Khurana

First Edition 2016
Reprint 2024

Published by **Satish Kumar Jain** and produced by **Varun Jain** for

CBS Publishers & Distributors Pvt Ltd

4819/XI Prahlad Street, 24 Ansari Road, Daryaganj, New Delhi 110 002, India.
Ph: 011-23289259, 23266838   Website: www.cbspd.com
                                   e-mail: delhi@cbspd.com

Corporate Office: 204 FIE, Industrial Area, Patparganj, Delhi 110 092
Ph: 011-4934 4934   Fax: 011-4934 4935
                         e-mail: publishing@cbspd.com; publicity@cbspd.com

Branches

- **Bengaluru:** Seema House 2975, 17th Cross, KR Road, Banasankari 2nd Stage, Bengaluru 560 070, Karnataka, India
  Ph: +91-80-26771678/79   Fax: +91-80-26771680   e-mail: bangalore@cbspd.com
- **Chennai:** 7, Subbaraya Street, Shenoy Nagar, Chennai 600 030, Tamil Nadu, India
  Ph: +91-44-26680620, 26681266   Fax: +91-44-42032115   e-mail: chennai@cbspd.com
- **Kochi:** 42/1325, 1326, Power House Road, Opp KSEB, Power House, Ernakulum Kochi 682 018, Kerala, India
  Ph: +91-484-4059061-65,67   Fax: +91-484-4059065   e-mail: kochi@cbspd.com
- **Kolkata:** 147, Hind Ceramics Compound, 1st Floor, Nilgunj Road, Belghoria, Kolkata-700056, West Bengal, India
  Ph: +033-25633055, 033-25633056   e-mail: kolkata@cbspd.com
- **Lucknow:** Basement, Khushnuma Complex, 7 Meerabai Marg (Behind Jawahar Bhawan), Lucknow-226001, UP, India
  Ph: +0522-4000032   e-mail: tiwari.lucknow@cbspd.com
- **Mumbai:** PWD Shed, Gala no 25/26, Ramchandra Bhatt Marg, Next to JJ Hospital Gate no. 2, Opp. Union Bank of India, Noorbaug, Mumbai-400009, Maharashtra, India
  Ph: 022-66661880/89   e-mail: mumbai@cbspd.com

Representatives

• Hyderabad	0-9885175004	• Jharkhand	0-9811541605	• Nagpur	0-8692091830
• Patna	0-9334159340	• Pune	0-9664372571	• Uttarakhand	0-9716462459

Printed at   HT Media Ltd, Greater Noida, UP, India

Foreword

While writing foreword for this book, *"Disorders of Uvea and Sclera"*, one of the eleven volume series the 'Modern System of Ophthalmology, (MSO)', by Prof AK Khurana, I feel pleasure and proud that books by the Indian authors are being well accepted at the world scenario. In fact this excellent MSO series is concise yet comprehensive and is well serving the academic needs of residents in ophthalmology. The book comprises two parts, one each, devoted to 'Disorders of Uvea' and 'Disorders of Sclera'. The text on disorders of uvea has been very thoughtfully organized into four sections covering comprehensively the basic aspects, inflammations, degenerations and dystrophies, and tumours of uvea.

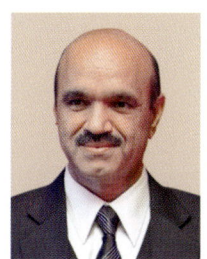

Dr Khurana has chosen, the dedicated ophthalmologists, Dr J Biswas, Dr Parthopratim, Dr Padmamalini, Dr Vishali Gupta, Dr Aruj K Khurana and Dr Bhawna Khurana as editors for this volume. I am delighted to know that three of the editors are from Narayana Nethralaya, Bengaluru. The contributors of different chapters are expert in the field and have included recent diagnostic and therapeutic modalities in the text matter. Further, the Editor-in-Chief has ensured that the text is in a lucid and easy to comprehend style and is supplemented with sufficient number of high quality clinical photographs, line diagrams, tables and flow charts.

I have known Dr AK Khurana as a highly sought after author whose books have been received with great enthusiasm by the undergraduate as well as postgraduate students. I am more than sure, like his other books, this volume of Modern System of ophthalmology (MSO series) will also serve as a highly useful resource for the residents and teachers in ophthalmology, as well as optometrists and general ophthalmologists alike. It will also serve as a handbook for fellows of uvea and retina. I congratulate and wish the entire editorial team and contributors a grand success for their wonderful endeavour.

Bhujang K Shetty
Chairman
Narayana Nethralaya
Bengaluru

Preface

Modern System of Ophthalmology (MSO) series comprises separate volumes on different subspecialties of ophthalmology. Each volume is planned with a very specific aim to cater to the needs of postgraduate students in ophthalmology.

Salient Features of MSO Series
- Each volume is edited by different editors, yet the layout and organization has been kept similar.
- Editors of different volumes are masters in their subspecialty with an uncanny knack of picking up the right perspectives.
- Text matter is designed to meet the needs of residents in ophthalmology with a comprehensive coverage in a concise manner. Text is complete and up-to-date with recent advances incorporated.
- Text is organized in such a way that the students can easily understand, retain and reproduce it. Various levels of headings, subheadings, bold face and italics given in the text will be helpful for a quick revision of the subject.

Disorders of Uvea and Sclera. Over the years uveitis has emerged as an important subspecialty in ophthalmology justifying the need for a simplified text on the subject. To make it a comprehensive volume on the disorders of uvea, even those disorders which are not dealt with by the uvea specialists, such as congenital anomalies and tumours of uveal tissue have also been included in this text. Further, since, uveitis and scleritis may co-exist not in frequently so disorder of uvea and sclera have been clubbed in this volume of MSO. An effort has been made in this volume to provide information on disorders of uvea and sclera keeping in view the requirements of trainee ophthalmologists in a more easily understood form. In a bid to simplify the text, at places the description looks more dogmatic than is warranted by the facts. This book has been organized into two parts: Part one: Disorders of Uvea, and Part two: Disorders of Sclera.

Part 1: Disorders of Uvea, has been arranged into four sections:

Section I: Anatomy, Physiology, Embryology and Congenital Disorders of Uvea, includes two chapters one on each aspect covered in this section.

Section II: Uveitis and Intraocular Inflammations, includes chapters one each on: Immune Mechanism, Etiopathogenesis and Pathology of Uveitis; Clinical Profile and Complications of Uveitis, (in this chapter different varities of uveitis have been described based on its anatomical classification, i.e. anterior, intermediate, posterior and panuveitis); Management of Uveitis; Infectious Uveitis (organized into various sub-chapters based on causative agents); Non-infectious Uveitis (includes sub-chapters on uveitis caused by known non-infectious agents and the idiopathic specific uveitis syndromes); Masquerade Syndrome; Retinal Vasculitis; and Post-Surgical Uveitis; Endophthalmitis and Panophthalmitis.

Section III: Degenerations and Dystrophies of Uvea, includes a chapter each on degenerations and dystrophies of iris, and choroid, respectively.

Section IV: Tumours of Uvea, includes a chapter devoted to tumours of iris, ciliary body, and choroid.

Part 2: Disorders of Sclera. This part has been organised into three chapters, one each on Anatomy and Physiology of Sclera, Inflammations of Sclera, and Staphylomas and Miscellaneous Scleral Conditions.

Editors of this volume Dr J Biswas, and Dr Parthopratim Dutt Majumder, from Sankara Nethralaya, Chennai, Dr Padmamalini Mahendradas from Narayana Nethralaya, Bengaluru and Dr Vishali Gupta from Advanced Eye Centre, PGIMER, Chandigarh are renownd uvea specialists. Dr Aruj K Khurana, trained at Sankara Nethralaya, Chennai and Narayana Nethralaya, Bengaluru has special interest in disorders of vitreo-retina and uvea. Dr Bhawana Khurana trained at Guru Nanak Eye Centre, MAMC, New Delhi and Narayana Nethralaya Bengaluru is keenly associated with the MSO series. This volume is outcome of hard work of the dedicated masters in this field.

Acknowledgement needs to be made to the selfless contributors of chapters for this volume and all others who have made this volume a reality. My sincere thanks are due to all of them. I want to express my gratitude to Prof CS Dhull, Head RIO, PGIMS, Prof Rakesh Gupta, Director, PGIMS, and Prof OP Kalra, Vice-Chancellor, UHS, Rohtak, for providing an atmosphere conducive to such academic activities. It is my pleasure to acknowledge the role of personalities namely Dr SS Badrinath, President Sankara Nethralaya, Chennai, Dr Bhujang Shetty, Chairman Narayana Nethralaya, Bengaluru, Dr Naresh Yadav, Head Vitreo-Retinal Services, Narayana Nethralaya, Bengaluru for their role in grooming the editorial team at some level.

The affection and moral support, in addition to editorial help, rendered by my wife Dr Indu Khurana, Senior Professor and Head, Department of Physiology, PGIMS, Rohtak, my daughter, Dr Arushi, MD, University of Connecticut, USA, and my son-in-law Dr Gurukripa Kowlgi, MD, University of Connecticut, USA, made my task untiring. My special thanks are due to dear friends, Prof R C Nagpal, Prof Amood Gupta, Prof Amar Agarwal, Dr MPS Sachdev, Prof S Sood, Dr Bhujang Shetty, Dr Rohit Shetty, Major General DP Vatas, Prof GS Bajwa, Prof Atul Kumar, Prof VP Gupta, Prof Vishnu Gupta, Prof BP Guliani, Prof MR Dogra, Prof Jagat Ram, and Prof KP Chaudhri, for their guidance and encouragement. I acknowledge with humble thanks, the respect, affection and cooperation received from faculty members of RIO, PGIMS, Rohtak, namely Dr SV Singh, Dr JP Chugh, Dr VK Dhull, Dr RS Chauhan, Dr Manisha Rathi, Dr Neebha Passi, Dr Manisha Nada, Dr Urmil Chawla, Dr Ashok Rathi, Dr Sumit Sachdeva, Dr Jitender Phogat and Dr Reena Gupta. I also acknowledge the enormous help received from Dr Shweta Goel and other residents of RIO, PGIMS, Rohtak. The enthusiastic co-operation received from Mr SK Jain, Managing Director, Mr YN Arjuna, Senior Director Publishing, Editorial and Publicity, and Mrs Ritu Chawla, Manager Production, CBS Publishers & Distributors, New Delhi, needs special acknowledgement. Mr Sanju, graphic artist, and Mrs Jyoti Kaur, DTP operator, need special mention because of their efforts to provide considerable beauty to this volume. In spite of the best efforts, a venture like this is unlikely to be error-free. Constructive criticism and suggestions from the readers are invited for further improvement in this volume.

AK Khurana
Editor-in-Chief

Editorial Board

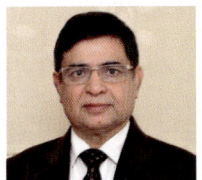
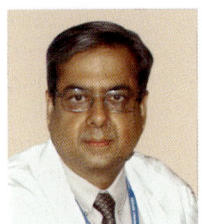
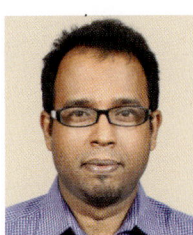
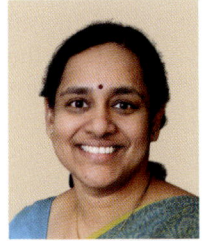
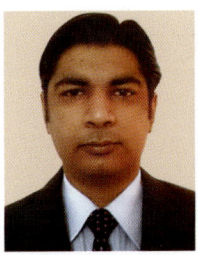
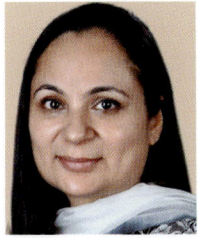
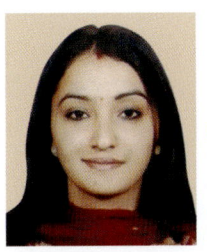

List of Contributors

AK Khurana MS, CTO (London)
Senior Professor
Regional Institute of Ophthalmology
Pt BD Sharma Postgraduate Institute of Medical
Sciences
Rohtak, Haryana

Parthopratim Dutta Majumder
Consultant, Department of Uveitis
and Intraocular Inflammation
Sankara Nethralaya
Chennai

Aruj K Khurana DNB, FICO
Fellow, Vitreo-Retina Services
Narayana Nethralaya
Bengaluru

Atul Kumar MD
Professor and Chief
Dr RP Centre for Ophthalmic Sciences
AIMS, New Delhi

Subina Narang MS
Associate Professor
Department of Ophthalmology
GMCH, Chandigarh

Kalpana Babu MS
Prabha Eye Clinic and Institue of Ophthalmology
Bengaluru

Pukhraj Rishi MS
Sankara Nethralaya
Chennai

Soumyava Basu MS
LV Prasad Eye Institute
Bhubaneswar

Amit Bhurmal Jain
Department of Vitreoretina
Sankara Nethralaya
Chennai

Radha Annamalai
Associate Professor of Ophthalmology and Senior
Consultant
Sri Ramachanda University
Chennai

Arushi Khurana MD
Chief Resident
University of Connecticut
USA

Jyotirmay Biswas
Director of Uveitis and Ocular Pathology Department
Sankara Nethralaya
Chennai

Padmamalini Mahendradas
Head, Uveitis and Ocular Immunology
Narayana Nethralaya
Bengaluru

Vishali Gupta MD
Advanced Eye Centre
Postgraduate Institute of Medical Education and
Research
Chandigarh

Bhawna Khurana MS, DNB, FICO
Fellow, Orbit, Oculoplasty and Oncology
Narayana Nethralaya
Bengaluru

S Sood MS
Professor and Head
Department of Ophthalmology
GMCH, Chandigarh

Indu Khurana MD
Senior Professor
Department of Physiology
PGIMS, Rohtak

Pooranchandra B Gowda MS
Narayana Nethralaya
Bengaluru

Ankush Kawali
Consultant
Uveitis and Ocular Immunology Services
Narayana Nethralaya
Bengaluru

Kavitha Avadhani
Consultant
Narayana Nethralaya
Bengaluru

Abhinav Dham MS
Sankara Nethralaya
Chennai

Gurukripa Kowlgi MD
Chief Resident
University of Connecticut
USA

Swetha Palla MS
Sankara Nethralaya, Chennai

Vikas Khetan MS
Senior Consultant
Department of Vitreoretina and Ocular Oncology
Sankara Nethralaya, Chennai

Shana Kansal Jain MS
Department of Ophthalmology
GMCH, Chandigarh

Hitesh Sharma
Senior Resident
Department of Uveitis and Intraocular Inflammation
Sankara Nethralaya, Chennai

Kanika Aggarwal MS
Advanced Eye Centre
Post Graduate Institute of Medical Education and
Research, Chandigarh

Avirupa Ghose
Senior Resident
Department of Uveitis
Aditya Birla Sankara Nethralaya, Kolkata

Sumi R Jayeswal MS
Sankara Nethralaya, Chennai

19 Shavanya MS
Sankara Nethralaya, Chennai

Shweta Goel MS
Regional Institute of Ophthalmology
PGIMS, Rohtak

Ruchi Vala
Vitreo-Retina Fellow
Narayana Nethralaya
Bengaluru

Debmalya Das MS
Associate Consultant
Department of Vitreoretina
Sankara Nethralaya
Chennai

Anjani Khanna MS
Department of Ophthalmology
GMCH, Chandigarh

Sarakshi Mahajan MS
Advanced Eye Centre
Post Graduate Institute of Medical Education and
Research
Chandigarh

Shajeera Sajid DNB
Prabha Eye Clinic and Institue of Ophthalmology
Benagluru

Neha Mohan Jain MS
Drishticone Eye Care
New Delhi

Suchitra Pradeep MS
Sankara Nethralaya
Chennai

Sukanya MS
Sankara Nethralaya
Chennai

Contents

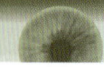

Part 1: Disorders of Uvea

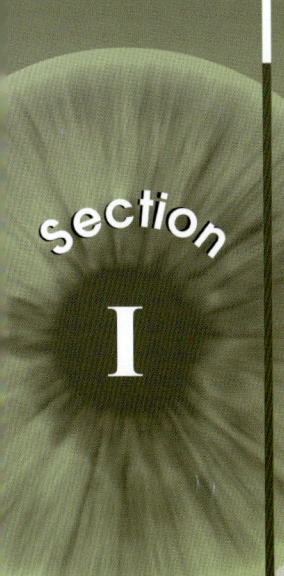

Anatomy, Physiology, Embryology and Congenital Disorders of Uvea

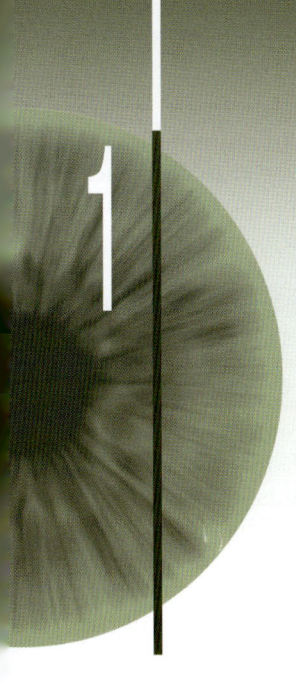

1 ANATOMY AND PHYSIOLOGY OF UVEA

ANATOMY OF UVEA
- Iris
- Ciliary body
- Choroid
- Blood supply of the uveal tract

PHYSIOLOGICAL CONSIDERATIONS
- Functions of uveal tissue
- Blood–ocular barrier
- Escanoids in the iris and ciliary body
- Detoxification and antioxidation in the anterior segment

ANATOMY OF UVEA

Uveal tissue constitutes the middle vascular part of the eyeball. From anterior to posterior, it can be divided into three parts, namely, iris, ciliary body and choroid. However, the entire uveal tract is developmentally, structurally and functionally one indivisible structure.

IRIS

It is the anterior most part of the uveal tract. It is a thin circular disc corresponding to the diaphragm of a camera. Its average diameter is 12 mm and thickness is about 0.5 mm. In its centre (slightly nasal), is an aperture of about 3–4 mm called the pupil, which regularises the amount of light reaching the retina. At the periphery, the iris is attached to the middle of anterior surface of the ciliary body. Iris is thinnest at its root and tears away easily from the ciliary body (iridodialysis) during blunt trauma to the eye. It divides the space between the cornea and lens into anterior and posterior chambers.

Macroscopic appearance

Anterior surface of the iris

It can be divided into a ciliary zone and a pupillary zone by a zigzag line called the collarette (which represents the attachment of papillary membrane) (Fig. 1.1). The collarette, which lies about 2 mm from the pupil margin, is the thickest region of the iris.

1. *Ciliary zone.* It is characterized by:
- *Radial streaks,* which are straight when pupil is small and wavy when it is dilated. These are due to underlying radial vessels.
- *Crypts* are depressions where the superficial layer of iris is missing. These are arranged in two rows—the peripheral crypts are present near the iris root and the central crypts are present near the collarette.

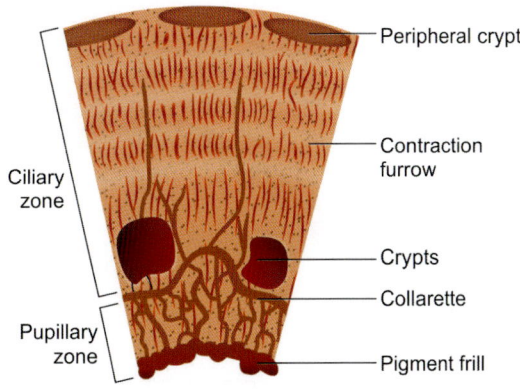

Fig. 1.1 *Gross appearance of anterior surface of the iris.*

- *Contraction furrows* are the faint lines concentric to the collarette. These are more marked on the outer part of the ciliary zone and become prominent when the pupil dilates.

2. *Pupillary zone.* This part of the iris (about 1.6 mm wide) lies between the collarette and pigmented pupillary frill. It is relatively smooth and flat.

Pigment frill is a fringe of black pigment present at the pupillary margin. It represents the anterior end of optic cup. It is due to the slight extension of the posterior pigmented epithelium of the iris around the edge of the pupil.

Posterior surface of the iris

It is dark brown or black in colour. It looks smooth with naked eye. However, when seen under magnification, it presents following radial and circular furrows and folds:

- *Schwalbe's contraction folds* are numerous little radial furrows which commence 1mm from the pupillary border.
- *Schwalbe's structural furrows* start about 1.5 mm from the pupillary border. These are narrow and deep to start with and become wide and shallow as they approach the ciliary margin.
- *The circular furrows* are finer than the radial ones. These cross the structural furrows at regular intervals. These are more marked near the pupil and are formed due to difference in the thickness of the pigmented epithelium.

Microscopic structure

The iris consists of four layers, which from anterior to posterior are as follows (Fig. 1.2):

1. Anterior limiting layer

It is the anterior most condensed part of the stroma. It consists of melanocytes and fibroblasts. Previously, this layer was called endothelial layer of the iris which was a misnomer. This layer is deficient in the areas of crypts and very thin at the contraction furrows. The definitive colour of the iris depends upon this layer. In blue iris, this layer is thin and contains few pigment cells. While in brown iris, it is thick and doubly pigmented.

2. Iris stroma

It forms the main bulk of the iris tissue and consists of loosely arranged *collagenous network* with mucopolysaccharide ground substance. In it, are embedded the sphincter pupillae muscle, dilator pupillae muscle, vessels, nerves, pigment cells and other cells which include lymphocytes, fibroblasts and macrophages.

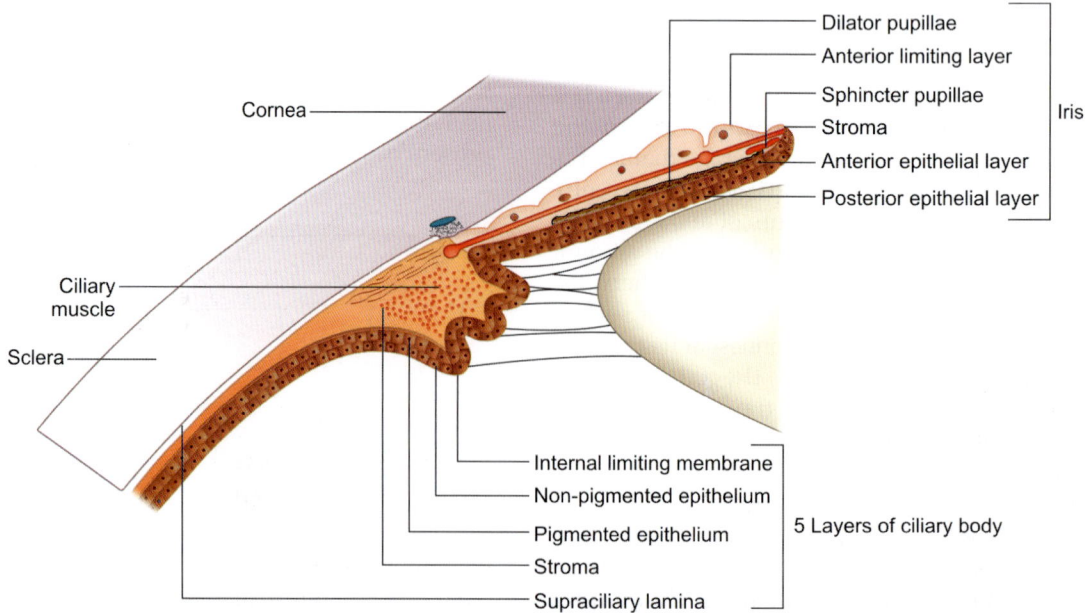

Fig. 1.2 *Microscopic structure of iris and ciliary body.*

- *Sphincter pupillae muscle:* It forms one millimetre broad circular band in the pupillary part of iris. It consists of flat bar of plain muscle fibres which are derived from the ectoderm. It is supplied by the parasympathetic fibres through the third nerve. It constricts the pupil.
- *Dilator pupillae muscle:* It lies in the posterior part of the stroma of ciliary zone of the iris. Its myofilaments are located in the outer part of the cells of anterior pigment epithelial layer. It is supplied by the cervical sympathetics and dilates the pupil.
- *The vessels:* These form the bulk of iris stroma. The radial vessels of the iris are the branches of circulus arteriosus major and are responsible for the radial streaks seen on the anterior surface of the iris. These radial vessels are straight when the pupil constricts and become wavy when the pupil dilates. The structural peculiarities of the iris vessels are:
  - Absence of internal elastic lamina and
  - Non-fenestrated capillary endothelium
- *Pigment cells* or melanocytes are branching elements with processes, which contain melanin granules. Clump cells are round pigment cells without processes. Their pigment granules are large, round and very dark.

3. Anterior epithelial layer

It is the anterior continuation of the pigment epithelium of retina and ciliary body. This layer is lacking in melanocytes, unlike the posterior layer, which is heavily pigmented. The basal processes of the cells of this layer give rise to the dilator pupillae muscle.

4. Posterior pigmented epithelial layer

It is the anterior continuation of the non-pigmented epithelium of the ciliary body which in turn is the continuation of the sensory retina (which stops at the ora serrata). This layer is derived from the internal layer of the optic cup. At the pupillary margin, it forms the pigmented frill and becomes continuous with the anterior pigmented epithelial layer. The pigment cells are of columnar type and certain round dark brown pigment granules.

CILIARY BODY

It is the forward continuation of the choroid at ora serrata. In cut section, it is triangular in shape. The anterior side of triangle forms the part of the angle of anterior and posterior chamber. In its middle, it is attached to the iris. The outer side of the triangle lies against the sclera with a suprachoroidal space in between. The inner side of the triangle is divided into two parts. The anterior part (about 2–2.5 mm) having finger-like ciliary processes is called *pars plicata* (corona ciliaris) and the posterior smooth part (about 5 mm wide temporally and 3 mm wide nasally) is called *pars plana* (orbicularis ciliaris) (Fig. 1.3).

Microscopic structure

From without inwards, ciliary body consists of following five layers (Fig. 1.2):

1. **Supraciliary lamina.** It is the outermost condensed part of stroma and consists of pigmented collagen fibres. Posteriorly, it is a continuation of the suprachoroidal lamina and anteriorly it becomes continuous with the anterior limiting membrane of the iris.

2. **Stroma of the ciliary body.** It consists of connective tissue of collagen and fibroblasts. Embedded in the stroma are ciliary muscle, vascular stroma, nerves, pigment cells and other cells.

Ciliary muscle. It is a non-striated muscle which occupies most of the outer part of the ciliary body. In cut section, it is triangular in shape. It consists of three parts:

- *The longitudinal or meridional fibres* take origin largely by tendinous fibres from the scleral spur and adjacent trabeculae and run posteriorly to insert into the suprachoroidal lamina as far back as equator or even beyond.
- *The circular fibres* occupy the anterior and inner portion of the ciliary body and run parallel to the limbus. These fibres lie nearest to the lens.
- *Radial fibres* are described as the obliquely placed fibres which become continuous with the circular fibres.

Actions: Main action of all the parts of the ciliary muscle is to slacken the suspensory ligaments

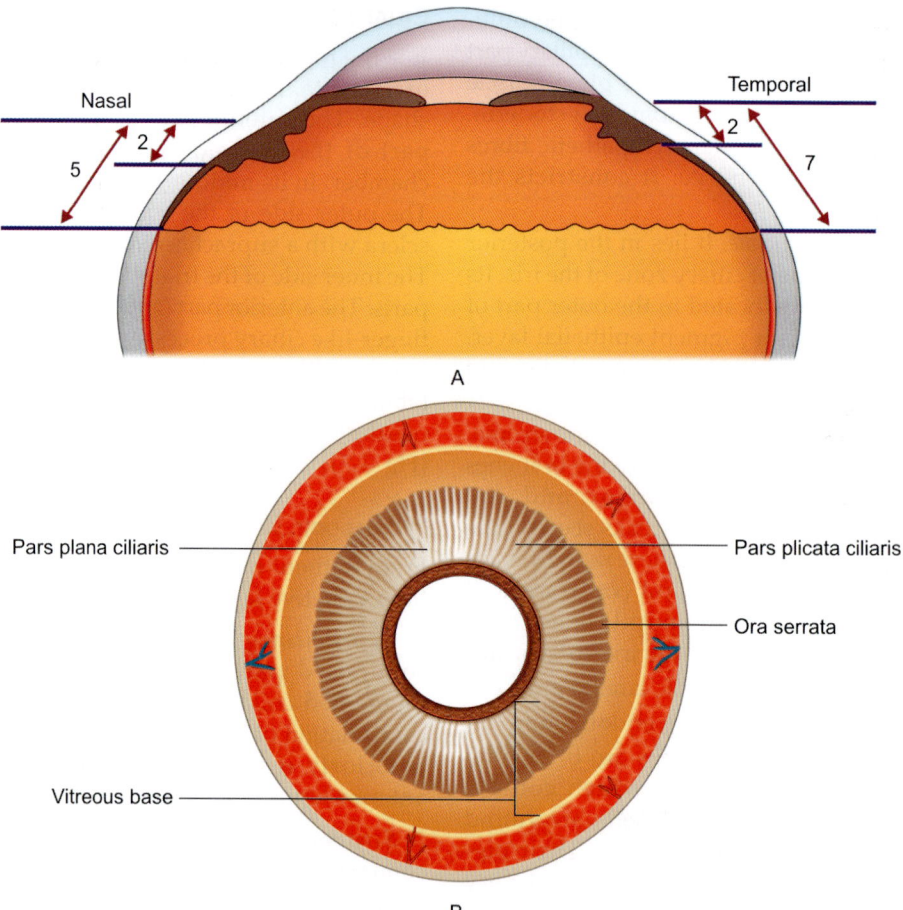

Fig. 1.3 *Region of the pars plana and pars plicata: A, As seen in the axial section of the eyeball; B, As seen from inside the eyeball posteriorly.*

of the lens and thus help in accommodation. Circular fibres act directly as a sphincter.

Radial fibres also act in the same way. Longitudinal fibres' mode of action is disputed. Some say these act by drawing the choroid forward. Due to their attachment to the scleral spur, these fibres also help in aqueous outflow.

Nerve supply: The ciliary muscle is innervated by the parasympathetic fibres from ciliary ganglion which reach the eyeball along the short ciliary nerves.

Vascular stroma of the ciliary body. The major arterial circle lies in the connective tissue stroma of ciliary body just in front of the circular fibres of the muscle. It is formed by anastomosis between the long posterior ciliary artery and anterior ciliary arteries and sends branches to the iris and ciliary body.

Vascular stroma forming ciliary processes is described separately.

3. Layer of pigmented epithelium. It is a forward continuation of the retinal pigment epithelium. Anteriorly, it is continuous with the anterior pigmented epithelium of the iris.

4. Layer of non-pigmented epithelium. It consists mainly of low columnar or cuboidal cells, and is a forward continuation of the sensory retina which stops at the ora serrata. It continues anteriorly with the posterior (internal) pigmented epithelium of the iris.

5. Internal limiting membrane. It lines the non-pigmented epithelium and is the forward continuations of the internal limiting membrane of the retina.

Ciliary processes

Ciliary processes are whitish finger-like projections from the pars plicata part of the ciliary body. They are about 70–80 in number and form the site of aqueous production. Each process is about 2 mm long and 0.5 mm in diameter.

Ultrastructure of the ciliary process

Each ciliary process is composed of three basic components: the network of capillaries, stroma and two layers of the epithelium (Fig. 1.4).

1. *The network of capillaries* occupies the centre of each process. Each capillary consists of a very thin endothelium with fenestrae or false pores (the site of increased permeability) which is lined by a basement membrane. Mural cells or pericytes are present within the basement membrane.

2. *Stroma of ciliary processes* is very thin and separates the capillary network from the epithelial layers. It consists of ground substance (containing mucopolysaccharides, proteins and solute of plasma), a few collagen connective tissue fibres and wandering cells.

3. *Two layers of epithelium* are arranged with their apical surfaces in apposition to each other.

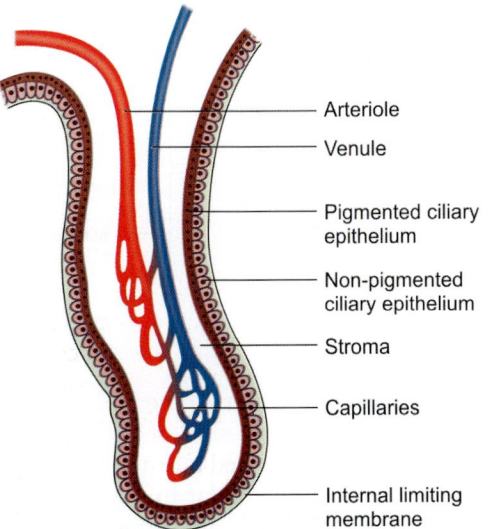

- Arteriole
- Venule
- Pigmented ciliary epithelium
- Non-pigmented ciliary epithelium
- Stroma
- Capillaries
- Internal limiting membrane

Fig. 1.4 *Microscopic structure of a ciliary process.*

The outer pigmented epithelium contains numerous melanin granules. The inner non-pigmented epithelium is characterized by mitochondria (M), zonula occludentes (ZO) and lateral and surface interdigitations (I). The tight junctions between the cells of this layer create part of the blood–aqueous barrier. Basement membrane lines the double cell layer and constitutes the internal limiting membrane (ILM) on the inner surface (Fig. 1.5).

CHOROID

Choroid is the posterior most part of the vascular coat of the eyeball. It extends from the optic disc to ora serrata. Its inner surface is smooth, brown and lies in contact with pigment epithelium of the retina. The outer surface is rough and lies in contact with the sclera. It is thicker posteriorly (0.22 mm) than anteriorly (0.1 mm).

Microscopic structure

From without inwards, the choroid consists of the following four layers (Fig. 1.6):

1. *Suprachoroidal lamina (lamina fusca).* It is a thin (10–34 mm) membrane of condensed collagen fibres, melanocytes and fibroblasts. It is continuous anteriorly with the supraciliary lamina of the ciliary body. The potential space between this membrane and sclera is called suprachoroidal space which contains long and short posterior ciliary arteries and nerves.

2. *Stroma of the choroid.* It consists of loose collagenous tissue with some elastic and reticular fibres. It contains plenty of pigment cells and other cells, like macrophages, mast cells, plasma cells and lymphocytes. Its main bulk is formed by vessels which are arranged in two layers: the outer layer of large vessels (Haller's layer) and the inner layer of medium vessels (Sattler's layer). It is difficult to separate the two layers. Large vessels are external and tend to diminish in size as we go towards the chorio-capillaris. The innermost vessels are arterioles which connect with the choriocapillaris. The outermost part next to suprachoroidal lamina mainly contains veins.

3. *Choriocapillaris.* It consists of a rich capillary network which receives most of its blood from

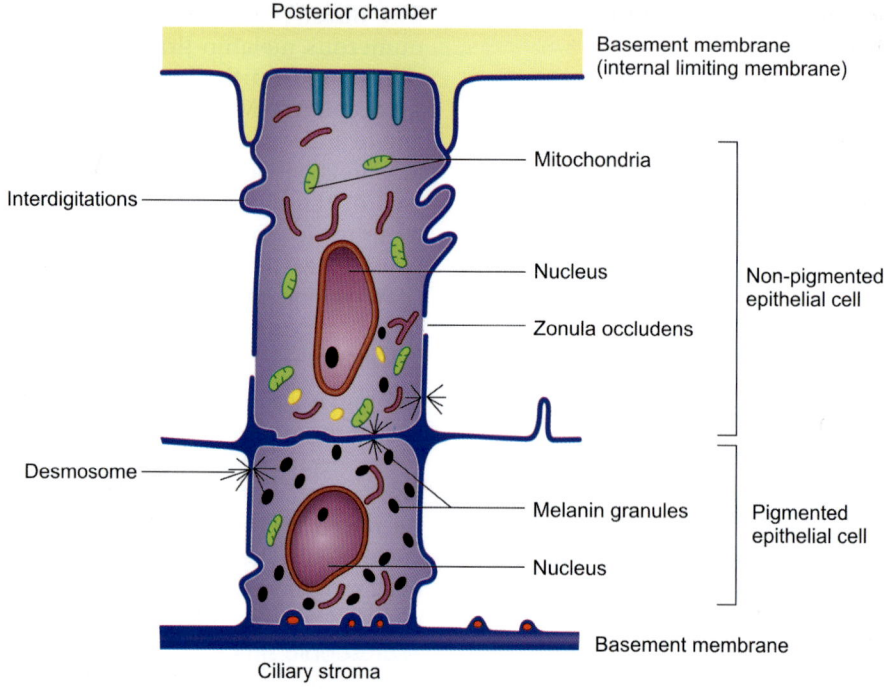

Posterior chamber

Basement membrane
(internal limiting membrane)

Mitochondria

Interdigitations

Nucleus

Non-pigmented
epithelial cell

Zonula occludens

Desmosome

Melanin granules

Pigmented
epithelial cell

Nucleus

Basement membrane

Ciliary stroma

Fig. 1.5 *Microscopic details of the cells of two layers of ciliary epithelium.*

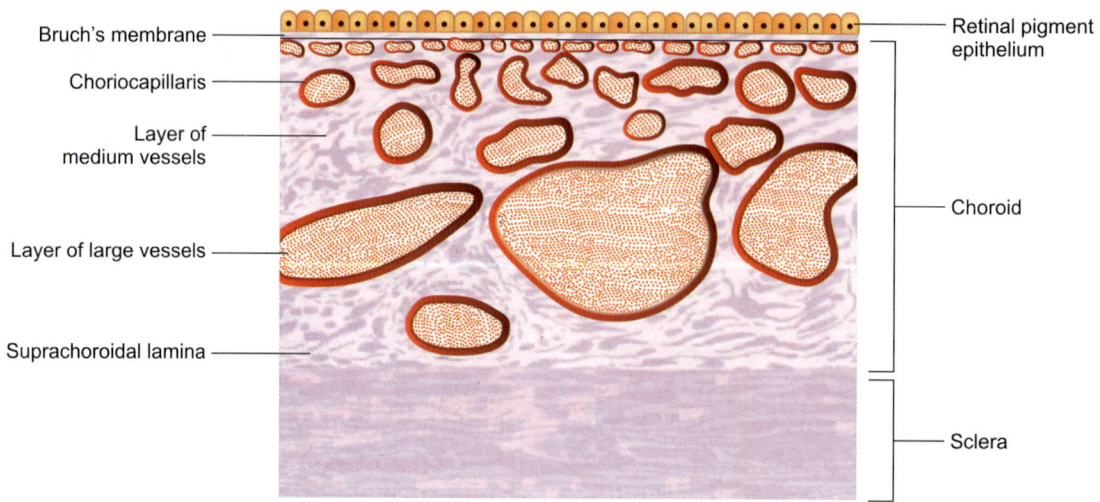

Bruch's membrane

Retinal pigment
epithelium

Choriocapillaris

Layer of
medium vessels

Choroid

Layer of large vessels

Suprachoroidal lamina

Sclera

Fig. 1.6 *Microscopic structure of choroid.*

the medium and large vessels of the stroma. It nourishes the pigment epithelium and the outer layers of sensory retina. These capillaries are fenestrated, have a wide limb (18 to 50 mm) and consist of endothelial cells joined together by zonulae occludentes. The endothelial cells are lined by a basement membrane which contains pericytes on the outer side of the capillaries. Choriocapillaris is divided into non-overlapping lobules in a fashion similar to that seen in the liver, and is not a freely anastomosing system, as previously believed.

4. *Basal lamina (Bruch's membrane or lamina vitrae).* Bruch's membrane is the innermost layer of choroid and is approximately 2–4 mm in thickness. It is a multilayered structure which lies between the choriocapillaris and pigment epithelium of the retina. On electron microscopy, it is described to consist of five layers:

- Basement membrane of the retinal pigment epithelium
- An inner collagen layer
- A middle elastic layer
- An outer collagen layer
- The basement membrane of the choriocapillaris.

Bruch's membrane becomes thickened with increasing age and produces hyaline excresences known as drusens.

BLOOD SUPPLY OF THE UVEAL TRACT

Arterial blood supply

The uveal tract is supplied by three sets of arteries (Fig. 1.7).

1. *Short posterior ciliary arteries.* These arise as two trunks from the ophthalmic artery. Each trunk divides into 10–20 branches which pierce the sclera around the optic nerve and supply the choroid in a segmental manner.

2. *Long posterior ciliary arteries.* These are two in number (nasal and temporal). These pierce the sclera obliquely on medial and lateral side of the optic nerve and run forward in the suprachoroidal space to reach the ciliary muscle, without giving any branch. At the anterior end of ciliary muscle, these anastomose with each other and with the anterior ciliary arteries to form the major arterial circle and also give branches which supply the ciliary body.

3. *Anterior ciliary arteries.* These are derived from the muscular branches of ophthalmic artery. These are 7 in number: 2 each from the arteries of superior rectus, inferior rectus and medial rectus muscles and one from that of lateral rectus muscle. These arteries pass anteriorly in the episclera, give branches to sclera, limbus and conjunctiva, and ultimately pierce the sclera near the limbus to enter the ciliary muscle where they anastomose with the two long posterior ciliary arteries to form the *circulus arteriosus major,* near the root of the iris. Several branches arise from the circulus arteriosus major and supply the ciliary processes (one branch for each process). Similarly, many branches from this major arterial circle run radially through the iris towards pupillary margin where they anastomose with each other to form 'circulus arteriosus minor.

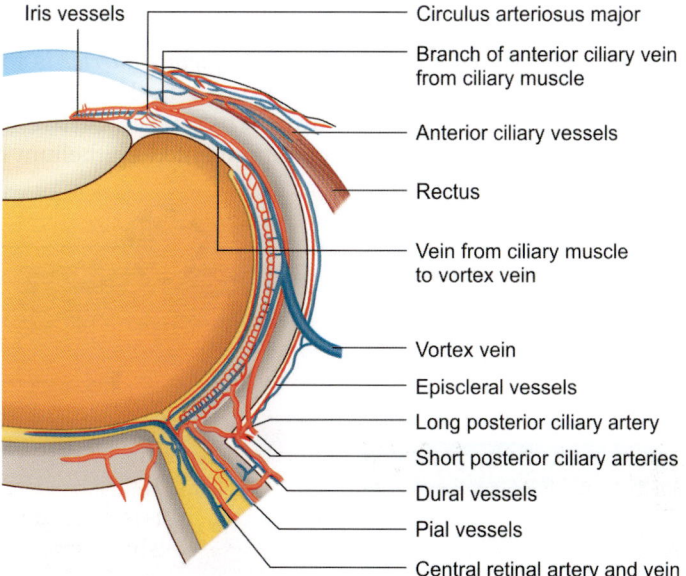

Iris vessels — Circulus arteriosus major

Branch of anterior ciliary vein from ciliary muscle

Anterior ciliary vessels

Rectus

Vein from ciliary muscle to vortex vein

Vortex vein

Episcleral vessels

Long posterior ciliary artery

Short posterior ciliary arteries

Dural vessels

Pial vessels

Central retinal artery and vein

Fig. 1.7 *Blood supply of uveal tract. The two inferior vortex veins open into the inferior ophthalmic veins.*

Venous drainage

Veins draining uveal blood are (Fig. 1.7):

1. *Anterior ciliary veins.* These are tributaries of the muscular veins. Since they carry blood only from the ciliary muscle, they are smaller than the corresponding arteries.

2. *Smaller veins from the sclera.* These correspond to the scleral branches of the short ciliary arteries. They only carry blood from the sclera and not from the choroid and are, therefore, smaller than the corresponding arteries.

3. *The venae verticosae (vortex veins or posterior ciliary veins).* These are usually 4 in number (superior temporal, inferior temporal, superior nasal and inferior nasal). They pierce the sclera obliquely on each side of the superior rectus and inferior rectus muscles, about 6 mm behind the equator of the globe. Of these, superior temporal vein is most posterior (8 mm behind the equator) and inferior temporal is most anterior (5.5 mm behind the equator).

At their choroidal end, the vortex veins have an ampulliform dilatation.

Venae verticosae drain blood from:

- Whole of the choroid
- Receive small veins from optic nerve head
- Sometimes small veins from retina also join it
- Anterior tributaries come from the iris, ciliary processes, ciliary muscle and anterior part of the choroid. There is no major venous circle corresponding to major arterial circle

Oblique scleral canals through which the vortex veins pass are about 4 mm long and directed posteriorly in such a way that the four veins appear to converge towards the apex of the orbit.

Superior vortex veins open into the superior ophthalmic vein directly or through its muscular or lacrimal tributaries.

Inferior vortex veins open into the inferior ophthalmic veins.

PHYSIOLOGICAL CONSIDERATIONS

FUNCTIONS OF UVEAL TISSUE

The uveal tissue performs the following physiological functions:

1. It is the source of blood flow to the ocular tissues.
2. It is the site of aqueous humour production and maintenance of intraocular pressure.
3. It constitutes the blood–aqueous barrier.
4. Musculature of the ciliary body plays role in the process of accommodation.
5. Eicosanoids are synthesized in the iris and ciliary body.
6. Uveal tissues play role in the detoxification and antioxidation in the anterior segment.

BLOOD–OCULAR BARRIER

By virtue of blood–ocular barrier, the protein and other large molecular size substances are largely prevented from entering the cavities (anterior chamber, posterior chamber and in tear cavity) of the eyes. This mechanism is essential to maintain the clarity of the media of the eye.

Blood–ocular barrier consists of two parts— the posterior blood–retinal barrier and the anterior blood–aqueous barrier.

Blood–retinal barrier in turn consists of two parts—the inner and the outer. The inner blood–retinal barrier is composed of the tight junction of retinal capillaries, endothelial cells and the outer blood–retinal barrier consists of tight junctional complexes (zonula occludens and zonula adherans) which are located between adjacent RPE cells (Fig. 1.8).

Blood–aqueous barrier is formed by the tight junctions (zonula occludens and the zonula adherans) between the cells of the inner non-pigmented epithelium of the ciliary body

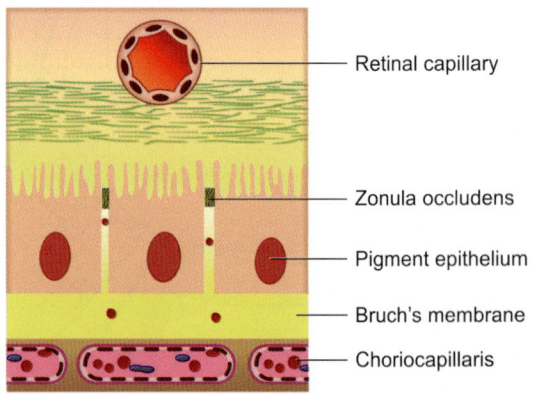

Fig. 1.8 *Blood–retinal barrier.*

- Retinal capillary
- Zonula occludens
- Pigment epithelium
- Bruch's membrane
- Choriocapillaris

(Fig. 1.5) and the non-fenestrated endothelium of the iris capillaries. However, the endothelial cells of iris capillaries are not joined by tight junctions and in inflammatory conditions they become leaky, causing an aqueous flare.

Note. The blood–ocular barrier is not absolute. Medium-sized, water-soluble substances may penetrate it but at much slower rate than their transit across capillary walls. Examples of such substances include urea creatinine and some sugars. Further, lipid solubility greatly facilitates the ability of a substance to penetrate the blood–ocular barrier.

Clinical applications of blood–ocular barrier

1. *Hyperosmotic agents,* like mannitol, penetrate the eye poorly because of the blood–ocular barrier, but are distributed fairly widely in the extracellular spaces of the body. Thus, water is drawn from the cells and the ocular fluids (vitreous more than the aqueous), resulting in a fall in the intraocular pressure.

2. *Ocular penetration of systemically administered antibiotics.* Only low molecular weight drugs, such as chloramphenicol, cephalothin and ampicillin can cross the blood–aqueous barrier. Very poor passage is allowed to large-sized molecules, such as penicillin, methicillin and erythromycin. Out of the borderline molecular weight drugs, those with high lipid solubility can pass easily, e.g. sulfonamides have the same molecular weight as sucrose but are 16 times more permeable due to their lipid solubility.

Breakdown of the blood–aqueous barrier
Factors interrupting blood–aqueous barrier

The blood–aqueous barrier is rather fragile. Certain conditions which can disturb the blood–aqueous barrier are listed below:

I. *Ocular trauma*
1. *Mechanical trauma*
   • Paracentesis
   • Corneal abrasion
   • Intraocular surgery
   • Stroking iris
2. *Physical trauma*
   • X-rays
   • Atomic radiation

3. *Chemical trauma*
   • Alkali
   • Irritants, e.g. nitrogen mustard

II. *Pathophysiologic factors*
1. Vascular dilatation
   • Histamine
   • Sympathectomy
2. Corneal and intraocular infections
3. Intraocular inflammations
4. Prostaglandins
5. Anterior segment ischaemia

III. *Pharmacologic factors*
1. Melano-stimulating hormone
2. Nitrogen mustard gas
3. Cholinesterase inhibitors
4. Cholinergic drugs
5. Plasma hyperosmolality

Effect of breakdown of blood–aqueous barrier on aqueous humour composition

• With the breakdown of blood–aqueous barrier, substances, such as proteins, that are normally almost completely excluded from penetration, appear in the aqueous humour in measurable amounts. Thus proteins and antibodies in the aqueous equilibrate with those in plasma to form plasmoid aqueous *(secondary aqueous).* Increased protein content in the aqueous humour is recognized clinically on slit-lamp biomicroscopy as a pronounced Tyndall beam.

• The ionic composition of the aqueous approaches that of simple dialysate of plasma.

• The rates of penetration of the smaller molecules, such as sucrose or p-aminohippurate (which were previously partly blocked from aqueous) are increased greatly. In fact, the rapid rate of entry into aqueous of such substances as fluorescein and Evans blue dye can be used as diagnostic indicators of barrier breakdown.

• Fibrinogen appears in the aqueous, which may allow the aqueous actually to clot.

EICOSANOIDS IN THE IRIS AND CILIARY BODY

Prostaglandins were first discovered in the eye in 1957 by Ambache, who demonstrated the biological activity in aqueous and named the factor 'irin'. Eicosanoids is the generic term to describe prostaglandins (PCs) and leukotrienes, both of which are metabolites of arachidonic acid. Prostaglandins are synthesized in great amounts after trauma or inflammation involving the iris/ciliary body, from arachidonic acid released by esterified sites in membrane phospholipids. Other neuropeptides are involved in this response. For instance, release of substance-P from the iris leads to receptor-mediated breakdown of PIP_2 and the formation of large amounts of arachidonic acid in the iris sphincter and synthesis of PGE_2. In the ciliary body, the cyclo-oxygenase pathway is also active in microsomes. PGE_2 is involved in miosis, while $PGF_{2\alpha}$ is involved in the control of intraocular pressure. Many other peptides are present in the iris/ciliary body and the aqueous including neuropeptide Y, vasoactive intestinal peptide, somatostatin and calcitonin gene related peptide (CGRP). Nitric oxide is also released during activation of iris/ciliary body tissues. Many of these peptides modulate normal iris/ciliary body functions, such as miosis and aqueous humour production. For instance, CGRP relaxes iris dilator smooth muscle via cAMP mechanisms. They also have other functions, such as immuno-suppressive role of VIP in ocular immune privilege.

Drugs that inhibit the cyclo-oxygenase pathway, such as indomethacin and aspirin, may be useful in ocular inflammation. However, steroids act at the level of phospholipase A_2 and may have a more global effect on the response. In addition, the lipo-oxygenase pathway is active in the anterior uvea with synthesis of leukotrienes B_4, C_4, and D_4, and the chemotaxis of polymorphonuclear leucocytes.

DETOXIFICATION AND ANTIOXIDATION IN THE ANTERIOR SEGMENT

The cytochrome P450 system—the major drug detoxification system in the eye

Microsomes contain a group of proteins known as cytochrome P450 proteins, which catalyze the transfer of a single oxygen atom to endogenous and exogenous substances destined for excretion and/or detoxification, such as steroids, phenobarbitone, etc. Their main effect is to convert hydrophobic compounds to hydroxy-lated hydrophilic compounds, which are then more easily metabolized.

The cytochrome P450 system is present in ciliary body (at about 5% of the concentration in liver) where it acts to detoxify many compounds. It does this by either converting the hydroxylated, highly reactive compound to a glucuronide via UDP-glucuronyl tranferase or by conjugating it to glutathione via glutathione-S-transferase. Most of the enzymes involved in the detoxification process have been identified and purified from the ciliary body, in particular the non-pigmented epithelium. There is considerable genetic variation in the induction of the cytochrome P450 system in the eye, perhaps explaining the variable toxic effects of drugs in individuals.

The ciliary body—the main source of antioxidant system in the anterior segment

Although, antioxidant systems exist in the lens and the cornea, the ciliary body is especially rich in antioxidant systems with the highest concentrations of catalase, superoxide dismutase, and glutathione peroxidase types I and II. Type I is selenium-dependent while type II is selenium-independent. Type I is closely linked to glutathione reductase whose main function is the reduction of oxidized glutathione (GSSH) produced by the detoxification of peroxides.

Hydrogen peroxide (H_2O_2) is present in normal aqueous, most of it derived from the non-enzymatic interaction between reduced ascorbate and molecular oxygen, and it is reduced to H_2O_2 by glutathione secreted by the ciliary epithelium. Most of these studies have been performed in experimental animals and it is not clear how relevant they are to the human eye. It has been suggested that oxidized ascorbate (via the superoxide anion) is more important in degrading H_2O_2 in humans. Melatonin, a neuropeptide involved in the biological circadian rhythm is also an H_2O_2 scavenger. A role for xanthine oxidase has also been suggested. H_2O_2 can induce norepine-phrine release from iris/ciliary body in the aqueous and has recently been implicated in cataract formation.

BIBLIOGRAPHY

1. Smelser GK. Electron microscopy of a typical epithelial cell and of the normal human ciliary process. Trans Am Acad Ophthal Otol 70: 738, 1966.

2. Davson H. The Eye-Vegetative Physiology and Biochemistry, Vol 12nd ed. New York, Academic Press, 1969.

3. Duke-Elder S. The Physiology of the Eye and of Vision, Vol IV System of Ophthalmology. St Louis, CV Mosby, 1968.

4. Shiose Y. Electron microscopic studies on blood–retinal and blood–aqueous barriers. Jpn J Ophthalmol 14:73, 1970.

5. Smith RS, Rudt LA. Ultrastructural studies of the blood–aqueous barrier. 2 The barrier to horseradish peroxidase in primates. Am J Ophthal 76:937, 1973.

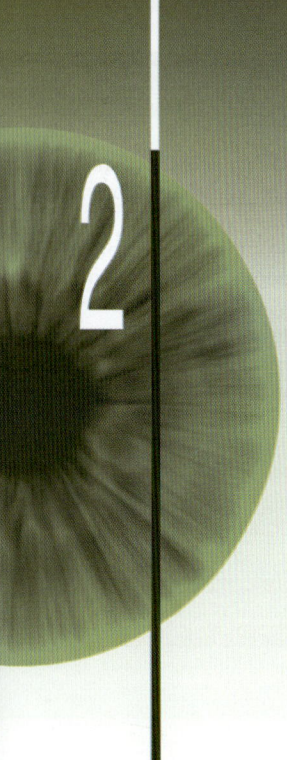

2

EMBRYOLOGY AND CONGENITAL DISORDERS OF UVEA

EMBRYOLOGY OF UVEA
- Formation of optic vesicle and optic stalk
- Formation of lens vesicle
- Formation of optic cup
- Changes in associated mesenchyme
- Formation of tunica vasculosa lentis
- Development of iris
- Developmnet of ciliary body
- Development of choroid
- Development of uveal vasculature

CONGENITAL DISORDERS OF UVEA
- Congente Coloboma of uveal tract
- Aniridia
- Albinism
- Heterochromia of iris
- Corectopia
- Polycoria
- Persistent pupillary membrane
- Congenital cyst of iris
- Iridotrabeculodysgenesis

EMBRYOLOGY OF UVEA

The development of the eyeball can be considered to commence around day 22 when the embryo has eight pairs of somites and is around 2 mm in length. The eyeball and its related structures are derived from the following primordial:

- An outgrowth from prosencephalon called optic vesicle (neuroectodermal structure).
- A specialised area of surface ectoderm called lens placode and the surrounding surface ectoderm.
- Mesoderm surrounding the optic vesicle.
- Visceral mesoderm of maxillary process.

Before going into the development of uveal tissue, it will be helpful to understand the formation of optic vesicle, lens placode, optic cup and changes in the surrounding mesoderm which play a major role in the development of the eye and its related structures.

FORMATION OF OPTIC VESICLE AND OPTIC STALK

The first evidence of primitive eye formation occurs during the third week of gestation. The region of neural plate (Fig. 2.1A), which is destined to form the prosencephalon, shows a linear thickened area on either side (Fig. 2.1B), which soon becomes depressed to form the optic sulcus (Fig. 2.1C). Meanwhile the neural plate gets converted into prosencephalic vesicle. As the optic sulcus deepens, the walls of the prosencephalon overlying the sulcus bulge out to form the *optic vesicle* (Fig. 2.1D, E). The proximal part of the optic vesicle becomes constricted and elongated to form the *optic stalk* (Fig. 2.1F, G, H).

FORMATION OF LENS VESICLE

As the optic vesicle grows laterally (during the third week of gestation), it comes in relation with the surface ectoderm. At about 27 days of gestation (embryo 4.0–4.5 mm), the area of the surface ectoderm overlying the optic vesicle

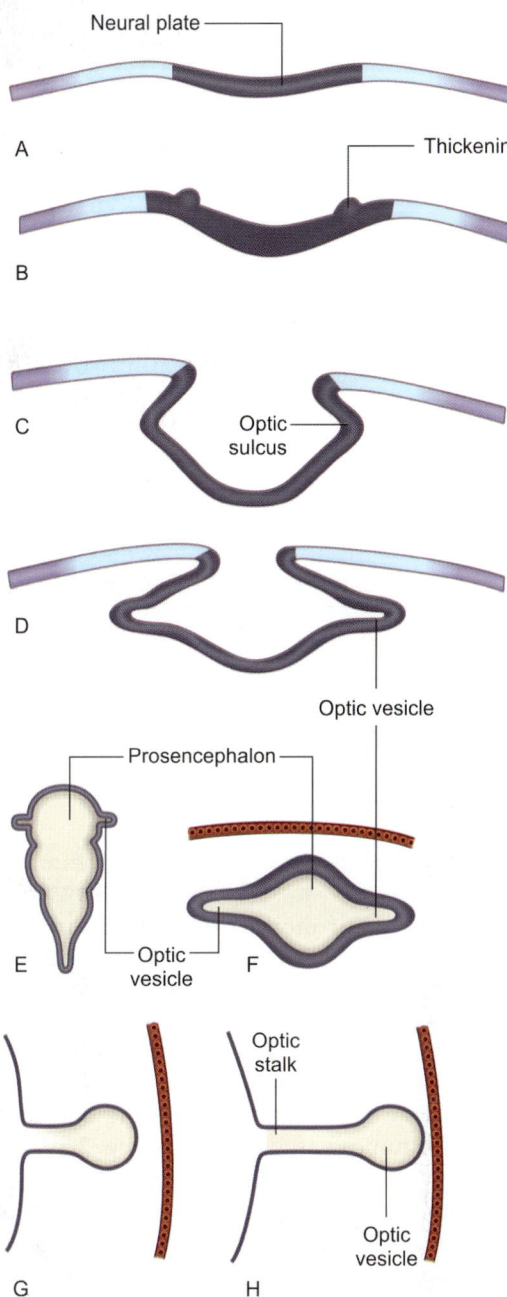

Fig. 2.1 *Formation of the optic vesicle and optic stalk.*

FORMATION OF OPTIC CUP

During the fourth week of gestation (embryo 7.6–7.8 mm), while the lens vesicle is forming, simultaneously the optic vesicle is converted into a double-layered *optic cup*. It appears from Fig. 2.2 that this has happened because the developing lens has invaginated itself into the optic vesicle. However, this is not so. The conversion of the optic vesicle to the optic cup is due to differential growth of the walls of the vesicle. The margins of optic cup grow over the upper and lateral sides of the lens to enclose it. However, such a growth does not take place over the inferior part of the lens, and, therefore, walls of the cup show deficiency in this part. This deficiency extends to some distance along the inferior surface of the optic stalk and is called the *choroidal* or *fetal fissure* (Fig. 2.3). This embryonic ocular fissure closes by 6th week of gestation. When the lips of the fissure fail to fuse by 6th or 7th week, typical colobomas result. By the end of 7th week of gestation, most of the basic structures of the eye are present. Thereafter, ocular development is mainly a process of differentiation and modification of various parts of the globe.

CHANGES IN ASSOCIATED MESENCHYME

The developing neural tube (from which central nervous system develops) is surrounded by mesenchyme. Mesenchyme is a loose tissue consisting of stellate, amoeboid mesenchymal cells embedded in a matrix rich in glycosaminoglycans.

Mesenchymal cells may be derived from serosal sources, namely mesoderm (dermatome or sclerotome component of the somite or lateral plate mesoderm) or neural crest. Thus this descriptive term mesenchyme does not imply an origin from any particular embryonic germ layer. The mesenchyme surrounding the neural tube subsequently condenses to form meninges. An extension of this mesenchyme also surrounds the optic vesicle, except at its apex, which is closely apposed to the surface ectoderm on the lateral side of the developing head. This mesenchyme may be derived from the cephalic neural crest and indeed from crest cells detaching from the outer surface of the optic

becomes thickened to form the *lens placode* (Fig. 2.2A) which sinks below the surface and is gradually converted into *the lens vesicle* (Fig. 2.2B, C). It is soon separated from the surface ectoderm at 33rd day of gestation (Fig. 2.2D).

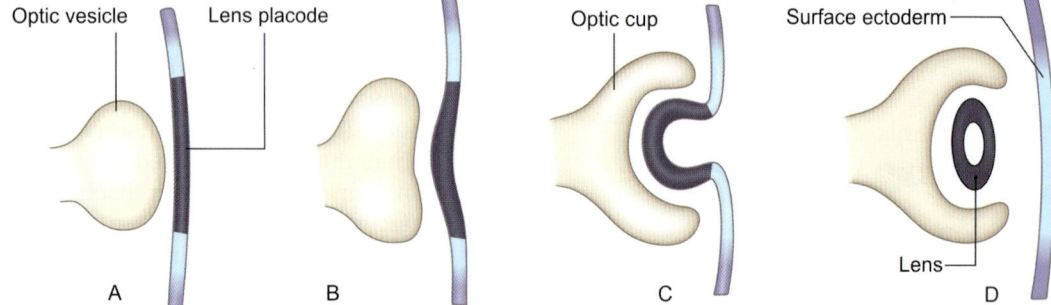

Fig. 2.2 *Formation of lens vesicle and optic cup.*

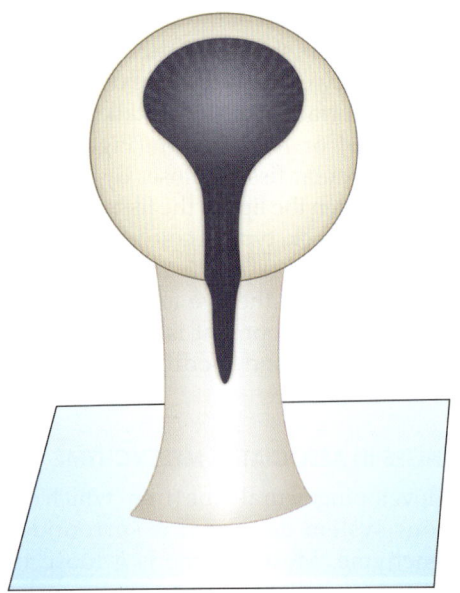

Fig. 2.3 *Optic cup and stalk seen from below to show the choroidal fissure.*

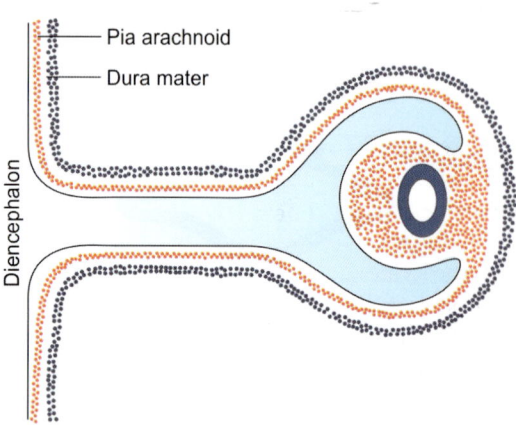

Fig. 2.4 *Developing optic cup surrounded by mesoderm.*

vesicle itself. Later, this mesenchyme differentiates to form a superficial fibrous layer (corresponding to dura), which will form the sclera and cornea and a deeper vascular layer (corresponding to pia-arachnoid) which will form stroma of uveal tissue (Fig. 2.4).

With the formation of optic cup, part of the inner vascular layer of mesenchyme is carried into the cup through the choroidal fissure. With the closure of this fissure, the portion of mesenchyme which has made its way into the eye through the fissure is cut off from the surrounding mesenchyme and gives rise to hyaloid system of the vessels (Fig. 2.5). The

fibrous layer of mesenchyme surrounding anterior part of optic cup forms the cornea. The corresponding vascular layer of mesenchyme becomes iridopupillary membrane, which, in the peripheral region, attaches to the anterior part of the optic cup to form iris. The central part of this lamina is pupillary membrane and also forms the tunica vasculosa lentis (Fig. 2.5).

In the posterior part of optic cup, the surrounding fibrous mesenchyme forms sclera and extraocular muscles, while the vascular layer forms the choroid and ciliary body.

FORMATION OF TUNICA VASCULOSA LENTIS

During embryonic and fetal development, the lens receives nourishment via an intricate vascular capsule, the tunica vasculosa lentis, that completely encompasses the lens by approximately 9 weeks. It is formed from the mesenchyme that surrounds the lens. Three components of tunica vasculosa are anterior

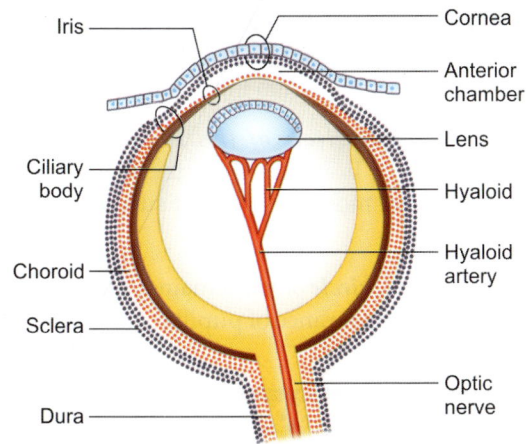

Fig. 2.5 *Derivation of various structures of the eyeball.*

pupillary membrane, capsulopupillary membrane and posterior pupillary membrane (Fig. 2.6). In the earliest stages of development, tunica vasculosa lentis receives an abundant arterial supply from the hyaloid artery. Later, this blood supply regresses, and the vascular capsule disappears before birth. For its nutrition, the lens now depends on diffusion from the aqueous and vitreous.

DEVELOPMENT OF IRIS

Pupillary membrane, as discussed above in tunica vasculosa, is formed by condensation of mesenchyme situated on the anterior surface of lens (Fig. 2.6).

- *Both layers of epithelium* of iris are derived from the marginal region of optic cup (neuroectodermal) (Fig. 2.5) which after having covered the ciliary muscle, extends on to the posterior surface of pupillary membrane.
- *Sphincter and dilator pupillae* muscles are derived from the anterior epithelium (neuroectodermal).
- *Stroma and blood vessels* of iris develop from vascular layer of mesenchyme present anterior to the optic cup. Towards the end of gestation, the central iris stroma (pupillary membrane) disappears forming the pupil. Sometimes a few strands of this tissue are left as *persistent pupillary membrane.*

DEVELOPMENT OF CILIARY BODY

- *Epithelial layers* of ciliary body develop from the two layers of anterior part of optic cup (neuroectoderm) (Fig. 2.5). The ciliary epithelium undergoes a convulating or folding movements to form about 70–75 ciliary processes.
- *Stroma of ciliary body,* including connective tissue, ciliary muscle and blood vessels are developed from the vascular layer of mesenchyme surrounding the optic cup.

DEVELOPMENT OF CHOROID

Choroid is mainly derived from the inner vascular layer of the mesenchyme that surrounds the

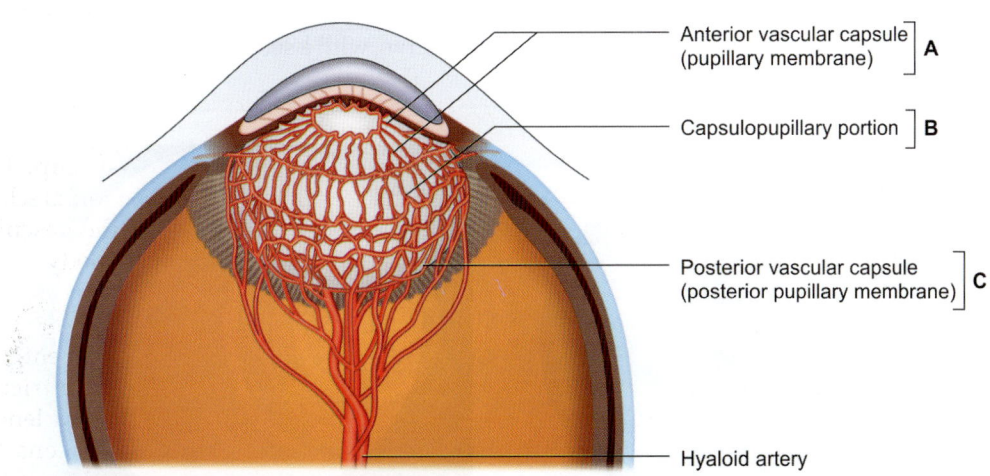

Fig. 2.6 *Three components of tunica vasculosa: **A,** Anterior pupillary membrane; **B,** Capsular pupillary membrane; and **C,** Posterior pupillary membrane.*

optic cup (Fig. 2.5). Choroid starts developing at the rim of optic cup and progresses posteriorly. Stroma and melanocytes of choroid originate from the neural crest. Choroidal stroma is invaded by choriocapillaris (fine vessels derived from mesoderm) during 4th to 5th week of gestation.

DEVELOPMENT OF UVEAL VASCULATURE

Primitive dorsal and ventral ophthalmic arteries bud inward from the internal carotid artery in the mesenchyme surrounding the optic vesicle late in the fourth week and join a loose reticulum of capillaries around the optic vesicle.

Hyaloid artery develops as a branch of primitive dorsal ophthalmic artery. After getting incorporated in the optic cup, the hyaloid system extends up to the lens and joins the tunica vasculosa lentis (Fig. 2.6). These vessels nourish the developing eye and disappear in the third trimester.

Stapedial artery, a transient vessel, arises from the carotid to supply the expanding orbit. Later, the distal part of stapedial artery is annexed to the ophthalmic artery.

Definitive ophthalmic artery is developed from the primitive dorsal ophthalmic artery at the sixth week of gestation, while the primitive ventral ophthalmic artery almost disappears, only a portion of it remains as the nasal long posterior ciliary artery.

Temporal long posterior ciliary artery, short posterior ciliary arteries and central reinal artery grow as buds from the ophthalmic artery.

Major arterial circle of iris is formed by a coalescence of branches from the long ciliary arteries in the mesenchyme that surrounds the optic cup.

Minor arterial circle of iris remains peripherally after the disappearance of pupillary membrane.

CONGENITAL DISORDERS OF UVEA

CONGENITAL COLOBOMA OF UVEAL TRACT

Congenital coloboma (absence of tissue) of iris (Fig. 2.7), ciliary body and choroid (Fig. 2.8) may be seen in association or independently.

Colobomas are formed by defects of closure of the optic cup that occur at 7–8 weeks of foetal life. They can present as a sectorial deficiency varying from the trivial to the gross. They are typically found inferonasally. Coloboma may be typical or atypical.

Typical coloboma

Typical coloboma is seen in the inferonasal quadrant and occurs due to defective closure of the embryonic fissure. Typical coloboma may be complete or incomplete.

Complete coloboma extends from pupil to the optic nerve, with a sector-shaped gap occupying

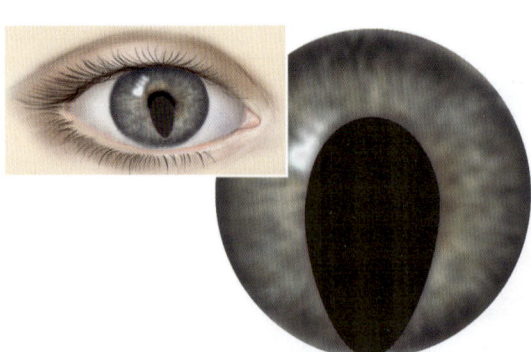

Fig. 2.7 *Typical coloboma of the iris.*

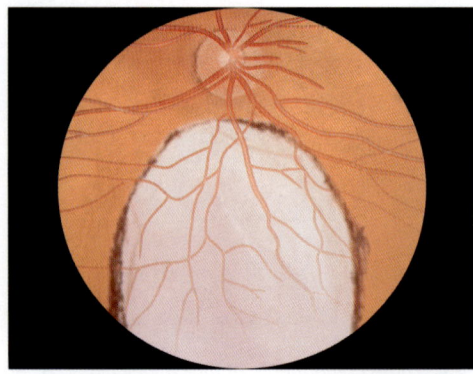

Fig. 2.8 *Coloboma of the choroid.*

about one-eighth of the circumference of the retina, choroid, ciliary body, iris and causes a corresponding indentation of the lens where the zonular fibres are missing.

Incomplete coloboma may involve the iris alone, or iris and ciliary body (more common), or iris, ciliary body and part of choroid (i.e. stops short of optic nerve).

Atypical coloboma

Atypical coloboma is occasionally found in other positions. It is usually incomplete.

ANIRIDIA

Aniridia (Fig. 2.9) refers to congenital absence of iris:

True aniridia, i.e. complete absence of the iris is extremely rare.

Clinical aniridia is more common presentation in which a peripheral rim of iris is present. A vestigial iris remnant can usually be seen as a frill on gonioscopy.

Genetics and associations. Aniridia occurs either as a familial autosomal dominant disease or sporadically. The autosomal dominant condition is associated with glaucoma, nystagmus, corneal opacities and photophobia, while sporadic cases usually have a high incidence of nephroblastoma (Wilms' tumour). This is associated with deletion of a tumour suppressor gene which has been identified on chromosome 11, analogous to the retinoblastoma gene on chromosome 13. All such children require regular screening by renal ultrasonography.

ALBINISM

Albinism is a hereditary condition. No apparent conditions seem to predispose a person to develop albinism. Albinos have a deficiency of melanin within the uveal tract and the disorder occurs in both systemic (autosomal recessive) or purely ocular forms (usually X-linked, but rarely recessive) when cutaneous pigmentation is normal.

Purely cutaneous albinoids have no ocular complications.

Oculocutaneous albinos, by hair follicle analysis, can be divided into those who have a complete absence of pigmentation (tyrosinase negative, Fig. 2.10), and those who are tyrosinase positive. *Tyrosinase positive subjects* can be more difficult to diagnose as they have more normal cutaneous and ocular pigmentation. Skin biopsy demonstrates structural anomalies in the melanosomes of X-linked patients.

Ocular manifestations

- *Skin, hair, and eye discolourations* are caused by abnormalities of melanin metabolism. However, this might not be as obvious in patients with ocular albinism.
- *Photophobia*, due to absence of pigment in iris.
- *Decreased vision* due to foveal hypoplasia, high refractive error, and/or nystagmus.
- Strabismus due to abnormal decussation of optic nerve fibres.
- *Nystagmus*—earlier onset of nystagmus correlates with degree of foveal hypoplasia.
- *History of easy bruising or recurrent infections* in patients with Hermansky-Pudlak syndrome and Chediak-Higashi syndrome, respectively.

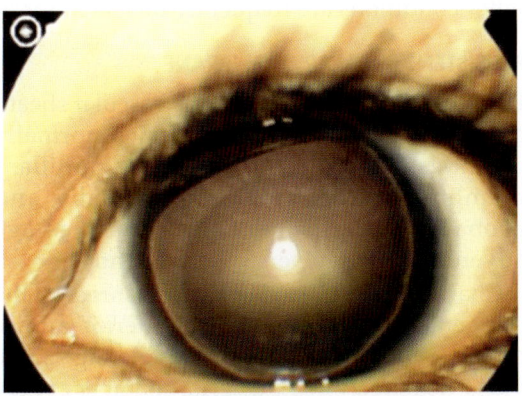

Fig. 2.9 *Aniridia.*

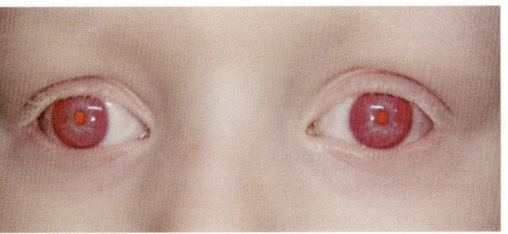

Fig. 2.10 *Oculocutaneous albinism.*

- *Decreased hearing* associated with some forms of X-linked ocular albinism.
- In addition to the above features, a curious anomaly of the optic chiasma in which the majority of optic nerve fibres from each eye decussate. This is thought to be caused by the absence of pigmented cells in the chiasma during embryogenesis which 'direct' the ingrowing axons.

Differential diagnosis

Oculocutaneous albinism and ocular albinism should be distinguished from other disease entities that can present with cutaneous and ocular hypopigmentation. These include the following:

- Aland Island eye disease (Forsius-Eriksson syndrome)
- Cross-McKusick-Breen syndrome
- Waardenburg syndrome
- Prader-Willi syndrome
- Angelman syndrome
- Vitiligo
- Congenital nystagmus
- Achromatopsia
- Piebaldism
- Kallmann syndrome
- Chondrodysplasia punctata

Foveal hypoplasia can be present in aniridia and retinopathy of prematurity.

Iris transillumination defects can be present in pseudoexfoliation syndrome, pigment dispersion syndrome, and uveitis.

Treatment

No specific medical treatment is available. Refractive errors should be corrected, and some patients benefit from bifocal lenses. If visual acuity is severely impaired, these patients can be helped with telescopic and other low-vision devices.

HETEROCHROMIA OF IRIS

Heterochromia refers to variations in the iris colour and is a common congenital anomaly. Heterochromia is a result of the relative excess or lack of melanin (a pigment). Eye colour, specifically the colour of the irises, is determined primarily by the concentration and distribution of melanin. The affected eye may be hyperpigmented (hyperchromic) or hypopigmented (hypochromic).

Heterochromia may be *congenital*, i.e. inherited, or caused by genetic mosaicism, or chimerism. *Acquired heterochormia* disease, or injury. Heterochromia of the eye is of two kinds:

- *Heterochromia iridum* is also called incomplete heterochromia in which colour of one iris differs from the other (Fig. 2.11A).
- *Heterochromia iridis* is also called partial heterochromia or sectoral heterochromia in which one sector of the iris differs from the remainder of iris (Fig. 2.11B).

Differential diagnosis. Congenital heterochromia must be differentiated from the acquired heterochromia as seen in heterochromic cyclitis, siderosis, Horner's syndrome and malignant melanoma of iris.

CORECTOPIA

Corectopia is the displacement of the eye's pupil from its normal, central position. It may be associated with high myopia or ectopia lentis. Medical or surgical intervention may be indicated for the treatment of corectopia.

POLYCORIA

Polycoria, associated with a genetic disorder is a pathological condition of the eye characterized by more than one pupillary opening in the iris. It may be congenital or result from a disease affecting the iris. Polycoria is extremely rare, and other conditions are frequently mistaken for it.

PERSISTENT PUPILLARY MEMBRANE

It represents the remnants of the vascular sheath of the lens, a fetal structure which normally disappear before birth. Persistant pupillary membranes are commonest in baby and probably undergo some absorption as age advances, but may persist permanently.

Characterized by stellate-shaped shreds of the pigmented tissue coming from anterior surface of the iris (attached at collarette) (Fig. 2.12). These float freely in the anterior chamber or may be attached to the anterior surface of the lens.

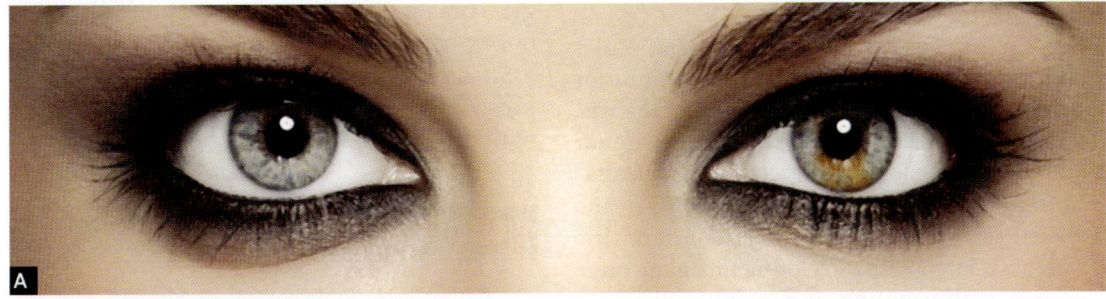

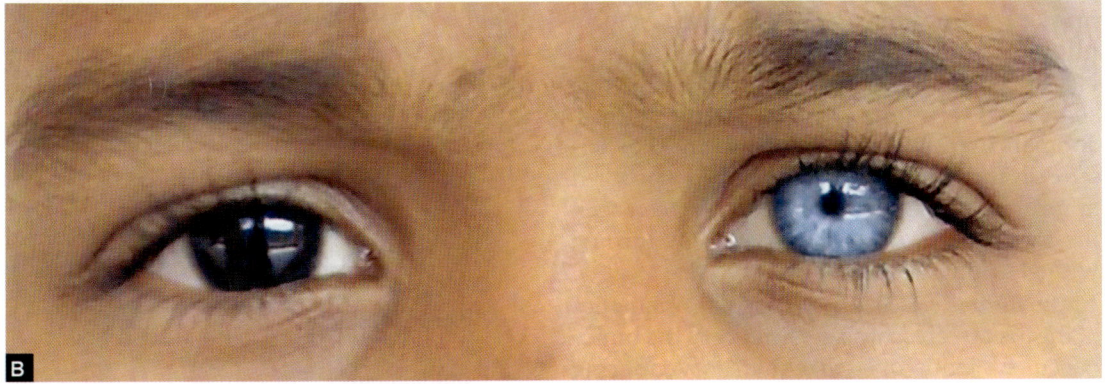

Fig. 2.11 *Heterochromia iridum (A) and iridis (B).*

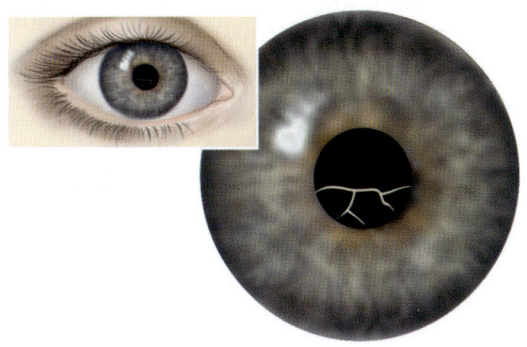

Fig. 2.12 *Persistent pupillary membrane.*

Such iris tags occur frequently and are of no pathological importance. Minute remnants of the pupillary membrane are very commonly seen in slit-lamp examination of adults. They can be differentiated from post-inflammatory synechia as they always come from the anterior surface of the iris from the region of collarette.

CONGENITAL CYST OF IRIS

An iris cyst, or uveal cyst is a small hollow structure either attached to iris or may sometime even float freely in the anterior chamber. An iris cyst is composed of single layer of epithelium and is filled with fluid.

Types. Congenital cyst of the iris is a rare anomaly and may arise either from the pigment epithelium or stroma of iris:

- *Cyst of pigment epithelium of iris* appears to failure of fusion of the two neuroepithelial layers of optic vesicles.
- *Stromal cyst of iris* is believed to be derived from the ectopic cells of the surface ectoderm from which the crystalline lens is developing.

Differential diagnosis of congenital cyst of iris needs to be made from the acquired iris cysts which include:

- *Implantation cyst* which occurs following perforating ocular injury or an intraocular surgery. The implantation cyst has characteristic pearly appearance.
- *Serous cyst of iris* may occur following closure of iris crypts associated with retention of fluid.
- *Parasitic cyst* of iris.

IRIDOTRABECULODYSGENESIS

Iris anomalies may occur in addition to trabecular malformation. They may involve the anterior stroma, iris vessels, or full thickness of the iris. The trabecular meshwork appearance is similar to that found in isolated trabeculodysgenesis.

• *Anterior stromal defects.* Hypoplasia of the anterior iris stroma is the most common iris defect associated with developmental glaucoma. There is malformation of the collarette with marked reduction of the crypt layer. The pupillary sphincter may appear prominent. Hypoplasia of the anterior iris stroma may be seen in Axenfeld's, Rieger's, and Peters' anomalies. In hyperplasia of the anterior iris stroma, there is a thickened, velvety, pebbled appearance. This condition has only been seen in association with Sturge-Weber syndrome with glaucoma.

• *Anomalous iris vessels.* Vascular anomalies of the iris can present as persistence of the tunica vasculosa lentis or as irregularly wandering superficial anomalous iris vessels. Tunica vasculosa lentis exhibits a regular arrangement of vessels looping into the pupillary axis in front of or behind the lens. Normal radial vessels on the iris surface are also prominent because of associated hypoplasia of the anterior iris stroma.

Anomalous superficial iris vessels may also wander irregularly over the iris surface with an often distorted pupil. The iris surface has a whorled appearance and the anterior iris stroma is often hypoplastic. Anomalous iris vessels are seen most frequently in eyes that present with glaucoma and cloudy corneas at birth, and are not associated with any particular syndrome.

• *Structural iris defects.* These defects may present as full-thickness holes through the iris with or without sphincter involvement.

BIBLIOGRAPHY

1. Barber AN. Embryology of Human Eye. CV Mosby, St. Louis, 1955.

2. Duke Elder S. System of Ophthalmology, Vol-III, Part-I, 1st edition, Henry Kimpton, London, 1964.

3. Kherani F, Robb RM. Congenital and developmental abnormalities of the eye, orbit, and ocular adnexa. In: Albert DM, Miller JW (eds). Principles and Practice of Ophthalmology, Elsevier, ISBN 978-1-4160-0016-7, Philadelphia, 2008, pp. 4177–83.

4. Kozart DM. Embryology of the human eye. In: Schcie HG, Albert DM (eds). Textbook of Ophthalmology, 9th edition, 1977, pp. 79–92, WB Saunders Company, London.

5. Levin AV. Congenital eye anomalies. Pediatr Clin North Am, vol 50, no.1, (February 2003). 1954, pp. 56-76, ISSN 0031-3955.

6. Mann Ida. Development of Human Eye, 3rd edition, British Medical Association, London, 1964.

7. Moore KL, Persaud TVN. The Developing Human, 6th edition, 1998.

8. Nema HV, Singh VD, Nema N. Congenital anomalies of the eye and its adnexa, 2nd edition. Jay Pee Brothers, New Delhi, 1991, pp. 162–5.

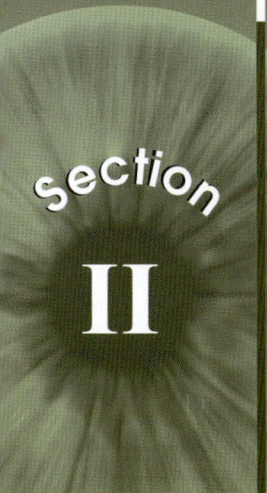

Uveitis and Intraocular Inflammations

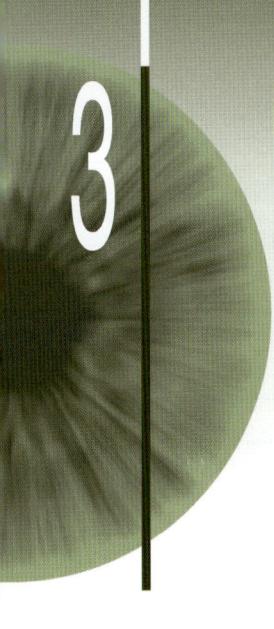

IMMUNE MECHANISMS, ETIOPATHOGENESIS AND PATHOLOGY OF UVEITIS

3.1 General Immunology

3.2 Ocular Immune Mechanisms and Etiopathogenesis of Uveitis

3.3 Pathology of Uveitis

3.1 GENERAL IMMUNOLOGY

Immunity and Hypersensitivity: An Overview
Introduction
Architecture of immune system
• Mononuclear phagocytic system
• Lymphoid organs
- Central lymphoid organs
- Peripheral lymphoid organs
Immunity
• Innate
• Acquired
- Active
- Passive
Antigens
• Definition
• Some facts about antigenicity
• Histocompatibility antigens
Antibodies
• Structure of antibody
• Types of immunoglobulins
Development of immune response
• Humoral immunity
• Cellular immunity
• Mediator systems that amplify immune response
Other immune mechanism-related aspects
• Immune tolerance
• Immune modulation
• Autoimmunity
• Hypersensitivity

IMMUNITY AND HYPERSENSITIVITY: AN OVERVIEW

INTRODUCTION

Pathogenesis of uveitis is a complex phenomenon. Before discussing etiopathogenesis of uveitis, it will be worth while to review the immunity and hypersensitivity mechanisms, in general as well as, the special ocular immune characteristics.

Immunity refers to resistance of the body to pathogens and their toxic products. Various aspects in relation to the immune mechanisms which need detailed discussion are introduced briefly:

Types of immunity. Immunity primarily is of two types:
• *Innate immunity* which is present by birth, and
• *Acquired or adaptive immunity* which is achieved during the lifetime by the individual.

Antigens. Antigens are substances that can stimulate an immune response in the body.

Antibodies. Antibodies or immunoglobulins (Igs) are gamma globulins which are produced in response to antigenic stimulation.

Immune system. The immune system that constitutes the body's defence system consists of lymphoid organs, reticuloendothelial components and the various types of immunological cells distributed throughout the body.

Immune response. The immune system of the body responds to an antigen by two ways:

- *Humoral or antibody-mediated immunity (AMI)* which is mediated by antibodies produced by plasma cells, and
- *Cell-mediated immunity (CMI)* which is mediated directly by the sensitized lymphocytes.

Immune tolerance. Immune tolerance refers to the inability of a host to express a specific immunological response to an antigen.

Autoimmunity. Refers to the condition when the body's immune response gets directed towards its own tissues which are normally exempted as self.

Immunomodulation refers to process of modifying the body's immune response. It may be in the form of:

- *Immunoenhancement* (immunopotentiation), i.e. to enhance the antibody or cell-mediated immune response against an antigen, and
- *Immunosuppression*, i.e. to reduce the body's immune response against the antigens.

Hypersensitivity. Refers to an abnormal immune response which produces physiological or histopathological damage in the host.

ARCHITECTURE (COMPONENTS) OF IMMUNE SYSTEM

The immune system is a complex network of organs containing cells that recognize foreign substances in the body and destroy them. It is a system of many biological structures and processes within an organism that gives protection against pathogen or infectious agents, such as viruses, bacteria, fungi, and other parasites. The organs of the immune system are positioned throughout the body (Fig. 3.1.1). They are called lymphoid organs because they serve as a home to lymphocytes, small white

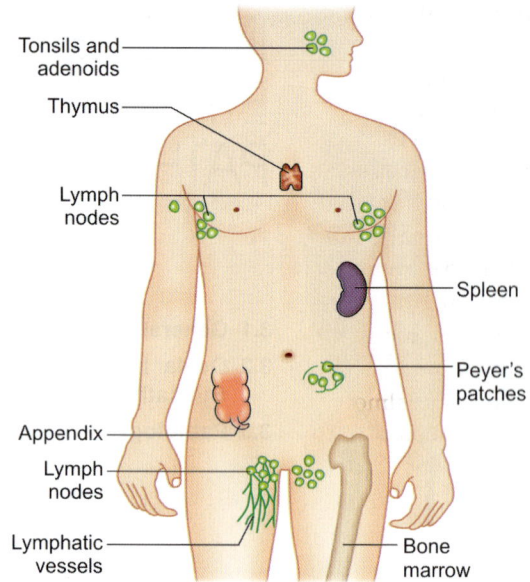

Fig. 3.1.1 *Organs of immune system.*

blood cells, that are the key players in the immune system.

The immune system consists of immunological cells distributed into two main components:
1. Mononuclear phagocytic system, and
2. Lymphoid component.

MONONUCLEAR PHAGOCYTIC SYSTEM

Mononuclear phagocytic system (MPS), also known as *tissue-macrophage system,* is the new name given to the system previously called as reticuloendothelial system (RES).

Formation of mononuclear phagocytic system

The monocytes enter the blood from the bone marrow and circulate for about 3 days. From the blood, the monocytes migrate into the tissue where they attain maturity, i.e. they increase in size and a large number of lysosomes and mitochondria develop in their cytoplasm. In this way, they acquire the ability to phagocytose and thus get converted to macrophages. The macrophages wander through tissues (*mobile macrophages*) and perform scavenger functions of eliminating microorganisms and other foreign particles that invade the tissues. Some of these macrophages become attached to certain tissues in the body (*fixed macrophages*) and remain there for several months. These tissue macrophages scattered in different parts of the body combinedly constitute the *tissue macrophage system* or the so-called *mononuclear phagocytic system (MPS)*. The tissue macrophage system includes the macrophages present at the following sites in the body:

- Macrophages lining the sinusoids of liver (Kupffer cells)
- Spleen
- Bone marrow (littoral cells)
- Lymph nodes
- Lungs (pulmonary alveolar macrophages or PAM, also called dust cells)
- Connective tissue (histiocytes)
- Pleura and peritoneum
- Subcutaneous tissue
- Bones (osteoclasts)
- Central nervous system (microglial cells).

Constituent cells of mononuclear phagocytic system

The term mononuclear phagocytic system (MPS) was coined in 1960 to include the following constituents:

- *Precursor cells of the monocyte* series from bone marrow.
- *Promonocytes* from the bone marrow.
- *Monocytes* from the bone marrow and blood.
- *Tissue macrophages* present in the above-cited sites in the body.

Role of MPS in the immune response

- The cells of MPS ingest and process the antigen entering the body. The processing of antigen is essential before an antigen can evoke cell-mediated immunity (CMI) or stimulate antibody formation in plasma cells.
- The cells of MPS have receptors for immunoglobulins and complements, so these are very efficient in phagocytosing the antigen–antibody complement complexes.

LYMPHOID ORGANS

The lymphoid component of the immune system consists of a network of lymphoid organs, tissues and cells and the product of these cells. Lymphoid organs can be classified into:

A. *Central or primary lymphoid organs*, which include:
  I. Thymus, and
  II. Bursa equivalent (fetal liver and bone marrow); and
B. *Peripheral lymphoid organs*, which include:
  I. Lymph nodes,
  II. Spleen and
  III. Mucosa-associated lymphoid tissues (MALT).

A. Primary (central) lymphoid organs

I. Thymus

The thymus gland is a complex lymphoreticular organ located in mediastinum just above the heart. It consists of two (right and left) encapsulated lobes joined together by a fibrous connective tissue.

Role of thymus in the immune system

- The main function of the thymus is development of cell-mediated immunity. The stem cells destined to form T lymphocytes leave the bone marrow and migrate to the thymus where they further differentiate.
- The thymus confers immunological competence on the lymphocytes during their stay in the organ. In the thymus, T lymphocytes are educated so that they become capable of mounting a cell-mediated immune response.
- The *immunologically competent lymphocytes* migrate from thymus into peripheral lymphoid organs as mature **T lymphocytes** which are precommitted to their function and antigen specificity. These are selectively seeded into paracortical areas of peripheral lymph nodes and into the white pulp of the spleen around the central arterioles. These regions are known as *thymus-dependent* areas.

Thus, T cells are formed in bone marrow and are educated in thymus. T cell-dependent antigens require compatible antigen presenting cells (APCs) for its recognition (Fig. 3.1.2A).

II. Bursa Equivalent

In humans, the **fetal liver and bone marrow** appear to be the equivalent of avian bursa of Fabricius.

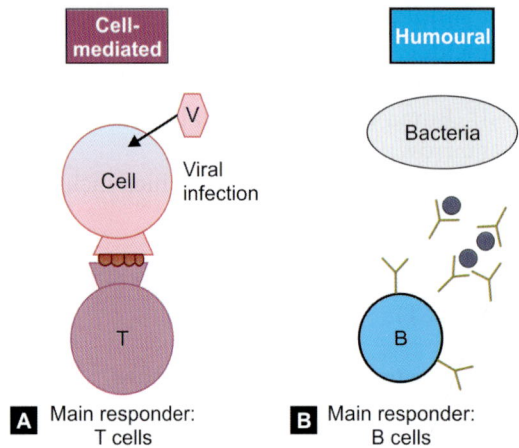

Fig. 3.1.2 *Role of T lymphocytes (A) and B lymphocyte (B) in defence mechanism.*

Bursa of Fabricius in birds is also a site of lymphocytic proliferation and differentiation. Immunocompetent lymphocytes produced in the bursa are called bursa lymphocytes or *B lymphocytes* or B cells. The mature B cells migrate from the bursa into outer or superficial cortex of the germinal follicles and medullary cords of lymph nodes and lymphoid follicles of spleen. These sites are known as bursa-dependent or thymus-independent areas. Following appropriate antigenic stimulation, B lymphocytes transform into plasma cells and secrete antibodies which constitute the humoural immunity or antibody-mediated immunity (AMI) (Fig. 3.1.2B). Surgical removal of bursa (bursectomy) from newly hatched birds destroys their subsequent ability to produce antibodies but does not affect their ability to produce cell-mediated immunity (CMI).

Since fetal liver and bone marrow appear to be the mammalian equivalent of the avian bursa of Fabricius, *so the bone marrow is the site not only of haemopoiesis but also of initial differentiation of stem cells to B lymphocytes.*

B. Peripheral lymphoid organs

I. Lymph nodes

The lymph nodes are small bean-shaped or oval structures which form part of the lymphatic network distributed throughout the body.

Functions of lymph nodes

1. *To mount immune response in the body.* It is the main function of lymph nodes. A bulk of antigens is processed and antibody production occurs in the lymphoid follicles
2. *To perform the function of active phagocytosis* for particulate material is another main function of the lymph nodes.

II. Spleen

The spleen is the largest lymphoid organ of the body.

Role in immune response. The spleen constitutes an important component of the defence system. It is an active site for production of T and B lymphocytes and antibodies. Blood-borne antigens entering the spleen are phagocytosed and processed by macrophages and fixed phagocytic mononuclear cells. Presentation of antigens, on the surface of such cells, to the splenic lymphocytes results in the formation of secondary follicles containing germinal centres of dividing and differentiating B cells which ultimately form antibodies. After splenectomy, antibody production continues to occur in other lymphoid organs but the antibody response is delayed and the antibody titre does not rise as high as in normal individuals.

III. Mucosa-associated lymphoid tissue

Mucosa-associated lymphoid tissue (MALT) refers to the lymphoid tissue distributed along the mucosa lining the alimentary, respiratory, genitourinary and other surfaces, e.g. conjunctiva which are constantly exposed to numerous antigens. Tonsils, adenoids and Peyer's patches of small intestine are known as gut-associated lymphoid tissues (GALT). Peyer's patches are small patches of organized lymphoid tissue along the intestine containing B lymphocytes (in germinal centre) and T lymphocytes. They play a primary role in defence against infectious organisms entering via the gastrointestinal tract (GIT).

IMMUNITY

Immunity refers to resistance of the body to pathogens and their toxic products. It can be classified as:

I. *Innate immunity*
  1. Non-specific, and
  2. Specific innate immunity:
     • Species,
     • Racial, and
     • Individual.
II. *Acquired (adaptive) immunity*
  1. Active acquired(adaptive) immunity:
     • Natural, and
     • Artificial.
  2. Passive acquired (adaptive) immunity:
     • Natural, and
     • Artificial.

INNATE IMMUNITY

• *Innate or natural immunity* is the inborn capacity of the body to offer resistance to pathogens and their toxic products. It is due to genetic and constitutional make up.
• It may be specific (against particular organism) or non-specific.
• Innate immunity may be:
  – *Species immunity*, i.e. resistance to a pathogen shown by all members of a species.
  – *Racial immunity*, i.e. resistance to a pathogen shown by only a particular race within a species.
  – *Individual immunity*, i.e. resistance to a pathogen shown by a particular individual within a race.

Mechanisms of innate immunity

1. **Mechanical barrier** against invading microorganisms is provided by the intact skin and mucosa in the body.
2. **Surface secretions** constitute one of the important mechanisms of innate immunity. These include:
• *Secretions* from the sebaceous glands of skin which contain both saturated and unsaturated fatty acids that kill many bacteria and fungi.
• *Saliva*, constantly produced in the mouth cavity, has an inhibitory effect on many microorganisms.
• *Gastric juice* and highly acidic environment of stomach may hydrolyse microbial invaders.
• *Tears* poured in the conjunctival sac mechanically wash away the particles and a hydrolytic

enzyme, lysozyme present in the tears, can destroy most of the microorganisms.
3. **Humoural defence mechanisms** provide innate immunity by the non-specific microbicidal substances present in the body fluids. A few examples are:
• *Lysozyme* is found in high concentration in most tissue fluids except CSF, sweat and urine. It is a mucolytic enzyme which kills microorganisms by splitting sugars of the structural mucopeptide of their cell wall.
• *Basic polypeptides* containing non-specific microbicidal activity include leukins, arginine- and lysine-containing proteins protamine and histone.
• *Complements* have lytic and several other effects on foreign substances.
• *Interferons* are antiviral substances produced by the cells stimulated by live or killed viruses. α and β interferons are part of innate immunity.
4. **Cellular mechanisms of defence** which provide non-specific innate immunity are:
• *Phagocytes*, i.e. neutrophils and the monocyte–macrophage system cells constitute the most important non-specific cellular defence against the invading microorganisms
• *Natural killer (NK) cells* refer to a subpopulation of lymphocytes which provide non-specific cellular defence against viruses, tumour cells and other infected cells.
• *Eosinophil* granules contain enzymes and toxic molecules that act against larvae of helminths.

ADAPTIVE (ACQUIRED) IMMUNITY

The resistance that an individual acquires during his lifetime is known as acquired or adaptive immunity. It is antigen-specific and may be antibody- or cell-mediated. It is of two types: active and passive.

1. Active immunity

Active immunity is acquired by the synthesis of antibodies (humoural immunity) and production of immunocompetent cells (cell-mediated immunity) by the individual's own immune system in response to an antigenic stimulation.

Active immunity can be induced naturally from a subclinical or clinical infection or artificially (by introducing antigens in the body in the form of vaccines and this process is called active immunization).

2. Passive immunity

Passive immunity refers to the immunity that is transferred to a recipient in a ready made form. Here, the individual's immune system does not play an active role.

Natural passive immunity is the transfer of ready-made antibodies from the mother as:
• *In a fetus,* the IgG antibodies are transferred from the mother through the placenta.
• *After birth,* immunoglobulins are passed to the newborn through breast milk. Human colostrum is rich in IgA antibodies which are resistant to digestion in stomach and small intestine.

Artificial passive immunity. Examples include injection of:
• Antitetanus serum (ATS),
• Antidiphtheric serum (ADS), and
• Antigas gangrene serum (AGS).

ANTIGENS

DEFINITION

Antigen. Antigens are substances that can stimulate an immune response in the body. Most antigens are proteins, but some are carbohydrates, lipids and nucleic acids. The specificity of an antigen is due to specific areas of its molecule called determinant sites or epitopes. The epitopes can bind to specific binding sites called paratopes of the antibody molecule (Fig. 3.1.3). A pure protein can have several

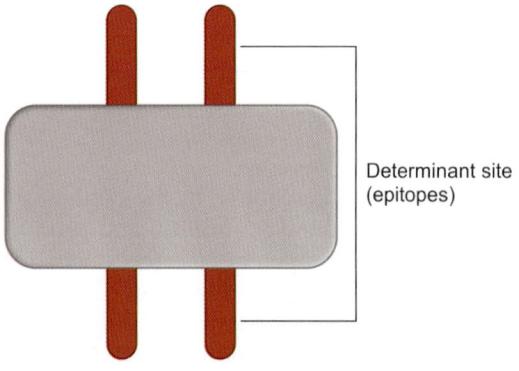

Determinant site (epitopes)

Fig. 3.1.3 *Structure of an antigen.*

epitopes and thus can stimulate formation of many distinct antibodies.

Hapten or incomplete antigen is a chemical substance of low molecular weight that cannot induce an immune response by itself. Nevertheless, haptens can produce the immune response when combined with larger molecules (usually proteins), which serve as carriers. For example, the atropine molecule is a hapten and does not produce an immune response, but when it combines with tear proteins it can excite immune response.

In contrast to complete antigens, haptens contain a single epitope.

SOME FACTS ABOUT ANTIGENICITY

Immunogenicity. Immunogenicity, i.e. ability of an antigen to stimulate an immune response is determined by:
• Size of molecule,
• Foreignness of molecules,
• Chemical structure of the molecule,
• Susceptibility of the substance to the tissue enzymes,
• Genetic constitution of the host, and
• Dosage, route and timing of administration.

HISTOCOMPATIBILITY ANTIGENS

Histocompatibility antigens refer to the antigens present on the plasma membrane of cells of each individual of a species. These antigens are encoded by genes known as histocompatibility genes which collectively constitute the major histocompatibility complex (MHC). These are located on the short arm of chromosome 6. MHCs present on the surface of leucocytes were previously known as human leucocyte-associated antigens (HLA) and now known as histocompatibility lymphocyte antigens (HLA). These have been studied extensively in organ transplantation. The major histocompatibility antigens in man and mouse are known as HLA and H_2, respectively. No two persons, except identical twins, have the same MHC proteins. No two persons can have the same MHC proteins on plasma membranes of their cells.

Classes of MHC gene

There are three subclasses of MHC genes: class I, II and III.

MHC class I. Molecules are found on the surface of virtually all the cells of the body excluding red blood cells. The MHC class I refers to the products of HLA-A, B, C, D, E, F, G.

MHC class II. Antigens are encoded by the HLA-DP, HLA-DQ and HLA-DR loci, all of which reside within HLA-D region of HLA complex. In man, MHC class II antigens are only found on immunologically reactive cells, such as B lymphocytes, monocytes, activated T lymphocytes and antigen presenting cells (APPCs) which include dendritic cells and macrophages. Some MHC class II molecules also express on CD4+ and CD8+ cells and act as APCs to themselves or autologous T cells.

MHC class III. There are over 20 genes. Some encode for the complement components of the classical (C_2 and C_4) and the alternative (properdin factor B) pathways, while others are involved in production of molecules of antigen processing.

HLA tissue typing

Histocompatibility typing or the so-called HLA tissue typing refers to detection of MHC class I and MHC class II antigens. HLA typing is used:

- To determine HLA compatibility prior to organ/tissue transplantation from one individual to another within a species,
- For paternity testing,
- For anthropologic studies, and
- For establishing HLA disease association.

ANTIBODIES

Antibodies or immunoglobulins (Igs) are gamma globulins which are produced in response to antigenic stimulation.

These react specifically with the antigens which stimulated their production. All antibodies are immunoglobulins but all immunoglobulins are not antibodies. Immunoglobulins (Igs) have been divided into five distinct classes or isotypes, namely, IgG, IgA, IgM, IgD and IgE.

STRUCTURE OF ANTIBODY

IgG has been studied extensively and serves as a model of basic structural unit of all Igs. An immunoglobulin is a Y-shaped molecule made of four polypeptide chains: two heavy (H) and two light (L). These are held together by disulphide bonds (Fig. 3.1.4).

TYPES OF IMMUNOGLOBULINS

On the basis of physiochemical and antigenic structure, five distinct classes of immunoglobulins are identified in human serum. These are IgG, IgA, IgM, IgD and IgE.

IgG

Distribution. IgG is the most abundant class of Ig in the body, constituting approximately 75% of the total body Igs. It is distributed equally between the intravascular and extravascular pools. It is also found in milk, saliva, nasal and bronchial secretions.

Production. A little IgG is produced during the early stage of primary response to antigen. But, it is the major form of antibody produced during secondary response in which the initial IgM production gives way to IgG production (class switch).

Subclasses. There are four subclasses of human IgG: IgG1, IgG2, IgG3 and IgG4, possessing distinct types of heavy chains known as γ1, γ2, γ3 and γ4, respectively.

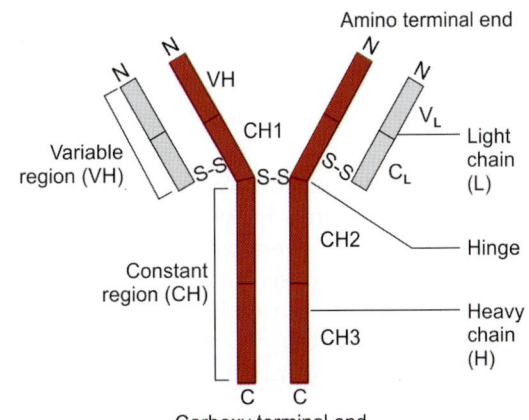

Fig. 3.1.4 *Basic structure of antibody showing the arrangement of heavy and light chains and its variables and constant domains.*

Placental transfer. IgG is the only class of Igs that can cross the placenta and is responsible for protection of the infant during the first few months of life. IgG is also found along with IgA, in milk during the first few weeks after birth, providing additional protection, if the infant is breastfed.

Binding characteristics of IgG are:

- Macrophages and monocytes bear Fc receptors (FcRs) which bind to the Fc portion of IgG1 and IgG3 in CH3 domain. Such binding permits these cells to exhibit antibody-dependent cellular toxicity (ADCC).
- IgG usually exhibits high affinity for antigens leading to efficient neutralization of toxins.
- Among NK null cells, a distinct subpopulation of cytotoxic cells has been recognized which also possess FcRs for Fc part of IgG; they are capable of lysing or killing target cells sensitized with IgG and are called killer cells.
- Platelets also possess FcRs for Fc portion of IgG leading to aggregation, degranulation and release of histamine.
- IgG is the only Ig which has the property to fixing guinea pig's skin. Thus, IgG participates in most immunological reactions, such as complement fixation, precipitation and neutralization of toxins and viruses.

IgM

Distribution. IgM constitutes about 10% of the total serum immunoglobulins. In contrast to IgG, IgM, because of its large size, remains almost exclusively in the serum and is not usually found extravascularly in body cavities or secretions.

Production. Phylogenetically, IgM is the oldest Ig class. It is the only Ig which is produced before birth. It is the predominant Ig produced during primary response. It appears early in the secondary response but its level does not rise significantly thereafter.

Placental transfer. Pentamer IgM is apparently too large to cross the placenta. As it cannot cross the placental barrier, the presence of IgM in a fetus or newborn indicates intrauterine infection. Its detection is, therefore, useful for the diagnosis of congenital syphilis, rubella and toxoplasmosis.

Binding characteristics. IgM contains 10 Fab fragments, and thus 10 antigen-binding sites. Therefore, theoretically, it can bind to 10 antigen molecules. However, practically, IgM is capable of binding to as few as five molecules of antigen.

- IgM is much more efficient than IgG in its ability to fix complement by the classical pathway promoting lysis and death of most Gram-negative bacteria. This greater efficiency is due to the fact that the complement may bind to several Fc regions of pentameric IgM simultaneously, thus initiating a complement cascade and target cell lysis with a single molecule.
- IgM causes effective agglutination but its opsonizing power is rather weak.

IgA

Distribution. IgA is the second-most abundant class constituting about 15% of human serum Igs where it exists as a *monomeric* Ig. Its more important form is the dimeric form, known as secretory IgA (SIgA). It is the predominant class of Igs in secretions, such as milk, tears, nasal secretions, saliva, lung secretions, genitourinary and gastrointestinal fluids.

Production. Secretory IgA is synthesized by plasma cells in the subepithelial tissues of the body.

Binding characteristics. IgA does not fix complement in the classical pathway but can activate the alternative pathway. It promotes phagocytosis and intracellular killing of micro-organisms.

Important note: SIgA coats the microbes and inhibits their adherence to the mucosal cells thereby preventing the entry into the body tissues. *Nisseria gonorrhoeae* which produces IgA protease can penetrate the mucosal barrier even in an immune person.

IgD

Distribution. IgD is present on the surface of B lymphocytes (which are destined to differentiate into antibody-producing plasma cells) and is known to act as antigen receptors for the B cells.

Placental transfer. It does not cross the placenta.

Binding characteristics. IgD does not bind complement.

Since it is present on the surface of B lymphocytes, it is involved in antigen recognition. Reaction of an antigen with surface immunoglobulin may lead to cell differentiation and antibody synthesis.

IgE

Production. IgE is chiefly produced in the lining of the respiratory and intestinal tracts.

Distribution and serum concentration. Mostly a person's IgE is fixed to the surface of mast cells and basophils. Its presents in extremely low concentration (0.00004 ng/ml) in the serum. However, the serum IgE levels are raised in atopic (type I hypersensitivity) conditions, like asthma and hay fever.

Placental transfer. It does not cross the placental barrier.

Binding characteristics. It does not fix complement.

- The Fc portion of IgE binds to the Fc receptors present on the surface of mast cells and basophils leaving antigen-binding sites free to react with specific antigen. When a specific antigen binds with such IgE, the reaction results in the degranulation of mast or basophil cells with the release of pharmacologically active substances, such as histamine, slow-reacting substances of anaphylaxis (SRS-A), mast cell chemotactic factor, eosinophil chemotactic factor, etc.
- IgE production is particularly known to be stimulated in parasitic infestation. It has been suggested that mast cell-bound IgE reacts with antigens on the parasite followed by release of histamine. This results in increased vascular permeability followed by influx of plasma and cells (particularly eosinophils) and destruction of parasite.

Specific functions of various immunoglobulins

- *IgG* protects the body fluids.
- *IgA* protects the body surfaces.
- *IgM* protects the bloodstream.
- *IgE* mediates type I hypersensitivity.
- *IgD's* role is not clearly known.

DEVELOPMENT OF IMMUNE RESPONSE

Development of an immune response implies development of acquired (adaptive) active, immunity in the body.

Components of adaptive immunity (Fig. 3.1.5) are:

- *Cellular components*—These are leucocytes which contain B and T lymphocytes, phagocytes and auxiliary cells (basophils, mast cells, platelets), and
- *Tissue cells* also known as *antigen presenting cells (APCs).*

Immune system of the body responds to an antigen by two ways:

- Humoural or antibody-mediated immunity (AMI), and
- Cell-mediated immunity (CMI).

HUMOURAL IMMUNITY

The humoural immunity is mediated by antibodies and so is also called antibody-mediated immunity (AMI). The antibodies are produced by plasma cells which in turn are produced by B lymphocytes.

Role of humoural immunity

The humoural immunity provides defence against most extracellular bacterial pathogens and viruses. The antibody response to stimulation by an antigen is of two types (Fig. 3.1.6):

- Primary humoural response, and
- Secondary humoural response.

i. *Primary response* refers to the response of the body's immune system to an antigen which is introduced into the body for the first time. Always there is a latent period varying from 4 days to

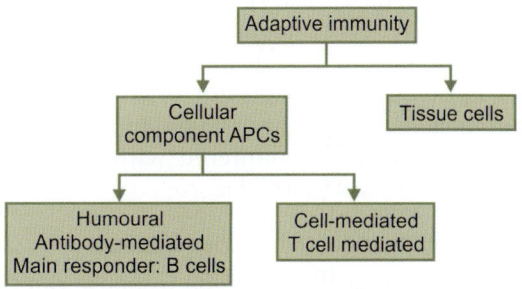

Fig. 3.1.5 *Components of adaptive immunity.*

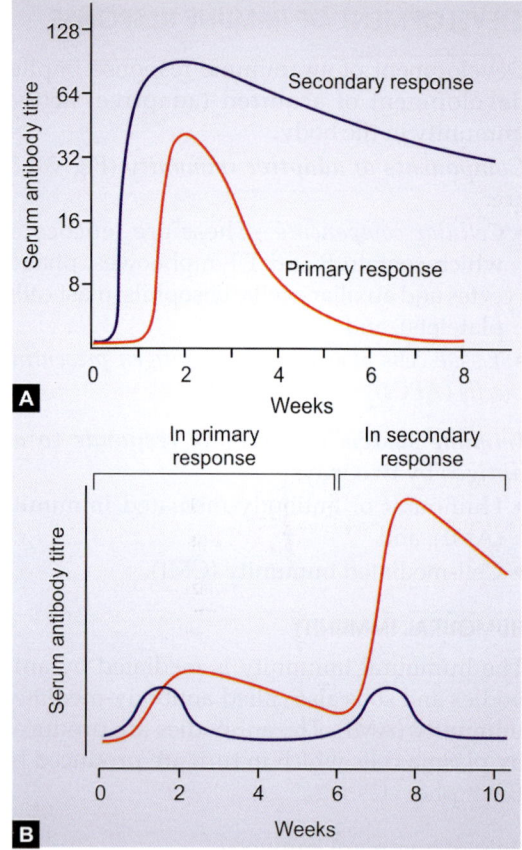

Fig. 3.1.6 *Response of body immune system to an antigen: A, Time course of antibody production in primary versus/ secondary response; B, Serum levels of IgM and IgG antibodies in primary and secondary response.*

4 weeks before the primary response in the form of a rise in the serum antibodies titre can be detected.

ii. *Secondary response* refers to the response of the body's immune system to an antigen which is introduced into the body on a second occasion. Such a response occurs more quickly and more abundantly. This is because of the fact that the immune system is liable to retain the memory of a prior antigenic exposure for long periods (immunological memory) and produce enhanced response when encountered with the same antigen for the second time.

Phases of humoural immune response

The development of immune response can be subdivided, using the concept of "*immune

response arc", into three phases (Figs 3.1.7 to 3.1.9):

- Afferent phase,
- Processing phase, and
- Effector phase.

I. Afferent phase

Afferent phase of immune response arc comprises transport, presentation and recognition of antigen to adaptive immune system.

1. *Antigen processing and presentation.* Once the antigen enters the body, it is phagocytosed by the macrophages (non-specific response). Phagocytosed material is broken down into polypeptide fragments. The antigen polypeptide fragments then combine with the MHC II present in the macrophages and move to the cell surface. This is called processing of antigen. The processed antigen is then presented to immuno-competent lymphocytes by the macrophages. So, the macrophages are also called antigen-presenting cells (APCs). Other antigen-presenting cells which can process and present the antigen to lymphocytes are:

- B lymphocytes themselves, and
- Dendritic cells present in the skin (Langerhans cells), thymus (medulla), lymph nodes (cortex and paracortex), spleen and other secondary lymphoid organs.

2. *Recognition of antigen by lymphocytes.* The lymphocytes possess the antigen recognition receptors. These include the membrane-bound (surface) immunoglobulins (mIgs or sIgs) in B lymphocytes and T cell receptors (TCRs) in the T lymphocytes. These receptors serve as specific

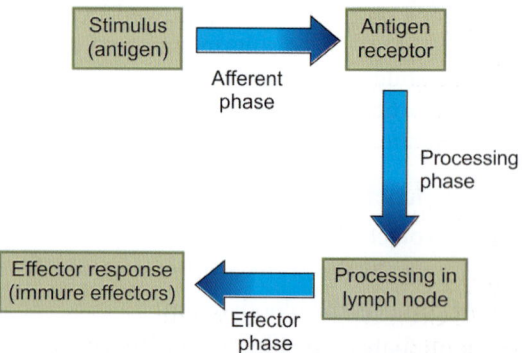

Fig. 3.1.7 *Phases of immune response arc.*

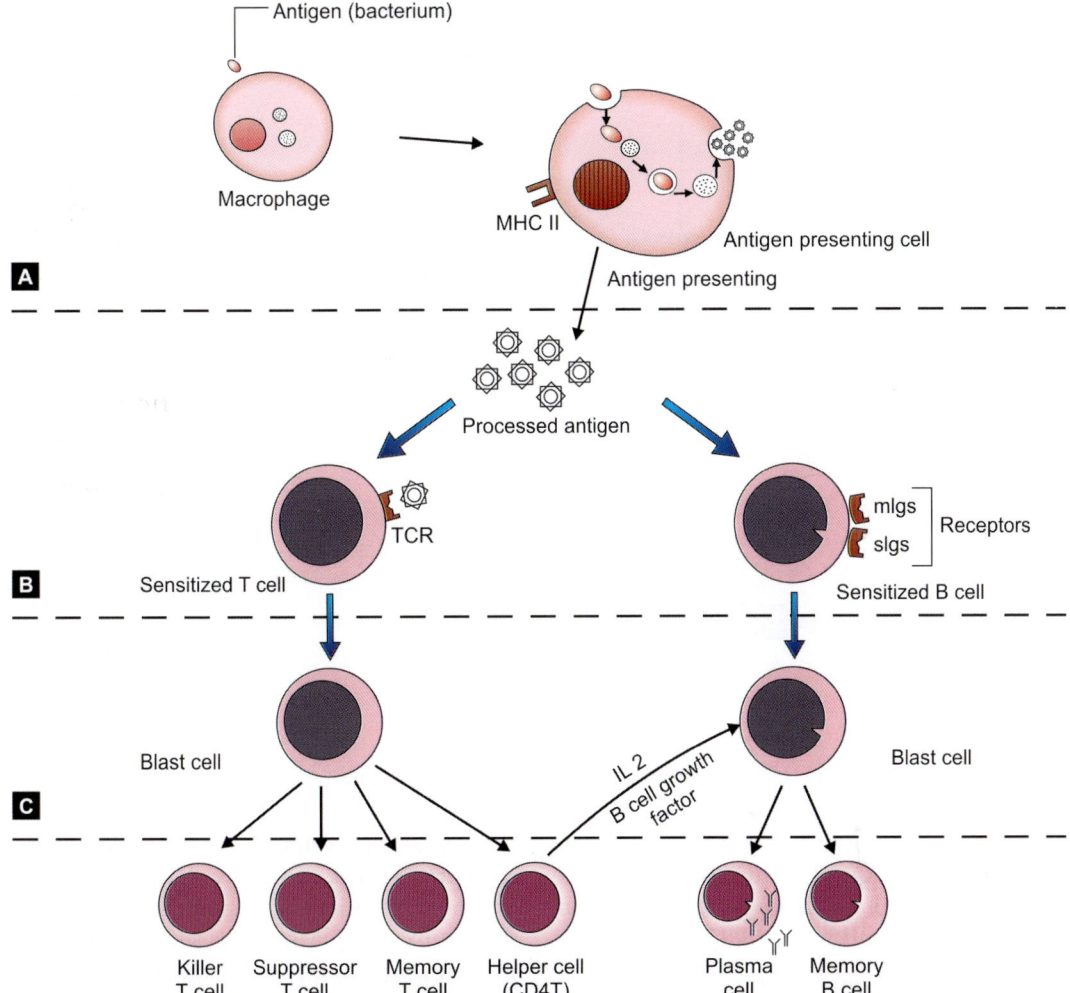

Fig. 3.1.8 *Broad outline of development of humoural immune response: A, Antigen processing and presentation to immunocompetent cells; B, Recognition of antigen by lymphocytes; C, Activation of lymphocytes (blast formation).*

surface receptors, recognizing and interacting with only a single antigenic determinant on the antigen presented to the lymphocytes. This process of binding of processed antigen to specific receptors on the surface of lymphocytes in technical terms is called *recognition of antigen by lymphocytes.* Thus, many million different T and B lymphocytes, each with the ability to respond to particular antigen, are present in the body.

Important note: The receptors on circulating T cell (TCRs) are mainly made of α and β polypeptide units, hence called α and β T cells. About 10% of T cell receptors (TCRs) have γ and

δ polypeptide units, and they are designated as γδ T cells.

II. *Processing phase*

Processing phase of immune response arc comprises activation or sensitization of lymphocytes. It involves conversion of antigenic stimulus into immunologic response

1. *Lymphocyte activation*

The lymphocytes that have combined with antigen are activated, i.e. the lymphocytes become larger and look like a lymphoblast. This is known as *blast transformation.* Activated B

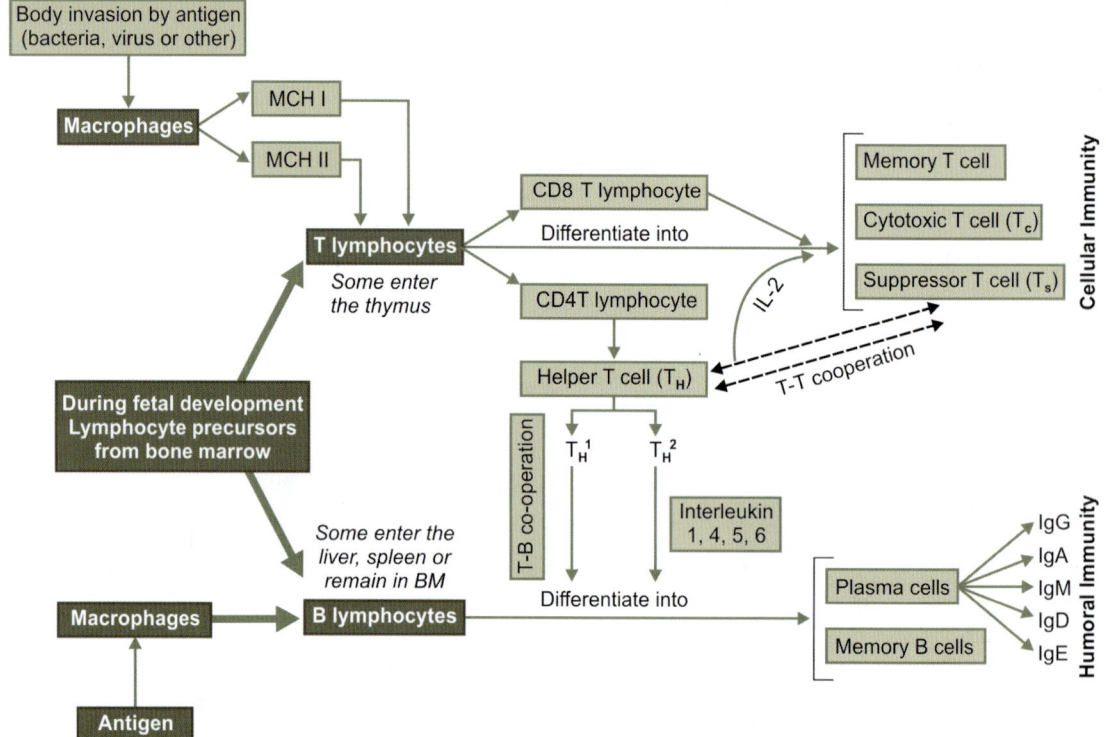

Fig. 3.1.9 *Summary of immune response.*

lymphocytes and helper T cells (CD4 cells) play a major role in humoural immunity. The macrophages liberate IL-1 and cause further activation of B lymphocytes and helper (CD4T) cells.

Activation of T lymphocytes. Activation of helper T cells by the processed antigen complex is essential for humoural immunity. The activated helper T cells secrete two substances: interleukins 2 (IL2) and B cell growth factor which further promote proliferation of B lymphocytes and their transformation into plasma cells. This phenomenon is called *T-B cooperation.*

Activation of B lymphocytes. After receiving cooperation from T helper cells (T-B cooperation), B lymphoblasts proliferate forming clones of cells that respond to this antigen (clonal selection). A clone is the population of cells descended by asexual reproduction from a single cell. The B lymphocytes proliferate and transform into two types:

• Plasma cells, and
• Memory B cells.

Role of plasma cells. When a B lymphocyte is converted to a plasma cell, its cytoplasm expands. It is filled with granular endoplasmic reticulum. The plasma cells secrete antibodies.

Role of memory B cells. A small portion of the activated B lymphocytes do not enlarge or undergo blast transformation. Instead, they only proliferate and transform into small-sized memory B cells, which occupy the lymphoid tissue throughout the body. Memory B cells have a long lifespan and remain inactive. When the body is exposed to the same antigen for the second time, they are able to recognize it become active, i.e. they are responsible for secondary response of antibodies.

2. Production of antibodies

The plasma cells so formed secrete antibodies which are also called immunoglobulins (Igs). Immunoglobulins are actually secreted form of antigen-binding receptors.

The rate of antibody production is very high, i.e. each plasma cell produces about 2000 molecules of antibodies per second. A plasma cell secretes an antibody of a single specificity of a single antibody class and a single light chain type. However, in a primary antibody response, a plasma cell produces IgM initially and later it may switch on to IgG production.

III. *Effector phase*

Effector phase is also known as inactivation of antigen or attack phase of immune response. This is the last phase of immune response and involves the inactivation of antigen by the antibodies. Antibodies act on the invading antigen in two ways:

1. *Direct attack on the invading agents*

Because of the bivalent nature of antibody and multiple antigen sites on most of the invading agents, antibodies can inactivate the invading agent by the following reactions:

- *Agglutination.* By this reaction, large number of particles (bacteria or red cells) with antigens on their surface are bound together to form a clump. Clumping increases the susceptibility to phagocytosis.
- *Precipitation.* In this reaction, the antigen–antibody complex forms an insoluble precipitate.
- *Neutralization.* Antibodies cover the toxic sites of antigen and neutralize them.
- *Cytolysis.* Antibodies attach to the membranes of cellular agents thereby causing rupture of cells.

2. *Attack on the antigen through complement system*

The complement system includes 11 enzymatic proteins which are named as C1 to C9, B and D. All these are present in the blood as plasma proteins. These are also present in the tissue fluid. The complement system acts in three ways (Fig. 3.1.10):

a. **Classical pathway.** This is activated by an antigen–antibody reaction. When an antibody binds with an antigen, a specific reactive site on the constant portion of the antibody becomes uncovered where the protein C1 binds and thus gets activated. The activated C1 in turn activates the other complements in a series of cascade reactions. The products of complement activation cause the following effects:

- *Opsonization.* Opsonization is the coating of antigen by antibody and complement. It helps the neutrophils and macrophages to phagocytose the antigen. The activated C3a product acts as an opsonin.
- *Lysis,* i.e. destruction of bacteria by rupturing the cell membrane. A membrane attack complex is formed by C5b–C6–C7–C8–C9. The cell lysis is brought about by the complement system by inserting proteins called *perforins* into the cell membrane. Perforins make holes in the cell membranes, resulting in free flow of ions and disrupting membrane permeability.
- *Agglutination,* i.e. clumping of bacteria and RBCs.
- *Chemotaxis,* i.e. attraction of leucocytes to the site of antigen–antibody reaction. Chemotaxis is enhanced by C5b–C6–C7 complex.
- *Neutralization,* i.e. covering the toxic sites of antigenic products.
- *Activation and degranulation of mast cells and basophils* is caused by C4b. This releases factors producing vasodilatation and chemotaxis. Vasodilatation increases capillary permeability; therefore, plasma proteins enter the tissues and antigenic products are inactivated.

The antibodies which can fix and thereby activate complements are IgM and IgG. IgA also fixes complements but does so by the alternative pathway and not by the classical pathway.

b. **Alternative pathway.** In the alternative pathway, the **complement system** is activated without an antigen–antibody reaction. The alternative or properdin pathway is initiated by binding of the factor I (a protein in circulation) with polysaccharide present in the cell wall of invading organism, i.e. bacteria (endotoxin) and yeast cell wall (zymogen). This binding triggers reactions that activate C3 and C5 which ultimately attack the antigenic products of invading organisms. *Properdin* (a circulating protein) stabilizes the activating enzyme complex that is why the alternative pathway is also called properdin pathway. Because this pathway does not involve an antigen–antibody reaction, it is one of the first-line of defence against invading organisms.

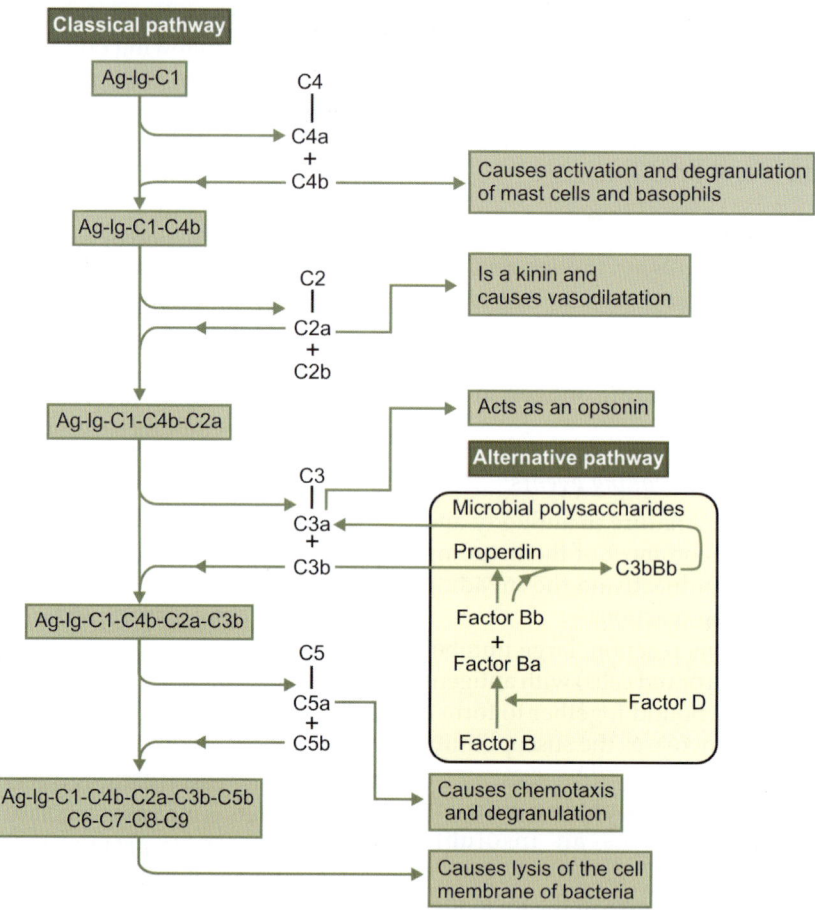

Fig. 3.1.10 *Broad outline of classical and alternative pathways of complement system.*

c. *Mannose-binding.* Lectin pathway of complement system is triggered when lectin binds to
mannose groups in bacteria.

CELLULAR IMMUNITY

The cellular immunity refers to specific acquired
immunity which is accomplished by effector T
cells and macrophages (Fig. 3.1.9). It is also called
cell-mediated immunity (CMI).

Types of T lymphocytes

They are classified on the basis of type and
function determined by surface receptors, as
below (Fig. 3.1.11):
- *Helper cells (Th cells) with CD4 markers* act with
  cells to produce antibodies. They also act
  with phagocytes. Helper T cells are divided
  into two types, i.e. T_H^1 and T_H^2, based on

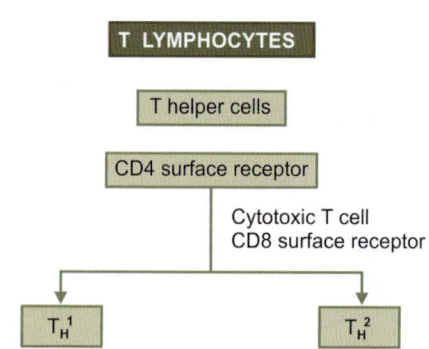

Fig. 3.1.11 *Types of T lymphocytes and their surface
receptors.*

production of various soluble mediators, like
cytokines.
- *Cytotoxic T cells* (Tc cells) kill viruses with CD8
  maker.

T cells have surface receptors (TCRs) for antigen recognition. This antigen receptor is disulphide glycoprotein. There are two types of TCRs:

- $\alpha\beta$ TCR—present in >95% peripheral T cells.
- $\gamma\delta$ TCR—present in <5% T cells.

Other cells included in T cell category

Natural killer cells. They are non-T and non-B lymphocytes. They do not produce immuno-globulins or T cell receptors. They constitute 15% of blood lymphocytes. These cells recognise and kill certain tumour cells and virus-infected cells.

Neutrophils. These cells are hallmark of acute inflammatory reaction. They ingest and kill invading organisms due to presence of granules. Types of neutrophils are:

- Azurophilic or primary granules
- Specific or secondary granules

Eosinophils. These cells phagocytose and kill ingested microbes. They play a pivotal role in immunity to parasites through extracellular release of toxin and termination or dampening of immune response through histamine and aryl sulphatase.

Mast cells. These cells function in the same way as basophils and release histamine. On interacting with allergen, they release IgE present on surface of mast cells.

Role of cellular immunity

1. Cellular immunity protects the host against fungi, most of the viruses and intracellular bacterial pathogens like *Mycobacterium tuberculosis, M. leprae* and *brucella*.
2. It participates in allograft rejection and graft versus host reaction.
3. CMI participates in delayed hypersensitivity reaction.
4. CMI is also associated with certain auto-immune diseases.
5. It provides immunological surveillance and immunity against cancer (tumour immunity).

Types of cellular immune response

Like humoural immune response, the cellular immune response is also of two types:

1. *Primary cellular response* which is produced by initial contact with a foreign antigen.
2. *Secondary cellular response* which is produced when the host is subsequently exposed to the same antigen. The secondary cell-mediated immune response is usually more pronounced and occurs more rapidly. Further, because of the availability of specific memory cells, an increased number of effector cells are produced in secondary response.

Phases of cellular immune response

The development of cellular immune response can be subdivided, using the concept of *'immune response arc'*, in three phases (Fig. 3.1.12):

- Afferent phase
- Processing phase and
- Effector phase

I. Afferent phase

Afferent phase of 'immune response arc' comprises transport, presentaion and recogni-tion of antigen to adaptive immune sysytem.

1. *Antigen processing and presentation.* An antigen entering the host body is phagocytosed and degraded into polypeptide fragments by the antigen-processing cells (APCs) which include macrophages and dendritic cells present in the peripheral lymphoid tissue. The antigen poly-peptide fragments then become associated with MHC antigen and are expressed on the surface of APC. Two modes of antigen processing are known:

- *Processing of phagocytosed material*, e.g. bacterial antigen is accomplished by combining with MHC-II molecules, and
- *Processing of antigen derived within the cell*, e.g. viral antigens synthesized in infected cell, is accomplished by combining with MHC-I molecules (probably in the endoplasmic reticulum).

2. *Recognition of antigen by lymphocytes.* T lymphocytes possess the antigenic recognition receptors known as *T cell receptors* (TCRs). These receptors serve as specific surface receptors recognizing and interacting with only single antigenic determinant on the antigen presented to lymphocytes.

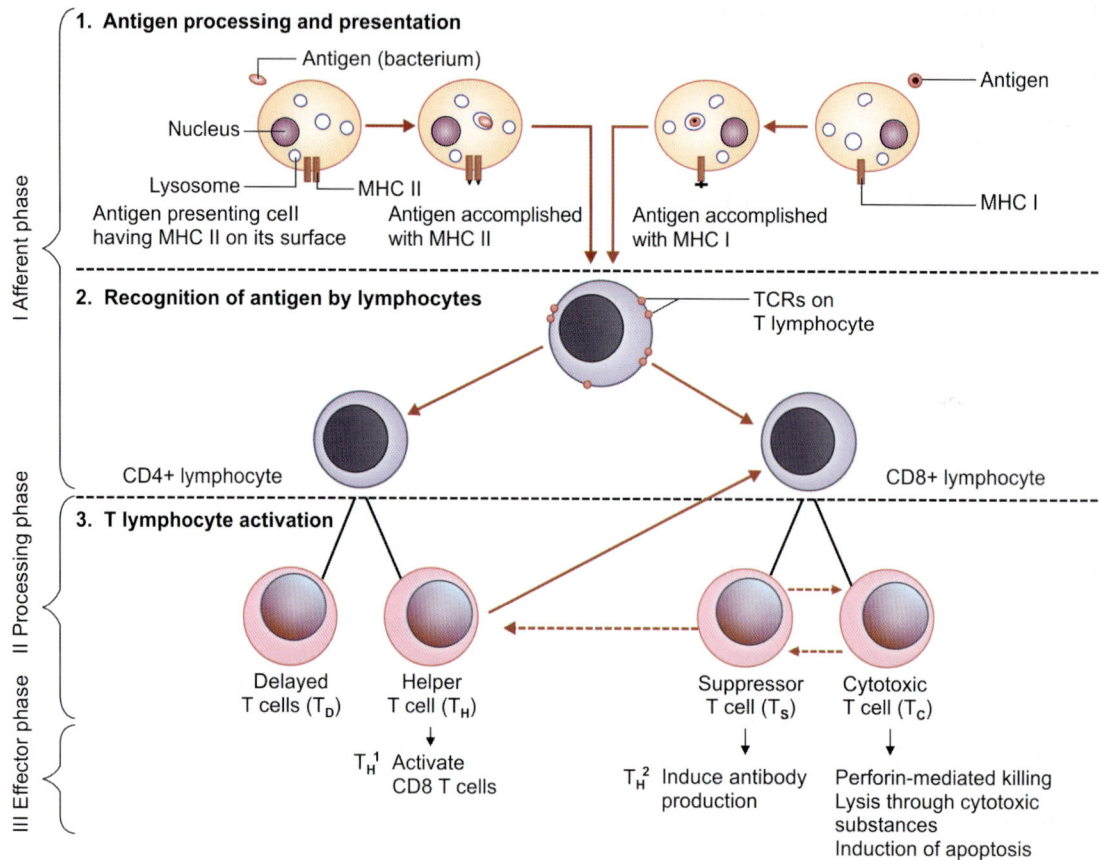

I Afferent phase

1. Antigen processing and presentation

- Antigen (bacterium)
- Antigen
- Nucleus
- Lysosome
- MHC II
- MHC I
- Antigen presenting cell having MHC II on its surface
- Antigen accomplished with MHC II
- Antigen accomplished with MHC I

II Processing phase

2. Recognition of antigen by lymphocytes

- TCRs on T lymphocyte
- CD4+ lymphocyte
- CD8+ lymphocyte

3. T lymphocyte activation

- Delayed T cells (T_D)
- Helper T cell (T_H)
- Suppressor T cell (T_S)
- Cytotoxic T cell (T_C)

T_H^1 Activate CD8 T cells

T_H^2 Induce antibody production

Perforin-mediated killing
Lysis through cytotoxic substances
Induction of apoptosis

III Effector phase

Fig. 3.1.12 Afferent, processing and effector phases of development of cellular immune response.

Compatibility of antigen presenting cells (APCs) and T cells is a pivotal step in antigen presentation. This recognition also called restriction is determined by major histocompatibility complex (MHC).

Mature T lymphocytes can be differentiated into two antigenic subtypes depending on the ensemble of their surface antigens: CD4+ and CD8+ cells.

- *CD8+ cells* recognize the combination of foreign antigen and class I MHC antigen, and
- *CD4+ cells* recognize the combination of foreign antigen and class II MHC antigen.

II. Processing phase

Processing phase of 'immune response arc' comprises activation and sensitization of lymphocytes. It involves conversion of antigenic stimuli into immunologic response.

T lymphocyte differentiation (activation). CD8+ type of T lymphocytes. After combining with foreign antigen-MHC-I complex are activated and differentiate into:

- Cytotoxic T cells (Tc cells), and
- Suppressor T cells (Ts cells).

CD4+ type of T lymphocytes. After combining with foreign antigen-MHC-II complex are activated and differentiate into:

- Helper T cells (T_H cells), and
- Delayed type hypersensitivity T cells (T_D cells).

T-T cooperation. The differentiation of T lymphocytes into T_h, T_c, T_s and T_D cells is interdependent. This interdependence is called T-T cooperation.

Release of differentiated T cells. The differentiated T lymphocytes so formed are released into the lymph and then enter the blood through which they are distributed throughout the body. They also pass out through capillary walls and enter in tissue fluid. From the tissue fluid, they enter back into the lymph, and then to lymphoid tissue and once again into blood. Thus, T lymphocytes circulate again and again throughout the body, sometimes lasting for months or years.

T lymphocyte memory cells are also formed. These spread throughout the lymphoid tissues of entire body. Therefore, on subsequent exposure to the same antigen, release of T cells occurs far more rapidly and much more powerfully than in the first response (secondary response).

III. *Effector phase*

Effector phase is also called as *'attack phase of cell-mediated immunity'*.

Role of cytotoxic T cells. Cytotoxic T cells (T_c cells) and natural killer cells (NK cells) are responsible for the attack phase of cell-mediated immunity.

Cytotoxic T cells have some receptor protein on their outer membrane. On the basis of their receptors and functions, cytotoxic T cells are divided into $\alpha\beta$ and $\gamma\delta$ ($\alpha\beta T_c$ and $\gamma\delta T_c$) cells. Cytotoxic T cells bind antigen-bearing cells (target cells) tightly and destroy them by the following mechanisms:

1. *Perforin-mediated killing.* The T_c cells after binding with the target cell secrete a hole-forming protein called perforin. The perforins literally punch round holes in the membrane of target cells in the presence of extracellular calcium (calcium-dependent lysis). The pores so formed cause cell death by disrupting cell homeostasis.

2. *Lysis through cytotoxic substances.* After binding with target cells, the T_c cells enlarge and release cytotoxic substances.

3. *Induction of apoptosis.* T_H cells secrete tumour necrosis factor β (TNF-β) which increases the Ca^{2+} permeability of antigen-bearing cell. The increased intracellular calcium activates enzymes that cause degradation of nucleus producing apoptosis.

Role of helper T cells (T_H cells). Helper T cells are of two types: $T_H{}^1$ and $T_H{}^2$.

Helper T^1 ($T_H{}^1$) cells play their roles by secreting three cytokines:
- Interleukin 2 (IL-2) secreted by helper T1 cells activates the CD8+ cells to differentiate into cytotoxic T cells and suppressor T cells (T-T cooperation).
- Interferon γ (IFN-γ) has the direct ability to kill antigen-bearing cells.
- Tumour necrosis factor-β (TNF-β) can induce apoptosis in antigen-bearing cells.

Helper T^2 ($T_H{}^2$) cells secrete interleukins 4, 5, 6, 10 and 13 and primarily with activation of B lymphocytes produce antibodies (T-B cooperation).

Role of suppressor T lymphocytes (T_s cells)
- Suppressor T cells regulate the activity of cytotoxic T cells. Thus, the cellular immune response is a balance between T_c cells and T_s cells.
- Suppressor T cells also play an important role in preventing the cytotoxic T cells from destroying the body's own tissue along with the invading organism.
- Suppressor T cells also suppress the activities of helper T cells.

MEDIATOR SYSTEMS THAT AMPLIFY IMMUNE RESPONSE

The effector response of immune system may directly induce inflammation; however, in most cases, these effectors instead initiate a process of inflammatory response. The molecules generated within the host that amplify inflammatory response constitute the mediator system. Most mediators act on target cells through the receptor mediated process, although some act as in enzymatic cascade that interact in a complex fashion. The mediator systems known so far have been categorized as below:
- Cytokines
- Plasma-derived enzyme system: Complement (*see* page 39), kinins, and fibrin.
- Vasoactive amines: Serotonin and histamine
- Lipid mediators: Ecosanoids, and platelets activating factors
- Reactive oxygen intermediates
- Reactive nitrogen products, and
- Neutrophils derived granules and products.

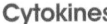

Cytokines

Cytokines are small protein molecules which act like hormones to regulate immune response.

Types, cell source and effects

Types, cell source and effects of various cytokines are summarized in Table 3.1.1. As shown in Table 3.1.1, the cytokines are secreted not only by lymphocytes and macrophages but also by endothelial cells, neuroglial cells and other types of cells. Broadly, cytokines can be grouped as:

I. Interleukins (IL). These are the principal cytokines and include IL-1 to IL-13 (Table 3.1.1).

Type of cytokine	Cell source	Effects
I. Interleukins (IL)		
IL-1 α and β	Macrophages and other antigen-processing cells (APCs)	i. B cell proliferation, ii. Igs production, iii. Stimulation of T cells, and iv. Inflammation fever.
IL-2	Activated helper cells ($T_H{}^1$), cytotoxic cells (T_c) and natural killer cells (NK)	i. Proliferation of activated T cell. ii. B cell proliferation, Igs expression.
IL-3	T lymphocytes	Growth of early progenitor cell
IL-4	$T_H{}^2$ and mast cells	i. Eosinophil growth and its function, ii. B cell proliferation, iii. Igs expression, iv. MHC class II expression, v. Proliferation of $T_H{}^2$ and T_c cells, and vi. Inhibition of production of inflammatory cytokines.
IL-5	$T_H{}^2$ and mast cells	Growth of eosinophils and its function.
IL-6	Activated $T_H{}^2$ cells APC and other somatic cells	i. Act with IL-I and TNF to stimulate T cells, ii. Proliferation of B cells and Igs production, and iii. Stimulates thrombopoiesis.
IL-7	Thymic and bone marrow stromal cells	Lymphopoiesis (T and B cells)
IL-8	Macrophages	Stimulates neutrophil activity and promote their accumulation.
IL-9	From cultured T cells	Stimulates haematopoietic and thymopoietic factors.
IL-10	Activated helper cells ($T_H{}^2$), TCD8, B lymphocyte and macrophages	i. Inhibition of cytokine production, ii. Stimulates B cells and antibodies production and its functions, iii. Suppresses cell-mediated immunity, and iv. Causes growth of mast cells.
IL-11	Stroma cells	Stimulates haematopoiesis and thrombopoiesis
IL-12	Macrophages and B cells	Stimulates proliferation of cytotoxic T cells and killer cells (T_c and NK).

Table 3.1.1 *Main characteristics of human interleukins and other immunoregulatory cytokines*

(Contd.)

Table 3.1.1 *Main characteristics of human interleukins and other immunoregulatory cytokines (Contd...)*

Type of cytokine	Cell source	Effects
IL-13	T_H^2 cells	Promotes cell-mediated immune response. i. B cell proliferation, IgG expression, class II MHC expression, ii. Proliferation of T_H^2, T_c cells and their function, and iii. Inhibition of production of inflammatory cytokines
II. Other cytokines TNF α	Activated macrophages	i. IL-I type effects, and ii. Causes vascular thrombosis and necrosis of tumour cells.
TNF β	Activated T_H^1 cells	Vascular thrombosis and tumour cell necrosis
Interferon (IFN α and β)	Macrophages, neutrophils and other somatic cells	i. Antiviral effects, ii. Stimulates class II MHC cells, and iii. Activation of macrophages and NK cells.
IFN-γ	Activated T_H^1 and NK cells	i. Antiviral effect, ii. Activation of class I MHC cells and class II MHC cells, and iii. Promotes cell-mediated immunity.
TGFβ	Activated T lymphocytes, platelets, macrophages and somatic cells	i. Anti-inflammatory effect by suppressing cytokine production and MHC-II cells, ii. Inhibits proliferation of macrophages and lymphocytes, iii. Proliferation of B cells, and iv. Healing (by stimulating fibroblast cells).

II. *Other cytokines* include:
- Chemokines,
- Growth factors,
- Colony-stimulating factors (CSF)
- Tumour necrosis factors (TNF-α and TNF-β) and
- Interferon

Chemokines are the substances that attract neutrophils and other white blood cells to the area of immune response or inflammation. About 40 chemokines have been identified. The receptors of chemokines are serpentine and act via G proteins. Chemokines also play role in growth and angiogenesis.

Mechanism of action

1. *Local effects.* Cytokines act in an *autocrine* (i.e. on the cell that produced them) or *paracrine* (i.e. on the cell close by) manner through their specific receptors.

Receptors of cytokines have been grouped under the *superfamily*. The superfamily includes receptors of:
- Cytokines,
- Haematopoietic growth factors,
- Prolactin, and
- Growth hormone.

The superfamily of receptors has been divided into three *subfamilies*:
- Subfamily I includes receptors for IL-4 and IL-7.
- Subfamily II includes receptors for IL-3, IL-5 and IL-6.
- Subfamily III includes receptors of IL-2 and other cytokines and related proteins, e.g. IL-2R and Tac antigen.

2. *Systemic effects.* Interleukin-1 (IL-1) affects the various body systems:

- *Central nervous system effect.* It causes fever, slow wave sleep, secretion of CRH and anorexia.
- *Metabolic effects.* It increases hepatic protein synthesis, excretion of sodium and decreases plasma zinc and iron level and also cytochrome P450. It also causes lactic acidosis.
- *Haematological effects.* It increases number of circulating neutrophils, colony-stimulating factors and non-specific resistance.
- *Vascular system effect.* It stimulates leucocyte adherence to the vessel wall, increases synthesis of prostaglandins, releases platelet-activating factor and increases the capillary permeability.

OTHER IMMUNE MECHANISM-RELATED ASPECTS

Some other aspects related to immune mechanisms which need to be elaborated are:

- Immune tolerance,
- Immune modulation,
- Autoimmunity, and
- Hypersensitivity.

IMMUNE TOLERANCE

Types of immune tolerance

Immune tolerance may be defined as a state of unresponsiveness to an antigen. It occurs in two forms: natural and acquired.

1. *Natural tolerance.* Refers to nonresponsiveness to a self-antigen. During embryonic development, when the immune system is immature, any antigen which comes in contact with the immature immune system is recognized as self-antigen. Therefore, it does not evoke any response in later life when body is exposed to the same antigen.

2. *Acquired tolerance.* Means unresponsiveness to a potential antigen. It is of further two types: general and specific.

i. *General immunological tolerance* results due to impairment of the immune system; hence, there is lack of responsiveness to potential antigens.

ii. *Specific immunological tolerance* arises when a potential antigen induces a state of unresponsiveness to itself and not to other antigens. This happens when an antigen becomes tolerogenic (tolerogen).

- In some instances, when an antigen is presented at particular concentration, it might induce specific immunological tolerance or unresponsiveness, whereas when presented at some other concentration, it promotes immunity. Therefore, an antigen that induces tolerance is referred to as *tolerogen*.
- Specific acquired tolerance has consequences for the host defences. Presence of tolerogenic epitopes on the pathogens compromises with the ability of the body to resist infections.

Mechanism of tolerance

Immunotolerance can arise by three possible mechanisms:

- Clonal deletion,
- Clonal anergy, and
- Suppression.

1. *Clonal deletion.* During embryonic life, clones of B and T cells are formed. These B and T cells possess receptors which recognize the antigens and are selectively deleted or eliminated and, therefore, not available to respond on subsequent exposure to that antigen in later life.

2. *Clonal anergy.* Clones of B and T cell receptors which recognize self-antigen might remain, but cannot be activated. This is referred as clonal anergy.

3. *Suppression.* Clones of B and T cells expressing receptors that recognize self-antigen are preserved and capable for recognition of an antigen when activated. However, an immune response might be inhibited through active suppression.

Factors influencing induction of tolerance

A number of factors influence induction of immunological tolerance. These are species, competency of the host, antigen and age of the host.

1. *Species.* Immunological tolerance varies from species to species. For example, species like rabbits and mice can be rendered tolerant more rapidly as compared to guinea pigs and chickens.

2. *Immunological competency of the host.* Also affects induction of tolerance. If degree of immunological competency of the host is high,

then induction of tolerance is very difficult. On the other hand, newborns and embryos are particularly susceptible for induction of tolerance because their immune system is immature and not very competent.

3. *Antigen.* Induction of tolerance also depends upon the antigen (i.e. its physical nature, dose and its route of administration).

4. *Age of the host.* As mentioned above, the immune system competency is related to the age of the host. Therefore, embryo and newborns can develop immune tolerance easily.

Tolerance to fetus

Fetus is genetically different from the mother and thus it should evoke an immune response in the mother. However, it usually never happens and it is considered to be the best example of immune tolerance.

Various factors which prevent an immunological response in a mother have been described.

Tolerance to lens crystallins

Lens proteins are immunologically privileged because they are isolated from fetal circulation early in the embryonic life (sequestered) and they may initiate an immunological sensitization after entering the aqueous humour. The so-called phacogenic uveitis, an immune-mediated phenomenon, thus may develop after a break in the lens capsule and sensitization to lens proteins. However, in practice release of lens proteins during cataract surgery almost always produce only a minimal reaction. Even though serum titre of antilens-crystalline antibodies often rise in patients after cataract surgery, effector T lymphocytes, pathognomonic antibodies, and true autoimmune uveitis rarely develop. Most investigators think that the protection against phacogenic uveitis is caused by the presence of an *active immunologic tolerance* and that the lens is not sequestered from the immune system. There exist both T and B lymphocyte tolerance to the lens crystallins.

T lymphocyte tolerance, nature and exact mechanism of T lymphocyte tolerance is not known, however, following suggestions have been made:

- *Colonal deletion of antilens T lymphocytes* is suggested by the detection of a crystalline protein and mRNA within the thymus.
- *Anergy,* after some experiment studies, is also suggested to play some role.
- *ACAID*-related ocular immune privilege may also provide an additional mechanism for tolerance by the generation of suppressor T lymphocytes.

B lymphocytes tolerance to lens proteins is probably indirect, controlled at the helper T lymphocyte. Functional lens specific B lymphocytes certainly exists, since antilens antibody can be identified in the serum of many normal persons and in most patients after cataract surgery. Further, antibody titre can be stimulated in all animals following cutaneous immunization with lens proteins. However, these loss of tolerance, as long as the antibody titers are predominated by non-complement-fixing isotypes observation, does not necessarily indicate phacogenic uveitis, though rare, but is known to occur following disruption of lens capsule (traumatic or surgical) or from leakage of lens proteins through lens capsule in mature or hypermature cataract. The exact mechanism of phacogenic uveitis although unknown, is thought to represent an autoimmune reaction to lens proteins. Experimental animal studies suggest that the altered tolerance to lens proteins leads to inflammation.

IMMUNE MODULATION

Immune modulation refers to modification of the immunological response. It can be either enhanced or suppressed.

Immune enhancement

Immune enhancement means there is increase in the response in terms of rate, intensity, duration and even induction of response to substances which were earlier non-immunogenic.

Immunological response can be potentiated by use of certain substances referred to as adjuvants.

Adjuvants. Adjuvants are the compounds which when introduced along with or mixed with an antigen, non-specifically enhance or modify the immune response to that antigen. The first adjuvant was discovered by Freund hence known as Freund's adjuvant. Their contribution in enhancement of response is basically achieved by two ways:

i. *More and prolonged production of antibodies, and*
ii. *Increasing the number of effector cells.*

Mechanism of action. Adjuvants act by the following ways:

• They alter the distribution and persistence of an antigen in the host.
• They stimulate lymphocyte number non-specifically.
• They activate macrophages.

Types. Adjuvants are of two main types:

i. *Incomplete adjuvants.* Substances, like aluminium hydroxide, aluminium phosphate and certain mineral oils (lanolin oil), act as incomplete adjuvants. When an aqueous solution of an antigen is mixed with mineral oil, an emulsion is formed, which serves as a depot for that antigen causing slow and prolonged release of the antigen.
ii. *Complete adjuvant.* The cell walls of certain bacteria, like tubercular bacilli and Gram-negative bacilli (e.g. diphtheria and of whooping cough), act as complete adjuvants because the constituents of the cell wall convert the soluble antigen into insoluble and particulate form which can be easily phagocytosed by macrophages. A typical example of a complete adjuvant is *killed Mycobacterium bacilli.*

Immune suppression

Immune suppression refers to reduction in the immunological response. It is of two types:

1. Specific immune suppression or immune tolerance

(See page 46).

2. Non-specific immune suppression

It is caused by immunosuppressive agents which inhibit the immune response of macrophages and B and T cells leading to either lowered phagocytosing capacity of the macrophages or production of antibodies and lymphokines.

Immunosuppressive agents refer to methods or substances causing immunosuppression. These have been grouped as physical, chemical and biological agents.

A. *Physical immunosuppressive agents* (methods):
1. *Irradiations.* This is the most common method for prolonged survival of transplants. Irradiations cause breakage in the nucleic acid chains of replicating cells.
2. *Surgical procedures,* like thymectomy, splenectomy and thoracic duct drainage.

• *Thymectomy.* Removal of fetal thymus gland ensures absolute depletion of mature T cells but the effect of thymectomy decreases with age. Therefore, this method is not usually applicable.
• *Splenectomy.* Though most of the antibodies are formed in the spleen, but splenectomy has little effect in adult life (because other peripheral organs—lymph nodes—can compensate for absence of spleen).
• *Thoracic duct drainage* is another method of immune suppression first used in humans during heart transplant. In this, the thoracic duct is cannulated and lymph is drained for many days, leading to decrease in size and weight of lymph node and depletion of lymphocyte (lymphopenia).

B. *Chemical methods* are non-specific suppressants and have limited effectiveness. This group includes the following drugs:
1. *Corticosteroids* suppress the immune response by the following ways:

• They impair the maturation of activated cells.
• They suppress the production of antibodies.
• Have an anti-inflammatory effect and diminish the responsiveness of B and T lymphocytes.
• They also inhibit production of IL-1 and IL-2.

Corticoids, though commonly used, have limited effectiveness due to their side effects, as prolonged use leads to hypertension, bone necrosis, cataract and mental disturbances.

2. *Cyclosporin or tacrolimus (FK-506)* has been widely used as an immunosuppressive drug in organ transplants. This acts by inhibiting the production of IL-2.

Normally, activation of T cell receptor increases intracellular calcium (Ca^{2+}) that activates calcineurin via calmodulin. Calcineurin in turn dephosphorylates the transcription factor NF-AT that moves into the nucleus and increases the gene coding activity for IL-2. The drugs cyclosporine (C_{sp}) and tacrolimus (Tcl) prevent dephosphorylation of NF-AT (Fig. 3.1.13). They also have adverse effects on the liver and kidney.

3. *Cytotoxic drugs,* such as *azathioprine* and *cyclophosphamide,* act on various stages of nucleic acid synthesis and thus prevent replication of lymphocyte.

Methotrexate, an antagonist of folic acid, produces competitive inhibition of an enzyme reductase (essential for synthesis of DNA). This drug is a known anticancer drug.

C. **Biological methods** include:

1. *Antigen-induced suppression.* This method is used for desensitization against an allergen. In this method, if the body is exposed to small doses of antigen for long time, then it can develop resistance to that antigen.

2. *Antibody-induced suppression.* This method of immunosuppression is used in pregnant mothers (Rh +ve) to prevent sensitization against Rh antigen (from fetus) by injecting anti-D after expulsion of placenta.

3. *Antilymphocytic serum* is used for depletion of T cell population. In this method, anti-lymphocytic serum is prepared from horse by injecting human lymphocytes.

The antibodies present in the horse serum destroy body T cell pool, but antibody production remains normal. The main drawback of this method is that the ability to fight against viral infection is tremendously decreased.

AUTOIMMUNITY

During fetal life, when many antigens are presented to the immune system, they are recognized as self-antigens and antibodies and cytotoxic T cells are not produced.

Therefore, tolerance to self-antigen is produced. However, sometimes body starts

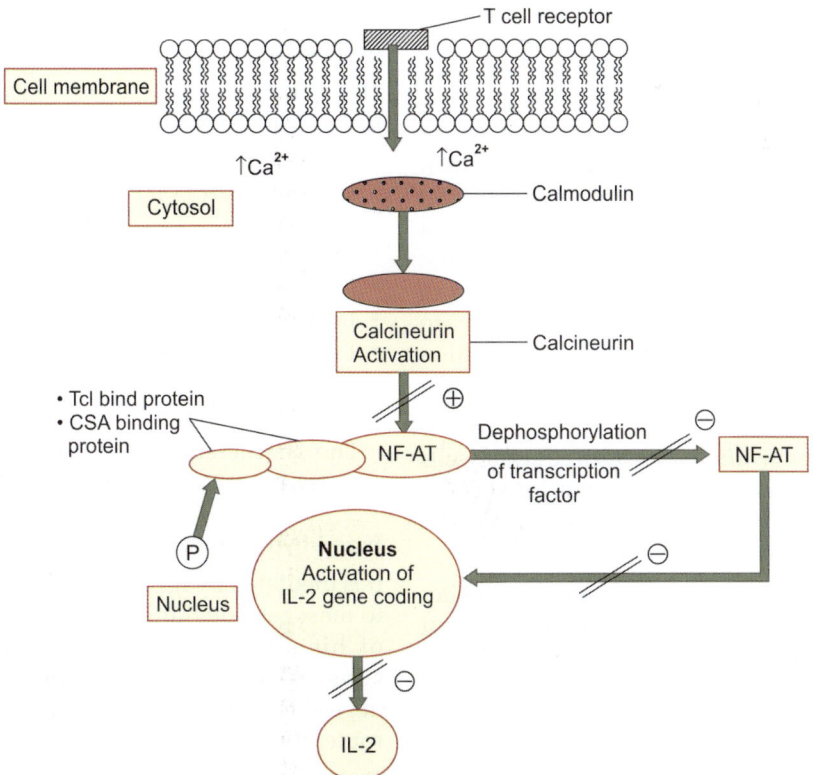

Fig. 3.1.13 *Mechanism of action of cyclosporin C and tarcolimus in T lymphocytes.*

producing antibodies or T cells against self-antigen (own cells or tissue) leading to an auto-immune disease. Therefore, autoimmunity may be defined as immune response to self-antigen.

Mechanism of autoimmunity

The possible mechanisms involved in development of autoimmunity are:

1. *Forbidden clones.* According to clonal selection theory, antibody-forming lymphocytes are formed against different antigens. In fetal life, lymphocytes are also formed against self-antigens, but get depleted. The clones of these cells are called forbidden clones and hence an immune response does not occur against self-antigen. However, persistence of these clones or their development in later life by some mutations leads to autoimmunity.

2. *Hidden antigen or sequestrated antigen.* Certain self-antigens are present in the close system and never exposed to the immune system during fetal life. These are known as hidden antigens or sequestrated antigens, e.g. *lens protein* being enclosed by its capsule does not come in contact with blood; therefore, immunological tolerance against such antigens does not develop. When such antigens in later life are somehow exposed to the immune system (accidental leak of lens protein during cataract surgery), this leads to an immune response and damages the other eye also. Another example of a hidden antigen is *sperm antigen*. Injury to testes or viral infections (mumps) leads to leakage of sperm proteins into the circulation and thus evokes an immune response against one's own testes and orchitis occurs.

3. *Neoantigen or altered antigen.* Certain cells of the body undergo alterations due to exposure to irradiations, drugs, sunlight, etc. and start producing an immune response.

4. *Cross-reacting antigen.* Although antibodies are highly specific for a particular antigen, but in some cases, they cross-react with other cells or body tissue. This phenomenon is called as molecular mimicry and these antigens are called cross-reacting antigens. For example, in rheumatic heart disease, the heart is damaged by antibodies formed against streptococci.

Molecular mimicry as a mechanism of auto-immune uveitis was suggested based on the observation that the primary amino acid sequence of a variety of foreign antigens (e.g. Baker's yeast histone, *E. coli*, hepatitis B virus, and certain murine and primate retroviruses) showed sequence homology to a pathogenic S-antigen. Further, T lymphocytes isolated from rats immunized with foreign substance cross-reacted with retinal autoantigen, providing evidence of molecular mimicry between self- and non-self-proteins.

5. *Mutations.* The body immune system becomes competent for self-antigen by certain mutations.

6. *Unbalanced activity of helper and suppressor T cells.* It has been observed that optimum antibody response always depends upon the balance activity of helper (T_H) and suppressor T cells. If somehow the activity of these cells is altered, i.e. overactivity of T_H cells and under-activity of Ts cells, then it may result in auto-immunity.

HYPERSENSITIVITY

Hypersensitivity is an abnormal response which produces physiological or histopathological damage in the host.

There are five types of hypersensitivity reactions:
- Type I (anaphylaxis or IgE-mediated)
- Type II (antibody-mediated cytotoxicity)
- Type III (immune complex-mediated disorders)
- Type IV (delayed type or T cell-mediated hypersensitivity)
- Type V stimulatory.

The characteristic features of each hypersensitivity reaction are given in Table 3.1.2.

Type I hypersensitivity or anaphylaxis

It is mediated by IgE antibodies and occurs due to mast cells degranulation resulting in release of histamine and many other vasoactive substances. Type I reaction (anaphylaxis) depends on the amount of histamine release and route of stimulating antigen.

Types. It occurs in two forms: local anaphylaxis and generalized anaphylaxis.

Table 3.1.2 *Characteristics of hypersensitivity reactions*

Characteristics	Type I	Type II	Type III	Type IV
1. Time of onset	1/2–8 h of reaction	5–12 h	3–8 h (peak 48–72 h)	24–48 h
2. Reaction mediators	IgE, histamine, serotonin, SRS-A, etc.	IgG, IgM and complement	IgG, IgM, neutrophils, eosinophils, lysosomal enzymes	T lymphocytes, macrophages and lymphokines
3. Response to intradermal injection of antigen (allergen)	Wheal and flare	—	Erythema and oedema	Erythema and induration
4. Passive transfer with	Serum	Serum	Serum	T cells
5. Samples	• Anaphylaxis • Asthma • Hay fever • Allergic with food and insect bite	• Transfusion reactions (incompatibility reaction) • Haemolytic disease of newborn • Drug-induced allergies	• Arthus reaction • Serum sickness	• Tuberculin test • Contact dermatitis • Graft rejection

- *Local anaphylaxis* occurs when an antigen called as allergen is administered locally in smaller dose. Examples of local anaphylaxis are asthma and hay fever.
- *Systemic or generalized anaphylaxis* is a shock-like condition. It occurs in individuals who are intensely allergic and when an antigen is administered in large amount or through systemic route.

Mechanism of type I hypersensitivity. In type I hypersensitivity reaction, the individual first comes in contact with an antigen and antibodies (IgE) are produced which get bound to mast cells or to fixed basophils. The specific IgE antibodies are fixed to mast cell surface by its Fc portion. After second exposure, the allergen passes on to these sensitized cells (IgE-fixed mast cells) and get attached on to the Fab site of IgE molecule attached to mast cell. Antigen–antibody binding triggers the degranulation of mast cells and releases pharmacologically active chemicals (histamine, serotonin, bradykinin and slow-reacting substances of anaphylaxis) causing vasodilatation, sensory nerve ending stimulation, etc. The individuals susceptible to type I hypersensitivity reaction are called *atopic* and reaction is known as *atopy*. Example of type I hypersensitivity includes allergic rhinitis and atopic dermatitis.

Type II hypersensitivity or antibody-mediated autotoxicity

It is an immediate reaction in which antigen-bearing cells are damaged. The mechanism involved in this reaction is either complement- or antibody-mediated cytotoxicity.

Examples. Type II hypersensitivity is most commonly seen in:
- Incompatible blood transfusion,
- Autoimmune haemolytic anaemia, and
- Haemolytic disease of the newborn. When antibodies react with the cells on which these antigens are present, i.e. RBCs get damaged.

Type III hypersensitivity (immune complex-mediated hypersensitivity)

Monocytes and macrophages are efficient in binding and removal of antigen–antibody complexes. When the body is exposed repeatedly to an antigen, which is not cell bound (free, small and soluble), then the body faces great difficulty, because the antigen–antibody complexes formation occurs in the serum and subsequently get deposited in the normal body tissue. Complement system is also activated (particularly C3a and C5a), which is cytotoxic for monocytes, macrophages and even nearby normal tissue where the antigen–antibody complexes are deposited. *Glomerulonephritis is* the best example of type III hypersensitivity reaction.

Type IV or delayed hypersensitivity

Delayed hypersensitivity is the cell-mediated reaction in tissues of a sensitized individual. The reaction is due to sensitization of T lymphocytes and not by antibodies or by B lymphocytes. The reaction starts after several hours (48–72 h). Two types of delayed hypersensitivity reactions are recognized: tuberculin (infection) type and contact dermatitis.

Tuberculin test. In this test, a small dose of tuberculin or purified protein derivative from *Mycobacterium tuberculosis* is injected intradermally in an individual sensitized earlier by tubercular protein by infection or by immunization.

Within 48–72 h, an inflammatory reaction of 5 mm diameter appears at the site of injection. The inflammatory reaction is recognized by erythema (increased blood flow) and induration (due to infiltration with large number of T lymphocytes and macrophages).

Contact dermatitis is type IV hypersensitivity reaction. Hypersensitivity against various chemicals in the forms of ointments, dyes, cosmetics, etc. is tested by *patch test.*

Patch test. In this test, a patch of an allergen is applied to the skin under a dressing. If itching occurs within 4–5 h and local reaction in the form of redness and induration appears within 24 h, then the test is positive.

Type V or stimulatory hypersensitivity

Over the last few years, type V hypersensitivity has been add to the original four types. In this reaction, an antibody can act as a stimulant to target cell or organ. An example is long-acting thyroid stimulatory (LATS) antibody, a feature of Graves' disease. The LATS antibody is directed toward a portion of TSH receptor in the thyroid and mimicks the function of thyroid stimulatory hormone.

BIBLIOGRAPHY

1. Elschnig A. Studien Zur sympathischen Ophthalmie.2. Die antigene Wirkung der Augenpigmentes, Albretche von Graefes Arch Ophthalmol 1910;76:509–546.

2. Foster CS, Streilen JW. Immune mediated tissue injury. In: Albert DM, Jakobiec FA (eds). Principles and Practice of Ophthalmolgy, 2nd ed. Philadelphia: Saunders; 2000 pp. 74–82.

3. Grencis RK. Th2-mediated host protective immunity to intestinal nematode infections. Philos Trans R Soc Lond Biol Sci 1997;352:1377–1384.

4. Riddell SR. Pathogenesis of cytomegalovirus pneumonia in immunocompromised hosts. Semin Respir Infect 1995;10:199–208.

5. Samson CM, Foster CS. Hypersensitivity: antibody mediated cytotoxic (type 2). Encyclopedia of life Sciences. London: John Wiley & sons.

6. Tonega S. The molecules of immune system. Sci Am 1985;253(4):122–131.

7. Unanue ER, Allen PM. The basis for the immuno-regulatory role of macrophages and other accessory cells. Science 1987;236:551–557.

8. Weigle WO. Immunologic tolerance and immunopathology. In: Dixon FJ, Fisher, DW eds. The Biology of Immunologic Disease, NY, 1983.

3.2 OCULAR IMMUNE MECHANISMS AND ETIOPATHOGENESIS OF UVEITIS

Special Immune Characteristics of Eye
- Special immune characteristics of conjunctiva
- Special immune characteristics of cornea and sclera
- Special immune characteristics of inner eye

Etiopathogenesis of Uveitis
Experimental Modles of Uveitis
- Experimental autoimmune uveitis
- Endotoxin-induced uveitis
- Disease-specific uveitis animal models

Etiological factors and pathomechanisms of uveitis
- Infectious uveitis
- Non-infectious uveitis
- Masquerade syndrome

SPECIAL IMMUNE CHARACTERISTICS OF EYE

Immune mechanisms play an important role in ocular inflammations. Therefore, it will be worth while to know about the general immunology (Chapter 3.1) and the special immune characteristics of the eye before discussing the pathomechanisms of uveitis. The special immune characteristics exhibited in the eye can be discussed as:
- Special immune characteristics of conjunctiva,
- Special immune characteristics of cornea and sclera, and
- Special immune characteristics of the inner eye.

SPECIAL IMMUNE CHARACTERISTICS OF CONJUNCTIVA

Characteristics of microenvironment of conjunctiva

- *Blood supply and lymphatics.* Conjunctiva is well vascularised and has good lymphatic drainage to preauricular and submandibular lymph nodes.
- *Adenoid layer* of conjunctiva, also called as lymphoid layer, consists of fine connective tissue reticulum in the meshes of which lie lymphocytes. This layer is most developed in the fornices. It is not present since birth but develops after 3–4 months of life. For this reason, conjunctival inflammation in an infant does not produce follicular reaction.
- *Resident APCs* include Langerhens cells, other dendritic cells and macrophages.
- *Resident effector cells* of conjunctiva include mast cells, T lymphocytes, B lymphocytes, plasma cells and rarely neutrophils.
- *Resident effector molecules* include all antibody isotypes, especially IgE, IgG sub-classes and IgA in tears.
- *Immunomediators.* Complement and kinogen act as immunomediators.

Immune regulatory system of conjunctiva

Mucosa-associated lymphoid tissue (MALT) constitutes the immune regulatory system for conjunctiva. The MALT in the body is present in the epithelial lining of conjunctiva, respiratory tract, gut and genitourinary tract. The MALT shares certain specific immunological features and this accounts for the disruption and homeing of effector T and B lymphocytes induced by immunisation at one mucosal site to all MALT sites.

SPECIAL IMMUNE CHARACTERISTICS OF CORNEA AND SCLERA

Characteristics of microinvironment of cornea

Microenvironment of cornea differs in the centre and periphery:
- *Lymphatics* are seen at the limbus only.
- *Vascularisation* is present at the limbus only.
- *Resident APCs* in the form of Langerhans cells are present only at the limbus. APCs, which are normally absent in central and paracentrals areas of cornea, can be recruited by various stimuli, such as mild trauma, certain cytokines (e.g. IL-1), or infections.
- *Resident effector cells* are normally absent in the cornea and sclera. However, if appropriate chemotactic stimuli are activated, the neutrophils, monocytes and lymphocytes can easily migrate through the stroma.

- *Resident effector molecules.* Plasma-derived enzymes (e.g. compliments), IgM, and IgG, are present in moderate concentration in the periphery, but only low levels of IgM are present centrally. The sclera has low antibody concentration.

Characteristics of immunoregulatory system of cornea and sclera

- *Cornea exhibits immune privilege* due to absence of vessels, lymphatics, and APCs from the central and paracentral areas. However, due to stimuli, both effector cells and effector molecules can ultimately infiltrate even the avascular cornea.
- *Anterior chamber-associated immune deviation* (ACAID) can also extend to the corneal endothelium.

SPECIAL IMMUNE CHARACTERISTICS OF INNER EYE

Characteristics of intraocular immunologic microinvironment

1. Absence of lymphatics

Like brain, placenta and testis, the inner eye does not contain well-developed lymphatics. This anatomic peculiarity may have a profound effect on the type of immune response elicited in the eye.

2. Role of circulating aqueous humour

Circulating aqueous humour makes a unique characteristic of the intraocular invironment as it:

- *Provides medium for intracellular communication* among cytokines, immune cells and resident tissue cells of the iris, cilliary body and corneal endothelial cells.
- *Provides medium for* antigen clearance through trabecular meshwork into the venous circulation, where they communicate with the spleen. Thus, the antigen inoculation into the anterior chamber results in efficient communication with the systemic immune system.
- *Provides a complex mixture of biological factors,* such as immunomodulatory cytokines, neuropeptides and compliments inhibitors, that can influence immunological events in the eye.

3. Partial blood–ocular barrier

Partial blood–ocular barrier makes another unique characteristic of the intraocular microinvironment:

- *Tight junctions between the pigments and non-pigmented ciliary epithelium* act as a more exclusive barrier, preventing passage of interstitial macromolecules into the aqueous humour. However, fenestrated capillaries of cilliary processes allow a size-dependent concentration gradient of macromolecules to penetrate the interstitial tissue.
- *Tight junctions between endothelial cells of retinal capillaries provide* inner blood–retinal barrier.
- *Choriocapillaris* are highly permeable to the macromolecules and allow transduction of most plasma macromolecules into the extravascular spaces of choroid and choriocapillaris.
- *Tight junctions between RPE cells* constitute the outer blood–retinal barrier between choroid and the retina.

4. Choroidal and retinal peculiarities

Choroidal and retinal peculiarities also contribute to special characteristics of intraocular microenvironment:

- *Relatively large blood flow and anatomical features of choroid* would act as a sort of trap for many blood-borne problems, most notably fungal disorders. Therefore, most fungal lesions begin as choroiditis.
- *High concentration of mast cells in the choroid* may be the one mechanism by which immunoreactive cells in the choroid could spread to other parts of eye. The release of immunoreactive factors by mast cells could help T cell egress and ingress from the compartment.
- *Retina, in addition to being richly invested with uveitogenic antigens, is also an extension of the brain,* which makes it particularly prone to certain neurotropic organisms, such as *T. gondii* and many viruses of the herpes family.

5. Resident ocular antigen-presenting cells (APCs) of uvea and immune system from important component of intraocular immunologic microenvironment

- *APCs present in the iris and ciliary body* include macrophages and dendritic cells. Few resident T lymphocytes and mast cells are also present in the anterior uvea, B lymphocytes, eosinophils and neutrophils are absent. Immune processing is unlikely to occur locally but APCs leave the eye through trabecular meshwork into venous circulation to ultimately home in the spleen. In the spleen, processing occurs that favors a Th 2 response and preferential activation of CD8 regulatory T lymphocytes.

- *Vitreous gel* can electrostatically bind charged protein substances and may thus serve as an antigenic depot as well as a substrate for the leucocytic cell adhesion. Hylocytes are macrophage-derived and may act as APCs.
- *Choroid and choriocapillaris.* The immunologic micrenvironments of choroid and choriocapillaris have not been well described.
- *Choriocapillaris are highly permeable* to macromolecules and allow transudation of most plasma macromolecules into the extravascular spaces of choroid and choriocapillaris.
- *Well-developed lymphatics are absent*, although choroid has abundant APCs.
- *Choroid and choriocapillaris are richly invested with certain potential APCs*, especially macrophages and dendritic cells. The density of mast cells is moderate in the choroid, especially around the arterioles; lymphocytes are present in only low density. Eosinophil and neutrophils appear to be absent.
- *Under various clinical or experimental conditions*, however, high density of T lymphocytes, B lymphocytes, macrophages and neutrophils can infiltrate the choroid and choriocapillaris.
- *Choroid can synthesise many different cytokines* that may alter the subsequent immune response.
- *Retinal pigment epithelium (RPE)* has many characteristics of macrophages, i.e. have capacity to migrate and engulf particles and have other characteristics that strongly suggest a capacity to participate in local immune response. RPE can be induced to express class III MHC molecules suggesting that RPE may also interact with T lymphocytes. RPE has been shown to produce cytokines (IL-6). Further, RPE cells in culture can act as APCs for S-Ag-specific T cells.

- *Microglia in the retina* (bone marrow-derived cell related to monocytes) also act as APCs. These cells are interspersed within all the layers of retina and can undergo physical changes and migration in response to various stimuli.

Immune regulatory system of the inner eye

Immunoregulatory systems of the inner eye are responsible for its immune privilege. Immune privileged sites in the body, other than eye are brain and testes. The modern concept of immune privilege refers to the observation that the tumour implants or allografts survive better within an immunologically privileged region, whereas a similar implant or graft is rapidly rejected by the immune mechanisms within the skin and other non-privileged sites.

Immunoregulatory mechanisms of inner eye include:
- Anterior chamber associated immune deviation (ACAID)
- Effector blockage
- Fas-Fas ligand interactions and programmed cell death (apoptosis)
- Anti-inflammatory or immunosuppressive cytokines
- Low-zone tolerance
- ACAID-like mechanism in vitreous humour
- ACAID-like mechanism in retina

Anterior chamber associated immune deviation

Anterior chamber associated immune deviation (ACAID) refers to transient depression of cell-mediated immunity (CMI) but an intact humoural response, i.e. antibody-mediated immunity (AMI) to certain antigens entering the eye. These include placement of following antigens in the anterior chamber:
- Alloantigens
- Hapten-specific suppressor T cell response to syngenic splenocytes that are coupled with azobenzene-arsonate (i.e. cell-bound antigens)
- Soluble antigen such as histocompatibility and tumour antigen.

Mechanisms of ACAID. Presence of an intact ocular-splenic axis is of prime importance in ACAID. It has been proposed that the *transforming growth factor B2 (TGF-B2),* present in the aqueous humour plays an important role in ACAID. In vitreo exposure of APCs (macrophages present in the anterior uvea) to the aqueous humour TGF-β2 converts these macrophages into ACAID inducing APCs, which leave through the trabecular meshwork into the venous circulation and ultimately in the spleen. In the spleen, these antigens secrete a chemokine (MIP-2), that will attract natural killer (NK) T cells. The NK-T cells inturn will secrete IL-10 and TGF-β, both associated with a Th2 response. The T cells responding to this environment become regulatory cells and suppress delayed hypersensitivity response (i.e. CMI) in the eye. In ACAID, the *afferent regulatory T cell* is a CD4+ cell, whereas the *efferent regulatory* is CD8+ T cell. The environment is such that the lymphoid cells in the eye will not produce IL-2 or express CD4+ which are important components of immune response.

Note. It has been suggested that in addition to TGF-β2, some other factors also might be playing role in the development of ACAID.

Clinically applied aspect. Role of ACAID in clinical situations still needs to be proved. However, in experimental studies, it has been proved that mice susceptible to IRBP-induced experimental autoimmune uveoretinitis (EAU) will not develop the disease of IRBP is injected into the eye before systemic immunization. This suggests that ACAID could be a mechanism by which nature attempts to limit the unwanted inflammatory responses in the anterior chamber. Thus ACAID may have a role in ocular tumours, as well as autoimmune and even infectious immune responses.

Effector blockade

Effector blockade refers to the immune regulatory mechanism in the anterior segment of eye exerted on the secondary effector phase of immune response arc. Infact, especially important to the clinicians is the capacity of a tissue site to sustain the secondary effector phase of immune

response arc, because the primary immune response arc in autoimmune disease might have occurred outside of the eye. Thus, Th1 delayed hypersensitivity T lymphocytes, cytotoxic T lymphocytes, natural killer cells, and complement activation appear to function less effectively in the anterior uvea than elsewhere. For example, the iris and cillary body are relatively resistant to induction of secondary purified protein derivatives delayed hypersensitivity response after primary immunization with mycobacteria in the skin.

Mechanisms of effector blockade are mutifactorial and include production of following factors:
• Immunomodulatory cytokines, produced by ocular tissues,
• Immunomodulatory neuropeptides, produced by ocular nerves,
• Functionally unique APCs,
• Compliment inhibitors in the aqueous humour, and
• Some other factors.

Fas-Fas ligand interactions and programmed cell death (apoptosis)

Fas ligand (FasL) or CD95 ligand is a type II membrane protein that belongs to the TNF superfamily and is found on the lymphocytes. It is constitutively expressed on the iris and corneal endothelium. FasL is normally expressed in the thymus and organs that appear to be able to limit immune response such as eyes, testes and brain. Other organs, such as liver and intestine, express this antigen only during severe inflammatory processes.

Apoptosis or programmed cell death of lymphocytes present in the iris can be triggered by FasL, thereby preventing the effector function of infiltering T lymphocytes.

Loss of this protective mechanism may occur prior to development of uveitis.

Fas-FasL works in concert with several factors.
• *One cofactor appears to be TNF.* Activated lymphocytes producing TNF will be more at risk of apoptosis.
• *Other mechanisms induce apoptosis* through IL-2 activation of lymphocytes. These highly

activated cells ultimately die a programmed cell death.

ETIOPATHOGENESIS OF UVEITIS

Etiopathogenesis of uveitis is not only a complex subject but ambiguous too. Because of the limitation of availability of tissue for study, most understanding on this subject is based on the animal models of uveitis. Therefore, for the purpose of understanding of this subject, the etiopathogenesis of uveitis can be discussed under two main heads:
- Experimental models of uveitis,
- Etiological factors, and pathomechanisms of uveitis.

EXPERIMENTAL MODLES OF UVEITIS

Over the years, several animal models of uveitis have been described by researchers to understand the pathomechanism of uveitis. These can be grouped as:
- Experimental autoimmune uveitis (EAU),
- Endotoxin-induced uveitis (EIU), and
- Specific uveitis animal models.

EXPERIMENTAL AUTOIMMUNE UVEITIS

Experimental autoimmune uveitis (EAU) is a well established animal disease model of human endogenous uveitis as both are T cell-mediated diseases (T_H^1). It can be induced in susceptible animals by immunisation with uveitogenic antigens.

Uveitigenic antigens

The concept that the eye harbours autoimmune inducing or uveitogenic materials has been suggested by many since the beginning of this century. Several antigens have been isolated that are capable of inducing ocular disease in rodents—in many respect similar to that seen in humans. The number of identifiable antigens capable of stimulating immune system makes the eye unique.

Uveitigenic antigens identified so far are:
- Retinal soluble antigen (arrestin), S-antigen
- Interphotoreceptor retinoid binding protein (IRBP)

- Rhodopsin and its illuminated form—opsin
- Recoverin
- Phosducin
- Bovine melanin protein
- RPE 65
- Tyrosinase

Note. EAU can be induced in a variety of species including rats, mice, monkey, guinea pigs and rabbits. Studies on EAU are available with all the above mentioned uveitogenic antigens. However, the S-Ag (Figs 3.2.1 and 3.2.2) and IRBP-induced models and these antigens themselves have been the best investigated to date.

Cellular mechanisms in EAU

It has been shown that depending on the model, EAU is driven by two effector arms, T_H^1 and

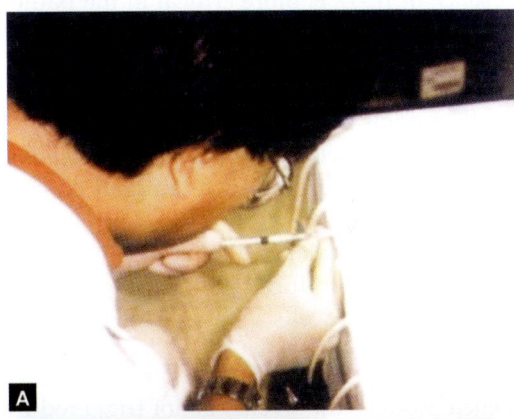

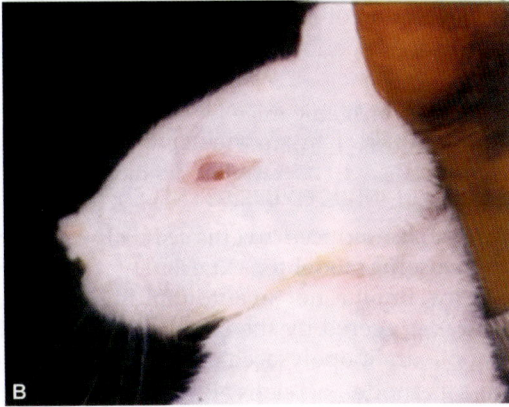

Fig. 3.2.1 *Experiment showing: A, Injection of retinal S antigen in foot pad of Lewis rat; B, Uveitis occurring after 14 days in the rat.*

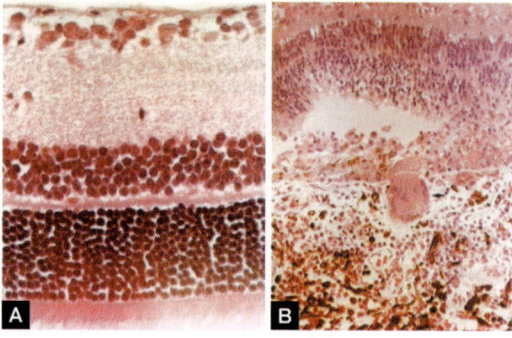

Fig. 3.2.2 *Histopathological changes of normal uveal tissue before (A) and after (B) retinal S antigen injection*

T_H^{17}, i.e. both IFN gamma and cytokine IL-17 are produced with very little IL-4. Though IFN gamma predominates over IL-17, but the studies also show that disease development can be stopped by neutralization of only IL-17 and not that of IFN gamma. This indicates that the presence of IL-17 is more critical in the pathogenesis of the disease.

Special models of EAU

Special models of EAU include:

• *Humanized models of experimental autoimmune uveitis* in human leucocyte antigen class II transgenic mice
• Experimental melanin uveitis
• Model of EAU induced with IRBP presented by the dendritic cells.

Spontaneous uveitic models

In such models, the uveitis is not triggered by the inoculation of the Ag, but develops spontaneously over a period. Examples of such models are:

• Human transgenic mice
• Autoimmune regulator knockout mice

ENDOTOXIN-INDUCED UVEITIS

• Endotoxin-induced uveitis (EIU) is another very useful model for experimental anterior uveitis. But it is not an autoimmune reaction, and is triggered by the injection of bacterial endotoxin lipopolysaccharide (LPS).
• In this model, a relatively fleeting anterior uveitis characterised mostly by an infiltration of polymorphonuclear cells and release of cytokine.

• This model has potential relevance because patients with ankylosing spondylitis and uveitis have been reported to have a higher incidence Klebsella organism in their stool or infection with other gram-negative bacterium during or shorty before the active portion of their disease than when their disease is quiet as compared with control subjects.

DISEASE-SPECIFIC UVEITIS ANIMAL MODELS

Disease-specific uveitis animal models which have evolved the understanding of some complex entities include:

• Experimental animal model of cytomegalovirus retinitis, and
• Experimental animal ocular tuberculosis model.

Experimental animal model of cytomegalovirus retinitis

Experimental animal model of cytomegalovirus (CMV) retinitis has been developed and used to study the use of *cytokine immunotherapy* in CMV retinitis.

Experimental animal ocular tuberculosis model

Key observations of the experimental model of ocular tuberculosis, developed in guinea pig by Rao et al, are:

• *Pulmonary tuberculosis* developed in all the exposed animals.
• *Ocular lesions* resembling the human disease, developed in 42% animals.
• *Ocular lesions included* primarily posterior uveitis followed by intermediate uveitis and limbal inflammation.
• *Granulomatous inflammation* was seen at all the sites.
• *Acid-fast bacilli* detectable by quantitative polymerase chain reaction (PCR) were seen at some sites.
• *Antitubercular therapy (ATT)* treated animals showed no granulomatous inflammation, indicating the importance of systemic ATT in the treatment of ocular tuberculosis.
• *Pathogenesis of retinal vasculitis* cannot be studied in this model owing to lack of retinal vasculature in the retina of guinea pigs.

ETIOLOGICAL FACTORS AND PATHOMECHANISMS OF UVEITIS

Despite a great deal of experimental research and many sophisticated methods of investigations, etiology and immunology of the uveitis is still largely not understood. Even today, the cause of many clinical conditions is disputed (remains presumptive) and in many others etiology is unknown. Conceptually, from the point of view of etiopathogenesis, the uveitis can be grouped as below:

- Infectious uveitis,
- Non-infectious uveitis, and
- Masquerade syndromes.

A. INFECTIOUS UVEITIS

Causative organisms

Depending upon the causative organism, the infectious uveitis can be sub-grouped as below:

1. *Bacterial uveitis*
- Tubercular uveitis
- Syphilitic and other spirochetal uveitis
- Laprotic uveitis
- Lyme disease
- Leptospiral uveitis
- Ocular nocardiasis
- Ocular bartonellosis
- Uveitis in whipple disease
- Rickettsial disease of eye

2. *Viral uveitis*
- Herpes simplex uveitis
- Herpes zoster uveitis
- Acquired cytomegalovirus
- Ocular involvement in AIDS
- Chikungunya uveitis
- Dengue uveitis.
- West Nile disease
- Rubella uveitis

3. *Fungal uveitis*
- Persumed ocular histoplasmosis syndrome
- Candidiasis
- Aspergillosis
- Cryptococcosis

4. *Parasitic uveitis*
- Toxoplasmosis
- Toxocariasis
- Onchocerciasis
- Cysticercosis
- Diffuse unilateral subacute neuroretinitis

Pathomechanisms of infectious uveitis

Modes of infection

Uveal infections may be exogenous, secondary or endogenous:

Exogenous infections wherein the infecting organism directly gain entrance into the eye from outside. It can occur following penetrating injuries, perforation of corneal ulcer and post-operatively (after intraocular operations). Such infections usually result in an acute iridocyclitis of suppurative (purulent) nature, which soon turn into endophthalmitis or even panophthalmitis.

Secondary infection of the uvea occurs by spread of infection from neighbouring structures, e.g. acute purulent conjunctivitis (pneumococcal and gonococcal), keratitis, scleritis, retinitis, orbital cellulitis and orbital thrombophlebitis.

Endogenous infections are caused by the entrance of organism from some source of infection situated elsewhere in the body, by way of the bloodstream. Endogenous infections play most important role in the inflammation of uvea.

Mechanisms of uveitogenic process

Once a microbial organism enters the body, the physiological function of the immune system, to provide defence against infections, is initiated. The defense against infection is mediated by two systems: the early *innate immunity* that clears the infection, or keeps it in check until the second system, the *adaptive immunity*, which is antigen-specific, develops (for details of innate and adaptive immunity see page 31).

Once the microorganism enters ocular tissue, an immune response is generated, which in general can be as below:

- *Gram-positive and gram-negative bacteria* produce an acute inflammatory response and abscess formation.
- *Acid-fast bacteria* produce granulomatous inflammation and caseation necrosis.

- *Fungi*, while targeting the choroid, produce chronic granulomatous or non-granulomatous inflammation and hypersensitivity reactions.
- *Viruses* tend to target the cornea and the retina.
- *Dead parasites* may cause an inflammatory reaction in the host.

Immune mechanisms involved in some infectious diseases are listed in Table 3.2.1. In certain circumstances, the immune responses are harmful, causing pathological outcomes, such as *hypersensitivity reactions* (see page 50) or *autoimmune reactions* (see page 49). The major outcome of both the useful and harmful immune responses is inflammation with ensueing local tissue damage. All components of the innate and adaptive immune system are involved in the pathogenic process of ocular inflammation.

Uveitogenic immune process

Uveitogenic immune processes involved in infectious uveitis, thus, include:

- Uveitis due to hypersensitivity reactions to microorganisms or their products
- Microbial-induced autoimmune uveitis
- Uveitis induced by exotoxins and other secretory products of bacteria, and
- Uveitis due to alternative pathway of inflammation induced by microbial cell wall.

1. Uveitis due to hypersensitivity reaction to microorganisms. Hypersensitivity, as described

Table 3.2.1 *Immune mechanisms involved in infectious diseases*

Infectious agent	Mode of defence
Bacteria and viruses	Neutralization IgG with complement and neutrophils. For gastrointestinal and respiratory infections: IgA, and alternative complement pathway
Pneumococci and encapsulated organisms	IgM, macrophages and complements
Mycobacteria, syphilic, fungi and virus	Cytotoxic T cell, perforin, macrophage and delayed hypersensitivity
Helminths	Intestinal IgE with mast cells

in detail on page 50, refers to an abnormal immune response which produces physiological or pathological damage in the host tissues.

Microbial allergic uveitis may occur due to hypersensitivity reactions to the microorganisms or to their proteins and toxins. A latent bacteremia or viremia causes sensitization of the uveal tissue with the formation of antibodies; and later when there is renewal of infections, the antigen reaches the uvea and results in severe antigen–antibody reactions.

2. Microbial-induced autoimmune uveitis. Pathogenic autoimmunity is assumed to be triggered by microbial infections by following two different mechanisms:

i. *Molecular mimicry.* Some experimental studies have revealed that uveitis induced by certain microbial molecules was similar to that induced by certain ocular antigens indicating thereby that the antibodies produced by antigens cross-reacted with uveal tissue. This phenomenon associated with cross-reacting antigens is called molecular mimickery.

ii. *Stimulation of innate immunity* has been suggested as another mechanism for triggering pathogenic autoimmunity by following microbial products:

- Endotoxins (bacterial lipopolysaccharide, i.e. LPS),
- Lipoteichoic acid in gram-positive bacteria,
- Lipoarabinomuraman in mycobacteria,
- Heat shock proteins of bacteria,
- Killed lysates of many gram-positive bacteria,
- Bacterial DNA, and
- Viral RNA.

Mechanism. The above microbial products are potent ligands for TLRs that are expressed on macrophages and other APCs and thus activate the innate immunity through TLR system. Stimulated APCs then release proinflammatory cytokines (IL-1, IL-6, and tumour necrosis factor, i.e. TNF), resulting in inflammation.

3. Uveitis induced by bacterial exotoxins and other secretory products. Some bacteria are known to secrete exotoxins and other products into the microenvironment in which the bacterium is growing. Many of these products are enzymes that, although not directly inflammatory, can cause tissue damage which subsequently results in inflammation.

Examples of such products are:

- *Collagenases* secreted by bacteria.
- *Hemolysin,* such as streptolysin O, which can kill neutophils by causing cytoplasmic and extracellular release of their granules.
- *Phospholipases,* such as the *Clostridium perfringes* alpha toxins, which kill cells and cause necrosis by disturbing the cell membrane.
- *Formyl peptide molecules (FMLP)* secreted by some bacteria act as potent triggering stimuli for innate immunity.

4. *Microbial cell wall stimulated alternate pathway for inflammation* can also induce uveitis. The alternate pathway for stimulation of immunity includes:

- *Complement system.* The complements are effector molecules used to amplify inflammation for both innate and adaptive immunities.
- *C-reactive proteins and alpha 2 macroglobulin* also act as alterative pathway for innate immunity. Alpha 2-macroglobulin is present in aqueous humour during uveitis and is synthesised by various ocular parenchymal cells of the eye as well.

Note. Like microbial cell wall, plastic surfaces of IOLs and traumatized tissues can also induce uveitis by alternate pathways.

B. NON-INFECTIOUS UVEITIS

Non-infectious uveitis is labelled when no specific infectious pathogen can be suspected clinically and isolated with the available investigations. Often the trigger or inciting event or agent that cause the inflammation is unknown or undetectable.

Mechanisms of non-infectious uveitis. Non-infectious uveitis may occur as:

- Autoimmune uveitis, or
- Immune-mediated uveitis

1. Autoimmune uveitis

Autoimmune uveitis is believed to be driven by aberrant immune recognition of self. For details about autoimmunity see page 49. Auto-immunity, i.e. immune response directed against the host, is a common phenomenon and in vast number of individuals does not lead to obvious disease. The term autoimmune disease is used when the autoimmune mechanisms lead to self tissue damage.

Mechanisms of autoimmune disease

Mechanisms of autoimmune disease may vary considerably depending upon the organ in question. Most understanding about patho-genesis of autoimmune uveitis has come from the 'experimental autoimmune uveitis' (EAU), which is an animal model of human uveitis (see page 57). In general, an autoimmune disease may be caused by any of the following mechanisms:

- *Effector T cell tolerance to antigen in question.* Such tolerance can occur, if small amounts of antigen are constantly circulating. This tolerance state is abrogated, however, if the effector T cell is now presented with a new moiety of the antigen, a situation which leads to disease expression.
- *Molecular mimicry.* In it, the offending agent mimics the body tissue(a phenomenon called cross-reacting antigens); and the antibodies formed against the offending agent also damage the host tissue.
- *Non-specific polyclonal activation of the immune system* by some immune stimulatory agents, may overwhelm the normal regulatory mechanisms and permit forbidden clones of cells to proliferate and cause tissue damage.

HLA associated uveitis

The etiological triggers in autoimmune uveitis are unknown. However, a strong association with HLA has been found in some different types of autoimmune uveitis. Human leucocytic antigens (HLA) is the old name for the histocompatibility genes which collectively constitute the histocompatibility complex (MHC). There are three subclasses of MHC gene; class I, II and III (For details see page 32). There are about 70 antigens in the human beings, on the basis of which an individual can be assigned different HLA-phenotype. There is growing evidence to suggest the role of HLA in uveitis, since a number of diseases associated with uveitis occur more frequently in persons with certain specific HLA phenotype.

Mechanisms of disease susceptibility in a specific HLA positive person is not known. Following hypotheses are in vogue:

- *HLA molecules act as peptide-binding molecules* for etiologic antigens or infectious agents.
- *Molecular mimicry* between bacterial antigens and an epitope of an HLA molecules (i.e. an antigenic site on the molecule itself) may be responsible for a cross-react effector response
- *T lymphocyte antigen receptor (gene)* may be the true susceptibility factor. This hypothesis is based on the fact that a specific T lymphocyte receptor uses a specific HLA hoplotype, so a strong corelation would exist between the HLA and T lymphocyte antigen receptor repertoire.
- *An innate cause unrelated to the role of HLA in adaptive immunity.* For example, transgenic mice genetically altered to express HLA-B51 molecule, which is associated with Adamentiades-Behcet syndrome, develops neutrophils with enhanced activation and perhaps exaggerated effector function.

Examples of HLA-associated diseases with uveitis include:
- Ankylosing spondylitis: HLA-B27
- Reiter's syndrome: HLA-B27
- Behcet's disease: HLA-B51
- Birdshot retinochoroidopathy: HLA-A29
- VKH syndrome: HLA- DR4, HLA-DR1
- Sympathetic ophthalmitis: HLA-DR4
- Sarcoidosis: HLA-B8, HLA-B13
- Persumed ocular histoplasmosis: HLA-B7, HLA-DR2
- Retinal vasculitis: HLA- B44
- Mutiple sclerosis: HLA-B7, HLA-DR2
- Intermedaite uveitis: HLA-B8, -B51,-DR2, -R15
- Juvenile rheumatoid arthritis : HLA-A2, -DR5, -DR8, - DR 11, -DR2.1

II. Immune-mediated non-infectious uveitis

Immune-mediated non-infectious uveitis is primarily an inflammatory reaction for which several mechanisms have been identified that trigger, and promote the development of this pathogenic process. These mechanisms include:
- Environmental factors, and
- Autologus (tissue damage) signals.

Environmental factors

The antigenic environmental factors circulating in the bloodstream sensitise the uveal tissue. Later, a renewal of activity leads to further dissemination of environmental antigenic factors which on meeting the sensitised ocular tissue excite an immune-mediated uveitis. Immune-related reactions which can excite uveal inflammation include:
- Innate immunity,
- Adaptive immunity, and
- Immune-related hypersensitivity reactions

Ocular inflammations occurring in different types of hypersensitivity reaction

Type I hypersensitivity or immediate hypersensitivity. Ocular inflammations associated with type I hypersensitivity are:
- *Atopic uveitis.* It occurs due to airborne allergens and inhalants, e.g. seasonal iritis due to pollens. A similar reaction to such material as danders of cats, chicken feathers, house dust, egg albumin and beef proteins has been noted.
- *Anaphylactic uveitis.* It is said to accompany the systemic anaphylactic reactions, like serum sickness and angioneurotic oedema.

Type II hypersensitivity or antibody-mediated autotoxicity. Ocular pemphigoid is reported to occur due to type II hypersensitivity with cytotoxic antibodies directed to the basement membrane of mucosal surface.

Type III hypersensitivity (immune complex-mediated hypersensitivity) reactions had been suggested as being one of the major immune mechanism leading to intraocular inflammatory responses, such as, Behcet's disease. However, more recent evidences suggest that it is not an important pathogenic mechanism for uveitis in humans. However, Type III hypersensitivity reaction appears to play a role, at least in part, in pathogenesis of phacoanaphylatic endophthalmitis.

Type IV hypersensitivity or delayed hypersensitivity also termed as 'cell-mediated immune (CMI) mechanisms', has been identified as the immunopathogenic mechanism in majority of animal models of uveitis. It is assumed that this reaction induced by T_H^1 lymphocytes is responsible for the most cases of intraocular inflammation in humans. Granulomatous inflammation seen in sarcoidosis, and sympathetic ophthalmitis is thought to be occurring due to type IV hypesensitivity.

Role of autologus (tissue damage) signals

Traumatic uveitis is known to occur following blunt or penetrating ocular trauma and surgical trauma from intraocular procedures, such as cataract extraction, trabeculectomy and vitreoretinal procedures.

Mechanisms. Following trauma or any other cause of tissue damage often there occurs accumulation of necrotic products at the site. As a result of tissue damage, and the ensuing enhanced release of sequestered self-antigen along with necrosis there occur activation of antigen-presenting cells (APCs). Once activated, the T cells enter the eye tissue where they are exposed to the target antigen, and initiate the pathogenic process. Thus the necrotic cells promote immunopathogenicity by stimulating 'damage signals' and proinflammatory process.

C. MASQUERADE SYNDROME

Masquerade syndrome refers to clinical presentation of uveal inflammation which are not due to immune-mediated uveitis entities. Such a clinical presentation, mimicking uveitis may be caused by neoplastic and certain non-neoplastic conditions.

Non-neoplastic masquerade syndromes

The non-neoplastic masquerade syndrome classically may occur in:
- Retinitis pigmentosa
- Ocular ischaemic syndrome
- Retinal detachment
- Intraocular foreign body
- Pigmented dispersion syndrome

Neoplastic masquerade syndromes

Some intraocular neoplasms which can present with features of uveitis include:

A. *Lymphoid malignances*
- Primary central nervous system lymphomas
- Secondary to systemic lymphomas
- Secondary to leukaemias
- Secondary to uveal lymphoid proliferation

B. *Non-lymphoid malignancies*
- Uveal melanomas
- Retinoblastoma
- Juvenile xanthogranuloma
- Metastatic tumours

Note: For details of masquerade syndrome see Chapter 8, page 358.

BIBLIOGRAPHY

1. Agarwal RK, Caspi RR. Rodent models of experimental autoimmune uveitis. Methods Mol Med 2004;102:395–419.
2. American Academy of Ophthalmolgy: Intraocular inflammation and Uveitis;section-9; edition 2009–2010;34–37,40–41,43,60–71.
3. Bansal S, Barathi VA, Iwata D, Agrawal R. Experimental autoimmune uveitis and other animal models of uveitis: An update. Indian Journal of Ophthalmology Vol 63, No 3, March 2015 pp 211–218.
4. Biswas J, Fogla R Rao, Jyotirmay Biswas. Retinal autoimmunity; Stephen J. Ryan; volume 1; Basic sciences and inherited retinal disease; 1989: 167–179. Sympathetic Ophthalmia following Cyclocryotherapy-Report of a case with histopathological correlation. 1996;27:1035–1308.
5. Borst DE, Redmod TM, Elser JE, Gonda MA, Wiggert B, Chader GJ, et al. Interphotoreceptor retinoid-binding protein. Gene characterization, protein repeat structure, and its evolution. J Biol Chem 1989; 264:1115–1123.
6. Buzdygon B, Philip N, Zigler JS Jr, Gery I, Zuckermann R: Identity of S-antigen and the 48 kilodalton protein in retinal rod outer segments, Invest Ophthalmol Vis Sci 26(suppl): 1985;293.
7. Caspi RR, Chan CC, Wiggert B, Chader GJ. The mouse as a model of experimental autoimmune uveoretinitis (EAU). Curr Eye Res 1990;9 Suppl:169–174.
8. Caspi RR, Roberge FC, Chan CC, Wiggert B, Chader GJ. Rozenszan LA, et al. A new model of autoimmune disease. Experimental autoimmune uveoretinitis induced in mice with two different retinal antigens. J Immunol 1988; 140:1490–1495.
9. Caspi RR. Understanding autoimmunity in the eye: From animal models to novel therapies. Discov Med 2014;17:15–62.

10. Chan CC, Caspi RR,ni M, Leake WC, Wiggert B, Chader GJ, et al. Pathology of experimental autoimmune uveoretinitis in mice. J Autoimmune 1990;3:247–255.

11. DeVoss J, Hou Y, Johannes K, Lu W, Liou GI, Rinn J, et al. Spontaneous autoimmunity prevented by thymic expression of a single self-antigen. J Exp Med 2006;203:2727–35.

12. Dick AD, Forrester JV, Liversidge J, Cope AP. The role of tumour necrosis factor (TNF-alpha) in experimental autoimmune uveoretinitis (EAU). Prog Retin Eye Res 2004;23:617–37.

13. Dix RD, Giedlin M, Cousins SW. Systemic cytokine immunotherapy for experimental cytomegalovirus retinitis in mice with retrovirus-induced immunodeficiency. Invest Ophthalmol Vis Sci 1997;38:1411–1417.

14. Faure JP. Autoimmunity and the retina. Curr Top Eye Res 1980;2:215–302.

15. Forrester JV, Liversidge J, Dua HS, Dick A, Harper F, McMenamin PG. Experimental autoimmune uveoretinitis: A model system for immuno-intervention: A review. Curr Eye Res 1992;11 Suppl: 33–40.

16. Gery I, Mochizuk M, Nussenblatt RB. Retinal specific antigens and immunopathogenetic process they provoke. In: Osborne NN Chader J (eds). Progress in Retinal Research, Oxford, Pergamom Press, 1998.

17. Gery I. Mochizuki M, Nussenblatt RB. Retinal specific antigens and immunopathogenic process they provoke. Prog Retin Res 1986;5:75–109.

18. Grey I, Nussenblatt RB, Chan CC, Caspi RR. Autoimmune diseases of the eye. In: Theofilopoulos AN, Bona CA, editors. The Molecular Pathology of Autoimmune Diseases. New York: Taylor and Francis; 2002, pp. 978–998.

19. Nussenblatt RB, Whitcup SM, Palestine AG. Uveitis: Fundamental Practice. 2nd ed. St. Louis: Mosby/Year Book; 1996.

20. Nussenblatt RRB. Bench to bedside: New approaches to the immunotherapy of uveitic disease. Int Rev Immunol 2002;21:273–289.

21. Peng Y, Han G, Shao H, Wang Y, Kaplan HJ, Sun D. Characterization of IL-17+interphtoreceptal retinoid-binding protein-specific T cells in experimental autoimmune uveitis. Invest Ophthalmol Vis Sci 2007;48:4153–4161.

22. Pennesi G, Mattapallil MJ, Sun SH, Avichezer D, Silver PB, Karabekian Z, et al. A humanized model of experimental autoimmune uveitis in HLA class II transgenic mice. J Clin Invest 2003;111:1171–1180.

23. Rahi AHS, Addison DJ. Autoimmunity and the outer retina. Trans Ophthalmol Soc.UK. 1983; 103:428–437.

24. Rao NA, Albini TA, Kumaradas M, Pinn ML, Fraig MM, Karakousis PC. Experimental ocular tuberculossis in guinea pigs. Arch Ophthalmol 2009;127:162–166.

25. Rao NA, Patchett R, Fernandez MA, Sevanian A, Kunkel SL, Marak GE, Jr. Treatment of experimental granulomatous uveitis by lipoxygenase and cyclo-oxygenase inhibitors. Arch Ophthalmol 1987;105:413–415.

26. Rao NA. Mechanism of inflammatory response in sympathetic ophthalmia and VKH syndrome. Eye. 1997;11:213–216.

27. Smith JR, Hart PH, Williams KA. Basic pathogenic mechanisms operating in experimental models of acute anterior uveitis. Immunol Cell Biol 1998;76:497–512.

3.3 PATHOLOGY OF UVEITIS

General Considerations
Pathological Characteristics of Uveitis
- Pathology of suppurative uveitis
- Pathology of non-suppurative uveitis
  - Pathology of non-granulomatous uveitis
  - Pathology of granulomatous uveitis

General Clinical and Histological Findings in Uveitis
Pathology of Some Uveitic Entities
- Sympathetic ophthalmia
- Phacogenic uveitis
- Toxocara granuloma
- Retinal vasculitis in SLE
- CMV retinitis

GENERAL CONSIDERATIONS

Inflammation of the uvea fundamentally has the same characteristics as any other tissue of the body, i.e. a vascular and a cellular response. However, due to extreme vascularity and looseness of the uveal tissue, the inflammatory responses are exaggerated and thus produces special results.

Pathologically, inflammations of the uveal tract may be divided into suppurative (purulent) and non-suppurative (non-purulent) varieties. Wood has further classified non-suppurative uveitis into nongranulomatous and granulomatous types. Although morphologic description is still of some value, the rigid division of uveitis by Wood into these two categories has been questioned on both clinical and pathological grounds. Certain transitional forms of uveitis have also been recognised. Some of these (e.g. phacoanaphylactic endophthalmitis and sympathetic ophthalmia) showing pathological features of granulomatous uveitis are caused by hypersensitivity reactions. While uveitis due to tissue invasion by leptospirae presents with manifestations of non-granulomatous uveitis. Nonetheless, the classification is often useful in getting oriented towards the subject of uveitis, its workup and therapy. Therefore, it is worthwhile to describe the pathological features

of these overlapping (both clinically and pathologically) conditions as distinct varieties.

PATHOLOGICAL CHARACTERISTICS OF UVEITIS

I. PATHOLOGY OF SUPPURATIVE UVEITIS

Purulent inflammation of the uvea is usually a part of endophthalmitis or panophthalmitis occurring as a result of exogenous infection by pyogenic organisms which include *Staphylococcus, Streptococcus, Pseudomonas, Pneumococcus and Gonococcus.*

Pathological reaction is characterised by an outpouring of purulent exudate and infiltration by polymorphonuclear cells of uveal tissue, anterior chamber, posterior chamber and vitreous cavity. As a result, the whole uveal tissue is thickened and necrotic and the cavities of eye become filled with pus.

II. PATHOLOGY OF NON-SUPPURATIVE UVEITIS

1. Pathology of non-granulomatous uveitis

Non-granulomatous uveitis may be an acute or chronic exudative inflammation of uveal tissue (predominantly iris and ciliary body), usually occurring either due to a physical and toxic insult to the tissue, or as a result of different hypersensitivity reactions.

Pathological alterations of the non-granulomatous reaction. As mentioned above, the inflammatory process in non-granulomatous uveitis can be acute and chronic.

- *In acute inflammation* (Fig. 3.3.1), the main infiltrating cells are polymorphonuclear neutrophils and macrophages accompanied by edema, vascular dilatation, and congestion. Marked dilatation and increased permeability of vessels, and breakdown of blood aqueous barrier leads to an outpouring of fibrinous exudate and infiltration of the uveal tissue, anterior chamber, posterior chamber and vitreous cavity. The inflammation is usually diffuse.

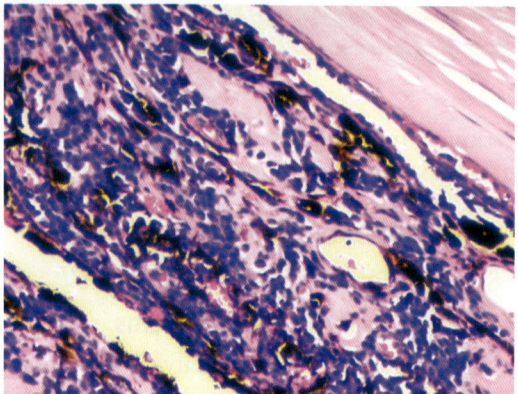

Fig. 3.3.1 *Histological picture in a case of non-granulomatous uveitis*

- *Tissue damage* can result in necrosis. In contrast, in chronic inflammation the main infiltrating cells are lymphocytes and macrophages with exudate, vascular congestion, and vascular obstruction. Tissue damage can result in necrosis and/or cellular proliferation, such as fibrosis and gliosis.
- *Chronic granulomatous inflammation* is a proliferative inflammation characterised by a cellular infiltrate of epithelioid cells and sometimes inflammatory giant cells, lymphocytes, plasma cells, polymorphonuclear leucocytes and eosinophils.

Gross and microscopic changes in uveal tissues and intraocular fluid cavities. As a result of these pathological reactions:

- Iris becomes waterlogged, oedematous, muddy with blurring of crypts and furrows. As a consequence, its mobility is reduced, pupil becomes small in size due to sphincter irritation and engorgement of radial vessels of iris.
- Exudates and lymphocytes poured into the anterior chamber result in aqueous flare and deposition of fine KPs at the back of cornea.
- Due to exudates in the posterior chamber, the posterior surface of iris adheres to the anterior capsule of lens leading to posterior synechiae formation.
- In severe inflammation, due to pouring of exudate from ciliary processes, behind the lens, an exudative membrane called *cyclitic membrane* may be formed.

Healing and structural changes. After healing, pin-point areas of necrosis or atrophy are evident. Subsequent attacks lead to structural changes, like atrophy, gliosis and fibrosis which cause adhesions, scarring and eventually destruction of eye.

2. Pathology of granulomatous uveitis

Granulomatous uveitis is a chronic inflammation of proliferative nature which typically occurs in response to anything which acts as an irritant foreign body, whether it be inorganic or organic material introduced from outside, a haemorrhage or necrotic tissue within the eye, or one of the certain specific organisms of non-pyogenic and relatively non-virulent character.

Common organisms which excite inflammation are those responsible for tuberculosis, leprosy, syphilis, brucellosis, leptospirosis, as well as most viral, mycotic, protozoal and helminthic infections.

Non-infectious granulomatous inflammation is also seen typically in sarcoidosis, sympathetic ophthalmitis and Vogt-Koyanagi-Harada disease.

Pathological reaction in granulomatous uveitis is proliferative in nature and is characterised by infiltration with lymphocytes, plasma cells and mobilisation and proliferation of large mononuclear cells which eventually become epithelioid and giant cells and aggregate into nodules.

Gross pathological changes include:

- *Iris nodules* which are usually formed near pupillary border (*Koeppe's nodules*) and some times near collarette (*Busacca nodules*).
- *Mutton fat KPs*. Similar nodular collection of the cells is deposited at the back of cornea in the form of mutton fat keratic precipitates and aqueous flare is minimal.
- *Necrosis* in the adjacent structures leads to reparative process resulting in fibrosis and gliosis of the involved area.

GENERAL CLINICAL AND HISTOLOGICAL FINDINGS IN UVEITIS

Clinical and histological findings in uveitis are described below and summarised in Table 3.3.1.

Table 3.3.1: *Signs of uveitis*	
Structure	*Signs*
Eyelid and skin	Vitiligo nodules
Conjunctiva	Perilimbal/diffuse injection
	Nodules
Corneal endothelium	Keratic precipitates
	Fibrin
	Pigments
Anterior chamber/	Inflammatory cells
posterior chamber	Flare
	Pigments
Iris	Nodules
	Posterior synechiae
	Atrophy
	Hetrochromia
Angle	PAS
	Nodules
	Vascularisation
Intraocular pressure	Hypotony
	Secondary glaucoma
Vitreous	Inflammatory cells
	Traction bands
Pars plana	Snowbanking
Retina	Inflammatory cells
	Retinal vasculitis
	CME
	RPE hypertrophy/loss, ERM
Choroid	Inflammatory infiltrate
	Nodules
	Atrophy
	Neovascularisation
Optic disc	Oedema
	Neovascularisation

Conjunctiva

- *Perilimbal vascular congestion* (ciliar flush) or diffuse injection of the conjunctiva or sometimes even episclera, is typical with acute anterior uveitis.
- *Perlimbal nodules* consisting of inflammatory cells may also be found in chronic uveitis sometimes.

Cornea

- *Corneal endothelial changes*, glaucoma, or both may be seen as sequelae of uveitis. This may result in chronic stromal and epithelial edema, finally resulting in bullous keratopathy.

Corneal bullae may rupture to become infected later on, forming corneal ulcer.

- *Keratic precipitates.* Cellular depositions consisting of mononuclear cells, mainly lymphocytes and plasma cells may be found on the corneal endothelium. These deposits are called as keratic precipitates. When newly formed, they tend to be white and smoothly round, but they soon become crenated (shrunken), pigmented or glassy. Large yellowish keratic precipitates (KPs) are described as mutton fat KPs. These types of KPs are usually associated with granulomatous type of inflammation.
- *Calcium deposition on corneal epithelium* is usually found in chronic uveitis forming band keratopathy.

Anterior chamber

Anterior chamber cells are individual cells, such as WBCs, that are floating in the aqueous. The flare is constituted by proteins that have released through inflamed vasculature inside the eye.

Anterior chamber reaction associated with increased capillary permeability, can be described as:

- *Serous*, i.e. aqueous flare caused by protein influx,
- *Purulent*, i.e. polymorphonuclear leucocytes and necrotic debris causing hypopyon,
- *Fibrinous*, i.e. plasmoid or intense fibrinous exudate, or
- *Sanguinoid,* i.e. inflammatory cells with erythrocytes manifested by hypopyon mixed with hyphema.

Organisation of the inflammatory products or *haemorrhage*, or *iris neovascularisation*, may obliterate the angle of anterior chamber.

Iris

- *Iris may undergo atrophy and necrosis* along with loss of dilator muscle, stroma, and even sphincter muscle and pigment epithelium.
- *Peripheral anterior synechiae* may be formed in chronic anterior uveitis.
- *Rubeosis iridis* (neovascularisation of anterior surface of iris) may result in secondary anterior chamber angle synechiae.

- *Ectropion uvea.* Shrinkage of the fibrovascular membrane on anterior surface of iris may result in eversion of its pupillary border causing ectropion uvea.
- *Seclusio and occlusio pupillae.* The same membrane that binds the pupil down to surrounding structures usually grows across the pupil resulting in seclusio and occlusio pupillae. Also,shrinkage of the membrane between iris and lens may cause inversion of pupillary border resulting in *entropion pupillae.*
- *Total annular synechiae* may be formed, resulting in complete pupillary block leading to formation of iris bombe, peripheral anterior synechiae and secondary closed angle glaucoma. Such eyes often have reduced aqueous flow and hypotony may result in the face of completely closed angle.
- *Iris nodules.* These are collections of mononuclear inflammatory cells on the surface or stroma of iris.

Lens

Complicated cataract formation. Chronic uveitis frequently induces the lens epithelium to migrate posteriorly. The presence of aberrant cells under the posterior lens capsule produces a posterior subcapsular cataract.

Ciliary body

- *Ciliary processes or crests tend to become flattened and attenuated* and their cores get fibrosed with chronic inflammation.
- *Ciliay epithelium (non-pigmented, pigmented or both) may proliferate* and may sometimes proliferate massively.
- *Intraocular inflammation may organise and fibrose* behind the lens between portions of pars plicata of the ciliary body. Such a fibrous membrane spanning the retrolental space often incorporating proliferated ciliary epithelium and vitreous base is called a cyclitic membrane.
- *When a cyclitic membrane shrinks,* the vitreous base, pars plana and peripheral neural retina are drawn inward causing total ciliary body and neural retinal detachment.
- *Ciliary body degeneration* results in decrease in aqueous production leading to hypotony.

Vitreous chamber

- *Vitreous opacities and organisation.* Inflammatory products in the vitreous body may induce vitreous opacities and if severe, causes organisation of the vitreous.
- *Newly formed blood vessels* from the neural retina or optic disc, or both, may grow into vitreous compartment of the eye. These vessels usually grow between the vitreous and internal surface of the neural retina, along the posterior surface of a detached vitreous, or into cloquet canal.
- *The vitreous body may collapse* and become detached posteriorly.

Choroid

- *Focal or diffuse areas of atrophy or scarring* may develop subsequently following choroidal inflammation.
- *Chorioretinal scar.* Retinochoroiditis or chorioretinitis may destroy Bruch's membrane and retinal pigment epithelium. The choroid and retina may become fused by fibrosis and a chorioretinal scar or adhesion may result.

Retina

- *Perivasculitis.* Uveitis may frequently cause neural retinal perivasculitis with lymphocytes surrounding the blood vessels. If vasculitis is extensive, that can be noted clinically as vascular sheathing.
- *Cystoid macular oedema.* Inflammation involving the peripheral neural retina or ciliary body, may be accompanied by fluid collection in macular region causing cystoid macular oedema.
- *Chorioretinal scarring* may result from retinochoroiditis or chorioretinitis.
- *Hyperplasia and atrophy of RPE.* The retinal pigment epithelium is a very sensitive tissue and may undergo massive hyperplasia after inflammation. Retinal pigment epithelium may show alternating areas of mild hyperplasia and atrophy or may be associated with intraocular ossification.
- *Neural retina may get detached* secondary to subneural retinal exudation or haemorrhage.

PATHOLOGY OF SOME UVEITIC ENTITIES

SYMPATHETIC OPHTHALMIA

It is a bilateral diffuse granulomatous non-necrotising panuveitis following penetrating injury or surgery to one eye, followed by a latent period and the appearance of uveitis in the uninjured fellow eye (sympathising eye).

Signs and symptoms in the sympathising eye vary in severity and onset, ranging from minimal problems in near vision, mild photophobia and slight redness to severe granulomatous pan-uveitis.

- *Anterior segment findings.* Both eyes show mutton fat KPs, thickening of the iris from lymphocytic infiltration, posterior synechiae formation and elevated IOP due to trabeculitis or hypotony as a result of ciliary body shutdown.

- *Posterior segment findings* show moderate to severe vitritis with characteristic yellowish white choroidal lesions called as Dalen-Fuchs nodules. Peripapillary choroidal lesions and exudative retinal detachment may also develop (Fig. 3.3.2).

- *It is unclear whether the injury causes a de novo primary immunisation to self antigens*, perhaps because of externalisation of sequestered uveal antigens through the wound site, or if it somehow changes the immunological microenvironment of the retina and uvea. It is thought that the inflammatory effect or response is mediated by a Th1 delayed type of hypersensitivity response to uveal antigens. Histopathology shows diffuse thickening of choroid with abundance of lymphocytes with focal collection of epithelioid cells Fig. 3.3.2. Immunopathology shows early disease having predominance of CD4 cells, with late stage having predominance of CD8 cells. Activated macrophages are also numerous in granulomas.

- *A light and electron microscopic study was undertaken* in an effort to establish the origin of the "epithelioid" cells in Dalen-Fuchs nodules (Fig. 3.3.3) from an eye enucleated because of sympathetic ophthalmia (Fig. 3.3.4). The nodules were visible as minute (130–160 μm), round, grayish-white mounds in Bruch's membrane elevating the retinal pigment epithelium. By electron microscopy, the "epithelioid" cells had round to oval nuclei with abundant, relatively lucent cytoplasm containing parallel profiles of rough-surfaced endoplasmic reticulum, prominent Golgi lamellae, clusters of polyribosomes, and scattered mitochondria. Some cells within the nodules showed large membrane bound phagosomes containing laminated structures (Fig. 3.3.3). Examination of the nodules under ultraviolet light shows myriad of auto-fluorescent yellowish-orange dots consistent with lipofuscin.

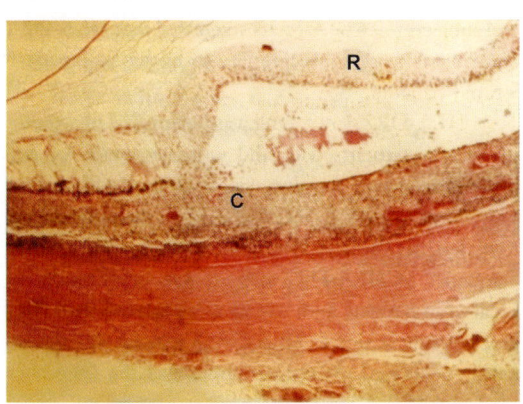

Fig. 3.3.2 *Microphotograph showing retinal detachment (R), diffuse thickening of the choroid in a case of sympathetic ophthalmia (haematoxylin and eosin, '100 X')*

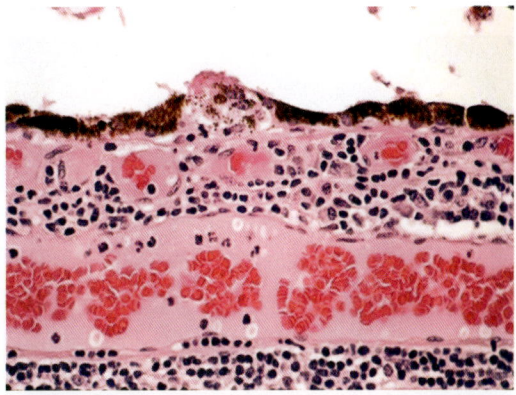

Fig. 3.3.3 *Microphotograph showing Dalen-Fuchs nodule with diffuse inflammation of the choroid in a case of sympathetic ophthalmia (arrow) (Courtesy: Dr Deepak Edward, USA)*

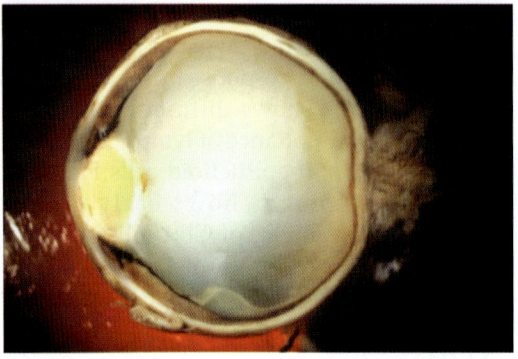

Fig. 3.3.4 *Enucleated globe of sympathetic ophthalmia.*

PHACOGENIC UVEITIS

It refers to intraocular inflammation induced by lens protein, usually after surgical or traumatic rupture of the lens capsule (Fig. 3.3.5).

Pathological features. Phacoantigenic uveitis is a form of lens-induced uveitis with three different zones of inflammation centred around the lens.

- *An inner zone of neutrophils* invading the lens substances.
- *A secondary zone of macrophages*, epithelioid cells, or giant cells surrounding the capsule at injury site.
- *An outer zone of fibrotic reparative* or granulation tissue infiltrated with non-granulomatous inflammation and plasma cells.

Phacogenic nongranulomatous uveitis was once referred to as phacotoxic uveitis because it was believed that the inflammation was caused by the release of toxic substances into the anterior chamber after disruption of the lens capsule. However, there is no evidence to support the hypothesis that lens proteins are directly toxic to ocular tissues. Most likely, this type of uveitis, represents a variant of phacoanaphylactic endophthalmitis..

Phacolytic glaucoma results from leakage of proteins through an intact lens capsule and is generally seen in the setting of a hypermature lens. Proteins that leak into the anterior chamber is engulfed by macrophages, which in turn cause blockage of the trabecular meshwork, resulting in the elevation of intraocular pressure, which is characteristic of this entity (Fig. 3.3.6). Retained lens material may elicit an ongoing inflammatory response, with cells and flare in the anterior chamber and posterior synechiae formation.

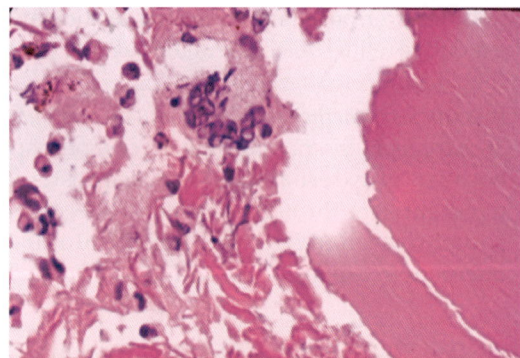

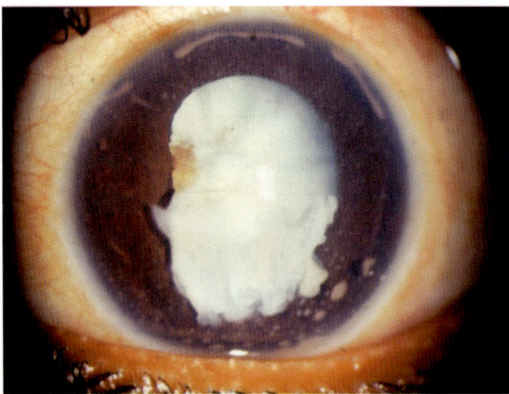

Fig. 3.3.5 *Phacogenic uveitis due to trauma to eye with fingernail.*

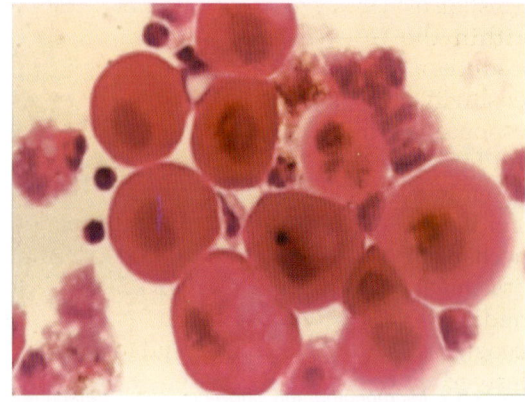

Fig. 3.3.6 *Macrophages with engulfed lens matter in lens-induced uveitis.*

Because lens-associated uveitis almost always occur in a severely traumatized eye, it has been suggested that the disease is initiated in eyes with atypical immunological microenvironment that allows a secondary afferent response to override immunological tolerance. The *effector phase* is believed to be through complement-fixing antibodies specific for crystalline lens, which are either produced locally by B lymphocytes or plasma cells within the eye, or leaked passively from the blood. Generation of anaphylatoxin C5a by complement activating immune complex within lens substances probably explains neutrophilic infiltration. Diffusion of anaphylatoxins into the anterior chamber results in a chemotactic gradient responsible for the zonal pattern.

Activated macrophages also seem to participate, because epithelioid and giant cells that are subsets of activated, differentiated macrophages are classic features. The mechanism for giant cell formation has not been totally resolved, but phagocytosis of immune complexes coated with complement can contribute to macrophage activation and giant cell formation.

TOXOCARA GRANULOMA

Toxocara canis is a nematode parasite that infects up to 2% of chidren worldwide. It may occasionally produce vitreoretinal inflammatory manifestations. The ocular immunology of this is not properly explained. However, animal models can be suggestive of its mechanism. The primary immune response begins in the gut after ingestion of viable eggs, which matures in larvae within the intestine. The primary phase produces a strong T_H^2-mediated delayed hypersensitivity response, leading to primary effector response that includes production of IgM, IgG and IgE antibodies. However, haematogenous dissemination of a few larvae may result from accidental avoidance of immune effector mechanism. This leads to choroidal or retinal dissemination followed by their invasion. A T_H^2-mediated T lymphocyte effector response recognises larval antigen there and release T_H^2-derived cytokines inducing eosinophil and macrophage activation, hence causing the characteristic eosinophilic granuloma in the eye.

In addition, antilarval B lymphocytes can infiltrate the eye and can induce production of IgE immunoglobulins.

RETINAL VASCULITIS IN SYSTEMIC LUPUS ERYTHEMATOSUS

Systemic lupus erythematosus (SLE) is a connective tissue disorder with multisystemic involvement. It primarily affects women of child-bearing age, and patients may have a typical macular rash (Fig. 3.3.7).

Pathogenesis of SLE is unknown. However, it is thought to be an autoimmune disorder characterised by B lymphocyte hyperactivity, polyclonal B lymphocyte activation, hyper-gammaglobulinaemia, autoantibody formation and T lymphocyte autoreactivity with immune complex deposition. All this leads to a stage of end-organ damage. Although rare, retinal vasculitis can develop in patients with SLE. It is suggestive that local immune complex formation plays a key role in its pathogenesis. DNA and histones released from injured cells become entrapped in the basement membrane of blood vessel wall, probably as a result of electrostatic binding by matrix proteins. Circulating cationic anti-DNA IgG autoantibodies permeate into vessel wall, bind the autoantigen and activate

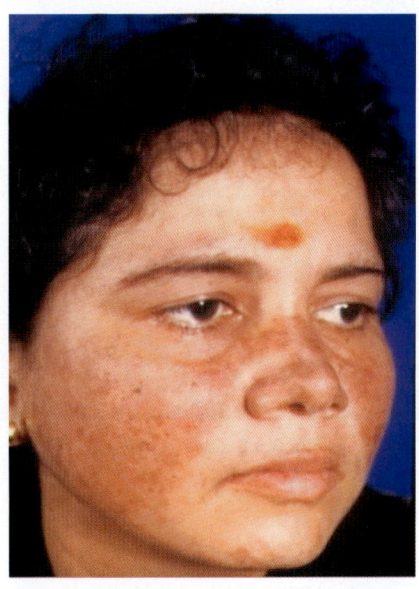

Fig. 3.3.7 *A-30-yr female with typical malar rash of SLE.*

the complement system. These cationic IgG antibodies are thought to have a strong affinity for anionic extracellular matrix and hence permeate tissues efficiently. The vascular sheathing in the retinal vessels is presumed to be caused by infiltration of neutrophils and macrophages in response to complement activation. Helper T cell lymphocyte responses and innate mechanisms may also contribute to its pathogenesis.

CYTOMEGALOVIRUS (CMV) RETINITIS

CMV retinitis (Fig. 3.3.8) is the most common cause of congenital viral infection, with clinical disease occurring among neonates and immunocompromised patients with leukaemia, lymphoma or conditions requiring systemic immunomodulation and also in patients with AIDS. The majority of most populations have serological evidence of prior CMV infection, typically thought to occur during childhood or after contact with infected children.

Pathophysiology of CMV infection is not clearly understood. The upper respiratory tract infection usually initiates primary afferent phase. The site of processing is not known. Innate effectors, like macrophages, natural killer cells and neutrophils, provide some antiviral

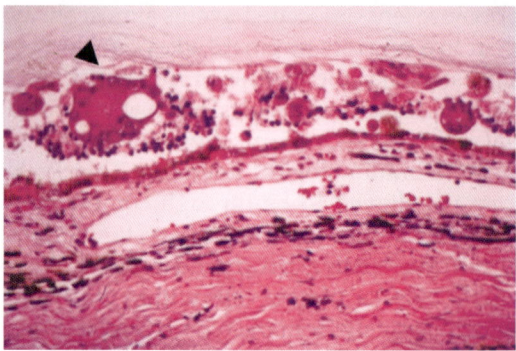
Fig. 3.3.9 *Arrow showing CMV inclusion body.*

activity. Some investigators, however, think that virus specific CD8 T lymphocytes are most important in controlling viral infection. Antibodies seem to limit reinfection.

Virus does not get completely cleared from the infected host during the primary infection, but remains in chronic stage as inclusion bodies (Fig. 3.3.9).

As long as the host immune response is intact, the virus does not replicate effectively to infect eye or other target organs. Immunomodulation allows the virus to reactivate into a productive infection. It infects neutrophils, macrophages and other leucocytes. The virus spreads through the blood to susceptible target sites, such as retina. It is believed that virus-specific CD8 T lymphocytes are the most effector cells in preventing spread. Natural killer cells might also be effective in this. CD4 T lymphocytes provides helper cytokines to fully activate CD8 T lymphocytes.

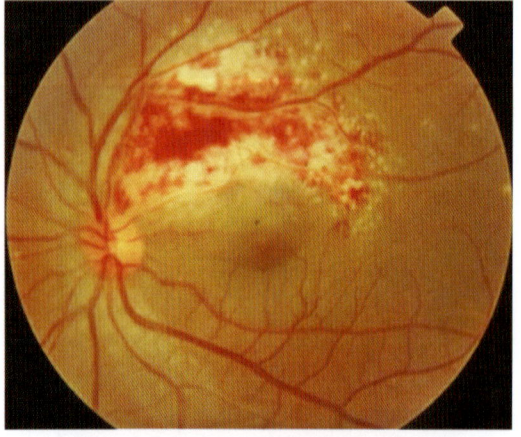
Fig. 3.3.8 *CMV retinitis.*

BIBLIOGRAPHY

1. Biswas J. Pathology of uveitis. Afro-Asian J Ophalmol 1992;9(3):206–209.
2. Biswas J, Krishnakumar S, Ahuja S. Manual of Ocular Pathology; first edition; 2010;52–53;102–103.
3. Myron Y, Ben SF. Ocular Pathology; fifth edition; 69–71.

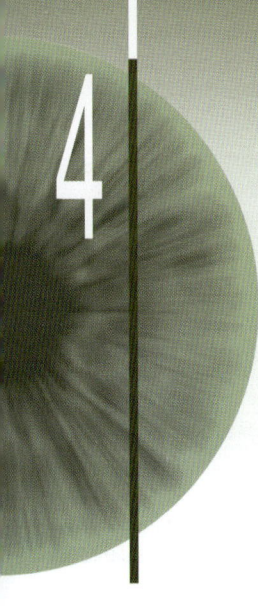

4

CLINICAL PROFILE AND COMPLICATIONS OF UVEITIS: A GENERAL OVERVIEW

4.1 UVEITIS: DEFINITION, CLASSIFICATION AND TERMINOLOGIES

Definition
Classification of uveitis
• Conventional classification
• IUSG classification
• SUN classification
• Etiological classification

DEFINITION

The term uveitis strictly means inflammation of uveal tissue only. However, clinically there is associated inflammation of the adjacent structures, such as retina, vitreous, sclera and cornea. Due to close relationship of the anatomically distinct parts of the uveal tract, the inflammatory process usually tends to involve the uvea as a whole.

CLASSIFICATION OF UVEITIS

Proper classification of uveitic entities is essential to avoid confusion and misinterpretation among ophthalmologists. Many classifications have been proposed for uveitis. Various available classification systems of uveitis are described briefly.

A. CONVENTIONAL CLASSIFICATIONS

I. Anatomical classification

1. *Anterior uveitis.* It is inflammation of the tissue from iris up to pars plicata of ciliary body. It may be subdivided into:
• *Iritis,* in which inflammation predominantely affects the iris,
• *Iridocyclitis* in which iris and pars plicata of ciliary body are equally involved, and
• *Anterior cyclitis,* in which pars plicata of ciliary body is predominantly affected.

2. *Intermediate uveitis.* It includes inflammation of pars plana and peripheral part of retina and underlying choroid. 'It is also called as pars planitis'.

3. *Posterior uveitis.* It refers to inflammation of choroid (choroiditis). Almost always there is associated inflammation of retina hence term 'chorioretinitis' is used.

4. *Panuveitis.* It is inflammation of the whole uvea.

II. Clinical classification

1. *Acute uveitis.* It has got a sudden symptomatic onset and the disease lasts for 3 months or less.

Table 4.1.1: *Difference between granulomatous and non-granulomatous uveitis*

Granulomatous uveitis	Non-granulomatous uveitis
Insidious onset and chronic course	Sudden onset and acute course
Absent or mild congestion	Severe episcleral congestion
Iris nodules (Keoppe's and Bussaca's nodules) are common	Iris nodules are uncommon
Medium to large keratic precipitates (Mutton fat KPs) are seen	Fine, small keratic precipitates are seen
Posterior segment involvement is common	Posterior segment involvement is uncommon

2. Chronic uveitis. It is frequently insidious and asymptomatic in onset. It persists longer than 3 months and is usually diagnosed when it causes defective vision.

3. Recurrent uveitis. This is characterised by repeated episodes separated by periods of inactivity of less than 3 months duration without treatment.

III. Pathological classification

One of the oldest classification of uveitis is *Woods classification* (also known as pathological or clinicopathological classification). This was proposed by Alan Churchill Woods. Uveitis is classified as granulomatous or non-granulomatous on the basis of the predominant clinical characteristics as given in Table 4.1.1.

1. Suppurative or purulent uveitts.

2. Non-suppurative uveits. It has been further subdivided into two group:

- Non-granulomatous uveitis
- Granulomatous uveitis.

B. IUSG CLASSIFICATION

International Uveitis Study Group (IUSG) classification of uveitis was originally devised by the International Uveitis Study Group, accepted at the XXV International Congress of Ophthalmology, and published in 1987. This classification is largely based on the anatomic position of the inflammation within the eye. Though this classification system permits the description of the physical location of the uveitis, it does not attempt to describe the course of the uveitis (Table 4.1.2).

Table 4.1.2: *IUSG classification of uveitis*

Anterior uveitis	Iritis, anterior cyclitis, irido-cyclitis
Intermediate uveitis	Pars planitis, posterior cyclitis, hyalitis, basal retino-choroiditis
Posterior uveitis	Focal, multifocal, or diffuse choroiditis, chorioretinitis, retinochoroiditis, or neuro-uveitis
Panuveitis	

C. STANDARDISATION OF UVEITIS NOMENCLATURE (SUN) CLASSIFICATION

Most recent and widely accepted version of classifying uveitis is the Standardization of Uveitis Nomenclature (SUN) Classification. This classification was proposed in a workshop in Baltimore, Maryland, USA in 2004 under the aegis of International Uveitis Study group to devise a set of uniform criteria for classifying and grading of uveitis. According to SUN classification, uveitis was divided into anterior, intermediate, posterior, and panuveitis according to their primary site of inflammation (Table 4.1.3).

Unlike the previous classification systems of uveitis, SUN classification has addressed various ambiguities of the uveitic nomenclature.

- *A clear consensus was reached to differentiate between pars planitis and intermediate uveitis.* According to SUN classification, the term "pars planitis" should be used only for idiopathic cases of intermediate uveitis that is in clinical entities where there is snowbank or snowball formation in the absence of an associated infection or systemic disease.
- *Panuveitis* term should be used for those situations, in which there is no particular

Table 4.1.3: *SUN classification of uveitis*

Type	Primary site of inflammation	Includes
Anterior uveitis	Anterior chamber	Iritis, iridocyclitis, anterior cyclitis
Intermediate uveitis	Vitreous	Pars planitis, posterior cyclitis, hyalitis
Posterior uveitis	Retina/choroid	Focal, multifocal, diffuse choroiditis chorioretinitis, retinochoroiditis, retinitis, neuroretinitis
Panuveitis	Anterior chamber, vitreous and retina or choroid	Panuveitis

predominant site of inflammation, but inflammation is observed in the anterior chamber, vitreous, and retina and/or choroid and noteworthy that structural complications, such as macular oedema or neovascularisation should not be considered in such cases.

- *Anterior and intermediate uveitis,* respectively, and not the panuveitis term is used, if there is more vitritis than anterior chamber inflammation in an iridocyclitis and more anterior chamber inflammation than vitritis in intermediate uveitis.
- *Retinal vasculitis* term should be used in cases with clinically visible inflammation with vascular changes. Retinal vasculopathy due to hypercoagulable states, etc. should not be considered as retinal vasculitis.

Descriptors of uveitis

Various descriptors for defining onset, duration, and course of uveitis have been proposed in SUN classification (Table 4.1.4).

Terminologies regarding activity of uveitis

Grading of cells and flare was also addressed in SUN classification. While grading cells in anterior chamber in inflammation, 0.5+ was advocated over the term "trace" and separate documentation of the presence or absence of a hypopyon was recommended. Though no consensus could be reached on a standard grading system for vitreous cells. The National Eye Institute system for grading vitreous haze was adopted in this classification. Based on these parameters, terminology regarding activity of a uveitic entity has been depicted (Table 4.1.5).

D. ETIOLOGICAL CLASSIFICATION

I. Infectious uveitis (non-purulent)

1. *Bacterial uveitis*
- Tubercular uveitis
- Laprotic uveitis
- Syphilitic and other spirochetal uveitis
- Syphilitic uveitis
- Lyme disease
- Leptospiral uveitis
- Ocular nocardiasis
- Uveitis in cat-scratch diseases
- Uveitis in Whipple disease
- Rickettsial disease of eye

Table 4.1.4: *SUN classification: Descriptors of uveitis*

Category	Descriptor	Description
Onset	Sudden	Acute onset
	Insidious	Slow onset
Duration	Limited	<3 months duration
	Persistent	>3 months duration
Course	Acute	Episode characterised by sudden onset and limited duration
	Recurrent	Repeated episodes separated by periods of inactivity without treatment <3 months in duration
	Chronic	Persistent uveitis with relapse in <3 months after discontinuing treatment

Table 4.1.5: *SUN classification: Activity of uveitis*

Term	Description
Inactive	Grade 0 cells (anterior uveitis)
Worsening activity	Two-step increase in level of inflammation (e.g. anterior chamber cells, vitreous haze) or increase from grade 3 to 4
Improved activity	Two-step decrease in level of inflammation (e.g. anterior chamber cells, vitreous haze) or decrease to grade 0
Remission	Inactive disease for 3 months after discontinuing all treatments for eye disease

2. *Viral uveitis*
- Herpetic uveitis
- Ocular involvement in AIDS
- Chikungunya uveitis
- Dengue uveitis
- West Nile disease
- Rubella uveitis

3. *Fungal uveitis*

4. *Parasitic uveitis*
- Toxoplasmosis
- Toxocariasis
- Cystecercosis
- Diffuse unilateral subacute neuroretinitis
- Onchocerciasis

II. Non-infectious uveitis

1. *Uveitis in juvenile idiopathic arthritis and systemic rheumatic disease*
- Juvenile idiopathic arthritis
- Systemic rheumatic disease and eye
- Rheumatoid arthritis (RA)
- Systemic lupus erytrematosus (SLE)
- Polyarteritis nodosa (PAN)
- Granulomatosis with polyangitis(GPA), i.e Wegener's granulomatosis)
- Systemic sclerosis (SS)
- Ankylosing spondylitis (AS)

2. *Ocular sacrcoidosis*

3. *Behcet's disease*

4. *Vogt-Koyanagi-Harada syndrome*

5. *Sympathetic ophthalmitis*

6. *Fuch's uveitis syndrome*

7. *Glaucomatocyclitic crisis*

8. *Phacogenic uveitis*
- Phacotoxic uveitis
- Phacoanaphylactic uveitis

9. *Traumatic and postsurgical uveitis*
- Traumatic uveitis
- Postsurgical uveitis
- Toxic anterior segment syndrome (TASS)
- Endophthalmitis

10. *White dot syndromes*
- Birdshot retinochoroidopathy
- Serpiginous choroidopathy
- Acute posterior multifocal placoid pigment epitheliopathy (APMPEE)
- Acute zonal occult outer retinopathy (AZOOR)
- Multiple evanescent white dot syndrome (MEWDS)
- Punctate inner choroidopathy (PIC)
- Acute retinal pigment epitheliopathy (ARPE)
- Acute idiopathic blind spot enlargemnt syndrome (AIBSES) Padmamalini
- Multifocal choroiditis and panuveitis (MCP) syndrome
- Subretinal fibrosis and uveitis (SFU) syndrome

III. Masquerade syndrome
- Non-neoplastic masquerade syndrome
- Neoplastic masquerade syndrome.

BIBLIOGRAPHY

1. Deschenes J, Murray PI, Rao NA, et al. International Uveitis Study Group (IUSG): clinical classification of uveitis. Ocular Immunology and Inflammation 2008;16:1-2.

2. Deschenes J, Murray PI, Rao NA, Nussenblatt RB. International Uveitis Study Group. International Uveitis Study Group (IUSG): clinical classification of uveitis. Ocul Immunol Inflamm 2008;16:1-2.

3. Jabs DA, Nussenblatt RB, Rosenbaum JT. Standardization of uveitis nomenclature for reporting clinical data. Results of the First International Workshop. Am J Ophthalmol 2005; 140(3):509–16.

4. Okada AA, Jabs DA. The standardization of uveitis nomenclature project: the future is here. JAMA Ophthalmol 2013;131(6):787–9.

5. Standardization of uveitis nomenclature for reporting clinical data. Results of the First International Workshop. Am J Ophthalmol 2005; 140:509–516.

6. Trusko B1, Thorne J, Jabs D, Belfort R, Dick A, Gangaputra S, et al. The Standardization of Uveitis Nomenclature (SUN) Project. Development of a clinical evidence base utilizing informatics tools and techniques. Methods Inf Med 2013; 52(3):259–65.

4.2 ANTERIOR UVEITIS

Definition and Etiopathogenesis
Definitions
• SUN classification
Etiopathogenesis
• Comon causes
Clinical Features
• Symptoms
• Signs
• Complication and sequelae
Diagnostic Approach
• Clinical diagnosis
• Investigations
• Differential diagnosis
Treatment of Anterior Uveitis
Non-specific treatment
• Cycloplegic drugs
• Corticosterodis
• NSAIDs
• Immunosuppressive drugs
• Physical measures
Specific treatment
Treatment of complications
• Monitoring the response of treatment

DEFINITION AND ETIOPATHOGENESIS

DEFINITION

Anterior uveitis refers to inflammation of iris and anterior part of ciliary body. It includes iritis, iridocyclitis and anterior cyclitis. The primary site of inflammation is the anterior chamber. It is commoner than posterior segment inflammation and is generally less sight-threatening and less serious, especially if treated early. Anterior uveitis normally causes reduction in the vision during the acute stage but it is the sequelae of anterior uveitis which can have long-lasting impact.

Inflammation confined to the anterior chamber is called *iritis*; if it spills over into the retrolental space, it is called *iridocyclitis*; if it involves the cornea, it is called *keratouveitis*; and if the inflammatory reaction involves the sclera and uveal tract, it is called *sclerouveitis*.

SUN working group definitions are given in Table 4.2.1 and 4.2.2.

ETIOPATHOGENESIS

Etiopathogenesis of uveitis is described in detail in Chapter 3.2.

Common causes of anterior uveitis are (Fig. 4.2.1):
• Idiopathic
• Seronegative HLA-B27-associated arthro-pathies
• Juvenile idiopathic arthritis
• Herpetic uveitis
• Sarcoidosis
• Fuchs' heterochromic iridocyclitis

Table 4.2.1 *SUN classification for anterior uveitis*

Type of uveitis	Site of inflammation	Subtypes
Anterior	Anterior chamber	Iritis Iridocyclitis Anterior cyclitis

Table 4.2.2 *SUN working group classification: Onset, duration and course*

Category	Type	Definition
Onset	Acute	
	Insiduous	
Duration	Limited	≤3 months
	Persistent	>3 months
Course	Acute	Sudden onset with limited duration
	Recurrent	Repeated episodes separated by periods of inactivity without treatment ≥3 months duration
	Chronic	Persistent uveitis with relapse in <3 months after discontinuing treatment

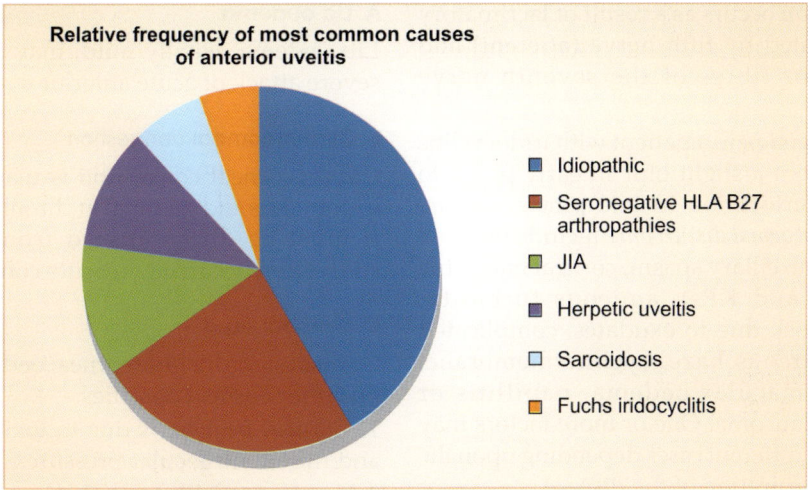

Fig. 4.2.1 *Common causes of anterior uveitis.*

- Intraocular lens-induced persistent uveitis
- Posner-Schlossman syndrome
- Syphilis, tuberculosis, phacogenic uveitis
- Systemic rheumatic diseases, like rheumatoid arthritis, granulomatosis with polyangiitis (Wegener's), polyarteritis nodosa, systemic lupus erythematosus and relapsing polychondritis.

Common causes of chronic anterior uveitis are:
- Tuberculous uveitis
- Sarcoidosis
- Syphilis
- Herpetic uveitis
- Lepromatous uveitis
- Masquerade syndromes

CLINICAL FEATURES

Though anterior uveitis, almost always presents as a combined inflammation of iris and ciliary body (iridocyclitis), the reaction may be more marked in iris (iritis) or ciliary body (cyclitis).

SYMPTOMS

Clinically, it may present as acute or chronic anterior uveitis.

Main symptoms of acute anterior uveitis are pain, photophobia, redness, lacrimation and decreased vision.

In chronic uveitis, however, the eye may be white with minimal symptoms even in the presence of signs of severe inflammation.

Common symptoms of anterior uveitis include:
1. *Pain.* It is dominant symptom of acute anterior uveitis. Patients usually complain of a dull aching throbbing sensation which is typically worse at night. Varying degree of pain in anterior uveitis can be atributed to ciliary muscle spasm. Severe pain can be associated with raised intraocular pressure. The ocular pain is usually referred along the distribution of branches of fifth nerve, especially towards forehead and scalp.
2. *Redness.* It is a feature of acute anterior uveitis and occurs due to circumcorneal congestion, which is result of active hyperaemia of anterior ciliary vessels due to the effect of toxins, histamine and histamine-like substances and axon reflex.
3. *Photophobia* is commonly due to ciliary muscle spasm but anterior chamber cellular infiltration, corneal epithelial oedema and pupillary muscle involvement can also contribute.
4. *Blepharospasm* observed in patients with acute anterior uveitis is due to a reflex between sensory fibres of fifth nerve (which are irritated) and motor fibres of the seventh nerve, supplying the orbicularis oculi muscle.

5. *Lacrimation* occurs as a result of lacrimatory reflex mediated by fifth nerve (afferent) and secretomotor fibres of the seventh nerve (efferent).

6. *Defective vision* in a patient with iridocyclitis may vary from a slight blur in early phase to marked deterioration in late phase. *Factors responsible for visual disturbance* include induced myopia due to ciliary spasm, corneal haze (due to oedema and KPs), aqueous turbidity, pupillary block due to exudates, complicated cataract, vitreous haze, cyclitic membrane, associated macular oedema, papillitis or secondary glaucoma. One or more factors may contribute in different cases depending upon the severity and duration of the disease.

SIGNS

Slit-lamp biomicroscopic examination is essential to elicit most of the signs of uveitis (Fig. 4.2.2).

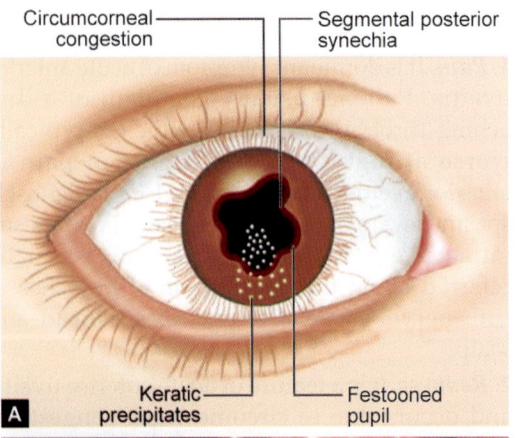

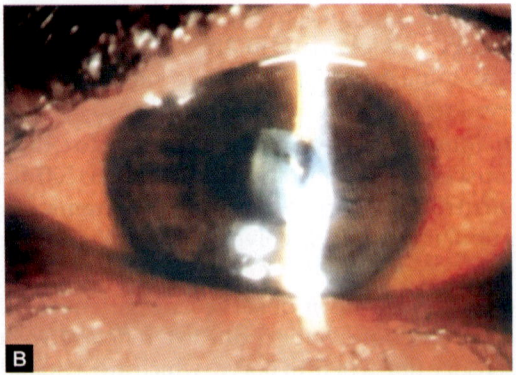

Fig. 4.2.2 *Signs of anterior uveitis: A, Diagrammatic depiction; B, Clinical photograph of a patient with acute anterior uveitis.*

A. Lid oedema

Lid oedema usually mild, may accompany a severe attack of acute anterior uveitis.

B. Circumcorneal congestion

Circumcorneal congestion is marked in acute iridocyclitis and minimal in chronic iridocyclitis. It must be differentiated from superficial congestion occurring in acute conjunctivitis.

C. Corneal signs

Corneal signs include corneal oedema, KPs and posterior corneal opacities.

1. *Corneal oedema* is due to toxic endothelitis and raised intraocular pressure when present.

2. *Keratic precipitates* (KPs) are proteinaceous–cellular deposits occurring at the back of cornea as endothelial dusting. Mostly, these are arranged in a triangular fashion (*Arlt's triangle*) occupying the centre and inferior part of cornea due to convection currents in the aqueous humour (Fig. 4.2.3). The composition and morphology of KPs varies with the severity, duration and type of uveitis. Following types of KPs may be seen:

• *Mutton fat KPs.* These typically occur in granulomatous iridocyclitis and are composed of epithelioid cells and macrophages. They are large, thick, fluffy, lardaceous KPs, having a greasy or waxy appearance. Mutton fat KPs are usually a few (10 to 15) in number (Fig. 4.2.3B).

• *Small and medium KPs* (fine or granular KPs). These are pathognomonic of non-granulomatous uveitis and are composed of lymphocytes. These small, discrete, dirty white KPs are arranged irregularly at the back of cornea. Small KPs may be numerous (Fig. 4.2.3C).

• *Old KPs.* These are sign of healed uveitis. Either of the above described KPs with healing process shrink, fade, become pigmented and irregular in shape (crenated margins). Old mutton fat KPs usually have a ground glass appearance due to hyalinization.

3. *Posterior corneal opacity* may be formed in long-standing cases of iridocyclitis.

D. Anterior chamber signs

1. *Aqueous cells.* It is an early feature of iridocyclitis. The cells should be counted in an

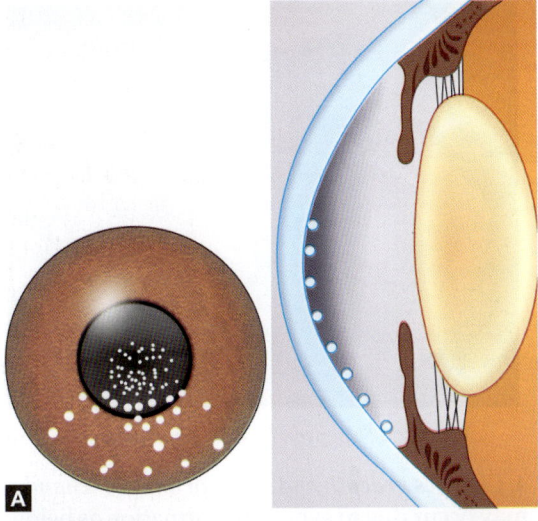

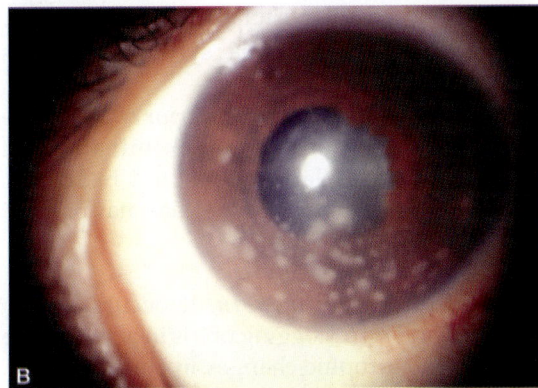

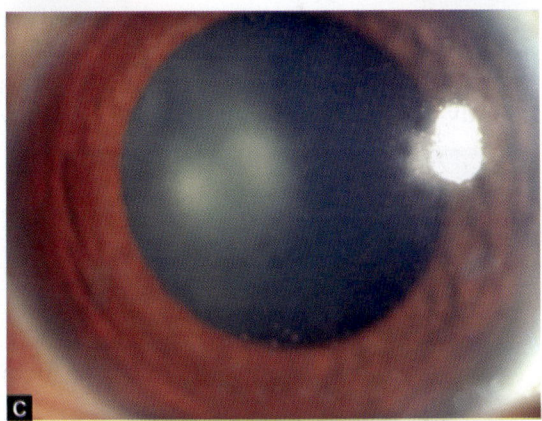

Fig. 4.2.3 *Keratic precipitates (KPs): A, Diagrammatic depiction; B, Clinical photograph of a patient with granulomatous anterior uveitis showing mutton fat KPs and broad segmental synechiae; C, Clinical photograph of a patient with non-granulomatous uveitis showing fine KPs.*

oblique slit-lamp beam, 1 mm long and 1 mm wide, with maximal light intensity and magnification, and graded as per 'Standardization of Uveitis Nomenclature (SUN)' working group as below:

Grade	Cells in field
0	<1
0–0.5	1–5
+ 1	6–15
+ 2	16–25
+ 3	26–50, and
+ 4	>50.

2. *Aqueous flare.* It is due to leakage of protein particles into the aqueous humour from damaged blood vessels. It is demonstrated on the slit-lamp examination by a point beam of light passed obliquely to the plane of iris (Fig. 4.2.4). In the beam of light, protein particles are seen as suspended and moving dust particles. This is based on the 'Brownian movements' or 'Tyndall phenomenon'. Aqueous flare is usually marked in non-granulomatous and minimal in granulomatous uveitis. The flare is graded from 0 to +4. Grade as per *SUN working group grading scheme*:

Grade	Description
0	None
+ 1	Faint, i.e. just detectable.
+2	Moderate (iris and lens details clear)
+3	Marked (iris and lens details hazy).
+4	Intense flare (fibrinous or plastic aqueous) (Fig. 4.2.4C).

3. *Hypopyon.* When exudates are heavy and thick, they settle down in lower part of the anterior chamber as hypopyon (sterile pus in the anterior chamber) (Fig. 4.2.5).

- *Dense immobile hypopyon,* slow to absorb due to high fibrin content, is seen in HLA-B27 acute anterior uveitis.

- *Hypopyon* in Behcet's syndrome has minimal fibrin and, therefore, shifts with the head position and is quick to absorb.

- *Haemorrhagic* hypopyon is a feature of uveitis associated with herpetic infection, trauma and rubeosis iridis.

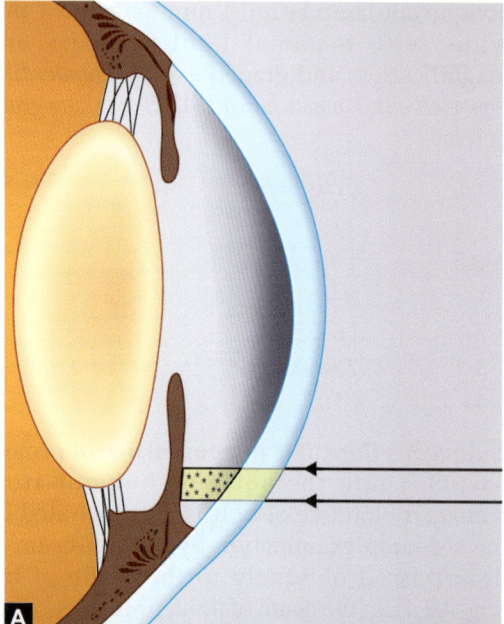

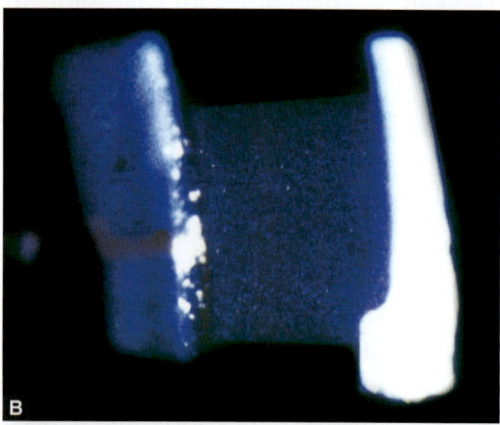

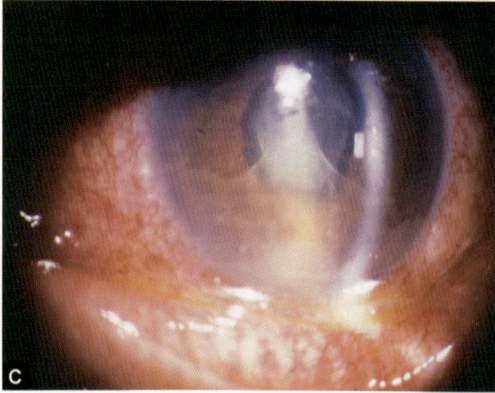

Fig. 4.2.4 *Aqueous flare: A, Diagrammatic depiction; B, Clinical photograph of the patient with aqueous flare; C, Fibrin in anterior chamber.*

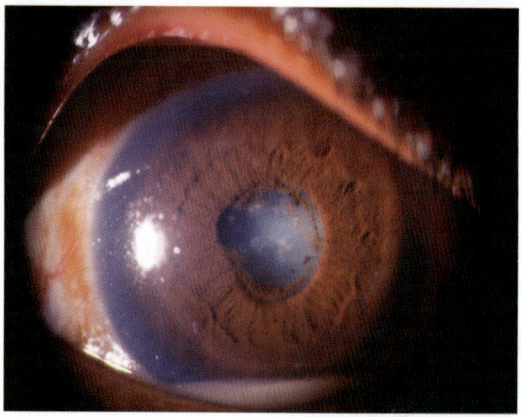

Fig. 4.2.5 *Hypopyon in acute anterior uveitis.*

4. *Changes in depth and shape of anterior chamber* may occur due to synechiae formation as below:
- Deep and irregular in total posterior synechiae.
- Funnel-shaped in annular synechiae with iris bombe formation.

5. *Changes in the angle of anterior chamber* are observed with gonioscopic examination. In active stage, cellular deposits and in chronic stage peripheral anterior synechiae may be seen.

E. Iris signs

1. *Loss of normal pattern.* It occurs due to oedema and waterlogging of iris in active phase and due to atrophic changes in chronic phase. Iris atrophy is typically observed in Fuch's heterochromic iridocyclitis and in herpes zoster iritis (Fig. 4.2.6).

2. *Changes in iris colour.* Iris usually becomes muddy in colour during active phase and may

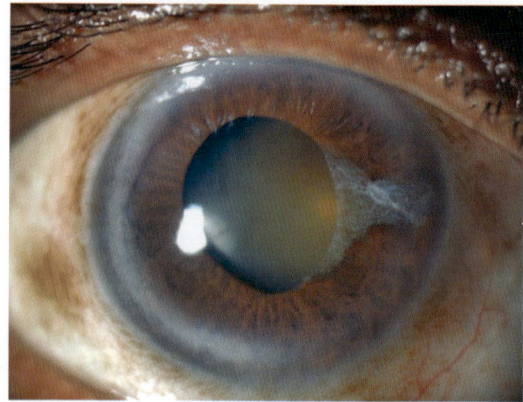

Fig. 4.2.6 *Iris atrophy in a patient with herpes zoster ophthalmicus.*

show hyperpigmented and depigmented areas in healed stage.

3. *Iris nodules* (Fig. 4.2.7). These occur typically in granulomatous uveitis.

- *Koeppe's nodules* are situated at the pupillary border and may initiate posterior synechia (Fig. 4.2.7A).
- *Busacca's nodules* situated near the collarette are large but less common than the Koeppe's nodules (Fig. 4.2.7B).

4. *Posterior synechiae*. These are adhesions between the posterior surface of iris and anterior capsule of crystalline lens (or any other structure which may be artificial lens, after cataract, posterior capsule left after extracapsular cataract extraction) or anterior hyaloid face. These are formed due to organisation of the fibrin-rich exudates. Morphologically, posterior synechiae may be segmental, annular or total.

- *Segmental posterior synechiae* refer to adhesion of iris to the lens at some points (Fig. 4.2.2).
- *Annular posterior synechiae* (ring synechiae) are 360° adhesions of pupillary margin to anterior capsule of lens. These prevent the circulation of aqueous humour from posterior chamber to anterior chamber (*seclusiopupillae*). Thus, aqueous collects behind the iris and pushes it anteriorly (leading to '*iris-bombe*' formation) (Fig. 4.2.8). This is usually followed by a rise in intraocular pressure.
- *Total posterior synechiae* due to plastering of total posterior surface of iris with the anterior capsule of lens are rarely formed in acute plastic type of uveitis. This results in deepening of anterior chamber (Fig. 4.2.9).

5. *Neovascularisation of iris* (rubeosis iridis) develops in some eyes with chronic iridocyclitis and in Fuchs' heterochromic iridocyclitis.

F. Changes in Pupil

1. *Narrow pupil*. It occurs in acute attack of iridocyclitis due to irritation of sphincter pupillae by toxins (Fig. 4.2.2B). Iris oedema and engorged radial vessels of iris also contribute in making the pupil narrow.

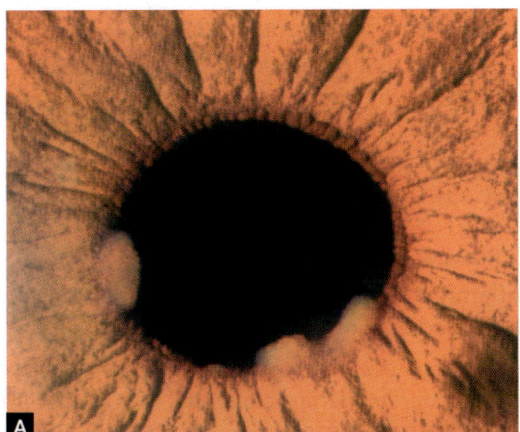
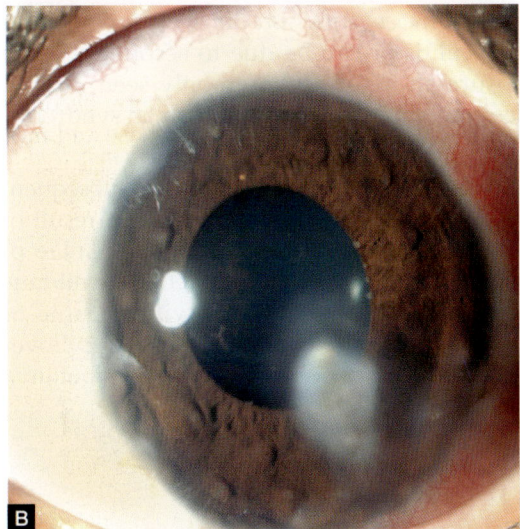

Fig. 4.2.7 *Iris nodules: A, Clinical photograph showing Koeppe's nodules at the pupillary margins in a patient with sarcoidosis; B, Busacca's nodules near collarette.*

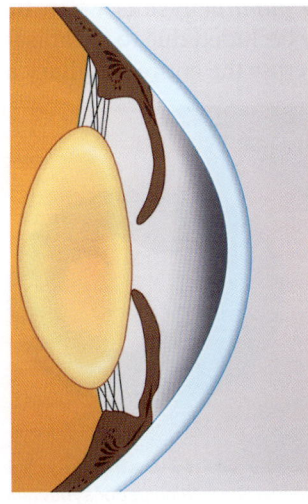

Fig. 4.2.8 *Annular posterior synechiae.*

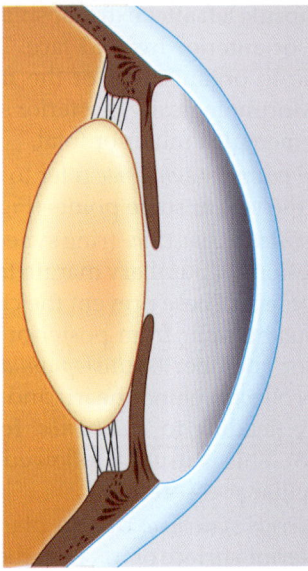

Fig. 4.2.9 *Total posterior synechiae causing deep anterior chamber.*

2. Irregular pupil shape. It results from segmental posterior synechiae formation. Dilatation of pupil with mydriatics (e.g. atropine) at this stage results in *festooned pupil* (Figs 4.2.2A and 4.2.10).
3. Ectropion pupillae (eversion of pupillary margin). It may develop due to contraction of fibrinous exudate on the anterior surface of the iris.
4. Pupillary reaction becomes sluggish or may even be absent due to oedema and hyperaemia of iris which hamper its movements.
5. Occlusio pupillae results when the pupil is completely occluded due to organisation of the exudates across the entire pupillary area.

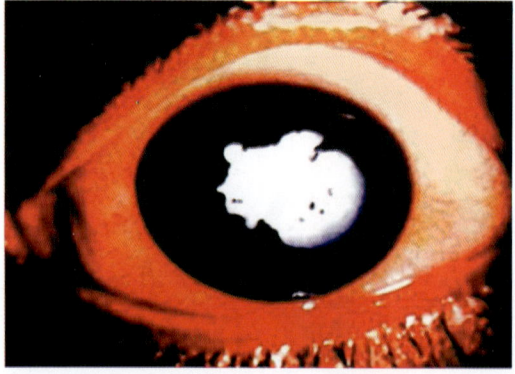

Fig. 4.2.10 *Iridocyclitis with posterior synechiae, festooned pupil and complicated cataract.*

G. Changes in the lens

1. Pigment dispersal on the anterior capsule of lens is almost of universal occurrence in case of anterior uveitis.
2. Exudates may be deposited on the lens in cases with acute plastic iridocyclitis.
3. Complicated cataract may develop as a complication of persistent iridocyclitis. Typical features of a complicated cataract in early stage are *'polychromatic luster'* and *'bread-crumb'* appearance of the early posterior subcapsular opacities. In the presence of posterior synechiae, the complicated cataract progresses rapidly to maturity (Fig. 4.2.10).

H. Changes in the vitreous and retina

1. Exudates and inflammatory cells may be seen in the anterior vitreous after an attack of acute iridocyclitis.
2. Cystoid macular oedema (CME) may occur, specially in chronic iridocyclitis.

I. Changes in the intraocular pressure

Inflammation can result in either increased or decreased intraocular pressure.

Acute attack of anterior uveitis with severe anterior chamber inflammation can lead to increase in intraocular pressure.

Raised intraocular pressure can be due to associated trabeculitis or can be due to secondary angle closure and is most commonly seen in viral keratouveitis or Posner-Schlossman syndrome.

Severe inflammation of the ciliary body may lead to decreased aqueous production and subsequent fall in intraocular pressure may be a result of the inflammation itself, or the sequelae of inflammation. Presence of cyclitic membrane over ciliary body in cases with chronic or recurrent intermediate uveitis with spillover anterior uveitis also leads to severe hypotony.

Uveitis with elevated IOP include:
• Posner-Schlossman syndrome
• Herpetic uveitis
• Toxoplasmosis
• Fuchs' heterochromic iridocyclitis
• Sarcoidosis

- Iridocyclitis with secondary angle closure glaucoma
- Secondary to treatment with steroids.

COMPLICATIONS AND SEQUELAE

1. *Complicated cataract.* It is a common complication of iridocyclitis as described above (Fig. 4.2.10).

2. *Secondary glaucoma.* It may occur as an early or late complication of iridocyclitis.

- *Early glaucoma.* In active phase of the disease, presence of exudates and inflammatory cells in the anterior chamber may cause clogging of trabecular meshwork resulting in the decreased aqueous drainage and thus a rise in intraocular pressure (*hypertensive uveitis*).

- *Late glaucoma in iridocyclitis* (post-inflammatory glaucoma) is the result of pupil block (seclusio pupillae due to ring synechiae formation, or occlusio pupillae due to organised exudates) not allowing the aqueous to flow from posterior to anterior chamber. There may or may not be associated peripheral anterior synechiae formation.

3. *Cyclitic membrane.* It results due to organisation of exudates present behind the lens. It is a late complication of acute plastic type of iridocyclitis.

4. *Retinal complications.* These include cystoid-macular oedema, macular scar, macular hole, epiretinal membrane, exudative retinal detachment, secondary periphlebitis retinae, retinal scars and subretinal fibrosis.

5. *Band-shaped keratopathy.* It (Fig. 4.2.11) occurs as a complication of long-standing chronic uveitis, especially in children having Still's disease.

6. *Phthisis bulbi.* It is the final stage end result of any form of chronic uveitis in which the eye becomes soft, shrinks and atrophic.

DIAGNOSTIC APPROACH

Detailed systematic approach to a patient with anterior uveitis will comprise the following approach:

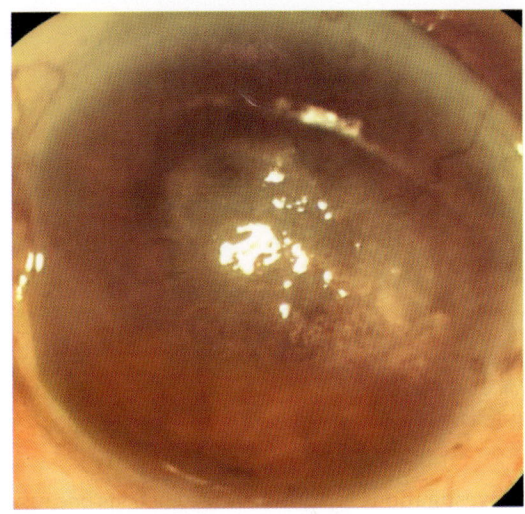

Fig. 4.2.11 *Band-shaped keratopathy.*

I. CLINICAL DIAGNOSIS

1. *Detailed history:* Uveitis work up starts with an elaborate history-taking. It is estimated that over 70% of diagnosis can be made on the basis of detailed medical history and meticulous clinical work up alone. Apart from a review of systems, the social history for pets, dietary history, sexual and drug history should be obtained in detail.

Certain demographic parameters can give a clue to etiology (Table 4.2.3).

2. *Ocular examination:* Careful examination of both the anterior and posterior segments is of utmost importance. The presence of corneal involvement in the form of keratitis or scleritis should be noted, since sometimes anterior chamber inflammation may be secondary to these conditions.

3. *Physical examination:* Anterior uveitis can be associated with dermatological, respiratory, rheumatologic, genital, gastrointestinal or neurological findings.

Note. Clinical approach for a case of uveitis is described in detail in Chapter 5.1.

II. INVESTIGATIONS

Before ordering investigations, a thorough *ocular* and *systemic examination*, as mentioned above, is required, which may provide clues to the underline disease.

Table 4.2.3 *Demographic parameter clue to etiology*

Parameters	Findings	Etiology
Age	Children	JIA, toxoplasmosis
	Young adults	Fuchs' heterochromic iridocyclitis, HLA B27 uveitis
	Old age	Herpetic uveitis, polyarteritis nodosa.
Gender	Male	HLA B27 associated uveitis, Reiter's syndrome, Behcet's disease.
	Female	Rheumatoid arthritis, JRA.
Race	Caucasians	Reiter's, ankylosing spondylitis.
	Blacks	Sarcoidosis
	Orientals	VKH.

Unilateral: Fuchs' uveitis, herpes zoster ophthalmicus, lens-induced uveitis.
Bilateral: Juvenile rheumatoid arthritis.

Investigations include a battery of tests because of its varied etiology. However, an experienced ophthalmologist soon learns to order a few investigations of considerable value, which will differ in individual case depending upon the information gained from a thorough clinical work up. Investigations in uveitis are described in detail in Chapter 5.2. However, a few common investigations required are mentioned here:

1. *Haematological investigations*
- *TLC and DLC* to have a general information about inflammatory response of body.
- *ESR* to ascertain existence of any chronic inflammatory condition in the body.
- *Blood sugar levels* to rule out diabetes mellitus.
- *Blood uric acid* in patients suspected of having gout.
- *Serological tests* for syphilis, toxoplasmosis and histoplasmosis.
- *Tests* for antinuclear antibodies, Rh factor, LE cells, C-reactive proteins antistreptolysin-0, ACE (for sarcoidosis).

2. *Urine examination* for WBCs, pus cells, RBCs and culture to rule out urinary tract infections.
3. *Stool examination* for cyst and ova to rule out parasitic infestations.
4. *Radiological investigations* include:
- *X-rays* of chest, paranasal sinuses, sacroiliac joints and lumbar spine.
- *CT scan* high resolution. CT scan of thorax should be considered for suspected sarcoidosis cases.
- *MRI scan* of head for suspected sarcoidosis, demyelination and lymphomas.

5. *Skin tests.* These include tuberculin test, Kveim's test for sarcoidosis, toxoplasmin test, lepromin test and pathergy test for Behcet's disease.

III. DIFFERENTIAL DIAGNOSIS

1. *Acute red eye.* Acute iridocyclitis must be differentiated from other causes of acute red eye, especially acute congestive glaucoma and acute conjunctivitis. The differentiating features are summarised in Table 4.2.4.

2. *Granulomatous versus nongranulomatous uveitis.* Once diagnosis of iridocyclitis is established, an attempt should be made to know whether the condition is of granulomatous or non-granulomatous type. The main clinical differences between the two are summarised in Table 4.2.5.

3. *Etiological differential diagnosis.* Efforts should also be made to distinguish between the different etiological varieties of iridocyclitis. This may be possible in some cases after thorough investigations and with a knowledge of special features of different clinical entities, which are described in respective chapters.

TREATMENT OF ANTERIOR UVEITIS

General goals of management of uveitis are:
- Relief of pain and photophobia
- Elimination of inflammation
- Prevention of structural complications such as synechiae, secondary cataract and glaucoma

Table 4.2.4 *Distinguishing features between acute conjunctivitis, acute iridocyclitis and acute congestive glaucoma*

	Feature	Acute conjunctivitis	Acute iridocyclitis	Acute congestive glaucoma
1.	Onset	Gradual	Usually gradual	Sudden
2.	Pain	Mild discomfort	Moderate in eye and along the first division of trigeminal nerve	Severe in eye and the entire trigeminal area
3.	Discharge	Mucopurulent	Watery	Watery
4.	Coloured halos	May be present	Absent	Present
5.	Vision	Good	Slightly impaired	Markedly impaired
6.	Congestion	Superficial conjunctival	Deep ciliary	Deep ciliary
7.	Tenderness	Absent	Marked	Marked
8.	Pupil	Normal	Small and irregular	Large and vertically oval
9.	Media	Clear	Hazy due to KPs, aqueous flare and pupillary exudates	Hazy due to oedematous cornea
10.	Anterior chamber	Normal	May be deep	Very shallow
11.	Iris	Normal	Muddy	Oedematous
12.	Intraocular pressure	Normal	Usually normal	Raised
13.	Constitutional symptoms	Absent	Little	Prostration and vomiting

Table 4.2.5 *Differences between granulomatous and nongranulomatous uveitis*

	Feature	Granulomatous	Nongranulomatous
1.	Onset	Insidious	Acute
2.	Pain	Minimal	Marked
3.	Photophobia	Slight	Marked
4.	Ciliary congestion	Minimal	Marked
5.	Keratic precipitates (KPs)	Mutton fat	Small
6.	Aqueous flare	Mild	Marked
7.	Iris nodules	Usually present	Absent
8.	Posterior synechiae	Thick and broad based	Thin and tenuous
9.	Fundus	Nodular lesions	Diffuse involvement

- Preservation or restoration of good visual function.

Principles of treatment in anterior uveitis are summarized in Fig. 4.2.12.

Detailed medical and surgical management are described in chapters 5.4 and 5.5, respectively.

Outlines of management of anterior uveitis are summarised below.

I. NONSPECIFIC TREATMENT

1. Cycloplegic drugs

Cycloplegic drugs are very useful and most effective during acute phase of iridocyclitis.

- Commonly used drug is 1% *atropine sulphate* eye ointment or drops instilled 2–3 times a day.

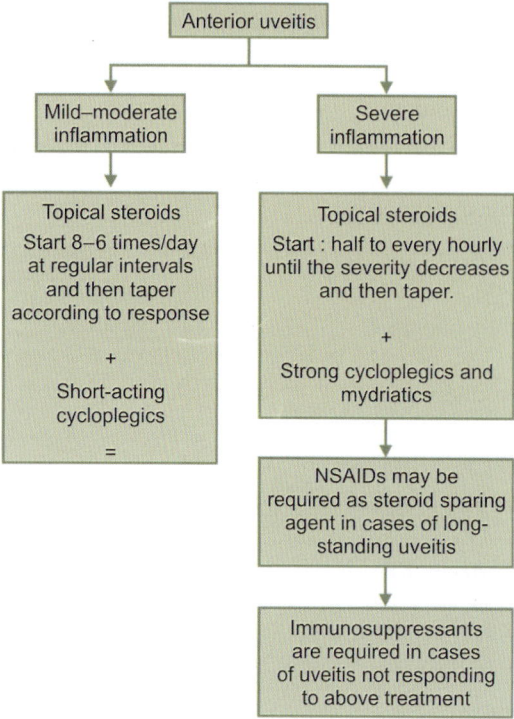

Fig. 4.2.12 *Treatment principles in anterior uveitis.*

- In case of atropine allergy, other cycloplegics like 2% *homatropine* or 1% *cyclopentolate* eye-drops may be instilled 3–4 times a day.
- Alternatively for more powerful cycloplegic effect, a subconjunctival injection of 0.25 ml in *mydricain* (a mixture of atropine, adrenaline and procaine) should be given.
- Cycloplegics should be continued for at least 2–3 weeks after the eye becomes quiet, otherwise relapse may occur.

Mode of action. In iridocyclitis, cycloplegic drugs out by following modes:

- Give comfort and rest to the eye by relieving spasm of iris sphincter and ciliary muscle,
- Prevent the formation of synechiae and may break the already formed synechiae,
- Reduce exudation by decreasing hyperaemia and vascular permeability, and
- Increase the blood supply to anterior uvea by relieving pressure on the anterior ciliary arteries. As a result, more antibodies reach the target tissues and more toxins are absorbed.

2. Corticosteroids

Topical steroids

Topical steroids are very effective in cases of iridocyclitis.

Mode of action. They reduce inflammation by their anti-inflammatory effect, allergic effect, and due to their antifibrotic activity, they reduce fibrosis and thus prevent disorganisation and destruction of the tissues.

- *Commonly used steroidal preparations* contain dexamethasone, betamethasone, hydrocortisone or prednisolone. The choice of topical steroid should be based on the severity of uveitis; in cases with severe AC reaction, topical steroid with strong potency, such as prednisolone acetate should be preferred whereas in cases with mild anterior uveitis, weak topical steroid, like flurometholone acetate can be used. In steroid responders, one should try and avoid steroid as far as possible and can use topical non-steroidal anti-inflammatory drugs (NSAIDs), like flurbiprofen or weak steroids or steroids with least propensity to raise IOP, such as rimexolone 1%. Periocular steroids may be required when there is associated posterior uveitis.

Route of administration. Locally, steroids are used as:
- Eyedrops 4–6 times a day
- Eye ointment at bedtime, and
- Anterior sub-Tenon injection is given in severe cases.

Systemic corticosteroids

When administered systemically they have a definite role in non-granulomatous iridocyclitis, where inflammation, most of the times, is due to antigen–antibody reaction. Even in other types of uveitis, the systemic steroids are helpful due to their potent nonspecific anti-inflammatory and antifibrotic effects.

Indications of systemic steroids in anterior uveitis:
- Anterior uveitis resistant to topical therapy
- Recurrent and bilateral anterior uveitis
- Occasionally prior to surgery
- Posterior/intermediate uveitis associated with spillover anterior uveitis.

Dosage schedules. A wide variety of steroids are available. Usually, treatment is started with high doses of prednisolone (60–100 mg) or equivalent quantities of other steroids (dexamethasone or betamethasone).

- *Daily therapy regime* is preferred for marked inflammatory activity for at least 2 weeks.
- In the absence of acute disease, *alternate day therapy regime* should be chosen.
- *Dose of steroids is decreased* by a week's interval and tapered completely in about 6–8 weeks in both the regimes.

Note. Steroids (both topical and systemic) may cause many ocular (e.g. steroid-induced glaucoma and cataract) and systemic side effects. Hence, an eagle's eye watchfulness is required for it.

3. Non-steroidal anti-inflammatory drugs (NSAIDs)

Non-steroidal anti-inflammatory drugs, such as aspirin, can be used where steroids are contra-indicated. Phenylbutazone and oxyphenbutazone are potent anti-inflammatory drugs of particular value in uveitis associated with rheumatoid disease. Naproxen is useful in patients with ankylosing spondylitis.

4. Immunosuppressive drugs

These should be used only in desperate and extremely serious cases of uveitis, in which vigorous use of steroids have failed to resolve the inflammation and there is an imminent danger of blindness.

- *These drugs are dangerous* and should be used with great caution in the supervision of a haematologist and an oncologist.
- *These drugs are specially useful* in severe cases of Behcet's syndrome, sympathetic ophthalmia, pars planitis and VKH syndrome.
- *A few available cytotoxic immunosuppressive drugs* include cyclophosphamide, chlorambucil, azathioprine and methotrexate.
- *Cyclosporine* is a powerful anti-T cell immuno-suppressive drug which is effective in cases resistant to cytotoxic immunosuppressive agents, but it is a highly renal toxic drug.

5. Physical measures

Dark goggles. These give a feeling of comfort, especially when used in sunlight, by reducing photophobia, lacrimation and blepharospasm.

II. SPECIFIC TREATMENT

Non-specific treatment described above is very effective and usually controls the uveal inflam-mation in most of the cases, but it does not cure the disease, resulting in relapses. Therefore, all possible efforts should be made to find out and treat the underlying cause. Unfortunately, in spite of the advanced diagnostic tests, still it is not possible to ascertain the cause in a large number of cases.

- Course of antitubercular drugs for underlying Koch's disease.
- Adequate treatment for syphilis, when detected should be carried out.
- When no cause is ascertained, a full course of broad-spectrum antibiotics may be helpful by eradicating some masked focus of infection in patients with non-granulomatous uveitis.
- Azithromycin or tetracycline or erythromycin should be considered to treat chlamydial infection in patients and their sexual partners with Reiter's syndrome having urethritis and iritis.

III. TREATMENT OF COMPLICATIONS

1. *Inflammatory glaucoma* (hypertensive uveitis). In such cases, drugs to lower intraocular pressure, such as 0.5% timolol maleate eyedrops twice a day and tablet acetazolamide (250 mg thrice a day) should be added, over and above the usual treatment of iridocyclitis. Pilocarpine and latanoprost eyedrops are contraindicated in inflammatory glaucoma.

2. *Postinflammatory glaucoma* due to ring synechiae is treated by laser iridotomy. Surgical iridectomy may be done when laser is not available. However, surgery should be performed in a quiet eye under high doses of corticosteroids.

3. *Complicated cataract* requires lens extraction with guarded prognosis in spite of all precautions. Presence of fresh KPs is considered a contraindication for intraocular surgery.

4. Retinal detachment of exudative type usually settles itself, if uveitis is treated aggressively. A tractional detachment requires vitrectomy and management of complicated retinal detachment, with poor visual prognosis.

5. Phthisis bulbi especially when painful, requires removal by enucleation operation.

MONITORING THE RESPONSE OF TREATMENT

Monitoring the response to treatment is an utmost important part of treatment and should include visual acuity and grading of cells and flare. The schedule of follow-up should depend on the severity of initial inflammation, potential for sequelae and type of therapy instilled. Patients should be carefully monitored for side-effects of corticosteroids and immuno-suppressives. Once the patient's condition has stabilized, follow-up should be every one to six months. The longer the eye is quiet, the longer can be the interval between follow-up visits.

BIBLIOGRAPHY

1. Abrams J, Schlaegel TF. The tuberculin skin test in the diagnosis of tuberculous uveitis. Am J Ophthalmol 1983;96:295-8.

2. Chang JH, McCluskey PJ, Wakefield D. Acute anterior uveitis and HLA-B27. Surv Ophthalmol. 2005;50:364-88.

3. Cunningham ET, Nozik RA. Uveitis: Diagnostic approach and ancillary analysis. In: Duane's Clinical Ophthalmology, Vol 37. Philadelphia: Lippincott-Raven: 1997, pp 1-25

4. de Groot-Mijnes JD, de Visser L, Rothova A, et al. Rubella virus is associated with Fuch's heterochromic iridocyclitis. Am J Ophthalmol 2006;141:212-4.

5. Goda C, Kotake S, Ichiishi A, et al. Clinical features in tubulointerstitial nephritis and uveitis (TINU) syndrome. Am J Ophthalmol. 2005;140:637-41.

6. Hogan MJ, Kimura SJ, Thygeson P. Signs and symptoms of uveitis. Am J Ophthalmol 1959; 47:155-70.

7. Kanski JJ. Juvenile arthritis and uveitis. Surv Ophthamol 1990;34:253-267.

8. Moorthy RS, Valluri S, Jampol LM. Drug-induced uveitis. SurvOphthalmol. 1998;42:557-70.

9. Myers TD, Smith JR, Lauer AK, Rosenbaum JT. Iris nodules associated with infectious uveitis. Br J Ophthalmol 2002;86:969-74.

10. Pavesio CE, Nozik RA. Anterior and intermediate uveitis. Int Ophthalmol Clin 1990; 30:244-51.

11. Rajaraman RT, kimura Y, Li S, et al. Retrospective case review of pediatric patients with uveitis treated with infliximab. Ophthalmology 2006; 113:308-314.

12. Rauz S, Stavrou P, Murray PI. Evaluation of foldable intraocular lenses in patients with uveitis. Ophthalmology 2000;107:909-19.

13. Ravalico G, Baccara F, Lovisato A, et al. Post-operative cellular reaction on various intraocular lens materials. Ophthalmology 1997; 104:1084-91.

14. Rosenbaum JT, Wernick R. Selection and interpretation of laboratory tests for patients with uveitis. Int Ophthalmol Clin 1990;30:238-43.

15. Smith RE, Nozik RA. Uveitis: A clinical approach to diagnosis and management, Baltimore, Williams and Wilkins: 1989: Ed 2.

16. Weinreb RN, Tessler H. Laboratory diagnosis of ophthalmic sarcoidosis. SurvOphthalmol 1984;28:653-64.

4.3 INTERMEDIATE UVEITIS

Introduction
- Historical prespective
- Definition

Etiopathogenesis and Pathology
- Idiopathic
- Systemic associations
- Pathology

Epidemiology and Clinical Profile
Epidemiology
Clinical profile
- Symptoms
- Signs
- Course, prognosis and complications

Diagnosis
- Clinical diagnosis
- Differential diagnosis
- Investigations

Treatment
- Kaplan approach
- Modified Kaplan approach

INTRODUCTION

Historical perspective

The disease has been variously named since its identification:
- *Cyclitis* by Fuch in 1908
- *Peripheral uveitis* by Schepen in 1950
- *Parsplanitis* by Welsh et al in 1960
- *Intermediate uveitis* by IUSG in 1987

Definition

Intermediate uveitis (IU) is characterized by ocular inflammation localized in the anterior vitreous and the vitreous base overlying the ciliary body and peripheral retina which is otherwise called pars plana.

The IUSG (International Uveitis Study Group) suggested following terms:

Intermediate uveitis to denote an idiopathic inflammatory syndrome, mainly involving the anterior vitreous, peripheral retina and the ciliary body with minimal or no anterior segment or chorioretinal signs.[1]

Pars planitis diagnostic term should be used only for that subset of intermediate uveitis where there is snow bank or snowball formation occurring in the absence of an associated infection or systemic disease. If there is an associated infection (e.g. Lyme disease) or systemic disease (e.g. sarcoidosis), then the term intermediate uveitis should be used.[2]

ETIOPATHOGENESIS AND PATHOLOGY

ETIOPATHOGENESIS

Idiopathic

Idiopathic, i.e. exact cause is unknown in 85% of cases.

Immunogenic predisposition is denoted by:
- Cell-mediated immunity
- Preponderance of T helper cells
- Increased sensitivity to retinal S-antigen
- Decreased level of complement C3
- Raised ICAM-1 and soluble IL-2 receptor
- Elevated level of novel protein (P36)
- HLA assossiation—A 28, DR 15

Systemic associations

Known causes or systemic associations, reported in 15% cases, include:
- *Infections.* Tuberculosis, syphilis, Lyme disease, cat scratch disease, hepatitis C.
- *Non-infectious disorders.* Sarcoidosis, multiple sclerosis, intraocular lymphoma, TINU syndrome.

PATHOLOGY

Peripheral snow bank in pars planitis shows exudates deposited on the peripheral retina and pars plana. Histological examination of this reveals a collapsed vitreous, blood vessels, fibroglial cells including fibrous astrocytes, and scattered inflammatory cells, mostly lymphocytes. Peripheral veins show lymphocytic cuffing and infiltration.[8]

EPIDEMIOLOGY AND CLINICAL PROFILE

EPIDEMIOLOGY

Prevalence of IU varies in different populations accounts for 2–31% of all uveitis presenting to tertiary eye centres in various parts of the world.

Age. It is predominantly seen in the third and fourth decade, though the disease affects patients in all age groups.[4,5]

Bilaterality is seen in 70–90% in the Western studies[5] and is 37.6% in a South India-based study.[4]

Gender. No definite gender predilection was seen. IU is not hereditary though it has been observed in families.

Human leucocyte antigen (HLA). Studies have shown common HLA haplotypes in a few families.[6] HLA-DR15-positivity and IU association is seen in multiple sclerosis, optic neuritis, and narcolepsy. IU accounts for 10–12% of all uveitis seen in children.

CLINICAL PROFILE
Symptoms

Asymptomatic. Patients with IU have very few complaints initially.

Mild symptoms. There may be mild blurring of vision, floaters and rarely, mild photophobia. In IU, unlike other uveitis conditions, the eye is white and quiet, rarely becoming red and painful. There is no gross diminution of vision at the initial stages. The benign nature of the disease can result in postponement of the patient's visit to the ophthalmologist. Patients typically complain of seeing floaters. Impairment of central vision in the initial stages is usually mild and mainly occurs due to cystoid macular oedema or early cataractous changes.

Severe vision loss can occur in the late stages due to chronic cystoid macular oedema, retinal detachment, complicated cataract and uveitic glaucoma.

Signs
Anterior segment signs

Most adult patients of IU have minimal anterior chamber inflammation. Intermediate uveitis associated with tuberculosis and sarcoidosis has mutton-fat keratic precipitates. Children otherwise develop anterior chamber reaction along with band-shaped keratopathy and posterior synechae. Occasionally, some patients may develop significant anterior chamber reaction with pain and photophobia and only later develop signs typical of intermediate uveitis.

Posterior segment signs

Vitritis is the hallmark of IU and is graded from trace to 4+. Cells are always present in vitreous in active IU. Absence of vitreous cellular activity precludes the diagnosis of active IU.

Snow or cotton ball opacities (Ant's egg). Inflammatory cells aggregate in vitreous are called snowballs (Fig. 4.3.1), some of which may coalesce.

Snow banking. Accumulation of yellow-grey exudates at the ora serrata with or without membrane formation is the characteristic feature of a subset of IU called pars planitis. Snowbanks are exudates on the pars plana, when present are usually found inferiorly, but may also extend 360 degrees of the retinal periphery (Fig. 4.3.2).

Snowbanking is usually associated with the more severe form of the disease, and warrants aggressive therapy. Not all patients with IU have snowbanks and its presence is not an absolute requirement for diagnosis of IU. Presence of snowbanks should guide one to look for associated neovascularisation because these areas are a source of potential vitreous haemorrhage.

Retinal changes in IU include tortuosity in arterioles and venules, sheathing of peripheral veins, neovascularisations and retinal detachments.[7]

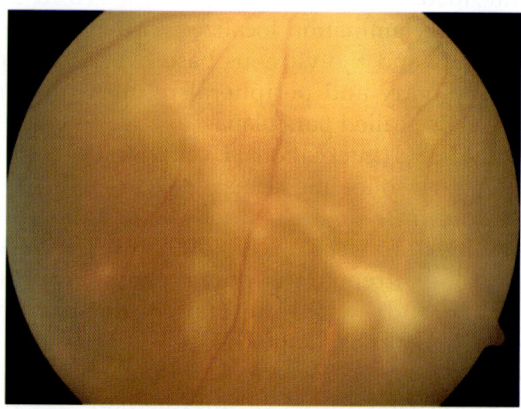

Fig. 4.3.1 *Snowball opacities.*

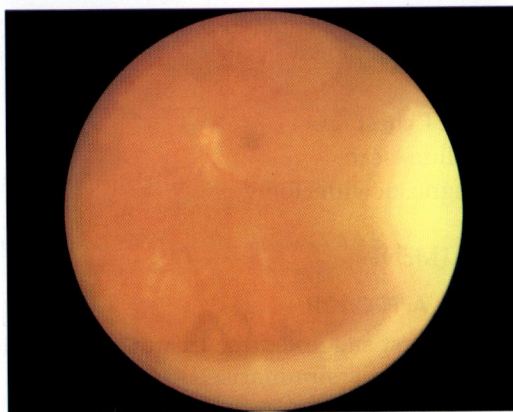

Fig. 4.3.2 *Snowbanking.*

Course, prognosis and complications

Course and prognosis

Prognosis is relatively good, if week treated.

Course is usually chronic with three distinct patterns:

- *Single, mild self-limiting episode* is seen in 10% cases,
- *Prolonged course without exacerbations* is seen in about 60% cases, and
- *Chronic smoldering course with multiple subacute exacerbations* is seen in about 30% cases.

Complications

1. *Cataract formation* is the commonest complication of IU. Inflammation along with associated steroid therapy hastens its formation. Posterior subcapsular cataracts are more common, sometimes associated with anterior subcapsular opacities also. The incidence of cataracts increases with the duration and severity of the disease.

2. *Raised IOP.* Active inflammation, steroid usage, increasing age, and number of years since diagnosis are significantly correlated with raised intraocular pressure (IOP) in patients with IU.[8]

3. *Macular oedema* is the most common complication of IU causing significant visual loss. Incidence varies from 12 to 51%. Like cataract their incidence increases with the duration and severity of the disease.

4. *Epiretinal membranes* occurred in 34–36% eyes, which was not related to duration of disease or chronic cystoid macular oedema (CME).[9]

5. *Peripheral neovascularisation* with and without vitreous haemorrhage was seen in 6.5% by Malinowski *et al.*[9]

6. *Periphlebitis* was seen in 13–26% patients.[10]

7. *Vitreous haemorrhage* from peripheral neovascularisation can occur in small percentage of patients, seen more commonly in pars planitis subset and children with IU.

Vitreous haemorrhage is also known to be associated with multiple sclerosis.[11]

8. *Retinal detachments* (RD) occurred in 2.2–51% eyes.[12] Exudative RD has been seen secondary to inflammation in IU. But the most common forms to be seen are vitreous traction secondary to long-standing vitreous inflammation and subsequent peripheral hole formation.

9. *Optic disc neovascularisation*, disc oedema and optic atropy have been reported.

10. *Poorly phthisis bulbi* treated IU can lead to total retinal detachments, proliferative vitreo-retinopathy or a cyclitic membrane causing ciliary body traction and hypotony eventually leading to phthisis bulbi.

DIAGNOSIS

CLINICAL DIAGNOSIS AND DIFFERENTIAL DIAGNOSIS

Clinical diagnosis is made from typical clinical features.

The patient's history should be directed on the duration of symptoms, the number of recurrences, and findings that might be associated with systemic disorders.

- *Fever, fatigue, or night sweats* are typical symptoms of sarcoidosis and tuberculosis.
- *Loss of sensitivity or paresthesias* of the hands, arms, or legs are suggestive of possible multiple sclerosis.
- *Signs of dermatitis* may point to Lyme disease, tuberculosis, or syphilis.
- *Arthritis of the knee* may suggest the possibility of Lyme's disease, and contact with cats may raise the possibility of Bartonella infection.[13]

Differential diagnosis need to be made from other ocular diseases which present, like intermediate uveitis which include:

- Fuchs' heterochromic iridocyclitis
- Toxocara granuloma
- Acute retinal necrosis
- Vogt-Koyanagi-Harada disease
- Endogenous endophthalmitis
- Vitritis associated with Eales disease.

INVESTIGATIONS

Laboratory investigations
- Total leucocyte count (TLC)
- Hemoglobin
- ESR
- Platelet count
- PPD
- Serum angiotensin
- Converting enzyme

Radiodiagnosis
- X-ray chest

Ancillary investigations
- FFA
- OCT
- HRCT chest
- Gallium scan
- Diagnostic vitrectomy

TREATMENT

KAPLAN APPROACH

Kaplan first suggested the treatment for IU in 1984 which is summarised in Table 4.3.1.[14] *Modified Kaplan approach* in the treatment of IU consists of following four steps:
- Step 1: Periocular steroids.
- Step 2: Oral steroids.
- Step 3: Immunomodulatory therapy.
- Step 4: Pars plana vitrectomy along with immunosuppressive therapy

Step 1: Periocular steroids

Periocular corticosteroids are the first line of management. They are indicated in unilateral

---

Table 4.3.1 *Kaplan approach for treatment of intermediate uveitis*

Management of non-infectious intermediate uveitis was well explained in a 4-step approach by Kaplan et al in 1984, which included:

Step 1 Corticosteroid therapy. Periocular corticosteroids usually constitute the first line of therapy. Intravitreal triamcinolone injections may be an alternative to periocular injections in severe refractory cases. Systemic corticosteriod therapy may be started, if local therapy is not effective.

Step 2 Cryotherapy or indirect laser ophthalmoscopy. If corticosteroid therapy fails, peripheral ablation of the pars plana snowbank with cryotherapy and/or indirect laser photocoagulation to the peripheral can be performed. Cryotherapy is doe by using a freeze-thaw technique to apply a double row of transconjunctival cryopexy to an area 1 clock-hour beyond all evidence of disease activity. Peripheral scatter laser photocoagulation burns may be placed confluently in 3 or 4 rows just posterior to the snowbank. Treatment may be extended to the equator posterior to the snowbank on each side.

Step 3. Pars plana vitrectomy with induction of posterior hyaloidal separation and peripheral laser photocoagulation of the pars plana snowbank may be perfomed, if cryotherapy fils and systemic IMT is contraindicated or not desired because of the risk of systemic side effects. Vitrectomy may be necessary to treat severe visual loss caused by dense vitreous cellular accumulation and veils, vitreal haemorrhage or traction, retinal detachment, CME, may reduce the need for high doses of maintenance oral corticosteroids in some patients.

Step 4 Systemic immunomodulatory agents, such as methotrexate, cyclosporine, azathioprine, mycophenolate mofetil, and cyclophosphamide may also be tried, and are indicated for treatment of bilateral disease.

However, individualisation of treatment should always be a priority rather than a rigid persistence with these 4-steps. Also with newer less toxic, better immunosuppressant available, the author frequently modifies the 4-step approach in his patients with good benefit noted. The modified approach has been outlined in the chapter on intermediate uveitis.

cases or bilateral cases with cystoid macular oedema. Local injection of depot preparation of a long-acting triamcinolone acetonide (40 mg/0.5 ml) is given through the posterior sub-Tenon route and can be spaced four weeks apart. Complications of periocular injections are increased IOP, cataract, aponeurotic ptosis and allergic reactions with conjunctival breakdown. Repeated injections may cause enophthalmos and orbital scarring.

Intravitreal triamcinolone (IVTA) may be an alternative to periocular injections in refractory cases though they carry the risk of retinal detachment, vitreous haemorrhage, IOP elevation and endophthalmitis. Cataract and glaucoma were the common side effects.[15]

Intravitreal injection for cystoid macular oedema in IU

Dexamethasone intravitreal implant (Ozurdex) is one of the most potent, with an anti-inflammatory activity that is six-fold greater than that of triamcinolone and 30-fold greater than cortisol. In the dexamethasone implant, the active drug is dispersed through a biodegradable copolymer of lactic acid and glycolic acid (PLGA), forming a matrix structure. Intravitreal bevacizumab (avastin) seems to be an effective, fast acting, and safe treatment in the management of inflammatory CME. The effect is transient, and reinjections may be necessary, although the time until reinjection is needed differs individually. The optimal dosage, number, and intervals of reinjections have to be better defined by additional studies and larger patient numbers.

Step 2: Oral steroids

If local therapy is not effective or bilateral severe disease is seen at presentation, oral corticosteroids are indicated. Oral prednisolone is started at 1 mg/kg/day with gradual tapering after one week and guided thereafter by the clinical response. Ideally, the disease should be controlled with 5 mg or less daily.

Step 3: Immunomodulatory therapy

This may be considered, if corticosteroid therapy fails to control the inflammation. Methotrexate, azathioprin, cyclosporine, mycophenolate mofetil, tacrolimus have been used in treating IU. Cyclophosphamide and chlorambucil have been used in refractory uveitis. Newer biologic agents can also be used.

Antimetabolites/antiproliferative drugs

Methotrexate (MTX), a folate analog which inhibits dihydrofolate reductase, is used at a dose of 7.5–25 mg per week oral/subcutaneous. Though its potential side effects are gastrointestinal (GI) upset, fatigue, hepatotoxicity and pneumonitis, it is effective and safe for chronic anterior and IU in children.[16]

Azathioprine, a purine nucleoside analog, alters purine metabolism. It is used at a dose of 50–150 mg per day in divided doses orally. Its potential side effects are GI upset, hepatotoxicity and bone marrow suppression.

Mycophenolate mofetil (MMF) acts by inhibiting purine synthesis, prevents replication of T and B lymphocytes by selectively inhibiting inosine-5-monophosphate dehydrogenase. It is used at a dose of 1–3 mg per day in divided doses orally. Diarrhoea, nausea, and GI ulceration are its potential side effects. GI disturbance was the commonest side effect seen. It has been found to be safe in children when used alongside oral corticosteroid. Galor *et al.* compared all the three antimetabolites in a cohort of patients with ocular inflammation which included patients with IU in all three groups, and concluded that time to control ocular inflammation is faster with mycophenolate than with methotrexate.[17]

Inhibitors of T cell signaling

Cyclosporine A (CsA): Inhibits NF-AT (nuclear factor of activated T cells) activation, and is used at a dosage of 2.5–5.0 mg/kg/day in divided doses orally. Known toxic effects are nephrotoxicity, hypertension, gingival hyperplasia, GI upset and paraesthesias.

Tacrolimus: Inhibits NF-AT activation, and is used at a dose of 0.1–0.2 mg/kg/day orally. Nephrotoxicity, hypertension and diabetes mellitus are its known potential complications. Tacrolimus efficacy for the treatment of uveitis is maintained long-term.

Biologic response modifiers: Newer anti-inflammatory drugs, like daclizumab, infliximab, eternercept, interferon alpha, are being increasingly used as first-line, second-line drugs in the management of refractory uveitis.

Daclizumab: Humanized monoclonal anti-IL-2 receptor alpha antibody. It binds to the alpha subunit of IL-2 receptor thereby suppressing autoreactive T cells. It is used at a dose of 1.0 mg/kg intravenous every two weeks for five doses. High-dose daclizumab can reduce inflammation in active uveitis and is well tolerated but there may be a potential increased risk of infection associated with immuno-suppression.

Step 4: Pars plana vitrectomy

Vitrectomy. Decreased inflammatory disease has been reported after pars plana vitrectomy (PPV) for chronic inflammation in patients with IU. PPV is an important means of correcting structural complications of uveitis, helps in decreasing inflammation in the anterior chamber and in the vitreous and in reduction of anti-inflammatory medication postoperatively. It helps in improving visual outcome and is beneficial in reducing CME.[18]

Cataract surgery. Cataracts are a frequent complication that result from both, chronic inflammation and corticosteroid therapy. Phacoemulsification and intraocular lens (IOL) implantation is safe in IU/pars planitis.[19] Visual acuity of 20/40 or better was seen in 88% of patients following cataract surgery and IOL implantation in whom control of inflammation for three months preoperatively was achieved.[20] Control of inflammation can be achieved with use of corticosteroids—topical, periocular, oral with or without immunosuppressive therapy.

SUMMARY

Definition. Intermediate uveitis is an anatomical classification including a diverse group of entities, poses a significant challenge to the ophthalmologists because a large proportion is still of undetermined etiology, its varied clinical course and tendency to involve the macula.

Clinical features of intermediate uveitis include:
- Minimal anterior chamber reaction
- Vitritis
- Snowbanking; snowball exudates
- Neovascularisation
- Tortuosity of arterioles and venules
- Sheathing of peripheral veins
- Retinal detachment

Diagnosis. Careful examination of the pars plana region in all cases of uveitis especially by indirect ophthalmoscopy and scleral depression can contribute to establish the diagnosis of intermediate uveitis.

Early diagnosis and proper treatment can usually salvage the vision in majority of eyes. When visual acuity deteriorates (less than 6/12) periocular or systemic steroids, immunosuppressive agents, intravitreal agents and vitrectomy are currently being used in the management of the disease in its various stages.

Most common complications are cataract, ocular hypertension, and cystoid macular oedema. Despite these complications, most patients retain good visual acuity, unless they develop persistent cystoid macular oedema, epiretinal membrane, or other macular changes. Longer duration of disease might potentially lead to chronic maculopathy and this may justify early and more aggressive treatment for associated macular oedema in IU.

REFERENCES

1. Becker M, Davis JL. Vitrectomy in the treatment of uveitis. Am J Ophthalmol 2005;140:1096–105.
2. Biswas J, Raghavendran SR, Vijaya R. Intermediate uveitis of pars planitis type in identical twins. Report of a case. Int Ophthalmol 1998;22:275–7.
3. Bloch-Michel E, Nussenblatt RB. International Uveitis Study Group recommendations for the evaluation of intraocular inflammatory disease. Am J Ophthalmol 1987;103:234–5.
4. Brockhurst RJ, Schepens CL. Peripheral uveitis. The complication of retinal detachment. Arch Ophthalmol 1968;80:747.
5. Galor A, Jabs DA, Leder HA, Kedhar SR, Dunn JP, Peters GB 3rd, *et al.* Comparison of antimetabolite drugs as corticosteroid-sparing therapy

for noninfectious ocular inflammation. Ophthalmology 2008;115:1826–32.

6. Ganesh SK, Babu K, Biswas J. Phacoemulsification with intraocular lens implantation in cases of pars planitis. J Cataract Refract Surg 2004;30:2072–6.

7. Herbert HM, Viswanathan A, Jackson H, Lightman SL. Risk factors for elevated intraocular pressure in uveitis. J Glaucoma 2004; 13:96–9.

8. Hogewind BF, Zijlstra C, Klevering BJ, Hoyng CB. Intravitreal triamcinolone for the treatment of refractory macular edema in idiopathic intermediate or posterior uveitis. Eur J Ophthalmol 2008;18:429–34.

9. Jabs DA, Nusenblatt RB, Rosenbaum JT. Standardization of Uveitis Nomenclature (SUN) working group. Standardization of uveitis nomenclature for reporting clinical data. Results of the First International Workshop. Am J Ophthalmol 2005;140:509–16.

10. Kaplan HJ. Intermediate uveitis (pars planitis, chronic cyclitis): a four-step approach to treatment. In: Saari KM, editor. Uveitis Update. Amsterdam: Experta Medica 1984, pp 169–72.

11. Kaufman AH, Foster CS. Cataract extraction in patients with pars planitis. Ophthalmology 1993; 100:1210–17.

12. Malinowski SM, Pulido JS, Folk JC. Long-term visual outcome and complications associated with pars planitis. Ophthalmology 1993;100:818–24.

13. Manohar Babu B, Rathinam SR. Intermediate Uveitis. Indian J Ophthalmol 2010;58:21–27.

14. Nusenblatt RB, Palestine AG. Intermediate uveitis. In: Uveitis: Fundamentals and clinical practice. Chicago: Yearbook Medical; 1989, pp. 279–88.

15. Paivönsalo-Hietanen T, Tuominen J, Saari KM. Uveitis in children: population-based study in Finland. Acta Ophthalmol Scand 2000;78:84–8.

16. Pederson JE, Kenyon KR, Green WR, et al. Pathology of pars planitis. Am J Ophthalmol 1978; 86:762–74.

17. Prieto JF, Dios E, Gutierrez JM, Mayo A, Calonge M, Herreras JM. Pars planitis: epidemiology, treatment, and association with multiple sclerosis. Ocul Immunol Inflamm 2001;9:93–102.

18. SR Rathinam, Namperumalsamy P. Global variation and pattern changes in epidemiology of uveitis. Indian J Ophthalmol 2007;55:173–83.

19. Thorne JE, Daniel A, Jabs DA, Kedhar SR, Peters GB, Dunn JP. Smoking as a risk factor for cystoid macular edema complicating intermediate uveitis. Am J Ophthalmol 2008;145:841–6.

20. Valentincic NV, Kraut A, Rothova A. Vitreous hemorrhage in multiple sclerosis-associated uveitis. Ocul Immunol Inflamm 2007; 15: 19–25.

4.4 POSTERIOR UVEITIS

Definition, Classification and Etiopathogenesis
- Definition
- Classifications
- Etiopathogenesis

Clinical Profile
- Symptoms
- Signs
- Clinical types

Diagnosis
- Clinical diagnosis
- Investigations

Treatment
- General considerations
- Specific treatment for infective posterior uveitis
- Nonsteroidal anti-inflammatory drugs
- Corticosteroids
- Immunosuppressive drugs

DEFINITION, CLASSIFICATION AND ETIOPATHOGENESIS

DEFINITION

According to SUN (Standardisation of Uveitis Nomenclature) working group[1] classification, posterior uveitis is defined as inflammation occurring in retina and choroid as the primary site (Table 4.4.1). Thus posterior uveitis can have inflammation involving structures, such as retina, vitreous, optic nerve head, retinal vessels along with choroidal inflammation. Posterior uveitis is commonly insidious in onset, though it can have an acute presentation. This sight-threatening condition has pathognomonic clinical features identifiable on clinical examination.

CLASSIFICATION

Posterior uveitis can be variously classified.

Pathological classification

1. Suppurative posterior uveitis
2. Non-suppurative posterior uveitis
   - Granulomatous posterior uveitis
   - Non-granulomatous posterior uveitis

Etiologicl classification

I. Infectious posterior uveitis
   - Bacterial
   - Viral
   - Fungal
   - Parasitic
II. Non-infectious posterior uveitis

Clinical classification

It is based on the extent of inflammation in the choroid and retina and includes following types (Table 4.4.1):

1. Choroiditis
   - Focal choroiditis
   - Multifocal choroiditis
   - Diffuse choroiditis
2. Chorioretinitis
3. Retinochoroiditis
4. Retinitis
5. Neuroretinitis

ETIOPATHOGENESIS

Posterior uveitis can occur due to infective (more common) a well as non-infective causes.

I. *Infective causes*
1. Toxoplasmosis
2. Toxocariasis
3. Tuberculosis (TB)
4. Syphilis
5. Bartonella

Table 4.4.1 *SUN working group classification of posterior uveitis*		
Type	*Primary site of inflammation*	*Subtypes (Based on clinical characteristics)*
Posterior uveitis	Retina/choroid	Focal, multifocal, diffuse choroiditis Chorioretinitis, retinochoroiditis retinitis, neuroretinitis

6. Viral (herpes simplex, varicella zoster, cytomegalovirus)
7. HIV-related eye diseases

II. *Non-infective causes*
1. Acute posterior multifocal placoid pigment epitheliopathy (APMPPE)
2. Multiple evanescent white dot syndrome (MEWDS)
3. Geographic helicoid peripapillary choroidopathy (GHPC)
4. Multifocal choroiditis (MFC)
5. Punctate inner choroidopathy (PIC)
6. Birdshot choroidopathy
7. Presumed ocular histoplasmosis syndrome (POHS)
8. Subretinal fibrosis and uveitis syndrome
9. Diffuse unilateral subacute neuroretinitis (DUSN)
10. Retinal pigment epithelitis (Krill's disease)
11. Sarcoidosis
12. Behcet's disease

Causes of different subtypes of posterior uveitis
Causes of different subtypes of posterior uveitis are mentioned along with the clinical profile.

Pathogenesis
Posterior uveitis may be caused by autoimmune conditions, infections, or rarely, trauma, but 50% of cases are idiopathic.

Non-infectious uveitis is usually immune-related inflammation. Many cases may be autoimmune.

Infectious uveitis nearly always results from haematogenous spread of infection from another part of the body to the highly vascular uvea.

Pathophysiology of uveitis depends on the specific etiology but in all types there is breach in the blood–eye barrier. The blood–ocular barrier, similar to the blood–ocular barrier normally prevents the cells and large protein entering the eye. Inflammation causes this barrier to breakdown, and WBCs enter the eye. Neutrophils predominate in acute uveitis cases, and mononuclear cells predominate in chronic uveitis.

Note. Some cases of intraocular inflammation masquerade as uveitis (masquerade syndromes) but other causes, such as malignancy (e.g. ocular-central nervous system lymphoma), must be ruled out.

CLINICAL PROFILE

SYMPTOMS
Choroiditis (non-suppurative inflammation) is a painless condition, usually characterised by visual symptoms due to associated vitreous haze and involvement of the retina. Therefore, small patches situated in periphery may be symptomless and are usually discovered as healed patches on routine fundus examination. On the contrary, a central patch produces marked symptoms which draw immediate attention.

Various visual symptoms experienced by a patient of choroiditis are summarised below:
1. *Defective vision.* It is usually mild due to vitreous haze, but may be severe as in central choroiditis.
2. *Photopsia.* It is a subjective sensation of flashes of light resulting due to irritation of rods and cones.
3. *Black spots floating in front of the eyes.* It is a very common complaint of such patients. They occur due to large exudative clumps in the vitreous.
4. *Metamorphopsia.* Herein, patients perceive distorted images of the object. This results due to alteration in the retinal contour caused by a raised patch of choroiditis.
5. *Micropsia* which results due to separation of visual cells is a common complaint. In this, the objects appear smaller than they are.
6. *Macropsia,* i.e. perception of the objects larger than they are, may occur due to crowding together of rods and cones.
7. *Positive scotoma,* i.e. perception of a fixed large spot in the field of vision, corresponding to the lesion may be noted by many patients.

SIGNS
I. *Anterior segment signs.* Usually, there are no external signs and the eye looks quiet. However,

fine KPs may be seen on biomicroscopy due to associated cyclitis.

II. *Vitreous opacities* due to choroiditis are usually present in its middle or posterior part. These may be fine, coarse, stringy or snowball opacities.

III. *Features of a patch of choroiditis* are as below.

1. *Active patch of choroiditis,* looks as a pale-yellow or dirty-white raised area with ill-defined edges. This results due to exudation and cellular infiltration of the choroid which hide the choroidal vessels. The lesion is typically deeper to the retinal vessels. The overlying retina is often cloudy and oedematous. There may be associated vasculitis.

It is important to differentiate between a lesions of choroiditis from retinitis (Table 4.4.2).

Choroiditis due to infectious etiology is usually associated with severe vitritis though it is often difficult to differentiate between infectious and non-infectious etiology clinically. Often choroiditis is associated with inflammation of the overlying retina and these lesions are known as chorioretinitis.

2. *Healed patch of choroiditis,* when active inflammation subsides, becomes more sharply defined and delineated from the rest of the normal area due to atrophy of choroidal tissue. The involved area shows white sclera below the atrophic choroid and black pigmented clumps at the periphery of the lesion (Figs 4.4.1 and 4.4.2). A healed patch of chorioretinitis must be differentiated from the degenerative conditions, such as pathological myopia and retinitis pigmentosa.

CLINICAL TYPES OF POSTERIOR UVEITIS

Posterior uveitis may manifest as:
• Choroiditis
• Retinitis
• Chorioretinitis
• Neuroretinitis
• Vasculitis

Choroiditis

Depending upon the number and location of lesions, choroiditis can be classified into three types: focal, multifocal and diffuse.

Focal choroiditis

Focal choroiditis also known as localised or circumscribed choroiditis. It is characterised by a single patch or a few small patches of inflammation localised in a particular area. Such patches of choroiditis are described by a name depending upon the location of the lesion which are as follows:

1. *Central choroiditis.* As the name indicates, it involves the macular area and may occur either alone (Fig. 4.4.1) or in combination with disseminated choroiditis. A typical patch of central choroiditis may occur in toxoplasmosis, histoplasmosis, tuberculosis, syphilis and rarely due to visceral larva migrans.

2. *Juxtacaecal or juxtapapillary choroiditis.* It is the name given to a patch of choroiditis involving an area adjoining the optic disc. One example is *Jensen's choroiditis* which typically occurs in young persons.

3. *Anterior peripheral choroiditis.* It implies occurrence of multiple small patches of choroiditis in the peripheral part of choroid (anterior to equator). Such lesions are often syphilitic in origin.

4. *Equatorial choroiditis.* It involves the choroid in the equatorial region only.

Common causes of focal (solitary) choroiditis include:
• Serpiginous choroiditis
• Tuberculosis

Table 4.4.2 *Choroiditis versus retinitis*	
Choroiditis	*Retinitis*
1. Appears as yellowish patches	1. Appears as a whitish patch
2. Relatively well-defined margins.	2. Ill-defined margins
3. Involved areas appear to be deep to the retinal blood vessels.	3. Associated with retinal oedema and overlying vitreous cells

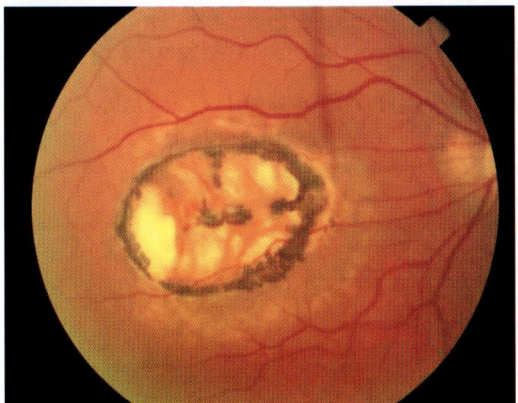

Fig. 4.4.1 *A healed patch of central chorioretinitis.*

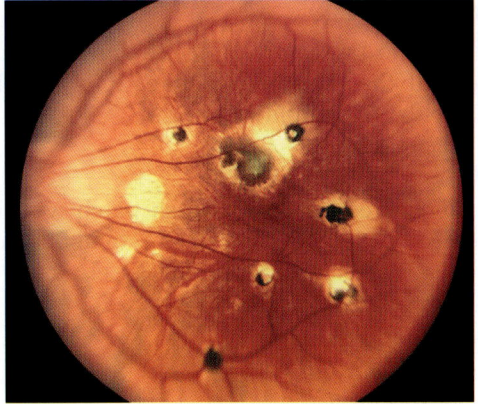

Fig. 4.4.2 *Healed lesions of multifocal choroiditis.*

- Sarcoidosis
- Onchocerciasis
- Toxoplasmosis (chorioretinitis)

Focal choroiditis (FC) can also be subdivided based on the presence or absence of vitritis into FC with vitritis and FC without vitritis.

Focal choroiditis with vitritis

- Toxocariasis
- Sarcoidosis
- Tuberculosis
- Nocardia
- Cat-scratch disease

Focal choroiditis without vitritis

- Tumours
- Serpiginous choroiditis

Multifocal choroiditis

Multifocal choroiditis also known as disseminated choroiditis is characterised by multiple but small areas of inflammation scattered over the greater part of choroid (Fig. 4.4.2). Such a condition may be due to syphilis or tuberculosis, but in many cases, the cause is obscure.

Common causes of multifocal choroiditis include:

- Multifocal choroiditis and panuveitis
- Acute posterior multifocal placoid pigment epitheliopathy (APMMPE)
- Multiple evanescent white-dot syndrome (MEWDS)

- Punctate inner choroidopathy (PIC)
- Presumed ocular histoplasmosis syndrome (POHS)
- Vogt-Koyanagi-Harada syndrome
- Birdshot retinochoroidopathy .

Multifocal choroiditis (MFC) can be divided based on presence or absence of vitritis into MFC with vitiritis and MFC without vitritis.

Causes of multifocal choroiditis with vitritis

- Birdshot retinochoroidopathy
- MCP
- Sympathetic ophthalmia
- VKH syndrome
- Sarcoidosis
- West Nile virus
- Cat-scratch disease
- Malignant masquerade syndromes
- Rubella
- Measles
- MEWDS

Causes of multifocal choroiditis without vitritis

- OHS
- PIC
- PORT
- Serpiginous choroiditis
- Acute retinal pigment epitheliitis
- Subacute sclerosing panencephalitis

Diffuse choroiditis

It refers to large spreading lesions involving most of the choroidal tissue. It is usually tubercular or syphilitic in origin.

Retinitis

Retinitis presents as a whitish patch with ill-defined border and associated retinal oedema. The lesion obscures the retinal vessels. It can be solitary or multifocal:

Focal retinitis
- Toxoplasmosis
- Onchocerciasis
- Cysticercosis
- Masquerade syndromes

Multifocal retinitis
- Syphilis
- HSV, VZV, CMV
- DUSN
- Candida infection
- Sarcoidosis
- Cat-scratch disease
- Masquerade syndromes

Chorioretinitis

All the causes of choroiditis can present as chorioretinitis.

Neuroretinitis

It can be due to following etiology:
- Idiopathic (25%)
- Cat-scratch disease
- Syphilis
- Leptospirosis
- Lyme disease

Characteristic features: Sudden, in onset painless, and variable loss of vision which is
- *RAPD* may or may not be present.
- *Papillitis with surrounding retinal* oedema involving the macula which later develops a macular star is the classical finding.

Vasculitis

The primary site of involvement is the retinal vessels seen as variable degree of sheathing, sclerosis and inflammatory vessel occlusion also. Vitritis is not so severe in primary vasculitic causes. Depending on the major vessels involved, it can be classified as:

Primary arteritic vasculitis
- Systemic lupus erythematosus
- Polyarteritis nodosa
- Syphilis
- ARN/PORN
- Churg-Strauss syndrome

Primary phlebitic vasculitis
- Sarcoidosis
- Multiple sclerosis
- Behcet disease
- Birdshot
- Retinochoroidopathy
- HIV paraviral syndrome
- Eales disease

Both arteritic and phlebitic vasculitis
- Toxoplasmosis
- Wegener's granulomatosis
- Chrohn's disease.

Complications

The complications depend on the etiology and include the following:

1. *Macular oedema* (also cystoid macular oedema): This can be acute (short-term) or chronic (long-term). Chronic macular oedema can persist in the absence of active uveitis and may be treated with steroid therapy or with immunosuppressants.

2. *Vitreous opacification.* Inflammation in uveitis may affect the vitreous gel. The result of this can be floaters or a more substantial obstruction of vision, if a lot of debris is present.

3. *Neovascularisation.* Specially seen with vasculitis.

4. *Choroidal neovascular membrane.* Toxoplasmosis, serpiginous choroiditis, VKH, PIC.

5. *Loss of visual field.* Inflammation may result in damaged areas of the retina to produce 'blind spots' or scotoma. These may be in the peripheral vision and hardly noticeable but if near the macula, the central vision can be significantly affected.

6. *Retinal detachment of different types* may occur:

- *Tractional:* RD in Eales' disease, toxocariasis.
- *Rhegmatogenous* RD in viral retinitis.
- *Exudative:* VKH, sympathetic ophthalmia, posterior scleritis.

DIAGNOSIS

CLINICAL DIAGNOSIS

History

Thorough history is a critically important step in evaluating any patient with uveitis. It allows the clinician to gain critical evidence. Specially important in posterior uveitis cases are the history of tuberculosis, exposure, history of oral and genital ulcers, prodromal symptoms of VKH, like headache, tinnitus, tingling sensation, history of neurologic problems, etc.

Systemic evaluation

Systemic evaluation is very important in posterior uveitis, specially respiratory system (tuberculosis, sarcoidosis), skin (sarcoidosis, leprosy, cat-scratch disease) and CNS (lymphoma).

Ocular examination

It is very important to examine the entire fundus with indentation, if possible. Posterior uveitis can have spillover AC cells and vitreous cells which needs to be documented. Sarcoidosis can have iris nodules, angle nodules along with posterior segment findings. Leprosy can have the characteristic iris pearls.

Fundus evaluation can reveal some caracteristic findings typical of some disease entities:

- *Sarcoidosis:* Skipped vascular sheathing, perivascular exudates resembling candle wax drippings.
- *Toxoplasmosis:* Focal retinochoroiditis adjacent to a previous scar along with overlying intense vitritis, *'headlight in fog'sign*. May also have arteriolitis which may involve the entire fundus, known as kyrieleis arteriolitis.
- *CMV retinitis:* Focal area of necrotising retinitis with areas of haemorrhage (pizza pie appearence) which then spreads in a bushfire pattern along the vessels.

- *ARN:* Areas of full thickness peripheral retinal necrosis which then become confluent, creating a scalloped margin which clearly delineates the normal and the necrotic retina.
- *PORN:* Initially the retinal necrosis involves the outer retina which then becomes full thickness and the lesions progress early towards the posterior pole. The necrotic retina has a perivascular clear zone as the macrophages are able to clear the perivascular necrotic material, giving a cracked mud appearance.
- *Tuberculosis and syphilis* can mimic any clinical presentation.
- *VKH* bilateral exudative RD and disc hyperemia should raise the suspicion of VKH, but multifocal CSR should always be ruled out.

INVESTIGATIONS

Ancillary investigations

Although a provisional clinical diagnosis can be reached in most cases of posterior uveitis, ancillary investigations assist in not only confirming the clinical diagnosis but also in cases of diagnostic dilemma.

Fundus photography and fundus fluorescein angiography

Fundus photography. Serial documentation of lesions with colour fundus photographs can assist in the follow-up of the disease with treatment.

FFA may be useful:
- *Confirming the activity* of a choroiditis/retinitis, e.g. a characteristic early hypofluorescence and late hyperfluorescence in case of active choroiditis.
- *To detect disease sequelae,* such as neovascularisation, capillary non-perfusion areas and vascular staining in cases of retinal vasculitis.
- *Behcet's disease* peripheral capillary ferning pattern is typical of and it can be found even in completely quiet eyes.
- *Subretinal abcess* has 'ring of fire' appearence in early phase due to central hypo- and peripheral hyperfluorescence. The central hypofluorescent area gradually becomes hyperfluorescent in later frames.

- Multiple pin point leakage in early frame with typical of VKH is pooling in late frames.
- *Cystoid macular oedema* (CME) FFA can reveal a typical flower petal pattern or pooling of dye in late phase in subretinal fluid with posterior uveitis.
- *FFA is most useful to detect* the presence, type and activity of choroidal neovascularisation (CNV) with is a vision-threatening complication associated with many posterior uveitic entities (e.g. toxoplasmosis, serpiginous choroiditis).

Indocyanine green angiography (ICG)

ICG is more helpful in case of deeper choroidal lesions, CNV and in the presence of haemorrhages.

- *ICS is especially useful in detection, identification* and follow-up of entities with deeper choroidal lesions, such as white dot syndromes where FFA may not be completely confirmatory.
- In ICG, the white dot syndromes characteristically present as multiple hypofluorescent areas, the cause of which is not clear. It can be due to focal choroidal vascular occlusion or due to inflammatory exudates blocking the fluorescence. The hypofluorescent dots are more numerous than clinically seen.
- ICG is not a good tool in choroiditis as it will present as a hypofluorescent area both in active or inactive choroiditis. In active choroiditis, surrounding choroidal vasculatures appear dilated.

Optical coherence tomography (OCT)

OCT is a non-contact imaging tool helpful in detecting and monitoring macular pathologies, such as CME, epiretinal membrane (ERM), CNVM, macular hole, etc. The conventional time domain OCT has a resolution of 10 microns while the newer spectral domain OCT (SD-OCT) has increased the resolution to 5 microns and gives a three-dimensional view enhancing its diagnostic potential. SD-OCT with enhanced depth imaging (EDI mode) is useful to measure the choroidal thickness which has implication in treatment of conditions, like VKH, sympathetic ophthalmia. The new modality, swept source OCT(SS-OCT), with its deeper depth and wider area of imaging has revolutionised the diagnosis of confusing diseases, like VKH, serpiginous choroiditis.

Ultrasound B scan (USG)

It is a very useful tool especially when the media is hazy, e.g. cataract or severe vitritis or vitreous haemorrhage.

- *Helps to differentiate rhegmatogenous and exudative retinal detachment* based on the shifting of fluid, which is more characteristic of an exudative retinal detachment.
- *Increased peripapillary choroidal thickness* can be a significant finding, which may be seen in Vogt-Koyanagi-Harada disease with significant posterior uveitic manifestations and in Posterior scleritis. Normal choroidal thickness is around 1.1 mm.
- *Presence of 'T' sign and/or Tenon's space widening* noted in USG-B scan is pathognomonic of posterior sclerits.
- *Intraocular tumours masquerading as uveitis* and elevated mass-like lesions, such as TB subretinal abscess, are easily diagnosed with USG.

Laboratory investigations

A tailored lab investigation relevant to the clinical entity in question is the right approach in identifying the etiology of a posterior uveitic entity. Laboratory tests are more useful in infective than non-infective conditions. Specific tests for each entity have been described later in the Chapter concerned.

Tuberculin skin test. Tuberculin skin test (TST), popularly known as Mantoux test, is a intradermal test based on the type IV hypersensitivity reaction for the diagnosis of latent TB.

Interferon gamma release assays. This test assesses the level of interferon γ in the serum in response to a specific tubercular antigen.

Serum ACE and serum lysozyme assay. Serum angiotensin converting enzyme (ACE) and serum lysozyme are often grouped together as both tests measure the same parameter, i.e. macrophage products produced by the sarcoid granulomas. However, ACE is normally secreted by pulmonary macrophages and vascular endothelium. That's why it is not pathognomonic of sarcoidosis and levels may also be raised in various conditions.

Chest X-ray and high resolution computerised tomography (HRCT) chest: They are useful in detecting characteristic hilar lymph node or pulmonary involvement in tuberculosis or sarcoidosis. HRCT chest is preferred due to higher sensitivity. HRCT has been found to be a useful boon in diagnosis.

Serum RPR and TPHA. In syphilitic uveitis, they are very sensitive. However, TPHA is a better choice as RPR can come false negative in 30% of such cases.

HLA typing

Some specific entities are mentioned only:

- HLA B51: Behcet's disease
- HLA A29: Birdshot chorioretinopathy
- HLA B7 and HLA DR2: POHS and APMPPE

Various serological tests. Diagnosis of ocular toxoplasmosis is almost always clinical. Laboratory diagnosis of this clinical entity is required in cases of atypical presentations, subclinical infections, etc. The serological diagnosis of ocular toxoplasmosis is confirmed by measurement of intraocular parasite-specific antibody production, which is an indirect proof of the presence of the parasite within the eye.

Various serological tests are available for the diagnosis of syphilis. In syphilitic infection, there is production of non-specific antibodies which react to cardiolipin. This forms the basis of traditional non-treponemal tests such as Veneral Disease Research Laboratory (VDRL) tests and rapid plasma regain tests. On the other hand, the treponemal tests, like fluorescent treponemal antibody absorption FTA-ABS, microhemagglu-tination-T. pallidum (MHA-TP) assays, detect antibodies against Treponema pallidum.

Ocular toxocariasis is diagnosed based on a positive history of contact with pets and suggestive ocular findings. Diagnosis is mainly clinical, although ELISA with toxocara excretory-secretory antigen (TES-Ag) has been shown to be highly specific for toxocara infection.

Pathological diagnosis

Biopsy. The important biopsy specimens in posterior uveitis are:

- Bronchoalveolar lavage.
- Lacrimal gland/conjunctiva/oral mucosa.
- Accessible nodules (e.g. iris).
- Vitreous biopsy (undiagnosed case/suspected PIOL).
- Chorioretinal biopsy.

Polymerase chain reaction (PCR). The polymerase chain reaction (PCR) is a technique of selectively amplifying a single or few copies of a piece of DNA, thereby generating millions or more copies of a particular DNA sequence. So, broadly PCR can be described as "molecular photocopier" or more simply it can be termed as "DNA replication in a test tube". In cases of diagnostic dilemma, intraocular fluid evaluation for polymerase chain reaction (PCR) and antibody titres help clinch the diagnosis.

TREATMENT

GENERAL CONSIDERATIONS

Non-infective posterior uveitis. Local and systemic steroids along with immuno-suppressives in select cases are the mainstay of treatment.

Infective conditions need to be treated primarily with the specific anti-infective agents along with anti-inflammatory therapy in the form of low dose steroids. In case of infective uveitis, systemic steroids need to be initiated at least 48–72 hours after start of specific anti-infective therapy and then stopped at least 1 week prior to stoppage of specific treatment.

SPECIFIC TREATMENT FOR INFECTIVE POSTERIOR UVEITIS

Infective posterior uveitis is a clinical diagnosis based on characteristic fundus picture and relevant positive history. Laboratory investigations are predominantly based on antibody testing against the specific antigen and PCR testing for the particular genome. Other tests to detect associated systemic condition may be required to clinch the diagnosis. It is important to treat the underlying systemic disease along with ophthalmic treatment.

Basic management approach to a case of infective posterior uveitis

- Identify the characteristic/typical fundus picture
- Confirm with specific investigations
- Treat the primary cause with appropriate anti-infective agent
- Use systemic steroids as additional anti-inflammatory therapy
- Avoid periocular/intravitreal steroids
- In diagnostic dilemmas, intraocular fluid evaluation for antibodies or PCR for identification of genome.

NON-STEROIDAL ANTI-INFLAMMATORY DRUGS (NSAIDs)

Before the development of corticosteroid, NSAIDs were the only available agent to treat intraocular inflammation. Indomethacin was the first topically used NSAID which was used extensively in treating ocular inflammation. However, *NSAIDs are of very little help while treating the posterior uveitis.*

CORTICOSTEROIDS

Oral steroids are given for systemic immuno-suppression and in severe ocular inflammation. Prednisolone is the most commonly used oral corticosteroid. Prednisolone acts in an hour or two and hence is the drug of choice in acute inflammation as the other immunosuppressive agents take a longer time to start their action. Oral prednisolone is used in a dose of 1–1.5 mg/kg body weight as an induction dose and based on the clinical response and the requirement of the patient, it can be tapered to lesser dosage.

Systemic corticosteroids can cause a number of side effects. The most common side effects are cushingoid face, hypertension, peptic ulceration, hyperglycaemia, psychosis, insomnia, osteoporosis, and electrolyte imbalance. Alternate day dosage regimen is an effective strategy to reduce the side effects of the drug to some extent.

Intravenous corticosteroids are sometimes needed in patients who need aggressive management of the inflammation, as in a patient with optic nerve involvement, severe VKH, sympathetic ophthalmia, serpiginous choroiditis or in case of panuveitis. The most commonly used drug is methylprednisolone. The usual dosage is 500 mg to 1 gm intravenous infusion with 0.9% normal saline or sodium lactate solution over 30 to 60 minutes daily for 3 consecutive days, followed by high dose of oral corticosteroids. Caution should be taken as intravenous methylprednisolone can cause cardiac arrhythmias and cardiovascular collapse. Intravenous methylprednisolone should be followed by high dose oral steriod or immunosuppressive agent.

Intravitreal implant, like fluocinolone acetonide sustained drug delivery devices (Retisert), releases the drug at the rate of 2 µg/day when implanted in vitreous cavity. This device has a high potency similar to dexamethasone. However, they are associated with rise of intra-ocular pressure and cataract formation. Another such device is Ozurdex. This device gradually releases 350–700 µg of dexamethasone over a prolonged period when inserted in vitreous cavity.

These are used primarily in corticosteroid-resistant cases or as steroid-sparing agents. Immunosuppressive options include antimetabolites, such as azathioprine, methotrexate, and mycophenolate mofetil, T cell suppressors, such as cyclosporine and tacrolimus, and cytotoxic agents including cyclophosphamide and chlorambucil.

IMMUNOSUPPRESSIVE DRUGS

Antimetabolites

These include the following:

1. *Azathioprine.* It is purine nucleoside analog (competitive inhibitor of purine synthesis), which interfere with adenine and guanine ribonucleotides by suppression of inosmic acid synthesis. This in turn interferes with DNA replication and RNA transcription. Azathioprine is a prodrug which is metabolized in liver and converted to its active form 6-mercaptopurine. It is used in Vogt-Koyanagi-Harada disease, sympathetic ophthalmia, Behcet's disease,

Wegener's granulomatosis in remission, chronic iridocyclitis, scleritis, and serpiginous choroiditis.

2. Methotrexate. It is folate analog. It inhibits the enzyme dihydrofolate reductase inhibiting the production of tetrahydrofolate which in turn inhibits formation of thymidylate, leading to inhibition of DNA replication and RNA transcription. It is mainly active against rapidly dividing immune cells. It is used in juvenile rheumatoid arthritis, children with pars planitis, sarcoidosis, and scleritis associated with connective tissue disorder.[11] Methotrexate is the first choice immunnosuppressant in paediatric uveitis.

3. Mycophenolate mofetil. Mycophenolate mofetil is derived from the fungus *Penicillium stoloniferum*. It inhibits purine metabolism. It inhibits the enzyme inosine monophosphate dehydrogenase, which in turn inhibits the synthesis of guanosine thereby affecting the proliferation of B and T lymphocytes. Mycophenolate mofetil is a prodrug which is metabolized in liver and converted to its active form mycophenolic acid. It is mainly used as alternative to azathioprine in Vogt-Koyanagi-Harada disease, sympathetic ophthalmia, Behcet's disease, Wegener's granulomatosis in remission, chronic iridocyclitis, scleritis, and serpiginous choroiditis.

T cell inhibitor

Cyclosporine. It works on T cell by binding to an intracellular peptide know as cyclophylin which results in blockage of transcription and production of interleukins, activation of CD4 and CD8 T cells and production of other lymphokines, such as interferon. Cyclosporine A is derived naturally from a fungus *Beauveria nivea*.

Cyclosporine is not a cytotoxic drug; it is a cytostatic drug, so inflammation may recur when the drug is stopped. For this rebound phenomenon, the drug is generally used for a long time.

BIBLIOGRAPHY

1. Anshu A, Chee SP. Diffuse unilateral subacute-neuroretinitis. Int Ophthalmol 2008;28:127–9.
2. Balansard B, Bodaghi B, Cassoux N, Fardeau C, Romand S, Rozenberg F. Necrotising retino-pathies simulating acute retinal necrosis syndrome. Br J Ophthalmol 2005;89:96–101.
3. Dreyer RF, Gass JD. Multifocal choroiditis and panuveitis. Arch Ophthalmol 1984;102:1776–84.
4. Kilmartin DJ, Dick AD, Forrester JV. Sympathetic ophthalmia risk following vitrectomy: should we counsel patients? Br J Ophthalmol 2000;84(5):448–449.
5. Margolis R. Diagnostic vitrectomy for the diagnosis and management of posterior uveitis of unknown etiology. Curr Opin Ophthalmol 2008;19(3):218–224.
6. Sudharshan S, Ganesh SK, Biswas J. Current approach in the diagnosis and management of posterior uveitis. Indian J Ophthalmol 2010; 58(1): 29–43.

4.5 PANUVEITIS

Definition and Causes
- Definition
- Causes

Clinical Features
- Symptomes
- Signs

Diagnosis
- Systemic evaluation
- Investigations
- Ancillary testing

Differential Diagnosis and Treatments
Differential diagnosis
- Infectious versus non-infections panuveitis

Treatment
- Medical treatment
- Corticosteroids
- Supportive therapy
- Immunosuppressive agents
- Newer agents
- Surgical treatment
- Vitrectomy
- Surgery for complications

DEFINITION AND CAUSES

DEFINITION

Panuveitis is a generalised inflammation of the whole of the uveal tract which also involves the retina and vitreous humour. According to Standardization of Uveitis Nomenclature (SUN) Classification, panuveitis is an intraocular inflammation where the primary site of inflammation is anterior chamber, vitreous and retina or choroid (Table 4.5.1).[1]

Diagnostic criteria. To establish the diagnosis of panuveitis, usually following clinical signs are required:
- *Presence of anterior chamber inflammation*, such as cells and flare in the anterior chamber, keratic precipitates, iris nodules, and posterior synechiae.
- *Presence of vitreous inflammation*, such as vitreous cells or vitritis.
- *Presence of inflammation of retina or choroid* or both, such as retinitis, choroiditis, retino-choroiditis, retinal vasculitis, choroidal granuloma, subretinal abscess, neuroretinitis, etc.

CAUSES

Common causes of panuveitis are tuberculosis, Vogt-Koyanagi-Harada (VKH) syndrome, sympathetic ophthalmia, Behçet's disease and sarcoidosis. Many cases seem to be idiopathic. Tuberculosis and VKH are the common causes of panuveitis in India.[2,3]

CLINICAL FEATURES

Symptoms

It is usually insideous in onset and has a chronic course. Common symptoms are:
- Gradual painless diminution of vision
- Blurring of vision
- Ocular pain
- Floaters
- Redness
- Photophobia

Signs

Many important findings can be present depending upon the type of uveitis: Granulomatous or non-granulomatous panuveitis.

Adnexal signs
- Subconjunctival granuloma
- Lacrimal gland enlargement
- Vitiligo
- Poliosis
- Periorbital skin nodules
- Perilimbal depigmentation (Sugiura's sign)
- Periocular viral vesicles and other lesions: Hutchinson's sign

Table 4.5.1 *Standardization of Uveitis Nomenclature (SUN) classification: Panuveitis*

| Primary site of inflammation | Anterior chamber, vitreous and retina or choroid. |

Anterior segment signs

- Keratic precipitates (granulomatous/mutton fat or non-granulomatous)
- Anterior chamber cells and flare
- Hypopyon
- Iris stromal nodules—Busacca nodules
- Pupillary margin nodules—Koeppe nodules
- Angle nodules—Berlin's nodules
- Peripheral anterior synechiae
- Posterior synechiae with/without iris bombe
- Complicated cataract
- IOP changes
- Signs of any previous ocular injury/surgery

Posterior segment

- Vitritis
- Snowballs/snowbanking/"string of pearls"
- Diffuse or focal retinitis or choroiditis
- Retinal vasculitis
- Perivenous sheathing ("candle wax drippings" or "taches de bougie")
- Multifocal cream-coloured chorioretinal lesions (Dalen-Fuchs nodules)
- Optic disc or choroidal granulomas
- Subretinal fluid/exudative retinal detachment
- Sunset glow fundus
- Choroidal tubercles
- Subretinal abscess or granulomas
- Pars plana membranes
- Cystoid macular oedema

DIAGNOSIS

SYSTEMIC EVALUATION

History

Many cases of panuveitis are associated with a systemic condition; so careful history taking can give a clue towards diagnosis:

- History of ocular injury
- History of respiratory illness/skin rashes/mouth ulcers/fever/arthralgia/hearing defects/meningismus
- Personal or family history of tuberculosis
- History of sexually-transmitted diseases (STDs)/immunocompromised status

Systemic examination

Various systemic features can give a clue towards diagnosis. Systemic features in various panuveitic entities are mentioned briefly.

1. *Tuberculosis*
- Constitutional symptoms (fever, weight loss)
- Respiratory complaints
- Enlarged lymph nodes
- Features of other systemic involvement

2. *Sarcoidosis*
- Constitutional symptoms (fever, weight loss, fatigue, night sweats)
- Respiratory complaints
- Bilateral hilar lymphadenopathy
- Skin lesions (erythema nodosum, lupus pernio)
- *Heerfordt's syndrome (uveo-parotid fever):* anterior uveitis, parotid gland enlargement, facial palsy and fever

3. *Vogt-Koyanagi-Harada (VKH) syndrome*
- *Neurological findings:* Meningismus, CSF pleocytosis
- *Auditory findings:* Sensorineural deafness, tinnitus
- *Integumentary (skin) findings:* Alopecia, poliosis, vitiligo

4. *Behcet's disease*
- Recurrent oral ulcerations
- Recurrent genital ulcerations
- *Skin lesions:* Erythema nodosum, cutaneous hypersensitivity, pseudofolliculitis, thrombophlebitis
- Arthritis
- *GI disease:* Intestinal ulcers
- Epididymitis
- Vascular diseases
- CNS symptoms

5. *Leprosy*
- Facial features: Saddle nose, ear deformities
- Skin lesions: Hypopigmented macules and papules, nodules
- Peripheral neuritis
- Limb deformities

6. *Syphilis*
- *Skin lesion:* Chancres, maculopapular or pustular rashes, gumma
- Lymphadenopathy
- Cardiovascular involvement
- Neurosyphilis
- Signs of congenital syphilis: Hutchinson's triad

7. *Juvenile idiopathic arthritis-associated uveitis*
- Systemic arthritis
- Skin rashes
- Lymphadenopathy
- Hepatosplenomegaly

INVESTIGATIONS

Panuveitis cases usually require extensive work up, laboratory investigations and other ancillary tests for coming up to a diagnosis. Still a large number of cases remain idiopathic and a specific diagnosis cannot be made up. These tests help in diagnosis, prognosis and studying the response to treatment.

Routine investigations. Some tests are required to be done routinely, like:
- Routine full blood counts including total and differential counts
- ESR
- Mantoux testing
- Chest X-ray or HRCT chest
- Interferon-gamma assay tests including quantiferon—TB gold test (QFT-G) and T-SPOT TB test.
  These tests mainly include testing for *tuberculosis* as it is an important and common cause of panuveitis in India.[2, 3]

Some disease specific tests can be done in cases of strong suspicion, like:
Sarcoidosis
- Definitive diagnosis requires tissue biopsy showing non-caseating granuloma
- Chest X-ray or HRCT chest
- Gallium scan (not done routinely)
- Serum angiotensin converting enzyme (ACE)
- Serum lysozyme
- Serum calcium and phosphorus
- Pulmonary function tests

Behcet's disease
- HLA-B51
- Positive pathergy test

Syphilis
- *Non-treponemal tests:* VDRL, RPR
- *Treponemal tests:* Fluorescent treponema antibody-absorption (FTA-Abs)
- *Lumbar puncture and CSF analysis:* In cases of neurosyphilis

Leprosy
- Slit skin smear test
- Full thickness skin biopsy

VKH
- Lumbar puncture and CSF analysis: CSF pleocytosis
- Tests for auditory functions
- HLA-DR4

Juvenile idiopathic arthritis-associated uveitis
- Serum ANA
- Rheumatoid factor (RF factor)

Wegener's granulomatosis
- Anti-neutrophilic cytoplasmic antibody (cANCA)

Newer tests include:
- *Polymerase chain reaction (PCR)* and reverse transcription PCR (RT-PCR) are used for qualitatively detect gene expression through creation of complementary DNA (cDNA) transcripts from RNA. They are used to diagnose various viral, mycobacterial, bacterial and protozoal causes of uveitis. It is a very simple, rapid, sensitive and specific test.
- *Real-time PCR (qPCR)* is used to quantitatively measure the amplification of DNA using fluorescent probes.

Other tests, like liver function tests and renal function tests, are done during the course of treatment, especially while giving immunosuppressive agents.

Ancillary testing

Some ancillary tests required with their indications are as below:

Slit-lamp photo and colour fundus photo
- Documentation
- Follow up

Fundus fluorescein angiography (FFA) and fundus autofluorescence
- Confirming diagnosis, like choroiditis, retinitis and vasculitis
- Confirming diagnosis in cases of VKH
- To see for cystoid macular edema (CME)
- To look for presence and extent of neo-vascularization (NVD or NVE) and capillary non-perfusion (CNP) areas
- To look for choroidal neovascular membrane (CNVM)

Indocyanine green angiography (ICGA)
- To confirm diagnosis and response to treatment in choroidal lesions

Optical coherence tomography (OCT) including SD-OCT and SS-OCT
To look for, quantify and response to treatment in cases of
- Cystoid macular edema (CME)
- Epiretinal membrane (ERM)
- Vitreomacular traction (VMT)
- CNVM
- Macular hole
   Measuring **choroidal thickness** especially using SS-OCT in cases of VKH and SO.

USG-B scan
- To look for posterior segment status in cases of complicated cataract, severe vitritis with no or poor view of fundus
- To look for choroidal thickness
- To look for "T sign"

Ultrasound biomicroscopy (UBM)
- For evaluation of ciliary body
- Useful in cases of chronic hypotony

DIFFERENTIAL DIAGNOSIS AND TREATMENT

DIFFERENTIAL DIAGNOSIS

Differential diagnosis of infectious and non-infectious causes is summarized in Table 4.5.2.

TREATMENT

Main goals in treatment of uveitis are:[4]
- Prevent vision-threatening complications.
- Relieve the patient's complaints.
- To treat underlying disease.

Modalities of management can be either medical or surgical.

Medical treatment

Medical treatment is the mainstay in panuveitis. It consists of:
- Corticosteroids
- Supportive therapy
- Immunosuppressive agents
- Newer agents

I. Corticosteroids

Corticosteroids are the drugs of choice in most cases. They can be given in various forms, like:
1. *Topical steroids.* They are useful for controlling inflammation of anterior segment. Prednisolone is the most effective agent. Others being dexamethasone, betamethasone and difluprednate. Rimexolone, loteprednol and fluorometholone are other lesser potent agents.
2. *Periocular steroids.* Posterior sub-Tenon (PST) injections of long-acting agents, like triamcilo-

Table 4.5.2 *Infectious versus non-infectious panuveitis*	
Infectious	*Non-infectious*
• Tuberculosis	• Sarcoidosis
• Syphilis	• Sympathetic ophthalmia
• Viral retinitis	• Vogt-Koyanagi-Harada disease (VKH)
• Presumed ocular histoplasmosis syndrome (POHS)	• Behcet's disease
• Diffuse unilateral subacute neuroretinitis (DUSN)	• Juvenile idiopathic arthritis associated uveitis
• Lyme disease	• Wegener's granulomatosis
• Toxoplasmosis	
• Leprosy	

none acetonide and methylprednisolone acetate, are giving using the Smith-Nozik technique. They are mainly indicated in cystoid macular oedema secondary to uveitis. Increase in intraocular pressure is an important complication of these injections and might require explanting them in very severe cases.

3. *Intravitreal steroids.* Triamcinolone acetonide (4 mg/0.1 ml) is mainly used as an intravitreal agent especially in cystoid macular oedema secondary to chronic uveitis. Cataract progression and raised intraocular pressure are the main complications.

4. *Intravitreal steroid implants.*
• *Retisert* is a non-biodegradable fluocinolone acetonide intravitreal implant; containing 0.59 mg of the drug. Following implantation (via pars plana incision and suturing) in the vitreous, the implant releases the active drug at a rate of 0.3–0.4 µg/day over a period of approximately 2.5 years.
• *Iluvien* is also a non-biodegradable injectable intravitreal implant with fluocinolone acetonide. It is small enough to be placed using an inserter with a 25-gauge needle and is expected to provide sustained delivery of fluocinolone acetonide for up to 3 years.
• *Ozurdex* is a biodegradable dexamethasone intravitreal implant and has a biodegradable copolymer of lactic acid and glycolic acid with micronized dexamethasone. This implant is placed into the vitreous cavity through the pars plana using a customized, single-use, 22-gauge applicator. The implant provides intravitreal dexamethasone for up to 6 months.

5. *Systemic steroids.* It is either oral or intra-venous form.
• *Oral steroids.* Oral prednisolone is the agent of choice. It is given in a dose of 1–1.5 mg/kg/day dose initially. It is the drug of choice in non-infective conditions, like SO, VKH, Behcet's disease. It is used as an adjunct in infective cases after specific treatment has been started.
• *Intravenous steroids.* Used in emergencies, like vision-threatening lesions encroaching macula or ONH. Intravenous methylprednisolone is given in a dose of 1 gram daily once for 3 consecutive days and under strict monitoring of blood sugar and blood pressure.

Side effects of systemic steroids should be explained to patient and consent obtained for the same. Common side effects include peptic ulcer, osteoporosis, increased blood sugar and increased blood pressure, infections, psychosis, renal and cardiac problems.

II. Supportive therapy

Cycloplegics, like atropine, homatropine and cyclopentolate, are used, which:
• Relieve ciliary spasm
• Prevent formation of synechiae
• Breakdown recently formed synechiae

III. Immunosuppressive agents

Many agents have been effective and the main indications are:
• Unresponsive cases
• Steroids sparing agents
• Patients intolerant to side effects of steroids
• Patients requiring chronic steroid therapy for >6 months in doses of more than 10 mg/day.

Conditions in which they are used as primary immunosuppressive therapy:
• Behcet's disease
• VKH
• Sympathetic ophthalmia
• JIA associated uveitis

Commonly used agents are:
Antimetabolites
• Methotrexate
• Azathioprine
• Mycophenolatemofetil

Alkylating agents
• Cyclophosphamide, chlorambucil

T cell inhibitors
• Cyclosporine, tacrolimus

Biologicals
• Infliximab
• Daclizumab
• Etanercept

IV. Newer agents

The main agents used are anti-tumour necrosis factor-α (TNF-α), cytokine receptor antibodies and interferon-α (INF-α). These agents have superior anti-inflammatory potential than conventional immunosuppressive agents. They are mainly used as second line agents in refractory uveitis and especially in Behcet's disease.[5]

B. Surgical treatment

Surgical management includes:

1. Vitrectomy. It can be used as therapeutic and diagnostic modality. It is mainly used in cases of dense vitreous opacities, epiretinal membrane, vitreomacular traction and tractional retinal detachment. Pars plana lensectomy along with vitrectomy prevents cyclitic membrane formation, completely removes cataractous lens along with posterior capsule and improves handling.[6]

2. Surgical treatment of complications, like cataract, glaucoma or combined.

REFERENCES

1. Jabs DA, Nussenblatt RB, Rosenbaum JT. Standardization of Uveitis Nomenclature (SUN) Working Group. Standardization of uveitis nomenclature for reporting clinical data. Results of the First International Workshop. Am J Ophthalmol 2005;140:509–16.

2. Singh R, Gupta V, Gupta A. Pattern of uveitis in a referral eye clinic in North India. Ind J Ophthalmol 2004; 52:121–5.

3. Biswas J, Narain S, Das D, Ganesh SK. Pattern of uveitis in a referral uveitis clinic in India. Int Ophthal 1996;20:223–8.

4. Biswas J, Rao NA. Management of intraocular inflammation: In: Ryan SJ, editor. Retina Vol.2. St. Louis: CV Mosby; 1989, pp 139–46.

5. Bodaghi B, Gendron G, Wechsler B, Terrada C, Cassoux N, Huongdu LT, et al. Efficacy of interferon alpha in the treatment of refractory and sight threatening uveitis: a retrospective monocentric study of 45 patients. Br J Ophthalmol 2007;91:335–9.

6. Soheilian M, Aletaha M, Yazdani S, Dehghan MH, PeymanGA. Management of pediatric Vogt-Koyanagi-Harada (VKH)-associated panuveitis. Ocul Immunol Inflamm 2006;14:91–8.

4.6 COMPLICATIONS OF UVEITIS

Anterior Segment Complications
- Corneal complication
- Anterior segment fibrosis and adhesions
- Inflammatory glaucoma
- Complicated cataract

Posterior Segment Complications
- Cystoid macular oedema
- Epiretinal membrane
- Retinal detachment
- Retinal ischaemia and neovascularisation
- Choroidal neovascular membrane

Phthisis Bulbi

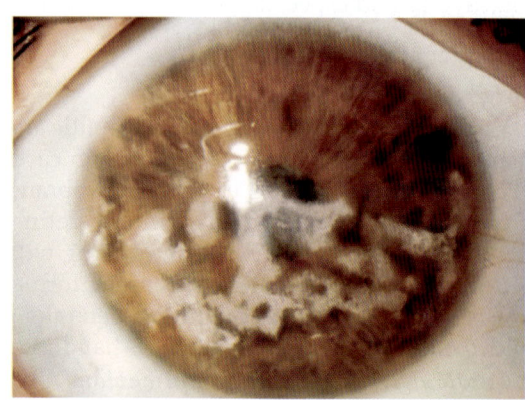

Fig. 4.6.1 *Band-shaped keratopathy.*

INTRODUCTION

The treatment of uveitis is often frustrating because of the complications associated with these intraocular inflammations. This chpter summarises these complications, many of them are sight-threatening and require effective and rapid treatment of the underlying intraocular inflammation.

ANTERIOR SEGMENT COMPLICATIONS

A. CONRNEAL COMPLICATIONS

I. Band keratopathy

Long-standing chronic iridocyclitis or intraocular inflammation, especially in children, can result in deposition of calcium hydroxyapatite in the cornea at the level of Bowman's membrane, giving rise to a condition known as band keratopathy (Fig. 4.6.1). Band keratopathy usually starts as grayish-white opacities at the periphery of the interpalpebral region. It is typically limited to the corneal periphery at the 3 o'clock and 9 o'clock positions. Gradually, the opacification spreads centrally and forms a complete band within the interpalpebral zone. Bowman's layer does not extend to the limbus, the reason a lucid interval is noted between the band keratopathy and the limbus. Small clear areas are noted in the band keratopathy, giving rise to characteristic "Swiss cheese" appearance. These small clear areas represent penetration or entry point of corneal nerves into Bowman's layer.

Profound band keratopathy can lead to diminution of vision in patients with chronic anterior uveitis, especially in children. Thus it is of paramount importance to treat vision robbing cases of band keratopathy in children with chronic anterior uveitis to prevent ambrosia.

Treatment

Treatment is as follows:

1. *Hypertonic saline.* (5% sodium chloride) may be of some use in early oedematous stage.
2. *Warm air* blown on the eyes (e.g. hair dryer) helps in reducing oedema.
3. *Intraocular pressure lowering drugs,* e.g. 0.5% timolol or others should be used to treat associated ocular hypertension.
4. *Bandage soft contact lenses* provide some relief from disturbing symptoms in bullous keratopathy stage.
5. *Penetrating keratoplasty* is the treatment of choice when the visual acuity is reduced markedly.

II. Corneal decompensation

Corneal decompensation in patients with uveitis is rare. It can be rarely seen in uveitis associated with corneal endotheliitis and in herpetic keratouveitis and is a well-recognized feature of chronic cytomegalovirus (CMV) anterior uveitis.

B. ANTERIOR SEGMENT FIBROSIS AND ADHESIONS

1. *Iridolenticular adhesion or synechia* following intense inflammation in anterior chamber is a common complication following recurrent attack of acute anterior uveitis.

2. *Fibrotic membrane.* In severe cases of inflammation, there can be formation of a fibrotic membrane over the pupil. This membrane can occlude the pupillary aperture and can obstruct the aqueous outflow, leading to the formation of iris bombe and acute glaucoma.

3. *Formation of peripheral anterior synechiae* in chronic anterior uveitis can also cause secondary glaucoma.

C. INFLAMMATORY GLAUCOMA

Glaucoma is a common complication of uveitis. The incidence of glaucoma is relatively more common in chronic than in acute uveitis.

During acute attack of uveitis, the IOP is often reduced because of ciliary body inflammation and increased uveoscleral outflow. With ongoing inflammation, various other mechanisms come into play, leading to increase the resistance to aqueous outflow and subsequent rise in IOP. Identifying the exact mechanism of glaucoma in uveitic patients is challenging.

Intraocular pressure can be raised by varied mechanisms in inflammations of the uveal tissue (iridocyclitis). Even in other ocular inflammations, such as keratitis and scleritis, the rise in IOP is usually due to secondary involvement of the anterior uveal tract.

Types of inflammatory glaucoma. Inflammatory glaucoma can be classified as below:
  I. *Non-specific inflammatory glaucomas*
    1. Open-angle inflammatory glaucoma
    2. Angle-closure inflammatory glaucomas
  II. *Specific hypertensive uveitis syndromes*
    1. Fuch's uveitis syndrome
    2. Glaucomatocyclitic crisis

I. Non-specific inflammatory glaucomas

These include all cases of inflammation of the uveal tract associated with raised IOP, other than the specific hypertensive uveitis syndromes, but inclusive of postoperative inflammation.

Based on the mechanism of rise in IOP, the inflammatory glaucoma can be:
• Open-angle inflammatory glaucoma
• Angle-closure inflammatory glaucomas

1. Open-angle inflammatory glaucoma

Clinically, the open-angle inflammatory glaucoma may manifest as:
• Acute, or
• Chronic entity.

Acute open-angle inflammatory glaucoma

Mechanisms of rise in IOP include:
• *Trabecular clogging* by inflammatory cells, exudates and turbid aqueous humour,
• *Trabecular oedema* due to associated trabeculitis, and
• *Prostaglandin*-induced rise in IOP.

Most cases of anterior uveitis are idiopathic, but uveitis commonly associated with open-angle inflammatory glaucoma include herpes zoster iridocyclitis, herpes simplex, kerato-uveitis, toxoplasmosis, rheumatoid arthritis, and pars planitis.

Clinical features. It is characterized by features of acute iridocyclitis associated with raised IOP with open-angle of anterior chamber IOP, usually returns to normal after acute episode of inflammation.

Management includes:
• *Treatment of iridocyclitis* by topical steroids and cycloplegics.
• *Medical therapy to lower IOP* by use of hyper-osmotic agents, oral acetazolamide and topical antiglaucoma medications (pilocarpine and prostaglandin agonists are contraindicated).

Chronic open-angle inflammatory glaucoma

Mechanisms of rise in IOP include:
• Chronic trabeculitis, and
• Trabecular scarring

Clinical features include:
• Raised IOP
• Open-angle on gonioscopy

- No active inflammation but signs of previous episode of uveitis are often present.
- Some chronic cases may also have signs of glaucomatous disc changes and field defects.

Treatment consists of:

- *Medical therapy* with topical beta blockers, and/or carbonic anhydrase inhibitors and alpha agonist may be useful. Preferably avoid pilocarpine and prostaglandin agonists.
- *Trabeculectomy* under cover of steroids may be tried, if medical treatment fails. The results are usually poorer than POAG, but can be improved by augmented trabeculectomy or tube procedures.
- *Cyclodestructive procedures* may need to be considered, if surgical treatment fails.

Note. Steroid-induced glaucoma may occur in some patients during treatment of uveitis and it needs to be considered as an differential diagnosis of open-angle inflammatory glaucoma. It is important to note that raised IOP due to steroids requires a reduction in the potency and frequency of topical steroids or even use of steroid sparing agents; whereas if raised IOP is due to uncontrolled inflammation, the dose of steroid needs to be increased.

Grant's syndrome

Grant's syndrome is a type of chronic secondary open-angle glaucoma (SOAG) with following key features.

Etiology. The condition is either idiopathic or could be associated with systemic conditions, such as sarcoidosis, ankylosing spondylitis, and rheumatic arthritis.

Mechanism of glaucoma is blockage of trabecular meshwork due to inflammatory trabecular oedema and blockage by inflammatory debris.

Clinical features include:

- *Clinical presentation* is similar to POAG with bilateral rise in IOP, with no complaints.
- *Eyes appear white and quite* with minimal inflammatory signs in the anterior segment.
- *Gonioscopy* reveals open-angle with grey to yellowish inflammatory precipitates present

over the trabecular meshwork, which is crucial in differentiating it from POAG.

Treatment consists of:

- *Topical antiglaucoma drugs* alone are not effective in lowering IOP.
- *Topical steroids.* IOP shows excellent response with disappearance of inflammatory precipitates and IOP returning to normal level within 1 to 2 weeks of therapy.

2. Angle-closure inflammatory glaucomas

i. Secondary angle-closure inflammatory glaucoma with pupil block

Mechanism. Pupillary block due to 360° synechiae or seclusio pupillae leads to iris bombe formation followed by appositional angle-closure (Fig. 4.6.2). If not treated, over the period PAS are formed causing synechial angle closure.

Clinical features include:

- Raised IOP
- Seclusio pupillae
- Iris bombe, and
- Shallow anterior chamber.

Management. It includes prophylaxis and curative treatment.

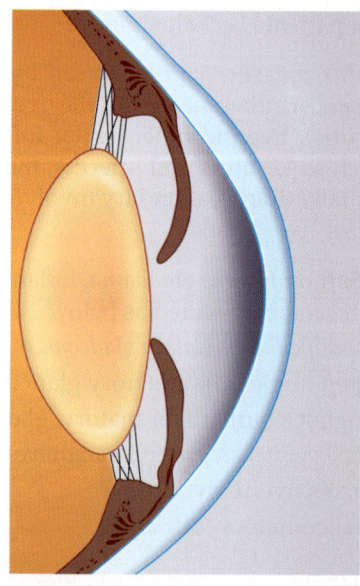

Fig. 4.6.2 *Diagrammatic depiction of pupillary block due to 360° synechiae leading to iris bombe formation and secondary angle-closure.*

1. *Prophylaxis*. Acute iridocyclitis should be treated energetically with topical steroids and atropine to prevent formation of synechiae.

2. *Curative treatment*. It consists of:
- *Medical therapy* to lower IOP (miotics are contraindicated).
- *Laser iridotomy* may be useful in pupil block without synechial angle-closure. Laser PI should be large (or multiple) than is necessary for primary acute angle-closure.
- *Surgical PI* may need to be considered when laser PI closes.

ii. Secondary angle-closure inflammatory glaucoma without pupil block

Mechanism. It occurs due to organization of the inflammatory debris in the angle, which on contraction pulls the iris over the trabeculum. It is followed by gradual and progressive synechial angle-closure with eventual elevation of IOP. Risk of synechial angle-closure increases in the presence of granulomatous inflammation and also in patients with pre-existing narrow angle. Also in cases of chronic uveitis with rubeosis iridis, there may occur fibrovascular growth at the angles leading to a decrease in the aqueous outflow.

Clinical features include:
- Raised IOP
- Shallow anterior chamber

- PAS with angle-closure (Fig. 4.6.3), and
- Signs of previous inflammatory episodes.

Treatment options are:
- *Medical therapy* with topical beta blockers, carbonic anhydrase inhibitors and alpha agonists may reduce IOP.
- *Surgical treatment* is required when medical therapy fails. Trabeculectomy with metabolites or drainage implants (tube shunts) may be required.

II. Specific hypertensive uveitis syndrome
Fuchs' heterochromic uveitis syndrome

Clinical features

Presenting symptoms include:
- *Gradual blurring of vision* due to posterior subcapsular cataract (PSC) is the most common presenting symptoms.
- *Floaters* and difference in the colour of the two eyes are other presenting symptoms.

Signs include:
1. *Keratic precipitates (KPs)* are typically fine stellate present all over the endothelium with filaments in between them, and possibly are pathognomonic of FUS.
2. *Anterior chamber signs*
   - *Aqueous flare* is usually faint.
   - *Aqueous cells* are never more than +2

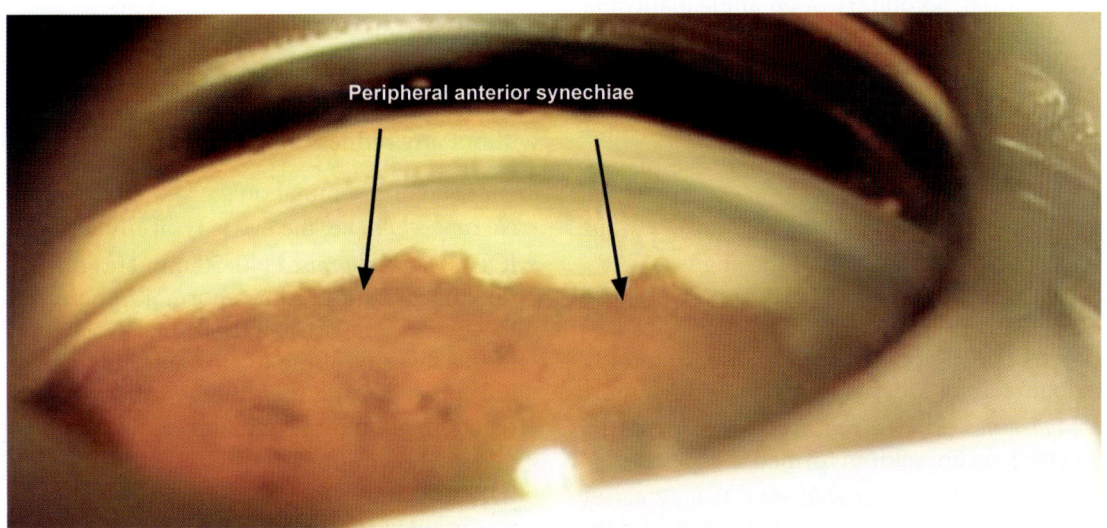

Fig. 4.6.3 *Gonioscopic picture depicting PAS with angle closure.*

3. *Iris signs* include:
- *Heterochromia iridis* is an important and common sign.
- *Diffuse stromal atrophy* gives rise to washed-out appearance (moth-eaten appearance). Radial iris vessel becomes more visible as stroma is atrophied.
- *Posterior pigment layer iris atrophy* is patchy and best detected by retroillumination as transillumination defects.
- *Iris nodules* may be present along the pupillary border.
- *Iris crystals.* Small, refractile iris crystals called Russell bodies can be seen on the surface of the iris. Russell bodies are aggregations of spherical immunoglobulin.
- *Rubeosis iridis* may be seen in the form of fine irregular fragile vessels on the iris surface. Recurrent hyphaema may occur as a result of bleeding from the fragile vessels (Amsler's sign).
- *Posterior synechiae* are conspicuously absent.

4. *Cataract* (posterior subcapsular cataract) is a common complication of Fuchs' uveitis syndrome having a chronic long-lasting course. Most of the time, blurring of vision due to posterior subcapsular cataract is the presenting symptom.

5. *Glaucoma in FUS* occurs in about 30% of the cases, with following key features:
- *Mechanism.* Secondary open-angle glaucoma, occurring probably due to trabecular sclerosis. Prolonged steroid use may also contribute in causation of glaucoma as well as cataract.
- *Raised IOP*, initially intermittent, later becomes constant. Occasionally, the IOP rise may be precipitated by cataract surgery.
- *Gonioscopy* reveals open-angle with ± twig-like neovascularization of the angle.

Treatment

Uveitis in FUS is typically resistant to steroids, though steroids are still used to provide comfort.
- *Mydriatics* are not required since posterior synechiae are seldom formed.
- *Posterior sub-Tenon injection of long-acting steroids* (triamcinolone) may be useful for the annoying floaters.

Glaucoma is treated similar to POAG. However, pilocarpine and prostaglandin analogous are avoided.
- *Medical therapy.* Glaucoma is resistant to hypotensive agents in many cases (with 73% failing to respond to maximal medical therapy).
- *Surgery* (trabeculectomy with antimetabolites or a drainage device) is the main line of treatment.

Posner-Schlossman syndrome

Posner-Schlossman syndrome (glaucomatico-cyclitic crisis) is characterized by recurrent attacks of unilateral acute rise of IOP. Both eyes may be involved at different times but very rarely contemporaneously.

Etiology

- *Cause of acute rise in IOP* is presumed to be acute trabeculitis, possibly secondary to HSV, CMV or *Helicobacter pylori*.
- *A direct correlation between elevated levels of prostaglandins* (prostaglandin E) in the aqueous humour and the level of IOP has been found during acute attacks of glaucomato-cyclitic crisis.
- Condition typically affects young adult males much more than females, 40% of whom are positive for HLA-BW 54.

Clinical features

Presenting symptoms include mild discomfort, haloes around light and slight blurring of vision without any redness and pain.

Signs seen on examination:
- *No congestion*, i.e. the eye is typically white.
- *IOP is markedly raised* (40–50 mm Hg) during the attacks, but becomes normal in between the attacks. The rise of IOP is out of proportion to the severity of the uveitis, and this rise in IOP precedes the identifiable inflammatory reaction, often by several days.
- *Cornea* shows epithelial oedema due to a high IOP, and fine KPs on the back. Fine keratic precipitates appear after 2–3 days of elevated IOP and resolve rapidly. Fresh precipitates

may appear with each episode of increased IOP.

- *Anterior chamber* shows few aqueous cells with minimal flare, no posterior synechiae.
- *Gonioscopy* reveals open-angle with no PAS (a differentiating point from other inflammatory glaucomas).

Course. The recurrent attacks are unilateral, however, about 50% patients do give history of bilateral attacks at times. The interval between the attacks becomes longer with time. Many patients develop chronic open-angle glaucoma as a result of damage to the trabecular meshwork caused by recurrent attacks.

Treatment

Uveitis is treated by:

- *Typical steroids* mainly.
- *Oral NSAIDs* may also be helpful.

Glaucoma may be treated by:

- *Topical antiglaucoma drugs,* such as beta blockers, alpha-2 agonists, and carbonic anhydrase inhibitors.
- *Oral acetazolamide* may be added according to IOP level.

Steroid-induced glaucoma

The therapeutic use of corticosteroids can lead to the rise of intraocular pressure (IOP). Increased IOP can occur as a consequence of any form of corticosteroid therapy—oral, intravenous, inhaled, topical, periocular, or intravitreal corticosteroid therapy. When treated with topical steroids for 4–6 weeks, 5% of the population demonstrate a rise in IOP greater than 16 mm Hg and 30% show a rise of 6–15 mm Hg. Children and older patients are at increased risk of developing increased IOP in response to corticosteroid. Also patients with pre-existing POAG, glaucoma suspect, or history of POAG in first-degree relative are important risk factors and any form corticosteroid should be used judiciously and under proper monitoring. There are variable reports on time taken to show rise of IOP in response to corticosteroid and varies with mode of administration of corticosteroid. The rise of IOP

usually occurs over a period of 4 to 6 weeks when used topically in majority of the patients. It is of paramount importance to understand that there is never a 'safe' period in patients on any form of corticosteroid, after which IOP monitoring becomes unnecessary. Usually IOP almost always returns to normal within days or weeks of disconnection of the corticosteroid treatment.

The primary mechanism of corticosteroid-induced ocular hypertension is increased aqueous outflow resistance. Corticosteroids are believed to induce physical and mechanical changes in the microstructure of the trabecular meshwork causing decreased outflow of aqueous humour.

How does steroid cause glaucoma?

- Increased glycosaminoglycan in trabecular meshwork
- Inhibition of phagocytic activity of meshwork cells
- Inhibition of prostaglandins

D. COMPLICATED CATARACT

Cause of cataract in uveitis

Cataract is one of the common complications of uveitis. Cataract formation in uveitic patient can be attributed to intraocular inflammation or as a side effect of the treatment with corticosteroid.

Intraocular inflammation

- Impaired nutrition to the lens
- Formation of inflammatory membrane over pupillary area

Corticosteroid-induced cataractogenesis

- Disulphide bond formation
- Increased cation permeability
- Decreased G6PD activity
- Binding of steroids to lens proteins
- Increased glucose concentration in lens

Clinical features

Posterior subcapsular cataract are most common, but complicated cataract with nuclear, cortical, and capsular opacities are also seen. Often they are associated with posterior synechiae and pupillary membranes.

Posterior cortical complicated cataract

Typically, the complicated cataract (Fig. 4.6.4) starts as *posterior subcapsular cortical cataract*. The opacity is irregular in outline and variable in density. In the beam of slit-lamp, the opacities have an appearance like *'bread-crumb'*. A very characteristic sign is the appearance of iridescent-coloured particles the so-called *'polychromatic lustre'* of reds, greens and blues. A diffuse yellow-haze is seen in the adjoining cortex. Slowly the opacity spreads in the rest of the cortex, and finally the entire lens becomes opaque, giving chalky-white appearance. Deposition of calcium is common in the later stages.

Anterior cortical complicated cataract

Anterior cortical complicated cataract may also occur in anterior segment lesion, such as glaucoma, hypopyon corneal ulcer and acute iritis. Earliest change is appearance of vacuole below the anterior capsule followed by opacities in the neighbouring cortical fibres and thickening of anterior capsule.

Note. Cataract can also obscure the view of the fundus, making the evaluation of posterior segment very difficult. Also it is very important to determine whether vision loss is due to the cataract or due to some pathologies in posterior segment prior to any surgical intervention.

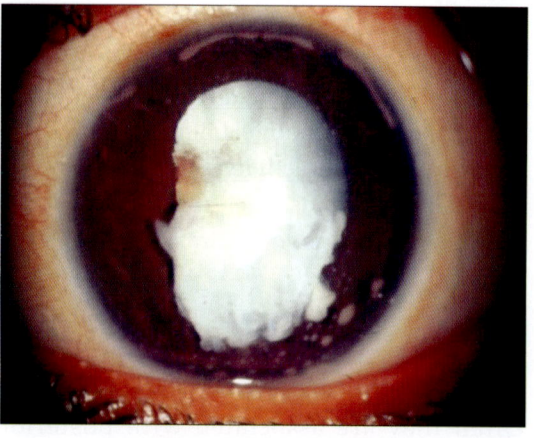

Fig. 4.6.4 *Complicated cataract.*

POSTERIOR SEGMENT COMPLICATIONS

1. CYSTOID MACULAR OEDEMA

Etiopathogenesis

Cystoid macular oedema (CME) is caused by cystic accumulation of intraretinal fluid in the outer plexiform and inner nuclear layers of the retina as a result of the breakdown of the blood–retinal barrier. It can complicate virtually any type of acute or chronic, anterior or posterior uveitis.

Common causes of uveitic CME are intermediate uveitis, pars planitis, Behçet's disease.

Exact pathogenesis of uveitic CME remains unclear. Usually CME develops when excess fluid accumulates within the retina of macular region (both extracellularly and intracellularly), which is primarily thought to occur following disruption of the blood–retinal barrier. This fluid accumulation disturbs cell function and retinal architecture. In uveitic eyes, this disruption of blood–retinal barrier is believed to occur with the release of inflammatory mediators.

Müller cells function as metabolic pumps and are thought to play an important role in keeping the macula dehydrated. Intracellular fluid accumulation in these Müller cells cause significant damage to the metabolic pump action of retina and further reduce macular retinal function. Vitreous traction at the macula also has been proposed as another causative factor for the development of uveitic CME.

Clinical feature

CME can cause profound visual loss and is one of the major causes of decreased vision in patients with uveitis.

Investigation

Fundus fluorescein angiography (FFA) is an important tool for the diagnosis and management of eyes with uveitic CME as it is more sensitive than clinical examination. However, patients' visual acuity has been found to correlate with the extent of macular thickening and not the severity of dye leakage on an FFA.

Optical coherance tomography (OCT). Thus, the gold standard of assessing and following up patients with uveitic CME is with serial optical coherence tomography (OCT).

2. EPIRETINAL MEMBRANE

Epiretinal membrane (ERM) is an avascular, fibrocellular membrane that proliferates on the inner surface of the retina and produces various degrees of visual impairment. Long-standing intraocular inflammation can lead to ERM formation, surface wrinkling and vitreomacular traction.

Pathogenesis

Epiretinal membranes contain glial cells, retinal pigment epithelial (RPE) cells, macrophages, fibrocytes and collagen fibres. ERM starts as small patchy areas of reflection from retinal surface which gradually progresses to form irregular, shiny sheet of membrane. In severe cases, it may lead to surface wrinkling and potentially to massive retinal folding.

Most of the time, these membranes are asymptomatic.

Clinical features

The most common presenting symptoms of ERM are decreased visual acuity, metamorphosis, micropsia and macropsia. The severity of symptoms is related to the involvement of macula and the thickness of ERM.

Signs. During biomicroscopical examination of fundus with a +90D or +78D lens, an ERM is seen as a glistening transparent, translucent membrane. Retinal changes associated with ERM can be surface wrinkling, vasculature distortion, cystoid macular oedema or pseudohole. Fundus examination with a blue filter is often helpful.

Grading. ERM has been classified into three grades:
- *Grade 1:* Cellophane membrane causing irregular wrinkling of the inner retina + no elevated edge of ERM.
- *Grade 2:* ERM with full-thickness retinal distortion + elevated edge of ERM elevated + less than half of ERM is opaque causing

obscuration of underlying retina and vasculature.
- *Grade 3:* Thick opaque membrane + half of the ERM opaque, causing marked obscuration and distortion of the underlying retina and vasculature.

Investigation

Fundus fluorescein angiography (FFA) has a limited role in diagnosis and follow-up of an ERM.

Optical coherence tomography (OCT) is very useful to monitor the progression of the membrane.

3. RETINAL DETACHMENT

Retinal detachment in uveitis can be of following types:
- *Exudative (serous) retinal detachment* can present as a part of the inflammatory process, e.g. Vogt-Koyanagi-Harada syndrome.
- *Rhegmatogenous or tractional retinal detachment* caused by traction secondary to intraocular inflammation, e.g. acute retinal necrosis syndrome.

Causes

Type of retinal detachment seen in uveitis and their common causes are listed in Table 4.6.1.

Table 4.6.1 *Common causes of retinal detachment in uveitis*

Type of retinal detachment associated with uveitis	Common causes
Exudative (serous) retinal detachment	Vogt-Koyanagi-Harada syndrome, sympathetic ophthalmia, posterior scleritis
Combination of rhegmatogenous and tractional retinal detachment	Toxoplasmic retinochoroiditis, pars planitis, Behçet's disease, Acute retinal necrosis syndrome, cytomegalovirus retinitis, ocular toxocariasis

Panuveitis and infectious uveitic entities are most frequently associated with combination of rhegmatogenous and tractional retinal detachment. Any substantial posterior uveitis can resutl into vitreoretinal traction which can lead to tractional retinal detachment. Rhegmatogenous detachment can supervene, if traction is adequate and it becomes very difficult to identify the sole mechanism of detachment in such cases. Usually vitreoretinal traction, resulting from intraocular inflammation, can often cause retinal elevations that are characteristically self-limiting with adequate control of inflammation. Tractional change is a characteristic feature of ocular toxocariasis. Retinal vasculitis has a tendency to produce traction specifically along the line of large retinal vessels. ARN and CMV retinitis frequently lead to retinal detachments that are difficult to repair because of multiple, large, posterior retinal breaks. Pars plana vitrectomy (PPV) and endolaser treatment with silicone oil tamponade are required to repair the detachment and remove the epiretinal membranes. When PVR is present, combined sclera buckling and PPV is often required. Thus, the prognosis in eyes with uveitis and retinal detachment is particularly poor. Also it is important to note that a chronic rhegmatogenous retinal detachment can often lead to development of intraocular inflammation.

Exudative retinal detachment is typically a feature of severe choroidal inflammation, for example, sympathetic uveitis or VKH syndrome and posterior scleritis.

Combined tractional and rhegmatogenous retinal detachment in uveitis

Abnormal vitreoretinal adhesions and tissue shrinkage are the two important components of retinal detachment in uveitis. In intraocular inflammation, abnormal adhesions exist between the vitreous and inflammatory fibrous or neovascular tissue. Shrinkage of fibrous tissue can result in the detachment of retina. Contraction of these fibrous bands can cause a retinal tear which in turn causes a rhegmatogenous detachment.

4. RETINAL ISCHAEMIA AND NEOVASCULARISATION

Intraocular inflammation can affect retinal circulation and sometimes can lead to vascular occlusion. The most important factor for development of retinal neovascularisation is retinal hypoxia which can result from vascular occlusion. Vascular occlusion is manifested clinically by capillary closure and loss of the retinal capillary bed.

Retinal angiogenesis, the pathophysiological process behind the process of neovascularisation, is controlled by the release of a complex family of stimulatory and inhibitory growth factors from hypoxic retina which stimulates neovascularisation on the retina, optic disc or choroid. The most important factor is vascular endothelial growth factor (VEGF) which targets mainly vascular endothelial cells but can also act on RPE cells.

Neovascularization most frequently arises at the disc or the capillary bed at the edge of an infarcted area of retina, most commonly from the wall of a thickened venule and often begin as a tuft of fine vessels. When these new vessels arise on or within one disc diameter of the optic nerve they are known as neovascularisation of the disc (NVD) and the new vessels arising one disc diameter away from the optic disc are called neovascularisation elsewhere (NVE).

All these new blood vessels lack barrier properties and rapidly and intensively leak fluorescein during angiography. These vessels are sight-threatening because they are fragile and tend to bleed to obscure the media. They are also associated with fibrosis and membrane formation which can lead to traction retinal detachment.

5. CHOROIDAL NEOVASCULAR MEMBRANE

Choroidal neovascular membrane (CNVM) is one of the most severe causes of visual impairment in patients with uveitis. A uveitic CNVM or inflammatory CNVM usually occurs adjacent to any post-inflammatory outer retinal or subretinal scar. CNVM secondary to uveitis can occur in both infectious and non-infectious uveitic entities. Common causes of inflammatory CNVM are listed in Table 4.6.2.

Majority of the inflammatory CNVMs are predominantly classical, and fundus fluorescein angiography is, therefore, excellent for diagnosis and monitoring.

Table 4.6.2 *Common causes of inflammatory CNVM*

Infectious uveitic entities	Non-infectious uveitic entities
Toxoplasmosis, toxocariasis, tuberculosis, viral retinopathies, presumed ocular histoplasmosis syndrome	Punctate inner choroidopathy (PIC), multifocal choroiditis (MFC), acute posterior multifocal placoid pigment epitheliopathy (APMPPE), Vogt-Koyanagi-Harada (VKH) disease, Behçet's disease, serpiginous choroiditis

PHTHISIS BULBI

Phthisis is the dreaded complication of uveitis. Long-standing inflammation can lead to deposition of exudates and cyclitic membrane over the ciliary body surface leading to diminished function or destruction of ciliary processes. This can result into decrease or cessation of aqueous production resulting in hypotony. The definition of ocular hypotony is debatable, but it can probably be considered when IOP reduces to less than 6 mm Hg. Patient experiences diminution in vision mostly due to massive fluctuating astigmatism and fundus examination can show macular choroidal folds with or without disc oedema often termed as hypotonous maculopathy. The collapsing of the scleral wall causes a wrinkling of the choroid and the retina which can be attributed to the cause of hypotonous maculopathy. If not treated, can lead to phthisis of the globe. A physical globe often assumes a quadrilateral shape because of the action of four recti muscles on a hypotonous eyeball.

Development of phthisis bulbi can be divided into three overlapping stages:

Stage of atrophic bulbi without shrinkage is the initial stage of loss of function of ocular tissues which occurs due to continued inflammation and loss of nutritional support. In this stage:

- Shape of globe is maintained.
- Vision is completely lost.
- Lens becomes cataractous.
- Retina develops serous detachment and atrophic changes.
- IOP is raised in early stages due to inflammatory glaucoma.

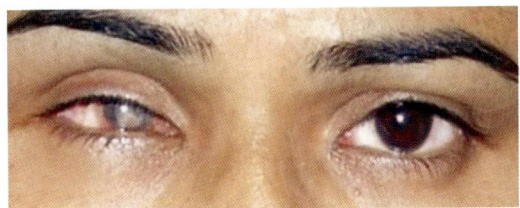

Fig. 4.6.5 *Phthisis bulbi.*

Stage of atrophic bulbi with shrinkage occurs due to continued ciliary body dysfunction. In this stage:

- IOP is lowered.
- Cornea becomes oedematous and vascularised.
- Anterior chamber is collapsed.
- Eyeball becomes smaller and square-shaped (maintained by four recti).

Atrophic bulbi with disorganisation is the final stage known as *phthisis bulbi* (Fig. 4.6.5). In this stage, due to continued disorganisation of ciliary body:

- IOP is markedly lowered.
- Size of eyeball is markedly decreased.
- Cornea becomes sclera like.

Histopathological examination at this stages reveals:

- Disorganization of all the intraocular tissues.
- Calcification may occur in Bowman's layer of cornea, lens and retina.
- Intraocular ossification (bone formation) may occur due to metaplasia in the retinal pigment epithelium, in the end stage of phthisis bulbi.
- Sclera becomes markedly thickened.

BIBLIOGRAPHY

1. AskMayoExpert. Uveitis. Rochester, Minn.: Mayo Foundation for Medical Education and Research; 2014.

2. Cunningham ET. Overview of uveitis. The Merck Manual Professional Edition. http://www. merck. com/mmpe/print/sec09/ch105/ch105a.html.

3. http://accessmedicine.mhmedical.com/ content.aspx? bookid=387 & sectionid = 40229324 & jumpsection ID = 40231264 & Resultclick = 2.

4. Parekh A, et al. Risk factors associated with intraocular pressure increase in patients with uveitis treated with the fluocinoloneacetonide implant. JAMA Ophthalmology. In press.

5. Riordan-Eva P, et al. Uveitis. In: Vaughan & Asbury's General Ophthalmology, 18th ed. New York: The McGraw-Hill Companies; 2011.

6. Rosenbaum JT. Uveitis: Etiology, clinical manifestations, and diagnosis. http://www. uptodate.com/home.

7. Rosenbaum JT. Uveitis: Treatment. http:// www.uptodate.com/home.

8. Uveitis. Natural Medicines Comprehensive Database. http://naturaldatabase.therapeutic research.com.

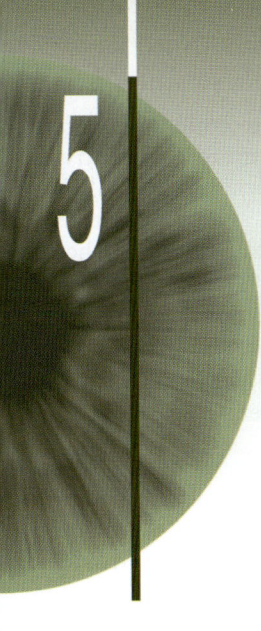

MANAGEMENT OF UVEITIS

5.1 CLINICAL APPROACH TO UVEITIS

Introduction
• Aims of clinical work-up

History Taking in Uveitis
History of presnet illness
• Demographics
• Diet, domestic and personal history
• Symptoms of uveitis
Past and family history
• Past history
• Family history

Systemic Work-up
• Systemic history
• Systemic examination

Ocular Examination
• Examination of lid and adnexa
• Examination of conjunctiva
• Examination of cornea
• Examination of anterior chamber
• Examination of pupil
• Examination of iris
• Examination of lens
• Evaluation of IOP
• Examination of vitreous
• Examination of fundus

Follow-up Examination

INTRODUCTION

Uveitis is a distinct ocular inflammation which encompasses a multitude of diseases. The underlying cause can be attributed to local ocular immune dysregulation, or may be part of a systemic disease. A meticulous approach to uveitis plays a pivotal role in the identification of etiology, anatomical localisation, and pathological involvement. In the diagnosis of uveitis, such as Fuchs uveitis syndrome, Vogt-Koyanagi-Harada disease, laboratory analysis can contribute little and examination can clinch the diagnosis. Besides diagnosis, a thorough clinical examination is critical to administer treatment and to judge the response in both infectious and autoimmune forms.

Aims of clinical work-up are to identify, if the uveitis is:
• Anterior, intermediate, posterior or panuveitis.
• Granulomatous or non-granulomatous
• Unilateral or bilateral
• Idiopathic, autoimmune or due to infection
• Associated with systemic disease
• Stage of the disease

- Severity if active or resolving
- Associated ocular complications

Key to a targeted and an efficient patient evaluation is a thorough history, physical examination, and review of systems. With this information, the practitioner can generate a differential diagnosis and a subsequent strategy for laboratory evaluation and treatment. A meticulous elicitation of history of the systemic status will help direct the examination and supplement the various laboratory tests.

HISTORY TAKING IN UVEITIS

An elaborate history taking is the corner stone of the management of a case of uveitis. It has been estimated that more than 75% of diagnoses can be made on the basis of the medical history and a thorough systemic examination. Because of frequent association of uveitis with rheumatologic, infectious diseases, it is very important to look beyond the eye and to perform a thorough physical examination and to obtain a meticulous history to clinch the diagnosis.

HISTORY OF PRESENT ILLNESS

1. Demographics

Age

Age is an important factor in history taking as few conditions are known to occur more predominantly in some age group:

- *Children:* Juvenile rheumatoid arthritis, retinoblastoma, toxocariasis, masquerade syndrome
- *Young adults:* Pars planitis, multiple sclerosis, and Fuchs' heterochromic iridocyclitis
- *Middle age:* Reiter's syndrome, ankylosing spondylitis, acute multifocal posterior placoid epitheliopathy, Vogt-Koyanagi-Harada syndrome, Behçet's disease
- *Old age:* Large cell lymphoma or choroidal melanoma, endogenous endophthalmitis, masquerade syndrome

Note. However, it should be kept in mind that certain diseases, like toxoplasmosis, sarcoidosis and tuberculosis, can be found at any age.

Gender

Uveitis associated with juvenile rheumatoid arthritis is found much more frequently in females, while uveitis associated with ankylosing spondylitis and Reiter's syndrome is usually seen in males. Most of the patients with Behçet's disease are males.
- *Male predominance:* Juvenile rheumatoid arthritis, rheumatoid arthritis
- *Female predominance:* Ankylosing spondylitis, Reiter's syndrome, Behçet's disease

Race

Conditions, like ankylosing spondylitis, Reiter's syndrome, and other HLA-B27-associated arthritides are common in whites and sarcoidosis occurs most commonly in blacks. Vogt-Koyanagi-Harada syndromes are most prevalent in Asians. In the Mediterranean countries, Behçet's disease is more common.
- *Asians:* Behçet's disease and VKH syndrome
- *Middle Eastern population:* Behcet's disease
- *African American:* Sarcoidosis and syphilis
- *Caucasians:* HLA B27, white dot syndromes and multiple sclerosis.

Geographical location

Geographical location of the patient often helps us in diagnosis of certain conditions as few clinical entities are more commonly seen in the some specific parts of the world. For example, Behcet's disease is more common in countries situated along the old Silk Road, a trade route used for centuries by Greeks, Romans and Chinese. Reported rates of the disease is higher the countries, situated along this route and highest in two ends of the old silk road – Turkey and Japan.

• *Tuberculosis*	Developing countries
• *Histoplasmosis*	Mississippi-Ohio-Missouri river valleys
• *Coccidioidomycosis*	Southwest United States, Central and South America
• *Birdshot choroiditis*	USA
• *Lyme disease*	USA
• *Behcet's disease*	Turkey, Iraq, Saudi Arabia, Iran, Afghanistan, Pakistan, Northern Chiana, Mongolia, The Koreas and Japan

2. Diet, domestic and personal history

- *Dietary habits.* A history of the ingestion of raw or undercooked meat in toxoplasmosis. Persons who ingest unpasteurized milk are at risk of contracting tuberculosis and brucellosis.
- *History of contact with pets* (cat, dogs and pigs) is important when considering a diagnosis of ocular toxoplasmosis, cat-scratch disease and toxocarian.
- *History of exposure to sewers or rodent urine* may give us a clue for the diagnosis of leptospirosis
- *Farmers* are far more prone to develop brucellosis than the general population.
- *History of sexual activity and preferences* is a must in suspected cases of human immuno-deficiency virus (HIV) infection, syphilis, etc.

3. Symptoms of uveitis

The symptoms in a case of uveitis depend on various factors. These are: part of the uveal tract involved, presentation and course of the uveitic entity (acute or chronic) and onset (sudden and insidious). For example, a case of anterior uveitis can present with an acute, chronic, or recurrent form. The severity of symptoms can range from very severe symptoms in a case of sudden onset acute uveitis to nil or minimal symptoms in a case of insidious-onset chronic anterior uveitis.

Ocular pain

The pain in iridocyclitis is due to ciliary spasm. The ciliary body is innervated by the trigeminal nerve, and pain caused by irritation of the nerve endings by the product of inflammation. The pain in uveitis can be variable and mostly described as a dull aching or a throbbing pain localized to the eye. Sometimes it can be associated with referred pain which seems to radiate over a larger area served by the trigeminal nerve.

Pain in scleritis is typically dull and boring in nature, exacerbated by eye movement, is worse at night often interfering with sleep, and characteristically wakens the patient from sleep.

Photophobia

Photophobia or intolerance to bright light is often accompanied by tearing (watering) and blepharospasm. Photophobia is usually caused by ciliary muscle spasm but can also be due to pupillary muscle involvement or corneal involvement.

Redness of eye

Redness of the eye in uveitis is primarily due to ciliary injection or circumcorneal injection, or "ciliary flush." It is manifested by a ring of dilated or engorged episcleral vessels radiating from the limbus.

Blurred vision and floaters

Anterior uveitis. Blurred vision is usually caused by ciliary spasm or in early stage cloudy media.

Intermediate uveitis most often presents with floaters and blurred vision. Floaters occur because of shadows cast by the products of inflammation in vitreous, like vitreous cells, debris, etc. Most common cause of decreased vision in these patients is cystoid macular oedema (CME).

Posterior uveitis usually presents with decreased vision, floaters, photopsias, metamorphopsia, scotomata, nyctalopia or a combination of these. The decreased vision may be due to the primary effects of inflammation involving retina and choroid, often directly affecting macular function or due to the complications of inflammation like CME, epiretinal membrane (ERM), retinal ischaemia, and choroidal neovascular membrane (CNVM).

PAST AND FAMILY HISTORY

- Previous episodes of uveitis, and type of treatment are important in recurrent uveitis.
- Past history of trauma or surgery would be useful in lens-induced uveitis or sympathetic ophthalmitis.
- Family history of infectious diseases may be positive in patient with infectious uveitis.

SYSTEMIC WORK-UP

SYSTEMIC HISTORY

A detailed history of various systemic diseases should be taken.

- *History of tuberculosis* should be taken in patients with vasculitis, choroiditis, etc.

• *Endogenous endophthalmitis* is more common in old patients with diabetes mellitus, renal failure and with patients on immuno-suppressant. It is of paramount importance to look for the evidence of septic foci, like boil, carbuncle, abscess, etc. in such patients.

Arthralgia

An elaborate history of joint pain should be taken especially in patients presenting with non-granulomatous uveitis. Information on type of joint involved, onset, timings and nature of the joint pain often provides useful clue to the diagnosis of a case of uveitis.

Uveitic entities with arthralgias include Behçet's disease, sarcoidosis, SLE, juvenile idiopathic arthritis (JIA), Lyme disease, syphilis, psoriatic arthritis, Reiter's syndrome, ulcerative colitis.

SYSTEMIC EXAMINATION

Skin lesions

Rashes can be seen in various conditions with uveitis. Malar butterfly rashes can be seen in patients with systemic lupus erythematosus (SLE). Thickening of skin can be seen in patients with scleroderma. Increased cutaneous sensitivity can be seen in various conditions including SLE, Behçet's disease. Acne-like eruptions are often seen in certain conditions, like Behçet's disease and it should be differentiated from similar skin lesions seen in patient on oral corticosteroid therapy.

• *Nodules.* Sarcoidosis, SLE, leprosy, Crohn disease, ulcerative colitis.
• *Rash.* Syphilis, Lyme disease, Reiter's syndrome, leprosy, sarcoidosis, herpes zoster, Behçet's disease, psoriasis, SLE, Kawasaki disease
• *Erythema nodosum.* Behçet's disease, sarcoidosis, acute posterior multifocal placoid pigment epitheliopathy (APMPPE), tuberculosis
• *Vitiligo, poliosis.* Vogt-Koyanagi-Harada (VKH) syndrome
• *Keratoderma blennorrhagicum.* Reactive arthritis

Hair loss and abnormalities

Hair loss and abnormalities may be associated with uveitis:

• *Hair loss* can be seen in patient with Vogt-Koyanagi-Harada (VKH) syndrome, SLE and syphilis.
• *Abnormalities,* like poliosis, are common in VKH patients and madarosis can be seen in leprosy patients.
• *Increased sensitivity to hair* is often complained by patients with VKH.

Examination of ear, nose and throat

Examination of ear, nose and throat is also important. Relapsing polychondritis is a rare small-vessel vasculitis which predominantly affect cartilaginous structures of the body, such as pinna of the ear, nasal cartilage, larynx and trachea. Relapsing polychondritis should be ruled out in patients with episcleritis and scleritis. Saddle nose deformity is characterised by a loss of height of the nose, because of collapse of the nasal bridge. Saddle nose deformity in a patient of uveitis should give rise to the suspicion of conditions, like Wegener's granulomatosis, leprosy, syphilis or relapsing polychondritis.

• *Bilateral ear pinna inflammation.* Relapsing polychondritis
• *Saddle nose deformity.* Syphilis, Wegener's granulomatosis (SLE), relapsing polychondritis
• *Sinusitis.* Sarcoidosis, Wegener's granulomatosis
• *Salivary/lacrimal gland swelling.* Sarcoidosis, lymphoma
• *Lymphadenopathy.* Lymphoma, HIV.

Gastrointestinal

Oral ulcer. Aphthous ulceration can be seen in patients with Behçet's disease, reactive arthritis, SLE, herpes simplex, Reiter's syndrome, ulcerative colitis, etc.

Gastrointestinal disorders. Though uncommon, uveitis can be associated with Crohn disease, ulcerative colitis.

Central nervous system

Neurological signs are common during prodromal stage of Vogt-Koyanagi-Harada syndrome (VKH) and can include neck stiffness, headache and confusion. Patients of VKH can have auditory symptoms, like tinnitus, dysacusis (difficulty in processing details of sound due to distortion in frequency or intensity), vertigo, etc. Similarly demyelinating diseases, like multiple sclerosis should be ruled out in cases with intermediate uveitis, retinal vasculitis, etc.

- *Headaches.* Vogt-Koyanagi-Harada syndrome (VKH), tuberculosis, herpes zoster, large cell lymphoma, cryptococcal meningitis, toxoplasmosis
- *Auditory/vestibular.* VKH disease
- *Cranial neuropathy.* Lyme disease, sarcoidosis, multiple sclerosis, syphilis, herpes simplex virus
- *Cerebral vasculitis.* Acute posterior multifocal placoid pigment epitheliopathy (APMPPE).

Pulmonary

Pulmonary involvement is common in various uveitic conditions, especially granulomatous uveitic entities. It is very important to elicit a proper history regarding symptoms, like hemoptysis, dyspnoea, cough, sputum, chest pain and fatigue.

- *Cough/breathlessness.* Tuberculosis, sarcoidosis, *Pneumocystis carinii*, Wegener's granulomatosis
- *Nodules/hilar adenopathy/infiltrates.* Ocular histoplasmosis, sarcoidosis (hilar adenopathy), malignancy, tuberculosis, *Pneumocystis carinii* pneumonia.

Genitourinary system

Examination of genitourinary system is important as many uveitic entities can have genitourinary involvement which can help one to clinch the diagnosis. However, history taking or examination of genitourinary system should be conducted tactfully so that the patient does not become embarrassed, or offended. Recurrent genital ulcer is a common feature of Behcet's disease, but urethritis is not common feature of the disease. Presence of urethritis in a uveitic patient with joint pain can give clue to the diagnosis of reactive arthritis (previously called Reiter's syndrome). Also circinate balanitis is a common feature of reactive arthritis. Circinate

balanitis is a form of skin inflammation where skin around the shaft and tip (glans) of the penis become inflamed and scale.

- *Genital ulcers.* Behçet's disease, Reiter's syndrome, syphilis
- *Hematuria.* Wegener's granulomatosis, polyarteritis nodosa (PAN), systemic lupus erythematosus (SLE)
- *Circinate balanitis.* Ankylosing spondylitis, Reiter syndrome
- *Nephritis.* PAN, Wegener's granulomatosis, tubulointerstitial nephritis and uveitis (TINU)

OCULAR EXAMINATION

A. External examination and examination of lid and adnexa

A careful examination of lid and adnexa can provide important clue in patients with uveitis.

- *Kaposi's sarcoma* may appear as purplish-red to bright-red and highly vascular with surrounding telangiectatic vessels in upper eyelid.
- *Enlargement of the lacrimal gland* can be seen in sarcoidosis.
- *Characteristic skin lesions or scar marks* can be seen in a case herpes zoster ophthalmicus (HZO). Herpes zoster ophthalmicus is defined as herpes zoster involvement of the ophthalmic division of the fifth cranial nerve. Skin lesion at the tip, side, or root of the nose is a strong predictor of ocular inflammation and corneal denervation in HZO and is known as Hutchinson's sign. The skin rash of HZO evolves through erythema, macules, papules, and finally pustulation and crusting. Periorbital oedema and ptosis may or may not be present. It should be noted that a minority of patients in HZO can have only ophthalmic symptoms and no skin lesions with dermatomal distribution pain (zoster non- herpete).

B. Examination of conjunctiva

- *Ciliary injection should be differentiated from conjunctival hyperaemia* (Table 5.1.1). Conjunctival hyperactive with discharge is usually seen in conjunctivitis. It is important to note that purulent conjunctivitis can be seen in Reiter's syndrome and psoriatic arthritis.

Table 5.1.1 *Ciliary injection versus conjunctival hyperaemia*

Ciliary injection	Conjunctival hyperaemia
Engorgement of episcleral vessels	Engorgement of anterior and posterior conjunctival vessels
Bright reddish violet in colour	Bright red in colour
Radially arranged blood vessels	Irregular branching vessels
Most intense near limbus	Most intense in fornix
Blood vessels do not move with conjunctiva	Moves with conjunctiva
Blood flow is from limbus to fornix	Blood flow is from fornix to limbus

- Ciliary injection or "ciliary flush," is manifested by a ring of dilated episcleral vessels radiating from the limbus. It should be distinguished from the deeper and more peripheral injection of scleritis and from the sectoral or diffuse injection of episcleritis. Also it is of paramount importance to differentiate ciliary injection of uveitis from conjunctivitis by the lack of involvement of the fornix and palpebral conjunctiva and absence of symptoms like discharge.
- *Perilimbal vitiligo* is often observed in patients with Vogt-Koyanagi-Harada syndrome and is known as *Suguira's sign.*
- *Subconjunctival haemorrhage* can be seen in patients with leptospirosis.
- *Nodules or any mass like lesion.* Nodular scleritis often associated with severe tenderness. Conjunctival nodules are often seen in patients with sarcoidosis. Sarcoid nodules are millet-shaped discrete solid nodules of variable size. They can be single or multiple
- *The sine qua non of scleritis* is the presence of scleral oedema and congestion of the deep episcleral plexus. Slit-lamp examination using red-free light is extremely helpful in determining the pattern and depth of episcleral vascular congestion and engorgement. In scleritis, the sclera assumes a violaceous hue. It is very important to examine patients in daylight with the unaided eye to note the subtle colour differences of the vessels. Also inflamed scleral vessels have a crisscross pattern. They are adherent to the sclera and cannot be moved with a cotton-tipped applicator. Engorged scleral vessels cannot be blanched with 10% phenylephrine, whereas phenylephrine easily blanches engorged vessels in the superficial episcleral and conjunctival plexuses. A tender nodule can indicate nodular scleritis which need systemic workup.

C. Examination of cornea

Keratic precipitates. Due to the convection current in anterior chamber, the circulating inflammatory cells can deposit in corneal endothelium which is known as keratic precipitates (KPs). KPs are normally deposited in inferior half of the cornea in base down triangle-shaped configuration (Arlt's triangle).

- *Mutton-fat or large KPs* can be seen in granulomatous uveitis.
- *Fine KPs* are seen in herpetic eye diseases and in other non-granulomatous conditions.
- *Stellate or star-shaped KPs* are seen in Fuch's heterochromic iridocyclitis.
- *Old KPs* are pigmented, have crenate margins.

Band-shaped keratopathy. Deposition of calcium hydroxyapatite in Bowman's layer can be seen in conditions, like chronic uveitis, and juvenile idiopathic arthritis. It typically begins at the periphery of the interpalpebral region and spread centrally. If visual axis is involved, it can cause marked diminution of vision. On slit-lamp examination, small clear dot-like areas are observed giving "Swiss cheese" appearance to band keratopathy. These clear small dot-like areas represent the location where corneal nerves penetrate Bowman's layer.

Scar or ulceration
- Cornea should be examined properly for superficial or deep scar, dendritic epithelial keratitis to detect keratouveitis.
- Stromal thinning and epithelial ulceration due to inflammation may be observed in

peripheral ulcerative keratitis (PUK). PUK may also be the first sign of a systemic necrotizing vasculitis, like rheumatoid arthritis, Wegener's grnaulomatosis, etc.

D. Examination of anterior chamber

Cells. Cells in the aqueous humour is generally seen after inflammation of the iris and ciliary body. Cells in the anterior chamber are counted using slit-lamp with a beam of 1 x 1 mm slit and graded according the SUN working group grading scheme (Table 5.1.2).

Table 5.1.2 *SUN working group grading scheme for cells in anterior chamber*

Grade	Cells in field of 1 mm by 1 mm slit beam
0	< 1
0.5+	1–5
1+	6–15
2+	16–25
3+	26–50
4+	> 50

- Polymorphonuclear leucocytes are the predominant cells in an acute case and in chronic cases, lymphocytes, plasma cells, monocytes and macrophages are seen.
- Larger cells are generally swollen macrophages or clumps of lymphocytes.
- Inflammatory anterior chamber cells are generally white in colour and should not be confused with pigmented cells. Pigmented cells can be iris pigments, dead erythrocytes, or macrophages filled with pigment like melanin.
- Iris pigments can be seen in the anterior chamber after dilatation and should be distinguished from cells.

Cells in aqueous humour migrate across the iris and ciliary vessels and depending on the nature and severity of inflammation, their numbers and types vary. In the aqueous, the cells are seen circulating due to the convection current.

Flare. In normal condition, aqueous humour is optically empty and if a slit-lamp beam is passed through, it cannot be seen. In case of inflammation, when breakdown of the blood–aqueous barrier occurs, there is increased protein content in the aqueous and if slit beam is obliquely aimed across the anterior chamber, the path of the beam can be seen, which is termed flare. Flare is graded according to the scheme proposed by SUN classification (Table 5.1.3).

Table 5.1.3 *SUN working group grading scheme for anterior chamber flaire*

Grade	Description
0	None
1+	Faint
2+	Moderate (iris and lens details clear)
3+	Marked (iris and lens details hazy)
4+	Intense (fibrin or plastic aqueous)

Flare is often the first sign of uveitis and it may persist despite adequate control of inflammation.

Flare can also be measured using a laser flare photometry, which quantifies anterior chamber protein by measuring light scattering of a helium–neon laser beam in the anterior chamber. (see Chapter 3)

Hypopyon. Often the inflammatory circulating cells particularly leucocytes can deposit at the bottom of the anterior chamber and can form hypopyon. Thus it is very essential to examine the area of the inferior limbus in uveitic patient. SUN classification has recommended that presence or absence of a hypopyon should be recorded separately while documenting a case of uveitis. It should be kept in mind that hypopyon frequently occurs in patients with endophthalmitis and should always be ruled out especially in patients who had undergone recent intraocular surgery.

Causes of hypopyon

- HLA-B 27 ant uveitis
- Ankylosing spondylitis
- Behçet's disease
- Endophthalmitis
- *Drugs:* Rifabutin

Hypopyon seen in Behçet's disease is mobile and often visible only during gonioscopy (microhypopyon). *Often retained lens fragments, tumour cells can* deposit in anterior chamber and mimic hypopyon. These are known as pseudohypopyon.

Hyphema. In some rare cases, erythrocyte can sediment in anterior chamber causing hyphema. The causes of hyphema are listed below.

Causes of hyphema
- Viral uveitis
- Trauma
- Malignancies
- Fuchs
- Chronic uveitis with rubeosis
- Any severe uveitis
- Post anterior chamber taps

E. Examination of pupil

- *Pupillary reaction* in acute cases of iritis or iridocyclitis becomes sluggish or abolished and constriction of pupil occurs.
- *Posterior synechiae* Often the exudates released during acute inflammation causes plastering of posterior surface of iris with anterior capsule of the lens. These iridolenticular adhesions are known as posterior synechiae.
  – *Festooned pupil:* Due to the application of cycloplegic topicals, often some parts of the posterior synechiae dilate thus making the pupil festooned-shaped.
  – In cases of severe anterior chamber inflammation, the pupillary margin may become plastered to the lens capsule which is called annular or ring *synechiae or seclusio pupillae.*
  – And if the pupillary aperture is blocked by the exudates forming a membrane over it, then it is called *occlusio pupillae.*
- Similarly adhesion between iris and the cornea near the anterior chamber angle can occur due to inflammatory process and known as peripheral anterior synechiae (PAS).

Note. Posterior synechiae can lead to pupillary block glaucoma and peripheral anterior synechiae can cause secondary angle closure glaucoma.

- *Afferent pupillary defect* is seen in patients with neuroretinitis.

F. Examination of iris

Iris pattern. In acute iritis or iridocyclitis, iris loses its normal pattern due to imbibition of inflammatory exudates in it and such iris is often called muddy iris.

Iris nodules. Accumulations of inflammatory cells in the iris or on iris surface can be clinically noted as iris nodule. Nodules seen in pupillary borders are known as Koeppe nodule and nodules on the iris surface is known as Busacca's nodule. Iris nodules are seen in granulomatous uveitis.

Heterochromia. Comparison of the colour of iris between two eyes can detect heterochromia of iris which can be either hypochromic (abnormal eye is lighter than fellow eye) as seen in Fuch's heterochromic iridocyclitis or hyperchromic (abnormal eye is darker than fellow eye) as seen in melanosis of iris.

Iris atrophy is a characteristic feature of herpetic uveitis. Herpes viruses generally produces sector iris atrophy due to a occlusive vasculitis

Causes of iris atrophy:
- Viral infections
- Anterior segment ischaemia
- Leprosy
- Syphilis
- Previous attacks of angle-closure glaucoma
- Iatrogenic (previous intraocular surgery)

Roseolae. In syphilis, dilated, hyperaemia of the iris vessels are noted which is known as roseolae

G. Examination of lens

Posterior subcapsular cataract is a common complication after long-standing uveitis as well as chronic corticosteroid therapy.

H. Intraocular pressure (IOP)

Hypotony. Patients with acute iridocyclitis have low IOP due to infiltration of the ciliary body by inflammatory cells which lead to reduction of aqueous production.

Raised IOP. Release of prostaglandin during inflammation can also cause reduction in IOP.
- Sometimes patients with uveitis can present with significant rise in IOP. Conditions like herpes simplex uveitis, herpes zoster uveitis, Posner-Schlossman syndrome, and toxo-

plasmosis can present with rise of IOP in acute cases.

- In case of long-standing uveitis, extensive membrane formation over ciliary body or ciliary body detachment can cause ocular hypotony and eventual phthisis bulbi.

Cause of rise of intraocular pressure in uveitis:
- Clogging of trabecular meshwork with inflammatory cells
- Inflammation of trabecular meshwork fibres ("trabeculitis")
- Peripheral anterior synechiae
- Pupillary block from posterior synechiae, and
- Corticosteroid-induced IOP rise (steroid responder).

I. Examination of vitreous

- *Cells in the anterior vitreous or retrolental space* should be looked for after pupillary dilation. Though there is no standard grading system for vitreous cells, documentation of this finding is important for follow-up of a uveitic case.
- *Vitreous should be carefully examined* with a 78/90D and also with indirect ophthalmoscope with indentation for snowball opacities, snow-banking in pars plana region and vitreous strands.
- *For classifying vitreous haze*, SUN classification has adopted the National Eye Institute system for grading vitreous haze with the provison that the designation "trace" be recorded as 0.5+ (Table 5.1.4).

J. Examination of fundus

Optic disc should be carefully examined with the help of slit-lamp biomicroscopy. Disc

Table 5.1.4 *SUN working group grading for vitreous haze*

Grade	Description
0	Nil
0.5+	Trace
1+	Few opacities, mild blurring
2+	Significant blurring, but still visible
3+	Optic nerve visible, no vessels visible
4+	Dense opacity obscures optic nerve head

hyperaemia, disc oedema, or optic neuritis is seen in various uveitic conditions. Glaucomatous damage to the optic disc due to secondary glaucoma, neovascularisation of the optic disc, optic disc granuloma and optic atrophy may also occur in uveitic patients.

Examination of retinal vasculature for vasculitis, vascular sheathing, and accumulation of inflammatory cells around vessels is important. Vascular sheathing is seen as white parallel lines along vessels. Sometimes inflammatory exudates are seen around the vessels in patients with sarcoidosis, known as candle-wax drippings. Also it is important to determine whether retinal veins, retinal arteries, or both are affected as it can help in differential diagnosis of the uveitic entity (Table 5.1.5).

Table 5.1.5 *Causes of involvement of retinal vessels in uveitis*

Arterial involvement (arteritis)	Venous involvement (phlebitis)
• Acute retinal necrosis	• Sarcoidosis
• Systemic lupus erythematosus	• Frosted branch angiitis
• Behçet's disease	

Patch of inflammation. Careful examination of the posterior segment can reveal inflammatory patches in the fundus. It is important to distinguish such leisons whether it involves retina or choroid or both (Table 5.1.6). Sometimes these lesions are associated with subretinal fluid or localized haze in vitreous.

Retinal detachment. Often a patient can present with a retinal detachment. Exudative retinal detachments can be seen in a number of ocular inflammatory diseases like Vogt-Koyanagi-

Table 5.1.6 *Retinitis vs choroiditis*

Retinitis	Choroiditis
• Appears as a whitish patch	• Appears as yellowish patch
• Ill-defined margins	• Relatively well-defined margins
• Superficial	• Deeper (deep to the retinal blood vessels)

Harada syndrome. One should be able to distinguish rhegmatogenous retinal detachment from such cases, which require a surgical management. Sequelae to vasculitis can lead to development of traction retinal detachment and should be dealt properly.

Macular lesions. Meticulous examination of the fovea with slit-lamp biomicroscopy often helps to identify cystoid macular oedema, choroidal neovascular membrane or sight-threatening inflammatory lesions, like serpiginous choroiditis. Cystoid macular oedema is a common in patients with uveitis which, if long-standing, can lead to formation of macular hole.

FOLLOW-UP EXAMINATION

The initial follow-up of uveitis patients should be scheduled between 1 and 7 days, depending on severity and should include visual acuity, IOP measurement, slit-lamp examination, assessment of cells and flare, indirect ophthalmoscopy and visual field examination using Amsler grid/automated perimetry. Fundus evaluation should be performed to look for complications, such as cystoid macular oedema, epiretinal membranes, macular holes, tractional bands, vitreous haemorrhage, secondary glaucoma or retinal detachment.

BIBLIOGRAPHY

1. Biswas J. Pathology of Uveitis. Afro-Asian Journal of Ophthalmology 1999;9:206–9.
2. Cunningham ET, Nozik RA. Duane's Clinical Ophthalmology. Vol. 37. Philadelphia: Lippincott-Raven; 1997. Uveitis: Diagnostic approach and ancillary analysis; pp. 1–25.
3. Cunningham ET., Jr Uveitis in children. OculImmunolInflamm. 2000;8:251–61.
4. Deschenes J, Murray PI, Rao NA, Nussenblatt RB. International Uveitis Study Group (IUSG): clinical classification of uveitis. Ocul Immunol Inflamm. 2008;16(1):1–2.
5. Diagnosis and treatment of uveitis. WB Saunders Company, Philadelphia 2002;731–812.
6. Harper SL, Chorich LJ, Foster CS. Diagnosis of uveitis. In: Foster CS, Vitale AT, editors. Diagnosis and Treatment of Uveitis. Philadelphia: WB Saunders; 2002. pp. 79–103.
7. Inungu J, Lewis A, Mustafa Y, Wood J, O'Brien S, Verdun D. HIV Testing among Adolescents and Youth in the United States: Update from the 2009 Behavioral Risk Factor Surveillance System. Open AIDS J. 2011;5:80–5.
8. Jabs DA, Johns CJ. Ocular involvement in chronic sarcoidosis. Am J Ophthalmol 1986;102:297.
9. Jabs DA, Nussenblatt RB, Rosenbaum JT. Standardization of Uveitis Nomenclature (SUN) Working Group: Standardization of uveitis nomenclature for reporting clinical data. Results of the first international workshop. Am J Ophthalmol 2005;140:509–16.
10. Nussenblatt RB, Palestine AG, Chan CC, Roberge F. Standardization of vitreal inflammatory activity in intermediate and posterior uveitis. Ophthalmology 1985;92(4):467–71.
11. Nussenblatt RB, Whitcup SM, Palestine AG. Examination of the patient with uveitis. Uveitis: Fundamentals and Clinical Practice, 2nd ed. St. Louis: Mosby; 1996; pp. 58–68.
12. Posterior Segment Intraocular Inflammation Guidelines. Edited by John V Forrester, Anabella Okada, David Ben Erza, Shigeaki Ohno. ISBN 90-6299-167-X
13. Rajapure V, Tirwa R, Poudyal H, Thakur N. Prevalence and risk factors associated with sexually transmitted diseases (STDs) in Sikkim. J Community Health 2013;38:156–62.
14. Rao NA, Forster DJ, Aigsburger JJ. General approach to the uveitis patient. The Uvea: Uveitis and Intraocular Neoplasms. Vol. 2. New York: Gower Medical Publishing; 1992, pp. 2.1–2.18.
15. Rathinam SR, Namperumalsamy P. Global variation and pattern changes in epidemiology of uveitis. Indian J Ophthalmol 2007;55:173–83.
16. Smith RE, Nozik RA. 2. Baltimore: Williams and Wilkins; 1986. Uveitis: Goals of Uveitis Management; A clinical approach to diagnosis and management; pp. 23–24.
17. Suttorp-Schulten Rothova A. The possible impact of uveitis in blindness: A literature survey. Br J Ophthalmology 1996; 80:844–8.
18. Yeh S, Grace A. Levy-Clarke, Nussenblatt RB. Introduction to Uveitis. Chap 90. In: Albert DM, Jakobiec FA, (Eds). Principles and Practice of Ophthalmology. Philadelphia:WB Saunders Co 2008;1:1113–23.

5.2 INVESTIGATIONS IN UVEITIS

Introduction
- Clinical workup checklist
- List of investigations in uveitis

Laboratory Investigations
- Haematological investigations
  - Routine blood investigations
  - Serological tests
- Urinalysis
- Stool examination for parasites

Skin Tests
- Mountoux test
- Histoplasmin skin test
- Kveim test
- Behçet's skin puncture test
- Cutaneous anergy

Radiological Tests
- X-rays
- CT scan

Nuclear Medicine Study
- Gallium study

Ancillary Test in Uveitis
- Funds autofluorescence
- Laser flare photometry and laser flare cell photometry
- Ultrasound biomicroscopy
- Fluorescein angiography
- Indocyanine green angiography
- Optical coherance tomography
- Ultrasonography
- Electrophysiological tests in uveitis

INTRODUCTION

Uveitis encompasses entities of varying duration, severity, location and above all a vast plethora of possible etiologies with quite similar and overlapping presentations. Examination of a patient with uveitis needs to be meticulous as the incidence of association with systemic disease is high.

The biggest challenge in uveitis is identification of the cause. One strategy used by nearly all clinicians is the formulation of a list of potential diagnoses and from a brief interaction with the patient, followed by a focused history and examination. Then appropriate investigations shorten the list of diagnostic possibilities.

Although a thorough clinical and systemic investigation is important. Investigations which include laboratory test, ancillary investigations like FFA, ultrasound, imaging studies like optical coherence tomography are often necessary to identify the cause of uveitis.

The list of investigations described here include a battery of tests because of its varied etiology. However, an experienced ophthalmologist soon learns to order a few investigations of considerable value which will differ in individual case depending upon the information gained from a through clinical workup.

Clinical workup and check list

Before ordering investigations, following should be ensured:
- Uveitis oriented history
- Complete ophthalmic examination
- Identification of anatomic location
- Extent of uveitis
- Overall systemic evaluation
- Compare with clinical characteristics of known uveitic entities
- Make short list of etiological possibilities
- Order 'tailored' laboratory tests to establish/rule out such etiology

List of Investigations in uveitis

Investigations in uveitis can be grouped as below:
- Laboratory investigations:
- Skin tests
- Radiological tests
- Nuclear medicine
- Ancillary tests
- Pathological tests (described in Chapter 5.3)

LABORATORY INVESTIGATIONS

- *Certain uveitic entities may not require laboratory tests* like Fuchs' heterochromic iridocyclitis, uveitis due to trauma, first attack of non-granulomatous acute anterior uveitis, an unequivocal case of Vogt-Koyanagi-Harada (VKH) syndrome and sympathetic ophthalmia.
- *No standard laboratory evaluation exists* for the patients with uveitis, except in screening for syphilis and possibly sarcoidosis because both of which can present in myriad of ways.
- *Certain laboratory tests can be done in general* to all uveitis patients. These are erythrocyte sedimentation rate (ESR), total and differential white blood cell count.
- *Tailored laboratory investigations relevant to the clinical entity* in question is the right approach in identifying the etiology of a uveitic entity.

Laboratory tests can be grouped as below:
  I. *Haematological investigations*
    A. *Routine blood investigations*
      - TLC and DLC
      - ESR
      - Blood sugar
    B. *Serological tests*
      - Antibody detection in infectious uveitis
      - Rheumatoid factor
      - Antinuclear antibody
      - Lupus anticogulant
      - Serological tests for syphilis
      - Toxocara serology
      - Serological tests for toxoplasmosis
      - Serological tests for herpetic group of viruses
      - Serological tests for HIV
      - Chalamydia serology
      - Borrelia titers in lyme disease
      - Leptospira antibodies
      - Bacterial serology
      - Brucellosis antibody test
    C. Other haemotological test
    D. Detection of major histocompatibility antigens
  II. *Urinalysis*
  III. *Stool examination*

I. HAEMATOLOGICAL INVESTIGATIONS

A. ROUTINE BLOOD INVESTIGATIONS

Routine blood tests are of limited value for the diagnosis of specific causes of uveitis. However, they are important when immunosuppressants are planned for the treatment of uveitis. They also provide a baseline to note therapeutic response and drug side effects.

1. *Total and differential counts* (TLC and DLC) sometimes could give clues to the etiology of the disease like:

- *Leucocytosis*, i.e. total count can be increased in bacterial infections
- *Eosinophilia* is seen in patients with sarcoidosis and parasitic infection
- *Lymphocytosis* is seen in tuberculosis and viral infections

2. *Erythrocyte sedimentation rate (ESR)* is raised in connective tissue disorders, sarcoidosis and also in infectious conditions such as tuberculosis, syphilis, etc.

3. *Estimation of the CD4/CD8 lymphocyte ratio* is an important haematological investigation in patients with suspected HIV infection. This ratio is said to have a sensitivity of 85% but a lower specificity.

Normal CD4 and CD8 count is above 400/cumm and 200–800/cumm, respectively. The CD4/CD8 ratio is usually 2.0 and in AIDS patient becomes reversed with a value of 0.5–1.0.

4. *Blood sugar leves* should be estimated to have baseline values and to rule out diabetis mellitus.

5. *Blood uric acid* should be estimated in patients suspected of having goute.

B. SEROLOGICAL TESTS

1. Antibody detection in infectious uveitis

Detection of specific antibodies to infectious agents with the various available laboratory tests helps us to click a diagnosis of infectious organism causing uveitis. *Facts which are very important to note before going to the individual antibody detection* laboratory methods include:

- *Infants are born with* very low levels of self-synthesized serum immunoglobulins and majority of an infant's IgG has been transferred transplacentally from mother.

- *IgG synthesis* in human usually begins about 2 months of age and normal adult levels of IgG is attained during late adolescence.
- *IgM is a relatively large molecule* to cross placenta, thus detectable IgM titles at any age indicates exposure to an infectious agent.

Tests available for antibody detection include:
- *Radioimmunoassay* (RIA)
- *Enzyme-linked immunosorbent assay* (ELISA)
- *Immunofluorescent assay* (IFA) systems: Indirect variants of this test are the fluorescent treponemal antibody (FTA) test used to detect syphilis and the indirect fluorescent antibody test for toxoplasmosis.
- *Complement fixation* (CF)
- *Agglutination and flocculation tests*
- *Indirect, or passive, agglutination* is used in the latex agglutination test for Toxoplasma spp., and to detect IgM rheumatoid factor.
- *Venereal Disease Research Laboratory (VDRL)* test for syphilis is a flocculation test, which combines the features of agglutination and precipitation tests to give a visible foaming rather than clumping reaction.

2. Rheumatoid factor

Rheumatoid factor is an autoantibody directed against the Fc region of IgG. Various immuno-assays are available for detection of rheumatoid factor.
- *The classic Rose-Waaler test* is haemagglutination test for rheumatoid factor in the serum, which depends on the ability of rheumatoid factor to agglutinate sheep erythrocytes coated with anti-sheep immunoglobulin.
- *The latex agglutination test*, in which latex particles coated with human IgG aggregate in the presence of IgM rheumatoid factor, can identify only the IgM isotype of rheumatoid factor.
- *Enzyme-linked immunosorbent assay (ELISA)* can measure IgG, IgA, and IgM rheumatoid factors. Oligoarticular rheumatoid arthritis may be associated with a negative test for IgM rheumatoid factor but a positive test for IgG rheumatoid factor.

3. Antinuclear antibody

Plasma cells, the activated B cells of patients with autoimmune diseases, produce antibodies directed against their own tissues. Antinuclear antibodies (ANA) are usually autoantibodies that are reactive with antigens in the nucleoplasm. These antibodies probably occur in the circulation of all human beings, but the employed test is only considered 'positive' if they occur at titres elevated significantly above the normal serum level. This test has limited value but probably most common test ordered to rule out systemic rheumatic disease.
- The presence of antinuclear antibodies in serum often warrants the presence of systemic collagen vascular disease, however, it can be found in normal individuals also.
- It is a sensitive screening test for systemic lupus erythematosus.
- Antinuclear antibody is a very useful investigations for juvenile idiopathic arthritis.

4. Lupus Anticoagulant

The lupus anticoagulant is an acquired serum immunoglobulin that prolongs several co-agulation measurements. Lupus anticoagulants are anti-phospholipid antibodies found in at least 10% of patients with systemic lupus erythematosus as well as in patients with infectious, drug-induced, malignant, and other autoimmune disorders, and otherwise healthy persons.

Despite the association with impaired co-agulation, thrombotic systemic and ocular disease occurs in lupus anticoagulant positive patients. Symptoms of disturbed vision may bring these patients to medical attention.

5. Tests for syphilis

Laboratory testing for syphilis is indicated in a broad variety of ocular diseases. Scrapings of mucocutaneous lesions to confirm a diagnosis of primary or secondary syphilis can be examined directly by phase-contrast or dark-field microscopy and confirmed by direct immunofluorescence, or DFATP, testing. In the absence of obvious superficial lesions, serology is required to make a diagnosis. These tests fall into two categories:

- Nontreponemal and
- Treponemal.

Nontreponemal or nonspecific antibody tests

Nontreponemal or nonspecific antibody tests measure IgM and IgG directed against a phospholipid antigen called cardiolipin, or diphosphatidylglycerol, produced coincidentally during luetic infections. These are also known as Wasserman, or reaginic, antibodies.

VDRL test is the simplest and most practical of these tests employing a slide microflocculation technique, and the RPR (rapid plasma reagin) circle card test. Positive tests are reported as the highest serum dilution producing a reaction. These nontreponemal tests are widely used for screening, as well as for quantitative assessment of treatment response. The quantitation VDRL titer is both helpful in diagnosis and in following the course of treatment. If positive, titers are low in primary syphilis, usually below 1:32, while in secondary syphilis it is virtually always greater than 1:32. A high or rising titer is essentially diagnostic of syphilis, despite the long list of diseases producing false-positive results. False-positive test results occur in 10 to 30% of the population, depending on a given laboratory's location.

The VDRL and RPR tests are, therefore, very sensitive but somewhat nonspecific. Following successful treatment of early syphilis, the titer declines approximately fourfold at 3 months, and eightfold at 6 months. Titers should be negative within 1 year of treatment of sero-positive primary syphilis, within 2 years for secondary syphilis, or within 5 years for late latent syphilis. If titers do not return to negative, persistent active infection or reinfection should be suspected, especially if the titer is greater than 1:4. If secondary syphilis is clinically suspected despite a negative nontreponemal test, a prozone phenomenon due to excess antibody might be responsible and additional dilutions should be ordered. The VDRL rises more slowly than the fluorescent treponemal antibody (FTA) test and thus may miss an early primary infection. Therefore, an FTA test should be obtained

whenever syphilis is clinically suspected, despite a negative VDRL test. The VDRL is the only test that can be reliably employed in evaluating cerebrospinal fluid.

Treponemal or specific tests

These include:
- *Treponema pallidum* immobilization test (TPI)
- Fluorescent treponemal antibody absorption (FTA-ABS) test
- Microhaemagglutination for *Treponema pallidum* (MHA-TP) test

In syphilis, as in all infections, it is best to use an antigen specific for the organism believed to be infecting the patient. These treponemal or specific tests measure antitreponemal IgG and remain positive throughout life; therefore, they cannot be used to distinguish between active or prior disease.

Treponema pallidum immobilization test (TPI), introduced in 1949, was the first treponemal test developed. Because of technical difficulty and poor standardization, it is rarely used now, although it has served as a valuable benchmark for the development of newer tests.

Fluorescent treponemal antibody absorption (FTA-ABS) test is an indirect immunofluorescent test found to be reactive in about 80% of patients with primary syphilis. The VDRL test is positive in only 50% of patients with primary syphilis, while both the FTA and VDRL tests are positive in all patients with secondary syphilis. The specificity of the FTA-ABS test is greatly enhanced by first absorbing the specimen with nonpathogenic treponemal strains. The FTA-ABS can be used to rule out a biologically false-positive nontreponemal test, although even this test is susceptible to false-positive reactivity, particularly in the presence of lupus erythematosus.

Microhaemagglutination with the MHA-TP test, or haemagglutination with the HATTS can also be performed for specific measurement of treponemal antibody. All of the specific treponemal tests are interpreted as reactive, borderline, or nonreactive. The automated MHA-TP is more rapid and less expensive than the FTA-ABS but may be less sensitive during primary and early secondary disease.

6. Toxocara serology

In this parasitic disease, the diagnosis does not rest on identification of the parasite. Since the larvae do not develop into adults in humans, a stool examination would not detect any Toxocara eggs. A presumptive diagnosis rests on clinical signs, history of exposure to puppies, laboratory findings (including eosinophilia), and the detection of antibodies to Toxocara.

Antibody detection tests are the only means of confirmation of a clinical diagnosis of visceral larva migrans (VLM), ocular larva migrans (OLM), and covert toxocariasis (CT), the most common clinical syndromes associated with Toxocara infections. *Enzyme immunoassay (EIA)* currently recommended serologic test for toxocariasis with larval stage antigen extracted from embryonated eggs or released in vitro by cultured infective larvae. The latter, Toxocara excretory–secretory (TES) antigens, are preferable to larval extracts because they are convenient to produce and because an absorption-purification step is not required for obtaining maximum specificity. Evaluation of the true sensitivity and specificity of serologic tests for toxocariasis in human populations is not possible because of the lack of parasitologic methods to detect Toxocara parasites. These inherent problems result in underestimations of sensitivity and specificity. Evaluation of the Toxocara EIA in groups of patients with presumptive diagnoses of VLM or OLM indicated sensitivity of 78% and 73%, respectively, at a titer of >1:32. When the cutoff titer for OLM cases was lowered to 1:8, sensitivity was increased to 90%.

7. Toxoplasmosis serology

About 40% of the adult population worldwide has been exposed to toxoplasmosis, but this can be much higher in areas where hygiene is poor or raw meat is routinely ingested. Infection leads to IgA, IgG, and IgM antibody production, which despite high titers is not necessarily protective. Complement fixation, latex agglutination, indirect haemagglutination, direct and indirect IFA, immunodiffusion, ELISA tests, and the Sabin-Feldman dye test have all been employed in the quantification of anti-toxoplasma titers.

Dye test was well documented and reliable, but it lacked standardization, required a great deal of technician time, required live Toxoplasma organisms, and was only available in a few centres.

ELISA and indirect IFA tests are now the most clinically useful. Titers may vary considerably among these tests, so laboratory methodology must be kept consistent when a suspected flare-up is evaluated by sequential serology. Nevertheless, any titer of specific anti-Toxoplasma antibody may be significant. State laboratories will often only report positive tests if a titer of greater than 1: 16 is found. There have been, however, cases of pathologically proven toxoplasmic retinitis in which serum antibody levels were positive only in undiluted specimens. The initial diagnosis of ocular toxoplasmosis is usually based on the characteristic focal, necrotizing retinal lesion; positive serum antibodies are used to confirm the clinical impression.

8. Serological tests for herpetic group of viruses

Human herpetic infections result from primary inoculation or reactivation of latent neural virions and include herpes simplex virus (HSV) types 1 and 2, varicella-zoster virus (VZV), cytomegalovirus (CMV), and Epstein-Barr virus (EBV).

Acute retinal necrosis syndrome or Kirisawa's uveitis entails anterior uveitis, vitreous inflammation, and progressive necrotizing vaso-occlusive retinitis with a poor prognosis for visual recovery. The disease may be unilateral or bilateral and generally occurs in otherwise healthy patients. Retinal necrosis syndromes have been attributed to HSV-1, HSV-2, CMV and VZV infections. Significant acute anti-herpes titer elevations, if present, can be useful in the diagnosis of active retinitis, as appropriate intravenous antiviral therapy should be started immediately. If CMV infection is implicated by acute serology in a patient started on empiric acyclovir without clinical improvement, a switch to ganciclovir may be indicated; CMV is far less sensitive to acyclovir than the other herpes viruses. Convalescent serum titers are often inconclusive and arrive from the laboratory long after the retinitis has taken its toll. Aqueous antibodies to HSV-1 in acute retinal necrosis syndrome may indicate local antibody production, antibody sequestration within the eye, or damage to the blood–ocular barrier.

Anti-HSV antibody clearly does not prevent reactivation of herpes labialis, and titers will often show no increase whatsoever with recurrent oral episodes. Seroconversion in paired sera may provide evidence of a primary HSV infection. In general, significant HSV titer rises occur only with primary infections.

Serodiagnosis of VZV infection

In the serodiagnosis of VZV infection, acute and convalescent phase sera should be tested in parallel in the same run. The value of VZV serology is limited somewhat by the fact that heterotypic antibody liter rises to VZV may occur in certain patients with HSV infection who have experienced a prior infection with VZV. This is most likely a heterotypic antibody response to common antigens in the two viruses. Thus a fourfold VZV titer rise is significant only in the absence of a concomitant HSV titer rise in the same specimens. Many clinicians will order paired sample testing for HSV-1, HSV-2, VZV, and CMV herpes virus types in appropriate patients.

Serodiagnosis of CMV infection

CMV recovery from urine, throat, or other body fluids is the preferred diagnostic method for congenital infection and may be of use in ocular disease.

Serodiagnosis in infants is complicated by the presence of transplacental maternal IgG. Although there are some technical difficulties with detection of CMV-specific IgM, this test is excellent for the rapid confirmation of an acute or congenital infection. Up to 20% of patients remain persistently IgM positive, indicating a latent CMV carrier state that regularly becomes re-established in host tissue. In suspected adult disease, a fourfold titer rise indicates a recent infection, due to either reinfection or reactivation. Since CMV titers can remain elevated for extended periods, elevated but unchanged acute and convalescent titers may indicate a recent infection in which the acute specimen was obtained relatively late in the patient's illness.

CMV antibodies are not helpful in the diagnosis of retinitis in patients with acquired immuno-deficiency syndrome (AIDS), especially since the clinical picture is so typical. Furthermore, CMV antibodies are very common in patients at risk for AIDS and CMV serum titers may be negative in AIDS patients despite the presence of CMV retinopathy.

CMV-positive titers should be confirmed by culture whenever possible. In acute CMV infections, characterized by fever, thrombocytopenia, hepatosplenomegaly, pneumonitis, and lymphadenopathy, virus is recoverable from most patients' urine and from 50% of throat swabs. Isolation from buffy coat cells, spun urine, saliva, subretinal fluid, or biopsy specimens can be diagnostic. Isolation, however, does not necessarily establish CMV as the responsible organism; asymptomatic viraemia has been described, and biopsy specimens often contain other pathogens, rendering the clinical interpretation tenuous. Direct specimen examination for CMV by exfoliative cytology, histopathology, immunofluorescence, electron microscopy, or DNA hybridization techniques can also assist in the diagnosis of CMV infection. Fresh spun urine should be passed through a membrane filter, and trapped cells should be stained with hematoxylin-eosin or Papanicolaou reagents. Characteristic large cells with prominent eosinophilic inclusions are seen in positive preparations. Similar cells are also rarely seen in HSV infections.

Serodiagnosis of EBV infection

EBV isolation is usually not clinically useful due to the ubiquity of EBV found in healthy persons, technical difficulties in culturing the organism, and a long incubation period.

Serologic studies are the method of choice. In primary infections with symptoms compatible with infectious mononucleosis, a positive heterophil antibody is diagnostic. This IgM antibody agglutinates sheep red blood cells but not guinea pig kidney.

A *slide spot test* is now used for screening and confirmed by the *Paul-Bunnell test*. The heterophil antibody rises rapidly, remains high, and then falls rapidly, generally after 4 weeks of illness.

9. Human immunodeficiency virus serology

Although the diagnosis of AIDS cannot be made in a person who is antibody-negative for human immunodeficiency virus (HIV), positive serology does not establish a diagnosis, as there are many healthy persons who are positive for the antibody. An *ELISA test* is available for routine documentation of HIV-specific antibodies, with informed consent required in nonmilitary settings. The screening tests for HIV antibodies are calibrated to be extremely sensitive, so a significant number of false-positive results occur. All positive tests should be confirmed with a *Western blot analysis*, in which purified, electrophoretically separated HIV antigens incubated with patient serum produce a characteristic pattern. Opportunistic infections such as *Mycobacterium tuberculosis, Treponema pallidum,* fungi, *Toxoplasma gondii,* and the herpes viruses define the syndrome and may cause uveitis. CMV retinitis is the most common form of ocular inflammation seen in AIDS and is a poor prognostic sign. A number of immunologic abnormalities have been documented in AIDS, including lymphopenia ($<600/mm^3$), a substantial reduction in the percentage of T cells ($<30\%$), and a reversed helper-to-suppressor T cell ratio (<0.5). T cell subsets can be accurately quantified with immunofluorescent labeling, flow cytometry, and cell-sorting techniques.

10. Chlamydial serology

Chlamydial organisms have been isolated from the joints and the anterior chamber from one patient with Reiter's syndrome. Although chlamydial urethritis and conjunctivitis have been implicated in the pathogenesis of Reiter's syndrome, the presence of antibodies is so common that an elevated titer is of minimal use. A significant convalescent IgG titer rise or high IgM titers might provide a clue to the cause of new-onset Reiter's syndrome in selected patients. The *microimmunofluorescence test*, an indirect antibody test using whole purified chlamydial elementary bodies, provides antibody titers with serotype specificities. Serotype-specific monoclonal reagents are now available for serologic testing in a research setting.

11. Borrelia titers in lyme disease

Either ELISA or indirect IFA tests for IgG and IgM directed against the tick-borne causative agent, *Borrelia burgdorferi*, are available through state laboratories and the CDC in Atlanta. Many patients with the classic cutaneous manifestation of early Lyme disease, erythema chronicum migrans, have *elevated IgM responses*. Sometimes, however, several weeks of illness are required before the levels of either IgM or IgG antibody become elevated. In these cases, testing of both acute and convalescent sera may increase the chances of obtaining a positive result. Because the antibody response may be aborted altogether by early antibiotic therapy, early Lyme disease cannot be documented in all patients. After the first 5 or 6 weeks of illness, almost all patients have an elevated IgG response, and virtually all patients with arthritis have elevated titers. Titers can be performed on the serum as well as the cerebrospinal fluid. Small amounts of *IgM rheumatoid factor* are produced at certain times in many patients with Lyme disease.

Relapsing fever is due to *Borellia recurrentis* or *Borellia novyi* infection and may be accompanied by uveitis. These Borellia species are transmitted by other members of the Ornithodoros tick family or by the human body louse. All of the Borellia spirochetes can be identified in Giemsa- or Wright-stained blood smears drawn during a febrile episode.

12. Leptospira antibodies

An *agglutination test* utilizing commercially available killed organisms is available through most state public health laboratories. A tentative diagnosis of ocular leptospirosis should not be made in the absence of serum antibodies to *Leptospira icterohemorrhagiae*, the major human pathogen. A titer of 1:400 or more is diagnostic. The organisms may be isolated from blood or urine in the early, febrile stages. Many mammals serve as reservoirs, where chronic renal infection leads to passage in the urine. Occasionally, small epidemics of Weil's disease are seen in sewer workers and others exposed to rat urine or contaminated water supplies. Signs and symptoms develop after an incubation period of 10 to 12 days and vary from a mild fever to severe illness, including jaundice, renal failure, and meningitis. Uveitis has not been a frequent component of the disease in the United States, but mild anterior iritis, membranous vitreous opacities, retinal and papillary haemorrhage, and chorioretinal exudate have been described.

13. Bacterial serology

Serologic testing for antibody responses to gram-negative and gram-positive organisms is not generally believed to be useful in the diagnosis of uveitis syndromes. The rare diagnosis of neisserial endophthalmitis is made by identification of organisms by culture and Gram's stain. Although serum antituberculous antibodies may be useful in identifying pulmonary tuberculous infection, tuberculous serology alone is not useful in isolated ocular tuberculosis. As focal extrapulmonary manifestations assume a greater proportion of tuberculous disease in the United States, ophthalmologists will have to rely more on clinical judgment, diagnostic therapeutic trials with anti-tuberculosis chemotherapy, a precise history, and skin testing rather than serology and the traditional chest roentgenogram in making a diagnosis of tuberculous uveitis.

14. Brucellosis antibody

Brucellosis has been incriminated as a cause of recurrent iritis, nodular choroiditis, and, rarely, a severe endophthalmitic panuveitis. A standard tube agglutination test with acute and convalescent titers should show a fourfold rise in order to establish a presumptive diagnosis of Brucella uveitis. Like leptospirosis, blood cultures may be positive in the early stages of the disease. Brucellosis is usually found in hoofed farm animals: goats, sheep, cattle, and swine. Pregnant animals are particularly susceptible and frequently abort. Human transmission occurs by direct contact with infected animals or consumption of unpasteurized milk. Acute symptoms include fever, chills, and weakness. Chronic infections are characterized by fever, malaise, depression, and abscesses in the bones, spleen, kidneys, or brain.

C. OTHER HAEMATOLOGICAL TESTS

C-reactive protein

Acute phase reactants are proteins that become elevated in response to stressful or inflammatory states such as infection, injury, surgery, trauma, or tissue necrosis. They include globulins, α1-antitrypsin, α1-acid glycoprotein, haptoglobin, ceruloplasmin, fibrinogen, and C-reactive protein (CRP). The CRP is a highly sensitive acute phase indicator and can be measured by ELISA or other immunologic methods. CRP has a molecular weight of 144 kd and reacts with numerous other substances, including DNA, nucleotides, various lipids, and polysaccharides, including the pneumococcal C-polysaccharide. There is still no consensus among physicians for the widespread use of CRP, because other clinical parameters may be just as sensitive, including fever, leucocytosis and the ESR. CRP has been used as a marker for disease activity in the seronegative spondyloarthropathies.

Angiotensin-converting enzyme

Angiotensin-converting enzyme (ACE) is produced by a variety of cells, including capillary endothelial cells, lung tissue, and activated monocytes, macrophages, and epithelioid cells found in noncaseating granulomas. ACE is a dipeptidylcarboxy-peptidase, catalyzing the conversion of the decapeptide angiotensin 1 to the pressor angiotensin 2, the cleavage of bradykinin to an inactive metabolite, and a number of other reactions. The serum ACE concentration is probably a reflection of the total amount of granulomatous tissue in the body. The normal level is 55 IU/litre. Serum ACE levels are elevated in about 75% of patients with active, untreated systemic sarcoidosis and about 40% of chronic, untreated patients. However, serum ACE level may be normal in active ocular sarcoidosis as the ocular granuloma load may not be enough to raise the serum concentration.

Lysozyme levels

Lysozyme, or muramidase, is a basic, cationic low-molecular weight enzyme present in tears, saliva, and nasal secretions. It reduces the local concentration of susceptible bacteria by attacking the mucopeptides in bacterial cell walls. Lysozyme originates from phagocytic cells and is normally present in serum at a concentration of 1 to 2 µg/ml. It is actively secreted by monocytes and macrophages. Lysozyme is also secreted by the sarcoid granuloma. In adults, serum lysozyme levels generally parallel elevated serum ACE levels, although lysozyme may be elevated with a normal ACE in occasional patients with sarcoidosis. The lysozyme test is nonspecific and may be elevated in other diseases, including tuberculosis, leprosy, osteoarthritis, and pernicious anaemia. In tuberculosis, lysozyme activity is elevated in over 50% of patients, while the ACE is elevated in only 10%. Serum lysozyme is depressed by systemic corticosteroid administration but, unlike serum ACE, is not normally higher in children when compared with adults. Also in patients on systemic ACE inhibitors, this test is of help. The serum lysozyme value may be elevated, however, in patients older than 60 yrs of age. So age must be taken into consideration when interpreting both ACE and lysozyme levels. Both ACE and lysozyme can be sensitive noninvasive tools in approaching a patient with granulomatous uveitis when the entire clinical presentation is carefully considered.

Lysozyme levels are elevated in tuberculous pleural effusion specimens and may prove to be a useful marker in aqueous paracentesis specimens taken from patients with presumed tuberculous uveitis. Most laboratories quantify lysozyme levels spectrophotometrically, but turbidometric, viscometric, immunologic, and bioassay methods are also available.

D. DETECTION OF MAJOR HISTOCOMPATIBILITY ANTIGENS

The human major histocompatibility complex, containing DNA encoding human leucocyte antigen (HLA) genes, is located on the short arm of chromosome 6. The HLA sites localize to heterodimeric (two different chains) cell surface molecules belonging to the immunoglobulin superfamily. Class I HLA molecules include the A, B, and C loci and are found on the surface of virtually every cell. Class II HLA molecules include the D, DR, DQ, and DP loci and are restricted to lymphocytes, macrophages, and other immunocompetent cells. Humans possess two haplotypes, usually inherited as a unit from each parent. Each haplotype has three class I and four class II alleles. Because HLA expression is codominant, it is theoretically possible to type two antigens at each of these seven loci unless the subject is homozygous for one or more loci or antisera are not yet available for a rare HLA type. There are currently 124 recognized HLA specificities.

The class I molecules provide a recognition target for lymphocytes responsible for cell-mediated immunity. Thus, class I antigens are recognized during graft rejection and they restrict the cytotoxic response against virus-infected cells to lymphocytes expressing the same class I antigens as the infected cells. Class II molecules are essential to antigen presentation and normal interactions between immuno-competent cells.

Genetically predetermined susceptibility to 530 distinct diseases has been linked to certain specific HLA markers in over 4,000 separate clinical studies. None of the HLA markers is, of course, specific for a given disease. The presence of an HLA antigen in a given patient, however, is suggestive of its associated disease and may provide the clinician with an additional clue in establishing a definitive diagnosis. The relative risk of 69.1 for HLA-B27 and ankylosing spondylitis, which was the first such association ever described, indicates that an HLA-B27-

positive white person is about 69 times more likely to develop ankylosing spondylitis than someone not carrying this antigen. The HLA-B27 antigen itself characterizes a unique clinical picture in uveitis, making it an important diagnostic tool, unlike the situation in rheumatologic practice in which HLA-B27 typing is less valuable. HLA-B27-positive patients with acute anterior uveitis are more likely to be younger at the age of onset, to be male, to show frequent unilateral alternating eye involvement, to have severe symptoms with each episode (including fibrinoid anterior chamber reactions), to have a higher incidence of ocular complications, to lack mutton-fat keratic precipitates, and to have an associated seronegative spondyloarthropathy.

The HLA type may also help define prognosis. In presumed ocular histoplasmosis syndrome, HLA-B7 is strongly associated with disciform macular lesions, but not with peripheral atrophic scars. HLA-DR2, however, is associated with both macular and peripheral scarring, suggesting a distinct genetic predisposition to macular neovascularisation in this disease.

Patients with pauciarticular juvenile rheumatoid arthritis are particularly prone to uveitis. HLA-DR5, which is associated with the early-onset form of this disease most frequently seen in girls, characterizes patients more likely to develop a chronic, bilateral disease associated with band keratopathy and the presence of antinuclear antibodies. HLA-B27, on the other hand, is associated with later-onset pauciarticular juvenile rheumatoid arthritis and concomitant uveitis similar to the classic HLA-B27 pattern. Uveitis occurs in 53% of patients with HLA-DR5 related early-onset juvenile rheumatoid arthritis found mostly in females and in 25% of patients with the HLA-B27-related, later-onset form usually found in males.

In general, HLA tests are not ordered on a routine basis and complete histocompatibility typing is never ordered as part of an evaluation for uveitis. Specific HLA types can, however, provide more information to the astute clinician who requires additional data to confirm a suspected diagnosis.

II. URINALYSIS

The urinalysis is also used to assess the general health status of the patient. A urine specimen is a cost-effective, painless liquid tissue biopsy of the urinary tract that rapidly provides a great deal of information. The urinalysis is a useful screening test for renal, genitourinary, metabolic, and hepatic diseases. Among the most significant conditions detected by chemical means in a macrourinalysis are proteinuria, glucosuria, ketonuria, and the presence of the pigments haemoglobin and bilirubin. A micro-urinalysis of centrifuged urine sediment should be performed on fresh or refrigerated specimens. White cells, red cells, urinary casts, and crystalluria can all be quantified under the microscope. The presence of a suspected infection can be rapidly confirmed by urine dip-stick nitrite and leucocyte esterase tests (Chemstrip, Boehringer-Mannheim Diagnostics, Indianapolis). A urine culture should probably be performed in all cases of presumed urinary tract infection including cases of suspected Reiter's syndrome with or without genitourinary symptoms. *Chlamydia trachomatis* may be isolated from the urethra, urine, conjunctiva, or rectum of patients with Reiter's syndrome, although iridocyclitis usually develops after the acute infectious phase. Only a few patients with Reiter's uveitis, however, have responded to tetracycline therapy.

Urine CMV cultures as well as CMV cytology are central to the diagnosis of CMV infection. Hypercalciuria is twice as common as hyper-calcaemia in sarcoidosis. Thus, a 24-hour urinary calcium determination may be helpful, however, inconvenient and nonspecific. Twenty-four-hour urine collections for uric acid can be a more sensitive screening test than serum uric acid in establishing a diagnoses of gout. Finally, the ova of *Endolimax nana* have been found in the urine of a patient with exudative chorioretinopathy.

III. STOOL EXAMINATION FOR PARASITES

Intestinal parasites are a rare cause of uveitis in the United States: for example, only one case of Ascaris ocular invasion has been proven.

Entamoeba histolytica, Escherichia coli, E. nana, and *Giardia lamblia* have been described as producing a cystic macular lesion. Although *Toxocara canis* and *T. cati* are recognized causes of uveitis, humans are not natural hosts. Ingested ova from contaminated soil or uncooked vegetables such as lettuce advance to the larval stage in the human intestinal epithelium, penetrate the portal vasculature and lymphatics, and spread to the liver, where eosinophilic granulomas may be produced. Some larvae survive, infect the lungs, enter the heart, and thereafter disseminate throughout the body. The larvae never mature in the human host; thus neither ova nor mature Toxocara parasites are found in human faeces.

SKIN TESTS

Intradermal injection of 0.1 ml of soluble antigens prepared from a number of infectious agents can be performed in the office during the initial visit.

MANTOUX TEST

The most useful test antigen is the tuberculin purified protein derivative (PPD). The standard dose is 5 TU (US tuberculin units) or intermediate strength, equivalent to 0.0001 mg (Aplisol, Parke-Davis, Morris Plains, NJ). Current lots of PPD are standardized for biologic activity against PPD-Seibert (PPD-S), a reference bulk lot prepared in 1940. Second strength (250 TU) can be given to patients who do not react to an initial 5-TU injection, whereas first strength (1 TU) should be given to patients who the clinician suspects may have a strong reaction and are therefore at risk for sloughing and ulceration at the injection site (Tubersol, in first and second strength, available through Squibb/Connaught, Princeton, NJ). There is no evidence of booster effects or repeated skin testing leading to conversion from negative to positive. Intracutaneous injection, the Mantoux test, is the most reliable test available. Injection of 0.1 ml of PPD antigen into the volar or dorsal surface of the forearm is made just below the skin surface with a short (1/2 inch) No. 27 gauge needle, bevel upward, to produce a discrete 6- to 10-mm wheal or bubble. The use of insulin syringes with intrinsic needles will avoid repeated waste of antigen extract in the needle hub of standard tuberculin syringes. If no bubble appears due to a deep injection, the test should be immediately reapplied at a site at least 5 cm away. Skin tests are read 48 to 72 hours following injection. Induration measuring 10 mm or more is considered positive (Fig. 5.2.1) this indicates a previous infection with *Mycobacterium tuberculosis*, although previous infection with *M. bovis* or photochromogenic mycobacteria may also produce a positive result. Patients may also develop coexistent erythema, a wheal and flare that usually fades after 12 to 18 hours, which is evidence of an immediate hypersensitivity to the same test antigen. Uveitis patients with induration less than 10 mm, or even erythema alone, have had favourable clinical responses to oral antituberculous therapy. On the other hand, patients with proven ocular tuberculous infection have had insignificant or negative PPD skin tests.

HISTOPLASMIN SKIN TEST

Although the use of histoplasmin skin testing in uveitis is no longer universally recommended, greater than 80% of patients with presumed ocular histoplasmosis syndrome have positive skin tests. Some authors believe that histoplasmin skin testing may increase the danger of activating a macular lesion in susceptible patients.

KVEIM TEST

Approximately 80% of patients with sarcoidosis react positively to skin testing with the Kveim antigen. This antigen is prepared from human

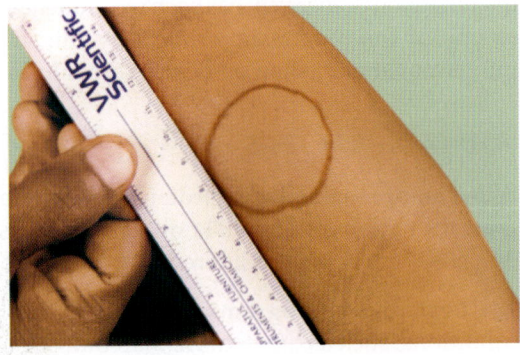

Fig. 5.2.1 *Mantoux reading.*

sarcoid granulomas, is difficult to obtain, requires several months of incubation followed by a biopsy at the injection site for histologic verification, does not have absolute specificity, and entails a risk of hepatitis or retrovirus transmission. False-positive and false-negative results may occur, limiting its usefulness.

BEHÇET'S SKIN PUNCTURE TEST

Patients with active systemic Behcet's disease show increased dermal sensitivity to needle trauma, owing to their unusual leukotactic tendency. The appearance of a pustule 24 to 36 hours after an intradermal needle puncture, with or without the injection of 0.1 ml of normal saline, is almost diagnostic for Behcet's disease. Erythema and infiltration may appear within a few hours, and occasionally a microabscess can be produced. This test may not be positive in patients with ocular manifestations when the systemic disease is in remission. No universal agreement on the usefulness of this test exists because only 10% of Behcet's patients demonstrate a positive response.

CUTANEOUS ANERGY

This is a phenomenon of reduced or absent cutaneous sensitivity to a given antigen to which the subject was sensitive before. In developing countries where Bacillus-Calmette-Guerin (BCG) vaccination is routinely performed, negative tuberculin test in a BCG-vaccinated patient or in a patient with a previously positive tuberculin skin test is of great value in diagnosis of sarcoidosis. This is the most well-known manifestation of anergy. It has been recommended as one of the diagnostic criteria by the first international workshop on ocular sarcoidosis.

RADIOLOGICAL TESTS

When an ophthalmologist orders a roentgenogram the radiologist should know exactly which diagnoses are being considered.

1. Chest roentgenograms are useful when conditions, such as tuberculosis, sarcoidosis, or histoplasmosis are suspected.

Active pulmonary sarcoidosis characteristically shows bilateral hilar adenopathy (Fig. 5.2.2) with or without parenchymal disease; hilar adenopathy characteristically precedes the onset of peripheral infiltrates. Chest roentgenographic abnormalities are found in about 80% of patients with ocular sarcoidosis.

Active pulmonary tuberculosis may reveal characteristic wedge-shaped segmental infiltrates, cavitary lesions, calcified granulomas, or diffuse parenchymal nodules accompanied by ipsilateral hilar enlargement. Lordotic views of the relatively oxygen-rich apices may demonstrate old scarring or concentrated active lesions due to the aerobic preferences of mycobacteria.

2. Ocular and orbital plane films may show calcification of various parts of the uvea; for example:

• Late degenerative choroidal changes
• Fine stippling in retinoblastoma, or intraocular calcification seen in retinopathy of prematurity and hyperparathyroidism.
• Intraocular foreign bodies can be identified and localized by plain films as well as ultrasonography and computed tomography.

3. Sacroiliac joint films should be ordered when ankylosing spondylitis or other seronegative spondyloarthropathies, such as Reiter's syndrome or psoriatic arthritis, are suspected. It is important to specifically order a sacroiliac series, not a lumbar spine series, since both a

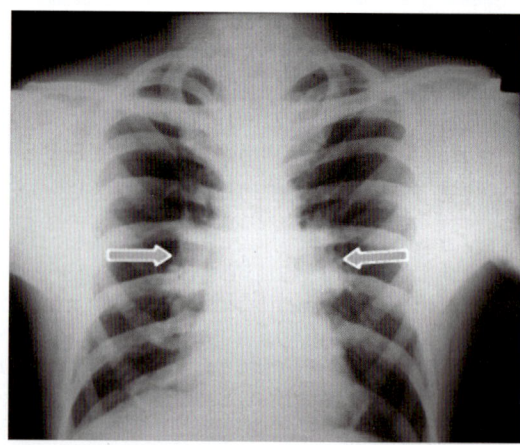

Fig. 5.2.2 *X-ray chest showing hilar adenopathy suggestive of sarcoidosis.*

straight anteroposterior projection and the more sensitive oblique tunnel view of the joints will be taken.

- *Sacroiliac disease* occurs in 20% of patients with Reiter's syndrome.
- When a patient has psoriasis with sacroiliitis (Fig. 5.2.3), iridocyclitis is also likely to occur, whether or not the HLA-B27 antigen is positive.

4. Painful, swollen joints can be X-rayed if juvenile or adult rheumatoid arthritis, Reiter's syndrome, or sarcoidosis is suspected.

- *In juvenile rheumatoid arthritis*, the knee is most commonly affected. Since children with pauciarticular manifestations develop the worst iridocyclitis, a routine knee roentgenogram is recommended, even though there is no clinically suspected arthritis.
- *In Reiter's syndrome*, the hands, feet, heels, and sacroiliac joints are most commonly affected.
- Weight-bearing joints are also afflicted.
- *In ankylosing spondylitis* and sarcoidosis. Permeating, lytic, and destructive bony changes are also seen occasionally in sarcoidosis.

5. Radiographic studies for cerebral calcification, although helpful, are nonspecific and do not differentiate between toxoplasmosis and CMV inclusion disease, as the roentgenographic findings can be the same for both infections. This is not surprising when one realizes that *Toxoplasma gondii* and CMV are both neurotrophic intracellular pathogens and may both be seen together within the same host cell.

6. Upper gastrointestinal small bowel series and barium enema roentgenograms may identify anomalies associated with uveitis, including Whipple's disease, Crohn's disease, ulcerative colitis, and abdominal abscess.

7. Paranasal sinus and dental films occasionally, may be of value in locating clinically suspected loci of infection in otherwise idiopathic uveitis.

8. CT scan chest is very useful in tuberculosis of the lung and also to delineate hilar lymphadenopathy in patients with sarcoidosis (Fig. 5.2.4).

NUCLEAR MEDICINE STUDY

GALLIUM STUDY

Gallium citrate scan can identify inflammatory disease and tumours throughout the body. Gallium is taken up by mitotically active liposomes of granulocytes. The actual scan is performed 48 hours following the intravenous injection of radiolabelled gallium citrate. For the purpose of sarcoid diagnosis, a limited scan of the head, neck, and chest is sufficient and less expensive than a total body scan. Although radiation doses are extremely minute, careful dosimetric consultation with a clinical radiation physicist should be undertaken before performing this test in pregnant women and young children.

- *Gallium scan is more sensitive than routine chest roentgenograms* for showing pulmonary involvement in sarcoidosis. It lacks specificity, however, as numerous other pulmonary diseases show abnormal uptake, including

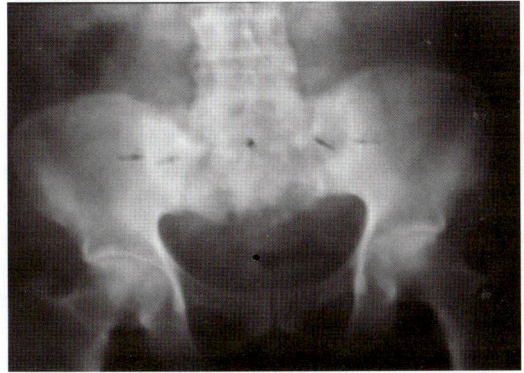

Fig. 5.2.3 *X-ray sacroiliac joint showing sacroiliitis.*

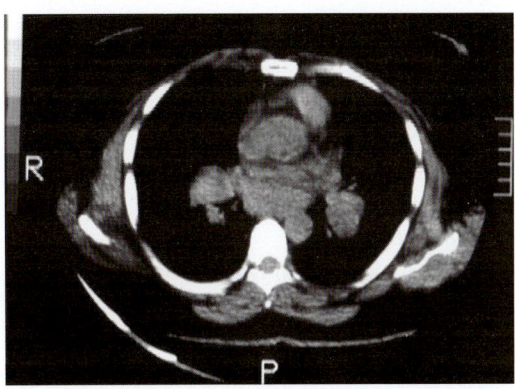

Fig. 5.2.4 *HRCT showing hilar adenopathy.*

tuberculosis, carcinoma, lymphoma, and silicosis.

- *Increased lacrimal gland uptake of gallium* occurs in over 80% of patients with active sarcoidosis, although this is also nonspecific; as many as 25% of patients with increased lacrimal gland uptake have no other evidence of the disease. Thus, gallium scans may lead to a false-positive diagnosis of sarcoidosis by physicians unfamiliar with these limitations.
- *When combined with determination of serum ACE and lysozyme levels, a skin test panel, chest roentgenogram, and other tests tailored* to a careful history and examination, the gallium scan can be instrumental in establishing a diagnosis of ocular sarcoidosis.

Technetium scans have been used in the diagnosis of Sjögren's syndrome and correspond well to minor salivary gland biopsy findings.

ANCILLARY TESTS IN UVEITIS

Recently, enormous progress has been achieved in investigational procedures for uveitis. A provisional clinical diagnosis can be reached in most cases of uveitis. Ancillary tests help in confirming the clinical diagnosis and are most useful in dilemmatic situations in diagnosis. Increased precision and accuracy in the assessment of the level and degree of inflammation and its monitoring goes parallel with the development of extremely potent and efficacious therapies.

Common ancillary tests used in uveitis include:
- Funds autofluorescence
- Laser flare photometry and laser flare cell photometry
- Ultrasound biomicroscopy
- Fluorescein angiography
- Indocyanine green angiography
- Optical coherance tomography
- Ultrasonography
- Electrophysiological tests in uveitis

FUNDUS AUTOFLUORESCENCE

Fluorescence is the capability of absorbing light at a specific wavelength and releasing it at a longer, less energetic wavelength. Autofluorescence is the natural and spontaneous emission of light by a substance.

Excitation wavelength used in fundus autofluorescence (FAF) imaging is generally, but not always, 488 nm (argon laser).

Modalities of FAF imaging could be near-infrared FAF and blue-light FAF imaging.

Source of fundus autofluorescence (FAF) is the lipofuscin of retinal pigment epithelial (RPE) cells. Lipofuscin is the lysosomal metabolic accumulate of non-dividing RPE cells. It accumulates with age and in some retinal disorders as a byproduct of light-related vitamin A cycling. Lipofuscin exhibits a characteristic autofluorescence when excited in ultraviolet (UV) or blue light. The level of autofluorescence represents a balance between accumulation and clearance of lipofuscin.

Normal FAF image of the posterior pole of the retina would show:
- *Optic nerve head or dark* because of the absence of RPE thus lipofuscin.
- *Retinal vessels* are hypoautofluorescent because of absorption of light by the blood.
- *Macular area*, the FAF signal is reduced at the fovea when compared with the surroundings. From the foveola, a distinct increase in the signal can be observed till the margin of the fovea, followed by a further gradual increase of AF toward the outer macula. This is caused by absorption by luteal pigments (i.e. lutein and zeaxanthin) in the neurosensory retina at fovea, especially foveola, and a possible spatial differences in melanin deposition.

Mechanism of autofluorescence

Amount of autofluorescence is dependent on the amount of fluorophores in any given area.
- *Inflammation* can alter the amounts of fluorophores during acute phases.
- *Autofluorescence (FAF) photography complements other methods of imaging, such as colour fundus photography.* Acute inflammatory changes can alter the size and number of fluorophore content of the RPE cells due to a number of factors including RPE cell dysfunction and

destruction. Inflammation induces a number of pro-oxidative pathways, which may increase the amount of fluorophores present.

- *Hypertrophy and reactive hyperplasia of the RPE* may increase the thickness of the RPE, contributing to the formation of autofluorescence.
- *Choroidal neovascularization* (CNV) associated with intraocular inflammation produces characteristic autofluorescence findings.
- *Secondary CNV* is often easily recognised by FAF because the surrounding hyperplastic RPE is hyper-autofluorescent and, hence, FAF neatly outlines the neovascularisation.
- *Following treatment, CNV may contract* and leave a zone of absent RPE result in hypo-autofluorescent in that particular area.
- *Areas of RPE with increased pigmentation* also show increased autofluorescence. With time, the areas start to become thinner, and RPE cells are reduced and the area appears darker during autofluorescence photography because of the lack of fluorophores.

Uses of autofluorescence

From autofluorescence imaging, we can estimate the extent of damage due to a particular disease, monitor its progression and can anticipate future complications.

Causes of altered fundus autofluorescence

I. Causes for an increased FAF signal

1. *Excessive RPE lipofuscin accumulation*
- *Lipofuscinopathies.* Stargardt disease, Best disease, pattern dystrophy, and adult vitelliform macular dystrophy
- *Age-related macular degeneration*

2. *Occurrence of fluorophores anterior or posterior to the RPE cell monolayer*
- Cystoid macular oedema
- Serous PED
- Druse in the subpigment epithelial space
- Older intraretinal and subretinal haemorrhages
- Choroidal vessel in the presence of RPE and choriocapillaris atrophy
- Choroidal nevi and melanoma

3. *Lack of absorbing material*
- Cystoid macular oedema (displacement of luteal pigment)

- Idiopathic macular telangiectasia type 2 (depletion of luteal pigment)

4. *Optic nerve head druse*

5. *Artefacts*

II. Causes for a reduced FAF signal

1. *Reduction in RPE lipofuscin density*
- RPE atrophy (geographic atrophy)
- Hereditary retinal dystrophies (such as RPE65 mutations)

2. *Increased RPE melanin content*
- For example, RPE hypertrophy

3. *Absorption from extracellular material/cells/fluid anterior to the RPE*
- Migrated melanin-containing cells
- Crystalline druses or other crystal-like deposits
- Fresh intraretinal and subretinal haemorrhages
- Retinal vessels
- Luteal pigment (lutein and zeaxanthin)
- Media opacities (vitreous, lens, anterior chamber, cornea)
- Fibrosis, scar tissue, borders of laser scars

Autofluorescence in some posterior uveitic conditions

Choroiditis, multifocal choroiditis, panuveitis syndrome

- *Clinically visible chorioretinal scars* are hypo-autofluorescent due to damage and destruction of the RPE cells. FAF lesions often outnumbers the number of chorioretinal scars seen clinically, correctly delineating the extent of involvement. The hypoautofluorescent spots are very small, and clinically visible scars appear to be composed of multiple smaller hypoautofluorescent spots.
- *Secondary choroidal neovascularisation* is visible as an area of hyperautofluorescence.

Serpiginous choroiditis

- *Active lesions* have been reported to be hypo-autofluorescent. At a very early stage, FAF showed increased autofluorescence and changes from a granular to a speckled pattern within a few weeks, and finally becoming hypoautofluorescent after a few months.

• *In reactivation phase*, the margins of the lesions shows hyperautofluorescence because of the activity of the RPE cells at the margin and deposition of lipofuscin (Fig. 5.2.5).

VKH

• *In acute VKH disease*, mild and uniform hyperautofluorescence is seen in the macula and hypoautofluorescence at the area of the serous retinal detachment and fluid pockets.
• *Following treatment*, FAF returns normal. In late presentation, FAF abnormality is scattered and widespread and never returns to normal pattern due to extensive damage to the RPE.

LASER FLARE PHOTOMETRY AND LASER FLARE CELL PHOTOMETRY

Laser flare photometry (LFP) provides a noninvasive, objective and quantitative measure of aqueous humour flare. It is used as a research and an adjunctive clinical tool.

Principle

The LFP is based on the principle that increased protein content of the aqueous humour causes scattering of light. A laser beam of light scans a measurement window projected into the anterior chamber and light scattered by protein particles in the aqueous humour is detected by a photomultiplier. The amount of scattered light in the measurement window is proportional to the concentration and size of the proteins in the aqueous humour.

Method

• *Laser flare-cell photometer* (LFCP) is used for LFP. A fixed volume (0.5 mm) is scanned two dimensionally by the laser beam. The result of aqueous humour flare expressed in photon counts per millisecond (ph/ms).
• *Seven measures are taken*. The highest and lowest values are discarded and the machine automatically calculates the mean and standard deviation of the remaining five readings.
• In healthy young adults, normal aqueous flare values are in the range of 2.5–4.5 ph/ms. Higher value can predict the risk of impending and recurrent attacks. LFP can be used for assessing vitreous haze also.

Uses

• Flare measured by LFP may reflect severity of inflammation during exacerbations and in presence of subclinical inflammation during quiescent periods.
• It may guide both immediate as well as long-term immunomodulatory treatment of panuveitis entities, like Bechet's disease, VKH, etc.
• Laser flare photometry may play an even more important role in monitoring therapy and predicting outcomes in children with uveitis.

Pit falls

• Particles, such as pigment, cannot be differentiated from inflammatory cells and may be counted as cells.

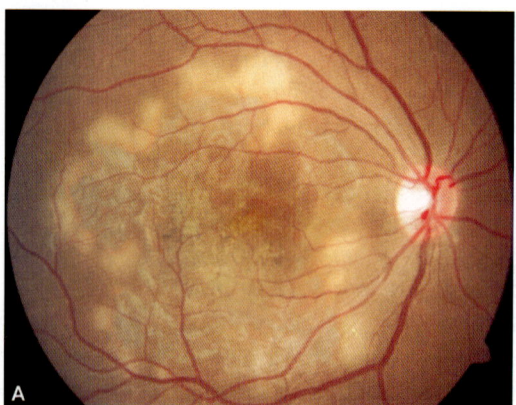

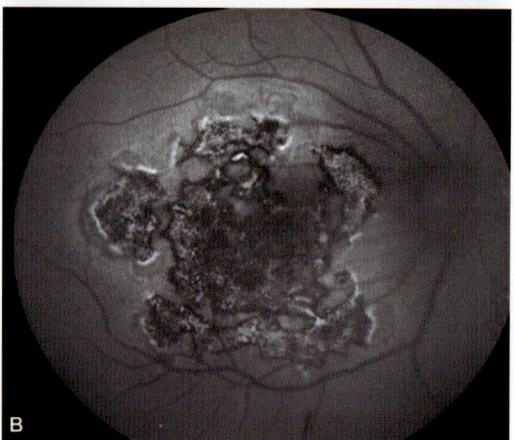

Fig. 5.2.5 *Fundus autofluorescence in serpiginous choroiditis showing hyperfluorescence of the active edge.*

- Differentiation between various cells, such as erythrocytes, ghost cells or leucocytes cannot be done either.

ULTRASOUND BIOMICROSCOPY

- *High frequency ultrasound biomicroscopy* (UBM) enables in vivo imaging of the anterior segment structures of the eye, including structures posterior to the iris plane that could not have been previously imaged by conventional ultrasonography.
- *Media opacities* (e.g. corneal opacity, cataract, pupillary membranes, etc.) do not preclude examination.
- *High-magnification and high resolution images* of the iridocorneal angle, posterior chamber, ciliary body, pars plana, vitreous base and peripheral retina and choroid can be obtained using the UBM.

Principle

The UBM uses high frequency transducers (50–100 MHz) incorporated into a B-scan ultrasound. The higher frequency transducers allow better resolution, but lower penetration of ocular tissues, thus are ideal for examination of superficial and anterior ocular structures. A real-time image can be displayed or stored.

Limitations

- Requires an experienced and technically skilled operator (the main disadvantage),
- It is time consuming, and
- The contact method might be uncomfortable for certain patients.

Method

Conventional UBM transducers are immersed in a cup filled with saline or a coupling media placed on the globe under topical anaesthesia with the patient in a supine position. Imaging with upright position is possible with advanced probes with built-in water bath.

Uses

It is a useful tool for detection of:

- *Ciliary body* inflammation, mass lesions and atrophy

- *Pars plana membranes*
- Exudates, zonular status
- Suspected cases of cyclodialysis cleft
- *Intraocular foreign* body at the angle of anterior chamber or pars plana, in hypotonous eye, and
- Other inflammatory and non-inflammatory conditions affecting pars plana and peripheral retina.

FLUORESCEIN ANGIOGRAPHY

Fundus fluorescein angiography (FFA) is an indispensable imaging tool for the diagnosis and monitoring of inflammatory diseases affecting the posterior segment of the eye.

Basic principles

The fluorescein dye is a small protein-bound (80%) molecule that absorbs light at 480–490 nm and emits at 530 nm. Remaining unbound dye (almost 20%) produces most of the fluorescence. Neither of the molecules (bound/unbound) can diffuse through the normal retinal vessel wall, the intact retinal pigment epithelium (RPE) or the large choroidal vessels. It diffuses freely through the fenestrated choriocapillaris.

Methodology

- *Fluorescein dye is injected* rapidly through intravenous route, usually through antecubital vein.
- *Blue excitation filter* (wavelength 465–490 nm) is used to project blue light. Blue light is then absorbed by unbound fluorescein molecules, and the molecules fluoresce, emitting light with a longer wavelength in the yellow–green spectrum (520–530 nm).
- *Barrier filter blocks* any reflected blue light so that the images capture only light emitted from the fluorescein molecules.
- *Images are acquired* in the digital media/film immediately after injection and continue for ten minutes depending on the pathology being imaged.

Phases of angiography

Fluorescein angiography has been divided into different phases:

1. *Choroidal flush*. The filling of the choroidal circulation is seen as the choroidal flush 10–12

seconds following injection. A patchy and mottled hyperfluorescence is seen as the choroidal lobules fill. Dye appears in the retinal circulation 1–3 seconds later.

2. Arteriovenous phase. The early arteriovenous phase involves the filling of the retinal arteries, arterioles and capillaries. This is followed by the late arteriovenous phase or laminar venous phase as the dye fills the veins in a laminar pattern.

3. Venous phase. It is characterised by the laminar flow in the retinal veins followed by venous filling. The peak phase with maximal fluorescence occurs at approximately 30 seconds and is characterised by complete filling of retinal veins.

4. Recirculation phase. During the recirculation of the dye, fluorescence gradually decreases with emptying of dye in the retinal vessels. Extravasated dye from the choriocapillaris stains the choroid and scleral rim of the optic disc.

After 10 minutes, the dye is no longer seen in retinal vessels. However, several structures including the optic nerve head, Bruch's membrane, and sclera are stained with the dye and continue to fluoresce.

Pathophysiological interpretations

There is no extravasation from the normal retinal vasculature. Abnormal patterns may be:

1. Hypofluorescence may be due to blockage or vascular filling defect in the choroidal or retinal circulation.

Blocked fluorescence may be caused by any opacity (vitreousopacity, blood, inflammatory infiltrate, fluid, pigment, etc.) that obscures the visibility of fluorescein in the choroid and/or in retinal circulation. Colour fundus photograph is sometimes required to differentiate between blockage and non-perfusion.

2. Hyperfluorescence may be caused by transmission (window) defects, abnormal retinal or choroidal vessels, leakage, staining or pooling of fluorescein.

- *Retinal pigment epithelial defects* cause transmission of choroidal fluorescence; thus hyperfluorescence (window defect) will have the same size and shape both in early and late phase.

- Pinpoint leaks of RPE are differentiated from window defects by their increasing size and change in shape with pooling of dye in the subretinal space.

- *Inflammation of the optic disc* causes hyperfluorescence due to dilated capillaries on the optic disc in the early phase and staining of the optic disc with leakage in the late phase.

- *Leaky abnormal vessels*, such as retinal neovascularisation (NVE or NVD) cause intense fuzzy hyperfluorescence due to profuse leakage of the dye.

- *Staining of retinal vessel walls* and retinal vascular leakage are the hallmarks of retinal vasculitis in FFA.

- *Leakage of dye* and pooling in the cystoid spaces at the macula give rise to a petalloid pattern of hyperfluorescence.

- *Diffusion of fluorescein into tissue* or material is defined as staining, which is a late phase phenomenon (during recirculation).

Uses of FFA in uveitis

Fluorescein angiography is especially useful in uveitis for the evaluation of:

- Optic disc inflammation,
- Macular oedema,
- Occlusive vasculitis, and
- Early detection of non-occlusive retinal vasculitis, neovascularisations, retinal pigment epithelial changes, disease activity in choroiditis and the source and pattern of leaks in exudative retinal detachment.

- *Inflammation of the retinal capillaries* can only be detected by angiography, so it has diagnostic importance in Behcet's disease and other vasculitis and intermediate uveitis.

- *In choroiditis, active lesions show early hypo- and late hyperfluorescence* (Fig. 5.2.6). It is due to oedema which blocks the initial dye but later leakage from the surrounding tissue cause hyperfluorescence.

- *In VKH*, in the acute uveitic stage, bilateral pinpoint RPE leaks and late pooling of dye in the subretinal space are the characteristic angiography findings. Similar findings are also seen in eyes with exudative retinal detachment associated with sympathetic ophthalmia and in posterior scleritis which is unilateral.

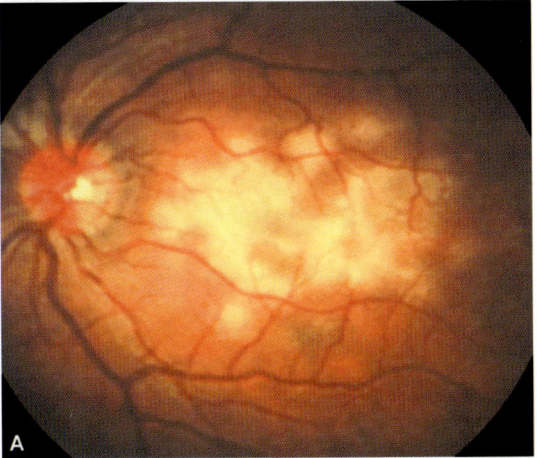

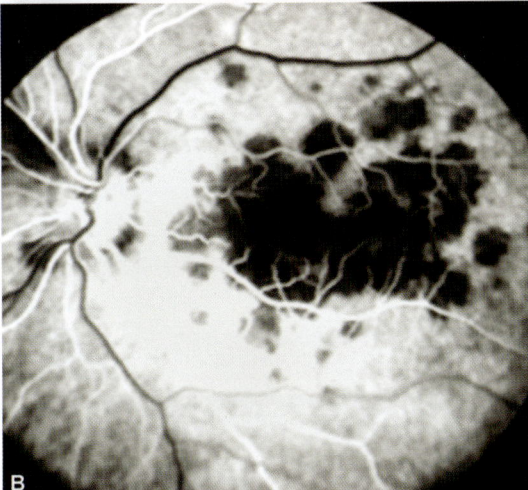

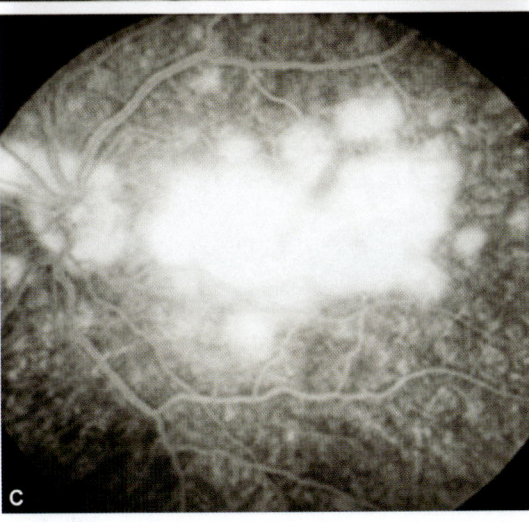

Fig. 5.2.6 *FFA in APMPPE showing early hypofluorescence and late hyperfluorescence of lesions.*

- *In active serpiginous choroiditis*, early hypo-fluorescence and late fuzzy staining are characteristic angiographic signs of an active lesion.

INDOCYANINE GREEN ANGIOGRAPHY (ICGA)

In the diseases which primarily involve the choroid and choriocapillaris, indocyanine green angiography is a better modality of investigation when compared with FFA.

Principle

Indocyanine green is a relatively large molecule than fluorescein with peak absorption of light at 795 nm and emission at 830 nm. Near infrared fluorescence of ICG allows access to the deeper structures. Almost all of the dye binds to serum proteins (80% binding globulins and α-lipoproteins). Therefore, the large ICG-protein complex does not leak from minimally inflamed retinal vessels. It leaks through the fenestrated choriocapillaris at a slower rate than fluorescein and slowly impregnates the choroid and is not readily washed out thus delineating the choroid and choroidal lesions. So the clinical interpretation of ICGA is mainly based on the changes in background choroidal fluorescence in pathologic conditions.

Phases of ICGA

Three main phases of ICGA have been defined:
1. *Early phase* (up to 3 minutes) characterised by filling of both the choroidal and retinal circulation, seen as superimposed vasculature.
2. *Intermediate phase* (8–12 minutes) characterised by maximum choroidal stromal background fluorescence.
3. *Late phase* (25–30 minutes) characterised by wash-out of dye from the circulation and a relatively dim choroidal background fluorescence.

ICGA in choroidal inflammations

- *Optic disc appears* dark throughout the phases of ICGA.
- *Choroidal vasculitis* may be seen as early stromal vessel hyperfluorescence, but it is best appreciated as fuzziness of choroidal vessels in the intermediate phase ICGA.

- *Hypofluorescent dots* have been described as an ICGA sign of active choroidal inflammation and they disappear after treatment.
- *Because of the infrared fluorescence of the ICG dye,* only heavy pigment deposition, thick blood or subretinal fluid can cause blockage of the background choroidal fluorescence.

Inflammatory choroidal vasculopathy and ICGA

Two types of inflammatory choroidal vasculopathy have been described based on the ICGA patterns.

Type 1 pattern represents *inflammatory choriocapillaropathies* or the white dot syndromes, including APMPPE, serpiginous choroiditis and multifocal choroiditis, where ICGA demonstrates patchy or geographic hypofluorescent areas, which may be associated with choriocapillaris non-perfusion. In multiple evanescent white dot syndrome (MEWDS), ICGA typically shows confluent hypofluorescence around the optic nerve and numerous dark dots throughout the posterior pole, which may not be appreciated on ophthalmoscopy or FA. In MEWDS, it was suggested that early hyperfluorescent lesions on FA associated with intermediate to late hypofluorescence on ICGA could represent RPE damage, while early hypofluorescent lesions on both FA and ICGA could represent perfusion disturbances of choriocapillaris or transient blockage caused by inflammatory lesions at the level of outer retina-RPE (Fig. 5.2.7).

Type 2 pattern represents more diffuse choroiditis with inflamed large vessels appearing fuzzy with the leakage of dye and dark dots associated with inflammatory foci in the choroid. Sympathetic ophthalmia, VKH, birdshot chorioretinopathy, sarcoidosis, tuberculosis and syphilis tend to exhibit the Type 2 pattern. While hypofluorescent dots, best appreciated in the intermediate phase, tend to have a uniform size and distribution in VKH, sympathetic ophthalmia and birdshot chorioretinopathy, a random distribution is usually observed in sarcoidosis and tuberculosis.

Several reports have shown that ICGA revealed choroidal lesions that were not detected by

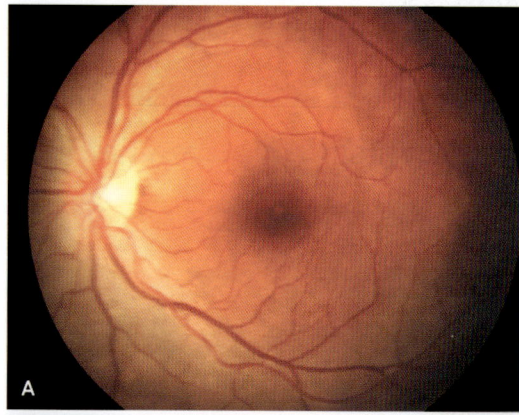

A

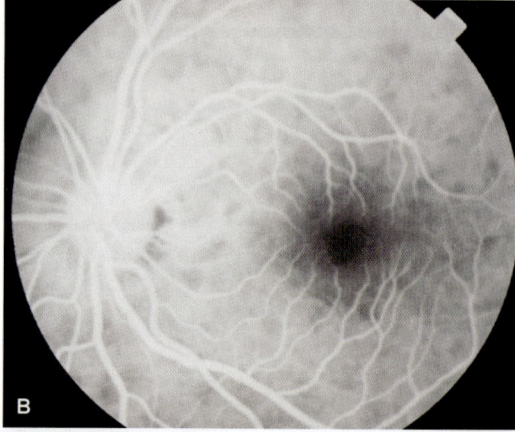

B

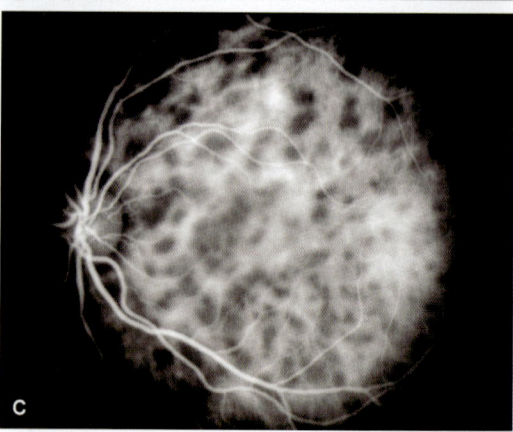

C

Fig. 5.2.7: *Fundus photo (A), FFA (B) and ICG (C) of a case of MEWDS showing better delineation of choroidal lesions in ICG.*

ophthalmoscopy or FA in a variety of chorioretinal inflammatory disorders, including ocular sarcoidosis, ocular tuberculosis, ocular syphilis, ocular toxoplasmosis, sympathetic ophthalmia, VKH disease, multifocal choroiditis, APMPPE,

MEWDS, serpiginous choroiditis, the choroidal involvement in birdshot chorioretinopathy, lupus choroidopathy and posterior scleritis. Also, indocyanine green angiography is an adjunct to FFA in the assessment of inflammatory choroidal neovascularisation, especially in eyes with occult membranes.

OPTICAL COHERENCE TOMOGRAPHY

Optical coherence tomography is a non-invasive, non-contact in vivo imaging of the retina and the optic nerve head.

Principle

It uses light to acquire high-resolution images of ocular structures. Measurements are obtained by directing a beam of light on to the tissues and measuring the echo time delay and magnitude of reflected or backscattered light using low coherence interferometry. A low-coherence, near-infrared light from a superluminescent diode light source is split into two beams, one goes to a reference mirror and the other to the retina. As the light comes back from the mirror and the eye, it creates an interference pattern, which then is analyzed by a photodetector. Cross-sectional images are generated by scanning the optical beam in the transverse direction, thereby yielding a two-dimensional dataset (B-scan) that can be displayed as a false-colour or grayscale image.

Scan protocol

For an optic nerve head or a macular scan with time domain (TD)-OCT, six radial line scans in a spoke-like pattern are centred on the optic nerve head or the fovea. Higher resolution spectral-domain OCT (SD-OCT) has entered clinical practice with reported resolution of 3–5 µm with improved visualization of retinal morphologic and pathologic features. Spectral-domain OCT technology relies on a spectrometer and high-speed camera and a fixed reference mirror.

Advances in OCT technology have been achieved by exploring ultrahigh-resolution (UHR) OCT, adaptive optics OCT, eye-tracking and Doppler OCT.

OCT interpretation

The currently available SD-OCT allow improved visualization of 4 bright lines in the outer retina, which represent the external limiting membrane (ELM), the photoreceptor inner and outersegment junction (IS/OS), the interdigitation of the photoreceptor outer segments (OS) and the RPE and the RPE-choriocapillary complex. All four layers are diagnostically useful in understanding the pathologies and structural changes of the retina in choroiditis. Integrity of ELM and IS/OS junction are important for vision.

Clinical applications

1. *Macular oedema.* Optical coherence tomography is suitable for detecting and monitoring uveitic macular oedema and provides important information about the type of macular oedema and any abnormality of the vitreoretinal interface. Different types of macular oedema of patients with uveitis are seen, like:

- *Cystoid macular oedema* (CME) with the presence of low reflective intraretinal cystic spaces separated by thin, high-reflective retinal tissue.
- *Diffuse macular oedema (DME)* characterised by increased macular thickness and the presence of small low-reflective areas with spongy appearance of the retinal layers.
- *Serous retinal detachment* is seen as a clear separation of the neurosensory retina from the RPE.

Epiretinal membrane (ERM) is an important feature of inflammation, which appears as a hyperreflective line adhering to the retinal layer. OCT also shows concurrent vitreoretinal traction. Higher resolution OCTs can also delineate choroidal layers.

2. *Iridocyclitis.* A peculiar finding described in eyes with active iridocyclitis using OCT is the occurrence of a ring-like pattern of retinal thickening outside the foveal centre in the inner ring and combined inner and outer rings. The macular thickening has been shown to have a significant correlation with active iridocyclitis.

3. *JIA.* Macular oedema and/or maculopathy in patients with juvenile idiopathic arthritis associated uveitis has also been observed by OCT.

4. *VKH disease.* VKH disease is the earliest and most extensively studied by OCT. Early studies involving the use of TD-OCT revealed that serous retinal detachments had two changes in structural patterns, namely, a true serous retinal detachment and an intraretinal fluid accumulation. Based on the observation that the subretinal septa dissolved immediately after pulse corticosteroid therapy, it has been concluded that the subretinal septa were composed of inflammatory products, such as fibrin which acts as a glue between outer segments, forming the membranous structure and the cystoid spaces characteristic of acute VKH disease. The mean choroidal thickness in the acute phase was significantly increased in the acute phase as compared with the convalescent phase of VKH and with normal eye.

5. *Sympathetic ophthalmia.* In patients with sympathetic ophthalmia (SO), OCT shows serous retinal detachment in the outer segment demarcated by the ELM and RPE, hyperreflective bands indicating fibrous septa within the serous detachment, disruption of the continuity of the RPE and IS/OS junction, and undulations and bumps on the RPE surface adjacent to the serous retinal detachment. OCT scans of Dalen-Fuchs nodules showed discrete nodules at the level of RPE that were associated with mild shadowing and overlying detachment of the neurosensory retina.

6. *Retinochoroidal toxoplasmosis.* Vitreoretinal morphology in patients with active ocular toxoplasmosis lesions shows hyperreflectivity of the retina at the site with active lesion and some degree of retinal RPE-choriocapillaris/choroidal optical shadowing. Incongenital toxoplasmosis macular structural changes consist of retinal thinning, RPE hyperreflectivity, excavation, intraretinal cysts and fibrosis.

7. *Multifocal choroiditis.* OCT shows choroidal and outer retinal involvement and the process extends into the inner retina leading to a circumscribed focal retinal thickening

8. *Serpiginous choroiditis.* The acute phase inflammation was limited to the deeper retinal and choroidal structures. There is an increased reflectance of the choroid and deeper retinal layers, along with disruption of the photoreceptor IS/OS junction in both active and inactive lesions.

9. *Birdshot chorioretinopathy.* OCT (ultra-high resolution) revealed disorganisation of inner retinal layers as well as photoreceptor and RPE atrophy. Decreased visual acuity was shown to be related with abnormal macular thickness and loss of the IS/OS junction, reduction in the total retinal thickness as determined by OCT. Restoration of retinal architecture following therapy has also been described based on OCT.

10. *APMPPE.* OCT shows hyperreflective area above the RPE in the photoreceptor layer in the early phase of the disease and nodular hyperreflective lesion on the plane of the RPE with mild underlying back scattering in the later phase of the disease.

11. *Acute zonal occult outer retinopathy (AZOOR).* OCT shows loss or irregularity of the IS/OS junction alone.

12. *Multifocal choroiditis and panuveitis (MCP).* Patients who had blind spot enlargement also had corresponding contiguous regions of IS/OS junction loss around the optic nerve head even in ophthalmoscopically normal areas between visible chorioretinal scars.

13. *MEWDS.* OCT described the widespread loss of the IS/OS junction during the acute phases.

14. *Anterior segment OCT (AS-OCT).* An adaptation of OCT technology for better visualisation of the anterior segment has been achieved using longer wavelength light of 1,310 nm as compared with 830 nm used for retinal imaging. Cross-sectional images of the anterior chamber were obtained using anterior segment OCT.

15. *In detecting AC cells in hazy media.* Hyperreflective spots in the anterior chamber could be quantified. Anterior segment OCT was able to detect anterior chamber cells in eyes with significant corneal oedema.

Limitations

Because the pigmented posterior layer of the iris prevents light transmission beyond this structure, the ciliary body cannot be visualised using anterior segment OCT scans.

ULTRASONOGRAPHY

It is a non-invasive, dynamic imaging modality for rapid evaluation of posterior segment structures in eyes with media opacities that obscures fundal examination. It is a useful adjuvant modality even in eyes with clear media to differentiate between inflammatory and non-inflammatory pathologies of the posterior segment.

Basic principle

The sound wave transmitted from a probe into the eye travels in ocular media of different densities. In ophthalmic ultrasound, both A-scan and B-scan ultrasonography are usually used in combination. A-scan/amplitude scan ultrasonography is a mono-dimensional scan and shows the distance between surfaces, as well as reflectivity characteristics (high/low reflective). The B-scan/brightness scan ultrasonography gives a two-dimensional cross-section image that shows the location, shape and extension of the lesion. Kinetic B-scan ultrasonography allows real-time assessment of movements of intraocular lesions. A three-dimensional ultrasonography is also possible with newer instruments. The sound reflected back to the probe from the interface of different media is known as an echo. Higher reflectivity produces stronger echo, which is seen as a high spike on the A-scan and brighter dots on the B-scan ultrasonogram. The sound waves are also absorbed by the media. Dense media absorbs more. Therefore, sound is both reflected and absorbed by dense media resulting in a weaker echo and even shadowing posterior to a dense medium. 10 MHz probe provides useful information on the vitreous cavity, retina, choroid, sclera, optic disc and periocular tissues. 20 MHz probe gives a better resolution and is useful for the evaluation of anterior vitreous cavity and lens.

Clinical applications

- *In the normal eye*, the vitreous is echolucent and the vitreoretinal interface produces a high spike.
- *Vitritis* causes diffusely distributed echoes of low reflectivity, which move freely.
- *Vitreous haemorrhage* produces moderate reflective mobile clump and membrane echoes.
- *Posterior vitreous detachment* is common in eyes with uveitis and appears as a mobile low reflective thin line.
- *Configuration of retinal detachment on ultrasonography* may suggest the underlying pathology. Traction retinal detachment appears as a tented hyperechogenic line (table top configuration) whereas exudative RD shows shifting fluid. Choroidal detachment shows an immobile thick line with higher reflectivity. But they do not appear posterior to equator.
- *Choroiditis.* Peripapillary choroidal thickness is an important measurement in choroiditis/posterior uveitis to understand activity. Choroidal thickening due to diffuse choroiditis has alow to medium reflectivity whereas diffuse posterior scleritis shows high reflective thickening of the posterior wall of the globe.
- There may be widening of the sub-Tenon space due to inflammatory oedema/fluid appearing as an echolucent zone posterior to the thickened wall and the posterior echolucent zone becomes continuous with the optic nerve giving rise to the T sign. It may be evident in diffuse posterior scleritis, sympathetic ophthalmia and VKH.
- *Focal retinochoroidal infiltrates or granulomas* may also be imaged by ultrasonography in the form of localized thickening or focal retinochoroidal elevation.
- *Malignant or benign intraocular tumours* have characteristic ultrasonographic features that differentiate them from inflammatory lesions.
- A high level expertise and quality imaging are essential for the use of ultrasonography as a diagnostic tool.

Limitations

- *It is an examiner-dependant procedure.* Technical skill and experience are important in the performance and interpretation of this imaging modality.

ELECTROPHYSIOLOGICAL TESTS IN UVEITIS

The electrophysiological examination includes the electroretinogram (ERG), visual evoked potentials (VEPs), electrooculogram (EOG), multifocal ERG (mfERG), and multifocal VEPs (mVEPs).

Electroretinogram

- *ERG is an electrophysiological examination* that reflects retinal electrical potential in response to a light stimulus.
- *Wave of ERG.* The a-wave is the first negative wave, and it is followed by the positive b-wave, which is further followed by a second negative wave—the c-wave. d-waves appear, only if the stimulus is applied for sufficient time.
- *Generation of wave.* a-wave is generated by the photoreceptors in the outer retina, b-wave reflects the responses of bipolar and Müller cells in inner retinal layers, c-wave is generated in the retinal pigment epithelium (RPE) and d-wave reflects the activity of "off" bipolar cells.
- *Evaluation of b:a wave ratio* is used as an index of inner to outer retinal function and the analysis of the waves gives information about the location of a retinal lesion.
- *Amplitudes and implicit times* of the waves are measured in ERG evaluation.
- *Flash ERG* represents the retinal electrical response to photic stimulation.
- *Pattern ERG* (PERG) is generated by a stimulus structure in the form of a black-and-white alternating checkboard or bars on a pattern monitor. The PERG wave consists of three components. The first, a small negative component, is N35, which is followed by a prominent positive component, P50, and finally a large negative component—N95. PERG is used primarily for the evaluation of the function of inner retinal layers and especially the ganglion cell layers of the retina.

Multifocal ERG. mfERG objectively evaluates the macula, allowing functional mapping of the central retina by selecting electrical responses from multiple retinal locations of the macular area, which are tested simultaneously.

Electro-oculography (EOG)

EOG is an electrophysiological test that examines the function of the outer retina and RPE, reflecting metabolic changes in the RPE and giving extra information about retinal function and supporting tissues. It is expressed as a ratio of the peak amplitude in the light to the minimum amplitude in the dark (light/dark or Arden ratio).

Visual evoked potentials

- *VEP is an electrophysiological examination* which objectively reflect the functional integrity of the whole visual pathway, from the photoreceptors in the retina to the visual cortex in the occipital lobe.
- *VEPs are generated* by the electrical activity in the entire visual cortex because of stimulation of the eye.
- *There are three types of stimuli:* The flash, the pattern reversal, and the pattern on/off. VEP examination is useful in the assessment of the visual function in uncooperative patients, in assessing visual pathway abnormality, prognosticating vision in patients with trauma and media opacity.
- *Limitation.* Since VEP reflects the entire visual pathway, an abnormal test does not provide the exact location of the dysfunction and over expression of the macular lesion.

Multifocal VEP. mVEP is an objective electrophysiological examination that evaluates the functional integrity of the visual pathway from the retina to the visual cortex.

Role of electrophysiological examination in posterior uveitis

Electrophysiological examinations have a role in different white dot syndrome entities, VKH, and retinochoroidal toxoplasmosis (Table 5.2.1).

Table 5.2.1 *Electrophysiological tests in some posterior uveitis entities*

Disease	VEP	ERG	EOG
1. MEWDS	In some cases: decrease of P100 amplitude P100 delayed	Acute phase: a- and b-wave amplitude reduced oscillatory potentials abnormal Resolved in recovery. mfERG sensitive indicator for recovery.	Abnormal
2. APMPPE	N/subnormal	Acute phase: Slightly abnormal values of a- and b-wave Recovery: Similar results, contrary to MEWDS	Acute phase: Highly abnormal Scar stage: Significantly improved
3. Birdshot chorio-retinopathy	Selective b-wave amplitude reduction most prominent finding, prolonged implicit times. Late stages: ERGs extinguished. They are useful in monitoring the disease severity and treatment monitoring	Abnormal	
4. Vogt-Koyanagi-Harada	Before treatment: Highly abnormal. During treatment, amplitude and latency initially improve significantly, but amplitude remains significantly decreased compared to normal for at least 1 year	MfERG: Useful test in guiding the therapy and detecting early retinal damage	
5. Behçet's disease	P100 significantly delayed (neuroBehcet, even before clinical signs)	Abnormal	Normal
6. Ocular syphilis	Significantly reduced	Before treatment extinguishing response, after treatment recovery	
7. Fuchs' heterochromic cyclitis		Patterned ERG and flash ERG abnormalities, reduced oscillatory potential amplitude	
8. Toxoplasma retinochoroiditis		Photopic and scotopic ERG abnormal	

BIBLIOGRAPHY

1. Becker MD, Rosenbaum JT. Essential laboratory tests in uveitis. Dev Ophthalmol 1999;31: 92–108.
2. Centers for Disease Control and Prevention. 2006 sexually transmitted diseases treatment guidelines. MMWR Recomm 2006;55 (RR11):1–85.
3. Chan CC, Shen D, Tuo J. Polymerase chain reaction in the diagnosis of uveitis. Int Ophthalmol Clin 2005;45(2):41–55.
4. Ciardella AP, Borodoker N, Costa DL, et al. Imaging the posterior segment in uveitis. Ophthamol Clin North Am 2002;15:281–96.
5. Kijlstra A. The value of laboratory testing in uveitis. Eye (Lond.) 1990;4(Pt 5):732–6.
6. Mahalakshmi B, Therese KL, Madhavan HN, Biswas J. Diagnostic value of specific local antibody production and nucleic acid amplicati on technique -Nested polymerase chain reaction (n PCR) in clinically suspected ocular toxoplasmosis. Ocular Immunology & Inflammation, 1744-5078, Volume 14, Issue 2, 2006, pp. 105–112.

7. Majumder PD, Sudharshan S, Biswas J. Laboratory support in the diagnosis of uveitis. Indian Journal of Ophthalmology 2013;61(6):269–76.

8. Ongkosuwito JV, Bosch-Driessen EH, Kijlstra A, Rothova A. Serologic evaluation of patients with primary and recurrent ocular toxoplasmosis for evidence of recent infection. Am J Ophthalmol 1999;128:407–12.

9. Rosenbaum JT, Wernick R. The utility of routine screening of patients with uveitis for systemic lupus erythematosus or tuberculosis. A Bayesian analysis Arch Ophthalmol 1990;108(9): 1291–3.

10. Sandler G. The importance of the history in the medical clinic and the cost of unnecessary tests. Am Heart J 1980;100(6 Pt 1):928–31.

11. Yamamoto S, Pavan-Langston D, Kinoshita S. Detecting herpesvirus DNA in uveitis using the polymerase chain reaction. Br J Ophthalmol 1996;80:465–8.

5.3 PATHOLOGICAL DIAGNOSTIC TESTS IN UVEITIS

Introduction
Biopsy Techniques used in Uveitis
- Aqueous and vitreous sample
- Iris and ciliary body biopsy
- Chorioretinal biopsy
- Fine needle aspiration biopsy

INTRODUCTION

Examination of a patient with uveitis needs to be very meticulous as the association with systemic autoimmune and infectious diseases is high. Some forms of uveitis, e.g. Fuchs' heterochromic iridocyclitis, serpiginous choroiditis can be diagnosed based on clinical picture alone. Ancilliary tests are also helpful in diagnosing an entity, like HLA-B27 related recurrent anterior uveitis. Importance of biopsy pathology in uveitis lies in certain situations, like masquerade syndrome:

- Vitreoretinal lymphoma and metastasis,
- Intraocular infections, and
- Undiagnosed, recalcitrant posterior uveitis.

BIOPSY TECHNIQUES USED IN UVEITIS

The following techniques with various modifications have been used in pathological diagnosis of uveitis:[1,2]

- Aaueous and vitreous sample collection
  - Anterior chamber paracentesis (keratocentesis).
  - Diagnostic vitrectomy and vitreous tap.
- Iris and ciliary body biopsy.
- Retinochoroidal biopsy.
- Fine needle aspiration biopsy.

AQUEOUS AND VITREOUS SAMPLE COLLECTION
ANTERIOR CHAMBER PARACENTESIS
Indications
- Masquerade syndrome.
- Hypopyon uveitis.
- Endophthalmitis.

- Lens-induced uveitis.
- Parasitic uveitis.

Technique
Anterior chamber paracentesis is a relatively safe outpatient technique.

Procedure
It should be done under aseptic precautions. Following steps can be followed:

- *Eye is anaesthetised* using topical proparacaine eyedrop for 3 times at 5 minutes interval and an universal eyelid speculum the patient is made to lies supine.
- *Separate the eyelids* and keep the lashes away from the ocular field. An antibiotic drop is instilled just before the procedure.
- *Tuberculin syringe* or 2 cc syringe with a 30 gauge needle is used for the paracentesis. However, if there is a fibrinous reaction in AC, a larger bore needle (25–26 gauge) should be used. In presence of a hypopyon in AC, the needle tip should be kept 1 mm away from the upper margin of the hypopyon.
- *Patient is asked to fixate at the ceiling*. The pupil preferably should be undilated as it reduces the risk of lens touch.
- *Needle is inserted*, bevel down, in an oblique fashion through the onset stroma, near the lower limbus to create a valvular, self-sealing AC entry.
- *One should stay over the peripheral iris tissue* at all times to avoid lenticular or endothelial touch. The plunger is slowly withdrawn to collect 0.1 to 0.3 ml of aqueous.
- *Needle is withdrawn* from the eye, the entry point is massaged with a cotton pledget, a drop of topical povidone iodine is applied
- *Eye* is patched with a sterile dressing, which is removed after 20–30 minutes.
- *Eye* is evaluated for any endothelial or lens touch and AC formation, topical antibiotic eyedrops are prescribed for 3 days and patient is re-evaluated after 1 to 2 weeks.

Complications

- Hyphema.
- Endothelial or lens touch.
- Wound leak.
- Iritis.
- Endophthalmitis.
- Needle track abscess.

VITREOUS TAP AND DIAGNOSTIC VITREOUS BIOPSY

Indications of vitreous biopsy

Vitreous biopsy is a useful adjunct to the systemic workup of the cases that constitute diagnostic dilemmas and in which intraocular inflammation is mostly confined to the posterior pole.[3] Such cases include:

- Chronic uveitis unresponsive to empirical treatment with systemic anti-inflammatory medications.
- Atypical clinical presentation.
- Inconclusive non-invasive laboratory work-up
- Acute sight-threatening disease.
- Endophthalmitis.[4]

Techniques

A vitreous specimen can be obtained by: Vitreous aspiration or pars plana vitrectomy.

Technique of vitreous aspiration

Vitreous aspiration can even be done in an office setting. As perforation of sclera is painful, the procedure is done using subconjunctival anaesthesia, by injecting 0.1 ml of 2% lignocaine over the area of needle insertion. 25 G needle is mostly used in uveitic eyes as the vitreous is liquefied due to the inflammation. In case of organised vitreous, 23 G needle can be used. The needle is attached to a 2 cc syringe along with a stopcock (Fig. 5.3.1). The needle is inserted 3.5 mm away from the limbus in a phakic eye and 3 mm in a pseudophakic/aphakic eye. 0.1–0.3 ml of vitreous is withdrawn in the syringe and manipulating the stopcock, an equal amount of antibiotic is injected.

Complications include:
- Retinal tear
- Refinal detachment
- Vitreous haemorrhage
- Endophthalmitis.

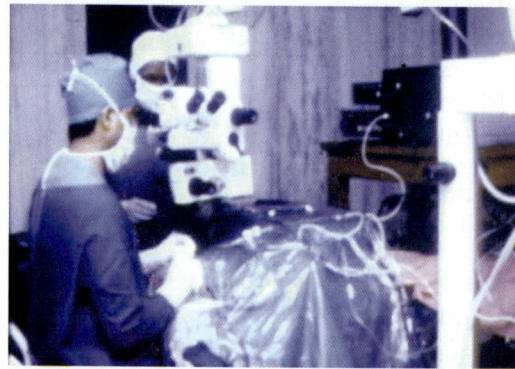

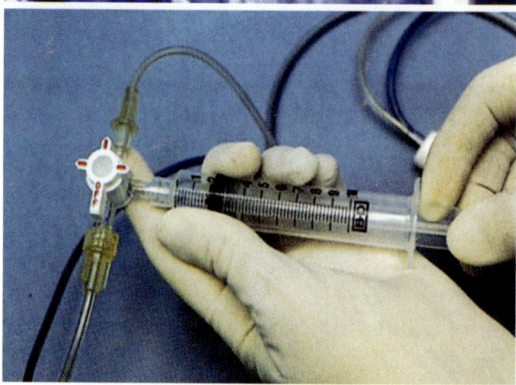

Fig. 5.3.1 *Vitreous biopsy sample being obtained using three-way stop-cock.*

Diagnostic pars plana vitrectomy

The procedure can be done under either general or topical anaesthesia. For vitreous aspiration, the one-port technique can be used. However, in eyes with uveitis, where there can be coexistent media opacities or intraocular inflammation, the three-port technique is preferable. Balanced salt solution (BSS) infusion is used to control the intraocular pressure during the procedure. Control of the pressure can minimise the risk of severe intraoperative hypotony as well as choroidal detachments and expulsive haemorrhage, all of which are more common in eyes with uveitis.[3] However, in diagnostic vitrectomy, the initial vitreous specimen is obtained undiluted (before the infusion port is opened); approximately 1.0 ml of vitreous is obtained directly from the vitrectomy cutter handpiece, with a cutting rate at 1200/minute, through an in-line stopcock and tubing attached to a syringe.[3,5,6] The infusion line is subsequently opened, and a standard, total vitrectomy is performed. Effort is taken to remove as much of the vitreous body as possible by harvesting material from all areas of the fundus including with scleral indentation.[3] Both the undiluted vitreous specimen and the vitreous washings from the subsequent total vitrectomy should be delivered immediately for cytopathological and microbiological analysis.[5,6]

Handling aqueous and vitreous samples

The following tests can be done using an aqueous or vitreous sample.

Microbiological analysis

The aqueous or vitreous specimen can be used for:
- Gram stain,
- KOH staining, and
- Culture.

Smears and stains. The smears and stains are very useful for rapid initial diagnosis of endophthalmitis but their role is limited. Gram stain is positive in 66% of culture proven cases.

However, positive smears can help the clinician choose the appropriate antibiotic for the organism before the results from the cultures are available.

Culture. Routinely, the culture media used for inoculation include blood agar, chocolate agar, thioglycollate broth, brain heart infusion agar, sabouraud dextrose agar, BHIB with gentamicin.

In case of vitreous specimen, cultures can be performed in both diluted and undiluted vitreous. Undiluted samples can be used directly for cultures or smears. Vitreous washings are initially passed through millipore filters. During filtration, microorganisms or any cellular elements concentrate on the filter surface. The filter is then cut under sterile conditions and used for culture.

Bacterial cultures should be kept for 5–14 days, if the presence of a slowly growing anaerobic bacterium (i.e. *Propionibacterium acnes*) is suspected.

Sensitivity of vitreous cultures has been estimated to be 50% and is much higher than that of aqueous.[7] Processing both diluted and undiluted vitreous increases the sensitivity of vitreous cultures to 57.4%.[8]

Molecular biologic study:
Polymerase chain reaction

This technique amplifies a specific locus on a DNA sample from a complex mixture of DNA. Approximately 0.05 ml of the sample should be preserved for this test, if viral infection, infectious or *P. acnes* endophthalmitis is suspected.

Nested PCR. In this technique, 2 pairs of primers are used for the same locus. If one locus gets wrongly amplified by a primer, there is very little chance it will get amplified by the second primer, so the proper locus only gets amplified, thus increasing the specificity of the procedure.[2]

Real-time PCR. In this technique, the load of the DNA copies is quantified in real-time by assessing the increasing fluorescence of a detector. So it allows both detection and quantification of a gene locus, thus giving evidence of active multiplication of an organism. Figure 5.3.2 demonstrates PCR test in a patient with chronic granulomatous uveitis.

Cytological analysis

The entire specimen is spinned down, the supernatant transpipetted, the pellet is resuspended in formalin or glutaraldehyde and then passed through 2 millipore filters. These filters can be used for staining including immunohistochemistry. Cytospin method can also be used[15] which involves the use of cytospin slides that are cleaned with alcohol and assembled with a slide filter card and sample delivery chamber, secured by a metal clip. Typically, up to 0.4 ml of fluid sample (3–5 drops) is added to the chamber together with an equal amount of cytospin collection fluid. After spinning at 1800 rpm for 2 minutes, slides are removed from the cytospin chamber, further fixed in cytology fixative (70% alcohol/formalin), and stained with haematoxylin and eosin.

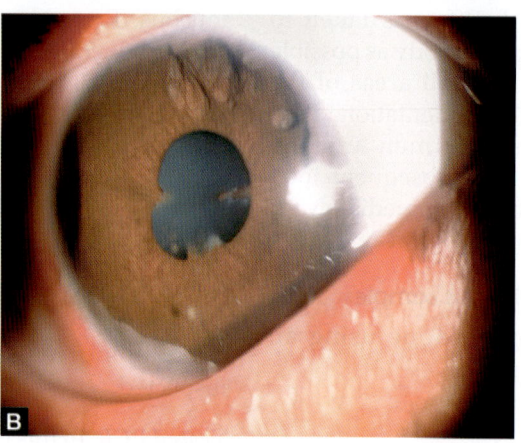

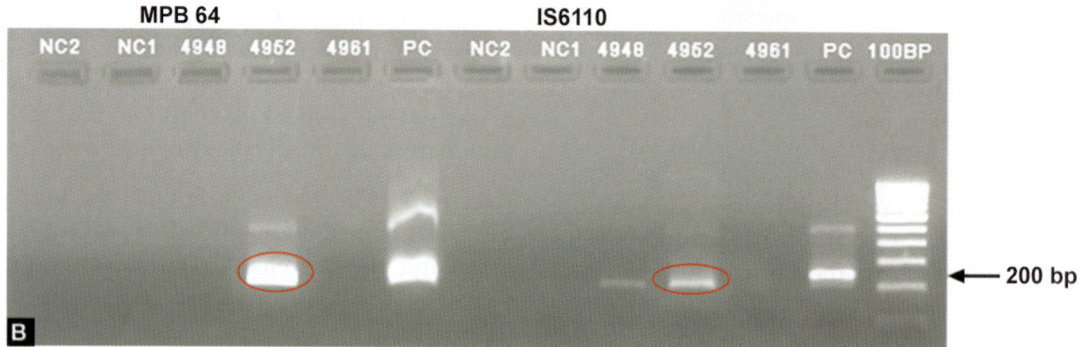

Fig. 5.3.2 *A, Clinical photograph of a patient with chronic granulomatous anterior uveitis with mutton fat KPs, broad posterior synechiae and peripheral anterior synechiae; B, PCR from aqueous tap positive for MPB64 and IS6110 genome confirming diagnosis of tuberculosis (PC: Positive control, 4962: Specimen well).*

Certain important findings on cytology are given below:

Aqueous aspirate

- *Phacogenic uveitis:* Macrophages engulfing lens particles, chronic inflammatory cells (Fig. 5.3.3).
- *Parasitic uveitis:* Eosinophils, polymorphs, sometimes parasite (Fig. 5.3.4).
- *Masquerade syndrome:* Malignant cells

Vitreous aspirate

- *Large cell lymphoma:* Large pleomorphic cells with round to oval nuclei with scanty cytoplasm, often with micronuclei (Fig. 5.3.5).
- *Phacoanaphylactic uveitis:* Lens fragments engulfed by macrophages, surrounded by epitheloid cells and giant cells.
- *Uveitis:* Heterogenous inflammatory infiltrate.

Antibody detection

The supernatant obtained after centrifugation can be used for antibody detection by ELISA.

This is specially useful for conditions, like toxoplasma or toxocara. The ocular antibody production should be analysed using Goldmann-Witmer coefficient.[9]

GW coefficient = Titre of aqueous antibody in serum globulin × Titre of serum antibody in aqueous globulin.

GW coefficient:
- 0.5–2 = No ocular infection.
- 2–4 = Probable ocular infection.
- > 4 = Diagnostic of ocular infection.

Flow cytometric analysis

This technique analyses the physical and chemical properties of particles or cells moving in a single file in a fluid stream. This technique is specially applicable for analysis of tumours, like retinoblastoma, leukaemia, lymphoma to give an idea about the variation in cell population in the tumors. This is used as an adjunct to histopathologic examination. Also, at

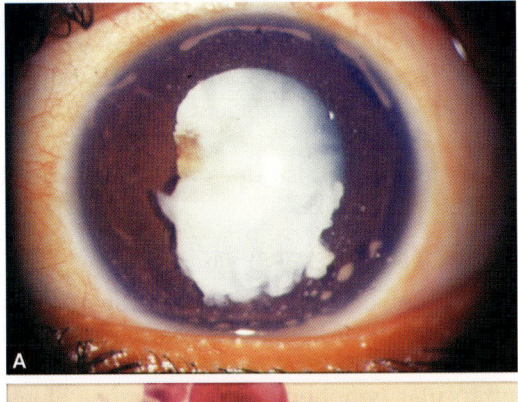

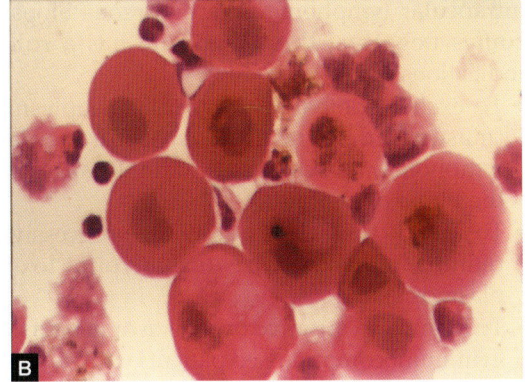

Fig. 5.3.3 *A, Granulomatous anterior uveitis in a case of traumatic cataract with ruptured anterior lens capsule; B, AC tap showing macrophages with engulfed lens matter.*

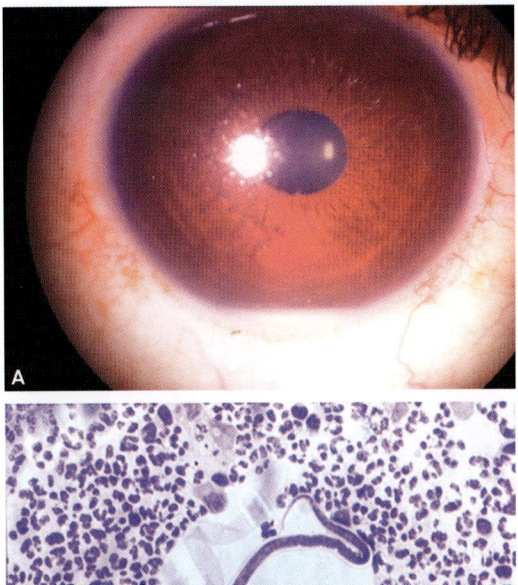

Fig. 5.3.4 *A, Hypopyon in anterior uveitis,not responding to topical steroid therapy; B, AC tap showing microfilaria along with chronic inflammatory cells.*

present, ratio between cytotoxic and helper T cells is used to analyse the pathology of ocular inflammation. In a study, CD22+ lymphocyte >20% in the cell population as found by flow cytometric analysis had a positive predictive value of 100% in diagnosis of intraocular lymphoma. A ratio of IL10/IL6 of >1 was found to have a sensitivity of 74.3% and specificity of 75% from vitreous biopsy in a study.[10]

IRIS AND CILIARY BODY BIOPSY

Indications

Indications are limited and include the following:

- Metastatic nodules or primary tumours of iris/ciliary body masquerading uveitis.
- Ruptured iris or ciliary body cysts.
- Granulomatous lesions of iris/ciliary body as seen in tuberculosis, sarcoidosis, certain fungal infection, like coccidioidomycosis to confirm the diagnosis.

Technique

A safe procedure has been described.[11] The *punch biopsies* can be performed as an ambulatory procedure under local anaesthesia. A clear corneal incision with a 3.2 mm angled slit knife is made close to the iris lesion. A viscoelastic is injected to fill the anterior chamber. A Kelly Descemet's membrane punch with a 1.0 mm diameter head and a 0.75 mm deep bite is inserted into the anterior chamber to lie over the iris lesion. The Kelly punch is placed with its mouth over the lesion and pressed down firmly before the punch is made. After taking a punch, the Kelly punch is kept closed and removed from the eye to be opened over a dry cellulose sponge . The viscoelastic is left in the anterior chamber. For a ciliary body biopsy, similar procedure can be used with the aid of visualisation by a direct goniolens.

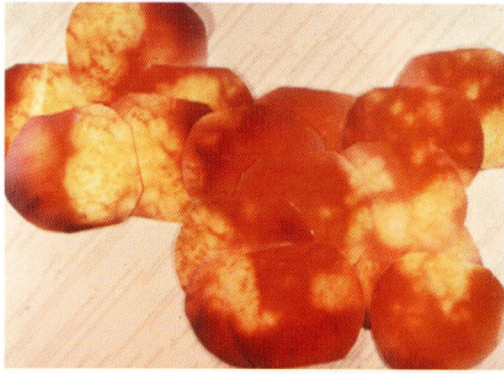

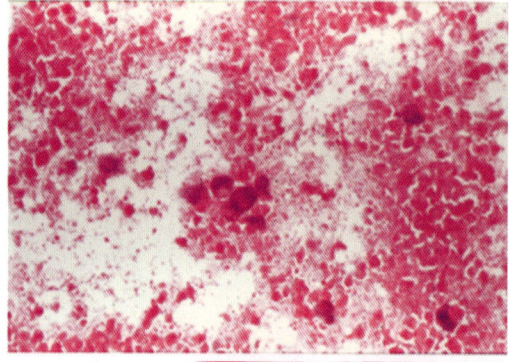

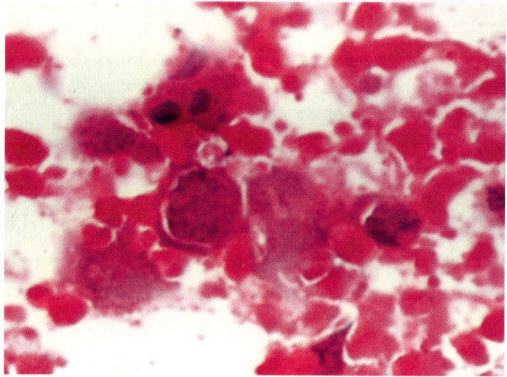

Fig. 5.3.5 *Colour fundus photograph of a 57-year-old female patient showing subretinal mass (extreme left). Vitreous biopsy showed large, pleomorphic cells with scanty cytoplasm in a necrotic background suggestive of large cell lymphoma.*

Complications

Bleeding, rise of IOP due to retained viscoelastic, corneal endothelial touch, exacerbation of inflammation.

Advantages

- FNAB, though can be used for solid tumours in this area, it actually yields an aspirate for cytopathology rather than a tissue sample.

Punch biopsy yields a tissue sample enabling both histologic and cytopathologic evaluation as well as architecture and level of infiltration.

- The tissue is also sufficient for special stains to aid in diagnosis.
- This technique also does not require much surgical expertise.

CHORIORETINAL BIOPSY

With the advent of new imaging systems, most of the choroidal lesions can be characterized. However, in atypical cases and in suspected intraocular lymphoma where vitreous biopsy comes negative, this technique has a role. Indications include:

- To exclude potential intraocular neoplasms (masquerade syndrome, e.g. intraocular lymphoma), which are primarily localised to the retina or choroid.
- To identify infective agents in progressive retinitis/retinal necrosis (e.g. atypical toxoplasmosis).
- To identify a causative organism or neoplasm in immunocompromised patients with uveitis.
- To aid in the diagnosis of uveitis with progressive sight-threatening chorioretinal lesions unresponsive to treatment.

Technique

Choroidal/chorioretinal biopsy can be done through an external or trans-scleral approach or an internal (Fig. 5.3.6) or transvitreal approach.

External approach

The surgical technique for performing an external chorioretinal biopsy is fairly straight forward.[12,13] First, provided that the fundus is clearly visible, laser photocoagulation is applied 1–3 days before surgery in a zone of the area to be biopsied. If the vitreous is too hazy, endolaser is placed immediately following vitrectomy. After a 360° conjunctival incision and isolation and tying of the rectus muscles, a three-port pars plana vitrectomy is performed (in addition to endolaser application in the area to be biopsied, if it was not placed prior to the surgery). The vitreous specimen (dilute and undilute) is sent for cytologic, microbiologic or flow cytometry analysis as required. A nearly full-thickness

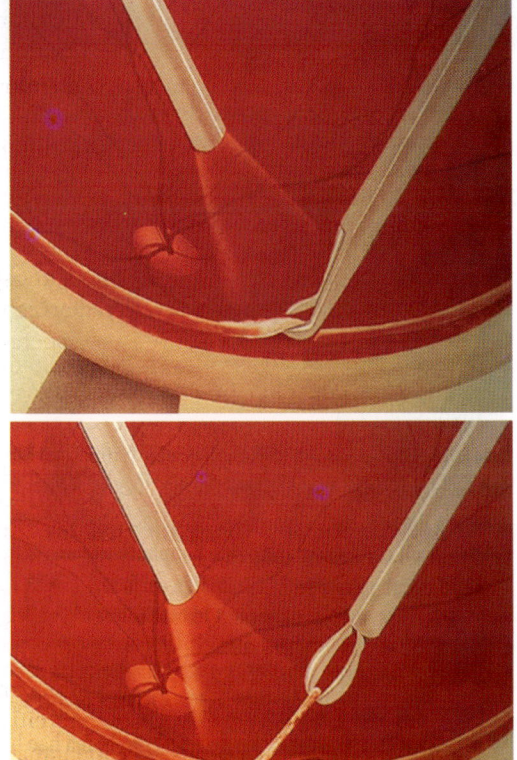

Fig. 5.3.6 *Technique of chorioretinal biopsy through internal approach.*

scleral flap is made, leaving one side attached to act as a hinge. When the flap of sclera is retracted, the surgeon is able to visualize the choroids, which is practically bare. Next, a penetrating diathermy is placed through the choroid and retina along the outer margin of the inner choroidal bed. Two incisions parallel to the limbus are made. Next, by inserting one blade of a 0.12 forceps through the incision, the full thickness of the choroid and retina may be grasped at one edge. Then, two more incisions, perpendicular to the limbus, are made with Vannas scissors, thereby yielding a block of chorioretinal tissue. Extreme care should be taken to grasp the full-thickness tissue only once with the forceps so that the architecture of the tissue remains intact. The scleral flap is then closed over the wound and is sutured closed followed by fluid-gas exchange.

Internal approach

Transvitreal retinochoroidal (endoretinal) biopsy is another approach by which chorioretinal tissue is acquired.[12,13] Briefly, in this technique, a standard three-port vitrectomy is performed (sending undiluted and diluted vitreous sample to the pathology lab for analysis) with endodiathermy used to outline an area of retina that is of interest. Intraocular scissors are introduced into the vitreous space and a small hole is created in the retina such that the area of interest is excised. With intraocular forceps, the retinal tissue is brought to the opening for the vitrector and is gently drained out of the eye using intraocular irrigation. In case of a retinal detachment, the specimen should be taken from the margin of attached and detached retina. Cassoux et al[14] also devised a technique of subretinal injection of sodium hyaluronate to induce a localized retinal detachment to collect the tissue specimen from the area of interest. The resultant bulging retina was subsequently excised by cutting around the perimeter with scissors and extricating the biopsy with forceps. Endolaser was then applied around the biopsy site.

Handling the specimen

The biopsy tissue is immediately processed by an ophthalmic pathologist in the operating room. It is generally divided into three portions. One-third of the tissue is fixated for routine histopathologic studies, including light and electron microscopic examinations. The second portion is snap frozen in optimal cutting temperature (OCT) embedding compound and is used for immunopathologic and molecular characterization. The third portion is sent for culture with the preference for viral and other microorganisms cultures and/or tissue culture. Sometimes, enough tissue may not be available for dividing in three parts and analysing. In that case, a frozen section analysis should at least be performed.

FINE NEEDLE ASPIRATION BIOPSY (FNAB)

Indications

Indications for FNAB are following:
- Cases of suspected infectious subretinal lesions mimicking as choroidal tumours.

- Patients with metastatic disease of choroid where primary is not known.
- Cases where patient refuses recommended therapy until histopathological confirmation is obtained.

Technique

Limbal route is used to approach anteriorly located lesions, like iris lesion.

For posterior segment lesions, two routes are available:

- *Pars plana approach.* In this approach, the needle is inserted through pars plana (3.5 mm from limbus) in the quadrant opposite to the lesion and passed through the vitreous to reach the lesion. For posteriorly located tumours, vitrectomy needs to be performed before aspiration.
- *Corneolimbal approach.* This technique is used in tumours with high risk of dissemination through needle track, e.g. retinoblastoma. The needle is passed through the limbus, then through the zonules to reach the vitreous. As it passes through multiple planes, the tumour cells are removed as the needle is removed from the eye.

Points to be remembered for biopsy in a case of intraocular lymphoma:[15]

- To stop the steroids before the diagnostic procedure to increase the yield.
- If a distinct mass lesion is there, biopsy from it is always preferable than do a vitreous tap.
- Vitreous tap may come negative due to apoptosis and degeneration of the lymphoma cells and due to increased inflammatory cell population. Doing a cytokine profile or cell culture can be considered in such cases.

Complications

- Bleeding from the needle track.
- Dissemination of tumour cells, though rare, can happen.
- Iatrogenic retinal perforation. In fact, when a choroidal lesion is biopsied in this technique, it is unavoidable and theoretically can cause a retinal detachment. But practically, the break is very small and it gets clogged by the blood clot from the underlying choroid.

REFERENCES

1. Van der Lelij A, Rothova A. Diagnostic anterior chamber paracentesis in uveitis: a safe procedure? The British Journal of Ophthalmology 1997; 81(11):976–9.
2. Biswas J, Annamalai R, Krishnaraj V. Biopsy pathology in uveitis. Middle East African Journal of Ophthalmology 2011;18:261–7.
3. Jeroudi A, Yeh S. Diagnostic vitrectomy for infectious uveitis. International Ophthalmology Clinics. 2014;54173–97.
4. Forster R, Abbott R, Gelender H. Management of infectious endophthalmitis. Ophthalmology 1980; 87:313–9.
5. Verbraeken H. Diagnostic vitrectomy and chronic uveitis. Graefes Arch Clin Exp Ophthalmol 1996;234:2–7.
6. Bovey EH, Herbort CP. Vitrectomy in the management of uveitis. Ocul Immunol Inflamm 2000;8:285–91.
7. Savitri S, Subhadra J, Muralidhar V et al. Sensitivity and predictability of vitreous cytology, biopsy and membrane filter culture in endophthalmitis. Retina 1996;16:525–9.
8. Donahue SP, Kowalski RP, Jewart BH, Friberg TR. Vitreous cultures in suspected endophthalmitis. Biopsy or vitrectomy? Ophthalmology. 1993; 100:1597–8.
9. Garweg JG, de Groot-Mijnes JD, Montoya JG. Diagnostic approach to ocular toxoplasmosis. Ocular Immunology and Inflammation. 2011;19255–61.
10. Wolf LA, Reed GF, Buggage RR, et al. Vitreous cytokine levels. Ophthalmology 2003;110(8): 1671–72.
11. Pe'er J, Blumenthal EZ, Frenkel S. Punch biopsy of iris lesions: a novel technique for obtaining histology samples. The British Journal of Ophthalmology 2007;91660–2.
12. Nussenblatt RB, Davis JL, Palestine AG. Chorioretinal biopsy for diagnostic purposes in cases of intraocular inflammatory disease. Dev Ophthalmol 1992;23:133–8.
13. Martin DF, Chan CC, de Smet MD, et al. The role of chorioretinal biopsy in the management of posterior uveitis. Ophthalmology 1993;100:705–14.
14. Cassoux N, Charlotte F, Rao NA, et al. Endoretinal biopsy in establishing the diagnosis of uveitis: a clinicopathologic report of three cases. Ocul Immunol Inflamm 2005;1379–83.
15. Finger PT, Papp C, Latkany P, Kurli M, Iacob CE. Anterior chamber paracentesis cytology (cytospin technique) for the diagnosis of intraocular lymphoma. The British Journal of Ophthalmology 2006;90:690–2.

5.4 MEDICAL MANAGEMENT OF UVEITIS

Introduction
- Objectives of treatment
- Ultimate goal of therapy
- Key issues in management
- Modalities of management

Mydriactics and Cycloplegics
- Preparation, action, salient features and side effects
- Mechanism of action
- Indications and choice of agent
- Essential practical points

NSAIDs
- Mechanism of action
- Preparations and uses
- Indications

Corticosteroids
- Mechanism of action
- Topical steroids
- Periocular steroids
- Systemic steroids
- Intravitreal steroids
- Steroid resoponsiveness

Immunosuppressive Agents
- Indications
- Mechanism of action
- Salient features
- Trials with immunosuppressive

Anti-VEGF Agents
- Mechanism of action
- Effects
- Advantages
- Disadvantages

INTRODUCTION

The final and most important challenge in uveitis is the management of uveitis. The management of uveitis not only includes management of the condition but also its associated sequelae. Ophthalmologist should make all attempts to preserve the structure and the function of the eye from the attack of uveitis.

Objectives of treatment are:
- Prompt and adequate control of intraocular inflammation

- To prevent the vision-threatening sequelae of the condition
- Treatment of the already present sequelae
- Minimize long-term complications of disease and its treatment

Ultimate goal of therapy is to prevent visual loss occurring from the structural and functional morbidities associated with uveitis.

Key issues in management are to decide whether uveitis is:
- Anterior, intermediate, posterior or panuveitis
- Acute or chronic, relapse or persistent
- Active or inactive
- Infectious or non-infectious
- Vision-threatening or not vision-threatening
- Associated with any complications due to uveitis
- Associated with any systemic condition.

Accurate diagnosis should be established before starting the treatment.

However, even in this modern era, it is not unusual to not get an accurate diagnosis of uveitis even after battery of investigations performed. The dependency on the clinical acumen of an ophthalmologist becomes the most important tool for managing the patient and the importance of the above mentioned questions rises further.

Further, individualisation of each case and condition helps us plan our management with better efficiency.

Modalities of management of uveitis
- *Medical therapy* form the mainstay of treatment
- *Surgical treatment* and when required
- *Adjuvant treatment* modalities, like laser photo-coagulation, cryotherapy, etc. may be required for an effective long-term control of the disease sequelae.

Medical therapy usually consists of:
- *Corticosteroids* (topical, periocular, intravitreal or systemic).
- *Cycloplegics* in the form of eyedrops or ointment.

- *NSAIDs* (topical or systemic). These are the mainstay agents to decrease the ocular inflammation, stabilize the disease process and reducing the complications associated with uveitis.
- *Other agents* are often added/substituted of uveitis is not controlled with conventional therapy include:
  - Immunomodulators
  - Biologic agents
  - Anti-VEGF therapy

Route and dosage of the medical therapy should be adjusted depending upon various patient-related factors, like age, systemic condition, effectiveness of the treatment, immune status, side effects of the treatment, etc.

MYDRIATICS AND CYCLOPLEGICS

Mydriatics and cycloplegics play a very important role in the management of patients with anterior chamber inflammatory response irrespective of the cause (infectious or non-infectious) or the actual site of inflammation (anterior, intermediate or posterior).

Various drugs that can be used under these categories are:
- *Cholinergic antagonists,* such as atropine (natural-atropa belladonna), homatropine (semisynthetic) and synthetics, like cyclopento-late, and tropicamide.
- α_1 adrenergic agonists, e.g. phenylephrine

PREPARATION, ACTIONS, SALIENT FEATURES AND SIDE EFFECTS

Dosage, preparations available, actions and side effects of commonly used mydriatics and cycloplegics are summarised in Table 5.4.1.

MECHANISM OF ACTION IN UVEITIS

- *Reduce the pain occurring from ciliary spasm* by producing paralysis of ciliary tones (cycloplegia).
- *Prevent the formation of posterior synechiae* from secondary iridocyclitis by pushing the lens–iris diaphragm posteriorly, thus decreasing the contact between pupillary margin and lens and also by keeping the pupil in motion.

- *Break the already formed synechiae* by constant mobilisation of the pupil.
- *Produce conjunctival and uveal arteriole dilation* and reduce permeability of the blood–aqueous barrier thus decreasing the access of inflammatory mediators to anterior chamber.

INDICATIONS AND CHOICE OF AGENT

Indications

- Anterior uveitis
- Intermediate uveitis or posterior uveitis with anterior spillover
- Posterior synechiae prevention and lysis
- Secondary glaucoma due to inflammation
- Secondary glaucoma due to ciliary block/ ciliary body rotation.

Choice of the agent and dosage

The choice of the agent and the dosage depends upon the severity, location and duration of uveitis.

- *For mild anterior uveitis*, 1% tropicamide 3 times/day or homatropine 2 times/day may be sufficient to relieve the ciliary spasm and also prevent synechiae.
- *Severe anterior uveitis* would need atropine 1–2% for 3 times/day to reduce ocular pain and fibrinous reaction. At times, the formed posterior synechiae has dense adhesions and frequent instillation of a potent mydriatic cylcoplegic would be needed. Also a *"dynamite cocktail"* (mixture of various dilating agents) may be applied near the site of dense adhesion or even a subconjunctival injection may be given.

ESSENTIAL PRACTICAL POINTS

- *Pigment binding of these agents decreases the initial bioavailabilty* (slow onset) but provides a longer duration of action by constant release of accumulated drug to the receptors. This should be kept in mind as Indian patients have dark iris compared to western counterparts.
- *Always be cautious about systemic side effects* when using atropine (eyedrops>> ointment). Also advice the patient about punctal occlusion, closing the eyes and instillation of eyedrops to avoid systemic absorption.

Table 5.4.1 Preparation, action, salient features and side effect of mydriatic-cycloplegic agents

Drug	Preparation	Mydriasis		Cycloplegia		Mydriasis (M) Cyclo-plegia (C)	Salient features	Side effects
		Maximum effect (min)	Recovery (days)	Maximum effect (hours)	Recovery (days)			
Atropine	Ointment (0.5%, 1%) Drops (0.5%, 1%, 2%, 3%)	30–40	7–10	1–3	7–12	M + C	Most potent, less effective in dark irides	Systemic toxicity–anti-cholinergic side effects, follicular or papillary conjunctivitis, IOP rise in open-angle glaucoma, precipitating acute angle-closure glaucoma
Homatropine	Drops (2%, 5%)	40–60	1–3	½–1	1–3	M + C	1/10 potent as atropine, good cycloplegia	Better tolerated than atropine. IOP rise in open-angle glaucoma more than atropine
Cyclopentolate	Drops (0.5%, 1%, 2%)	30–60	1	½–1	1	M + C	Chemoattractant to inflammatory cells–avoided in uveitis. No effect on IOP	Transient stinging, CNS side effects–ataxia, visual hallucinations, memory loss, disorientation
Tropicamide	Drops (0.5%, 1%)	20–40	¼–1	½	½ hr	M >> C	Shortest acting cycloplegic	Rare side effects due to short action. Hypersensitivity reaction, ACG in predisposed
Phenylephrine	Drops (2.5%, 10%)	20–60	¼	No cycloplegia	No cycloplegia	M only. No C	Maximal mydriasis. Decreases IOP	Transient pain, keratitis allergic keratoconjunctivitis, lid retraction due to Muller muscle action, rebound miosis. Tachycardia, hypertension, MI, subarachnoid haemorrhage

- *Long-term dilatation*, even during periods of remission may be helpful in patients with chronic uveitis, like JIA or sarcoidosis to reduce the morbidity associated with frequent, severe relapses. However, prolonged use may also lead to paralysis of accommodation. Hence caution to be maintained when using these agents.
- *Cautious use in patients with increased risk of ACG* to avoid precipitation of an acute attack.

NSAIDs

NSAIDs for ophthalmic use include:
- *Indoles:* Indomethacin
- *Phenylacetic acid:* Diclofenac, bromfenac
- *Phenylalkanoic acid:* Flurbiprofen, ibuprofen, ketorolac, naproxen, piroxicam
- *Aryl-acetic acid:* Nepafenac

MECHANISM OF ACTION

- *NSAIDs inhibit cyclo-oxygenase*, one of the two major enzymes responsible for the conversion of arachidonic acid to inflammatory mediators.
- *NSAIDs decrease the breakdown of the blood–aqueous barrier* and reduce the formation of aqueous humour proteins and prostaglandin 2 (PG-2).

Corticosteroids, which retard the release of AA by inhibiting phospholipase-A, inhibit both the cyclooxygenase and lipoxygenase pathway products. This phenomenon may explain the superior anti-inflammatory potency of corticosteroids as compared with that of NSAIDs and may provide the basis for therapeutic synergism when these agents are used together.

PREPARATIONS AND USE

The advent of the newer generation NSAIDs has widened their therapeutic potential. Apart from topical use of these drugs, systemic use has been one of the important mode of treatment in management of varied ocular conditions, like scleritis, postoperative pain, etc.

Commonly used topical preparation of NSAIDs are depicted in Table 5.4.2.

Nepafenac 0.1%: It is a prodrug. It penetrates the cornea six times faster than diclofenac. It is converted to amfenac in ocular tissues. This has an increased penetration into vitreous and subsequent increased delivery to retina.

Bromfenac 0.09%: Only NSAID approved for BD dosing; halogen attached to benzoyl side chain increases potency.
- *Side effects:* Excessive burning and stinging are most common adverse effects, which may influence patient compliance.
- *Corneal melt and infiltrates*, hyphema during ocular surgery are the other serious side effects of these drugs.
- *Systemic use is associated with side effects*, most commonly include dyspepsia and peptic ulceration. Thrombocytopenia, depression, tinnitus, nephrotoxicity, pruritus, asthma, etc. form some serious adverse effects of these drugs.

INDICATIONS OF NSAIDs

- Uveitis especially steroid responders
- Prevention of intraoperative miosis
- Postsurgical inflammation
- Prophylaxis and treatment of cystoid

Table 5.4.2 *Topical preparation and uses of NSAIDs*

Drug	Topical concentration	Uses
Flurbiprofen	0.03% solution	Cystoid macular oedema, maintenance of mydriasis
Diclofenac	0.1% solution	Cystoid macular oedema, maintenance of mydriasis, pain control post-LASEK/PRK
Ketorolac	0.5% solution	Cystoid macular oedema, maintenance of mydriasis, allergic and vernal conjunctivitis
Nepafenac	0.1% solution	Post-cataract surgery inflammation, CME
Bromfenac	0.09% solution	Post-cataract surgery inflammation, CME
Indomethacin	0.5%–1% suspension	Scleritis, pain

- Macular oedema
- Scleritis
- Episcleritis
- Prevents discomfort and pain post-surgery

NSAIDs are expanding their horizons in clinical ophthalmology. The introduction of newer NSAIDs has helped in the prevention and treatment of CME.

CORTICOSTEROIDS

MECHANISM OF ACTION

Corticosteroids form the epitome of management of any uveitis. Corticosteroids act by controlling the rate of protein synthesis at both cellular and molecular level. Corticosteroid enters the target cell by binding to a cellular receptor. Once inside the cell, it binds to a specific cytoplasmic steroid receptor protein, crosses the nuclear membrane to bind to DNA directly at sites known as glucocorticoid response elements (GREs). GREs either promote or inhibit production of specific mRNAs. This alters the rate of translation and production of specific protein products thus altering cell function. Figure 5.4.1 summarises the mechanisms of anti-inflammatory and immunosuppressive actions of corticosteroids.

Corticosteroid receptors have been identified in the iris, ciliary body, and adjacent corneoscleral tissue.

TOPICAL STEROIDS

These drugs form the mainstay in the management of anterior uveitis and other forms of uveitis with anterior spillover.

Preparations

Prednisolone acetate eyedrops provide greater theoretical anti-inflammatory effect than either dexamethasone or betamethasone.

Other corticosteroid eye preparations include fluorometholone, rimexolone, and loteprednol etabonate. Common topical preparation with their concentration are depicted in Table 5.4.3.

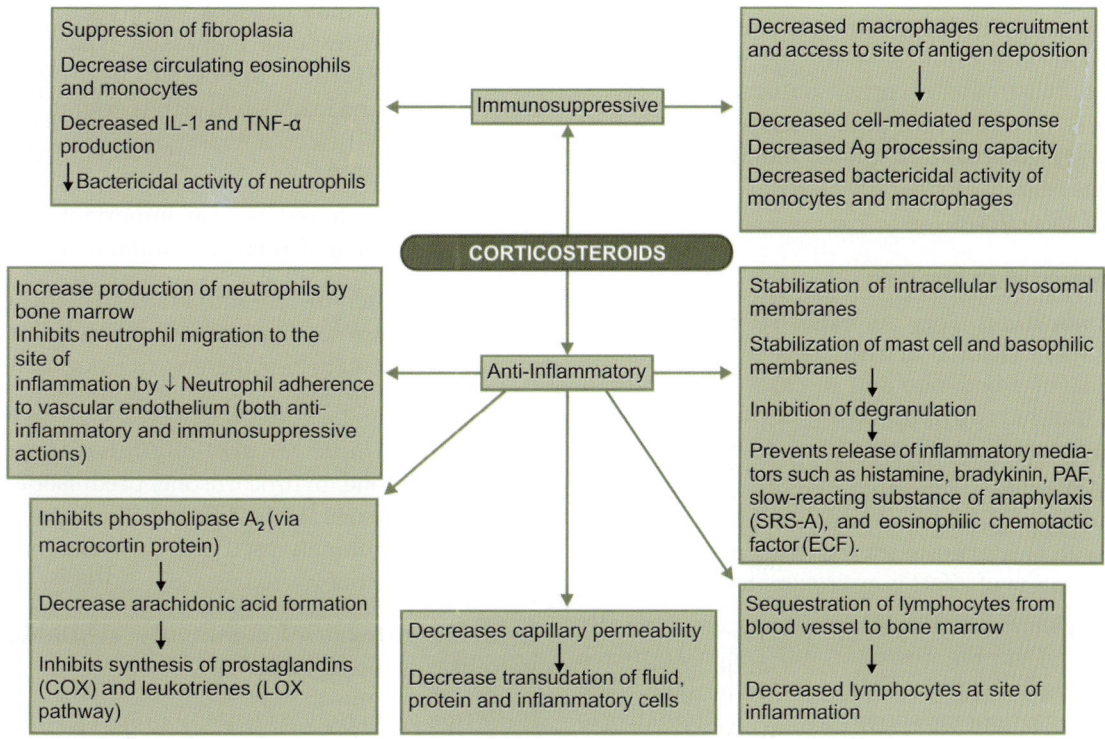

Fig. 5.4.1 *Mechanisms of anti-inflammatory and immunosuppressive actions of corticosteroids.*

Table 5.4.3 *Topical steroid preparations with concentration*

Medication with form	Concentration (%)
Prednisolone acetate suspension	1
Prednisolone sodium phosphate solution	0.125–1
Difluprednate emulsion	0.05
Betamethasone phosphate solution	0.1–0.5
Dexamethasone sodium phosphate solution	0.1
Dexamethasone alcohol suspension	0.1
Loteprednol suspension	0.2–0.5
Fluorometholone acetate suspension	0.1
Fluorometholone alcohol suspension	0.1
Rimexolone	1

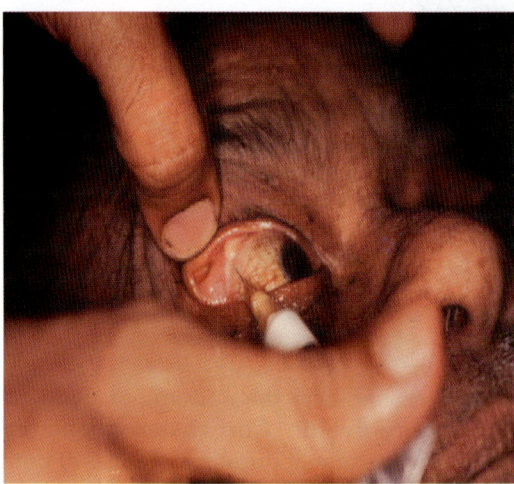

Fig. 5.4.2 *Technique of posterior sub-Tenon injection.*

Side effects of topical administration of steroids. Elevation of IOP, susceptibility to infections, impaired corneal or scleral wound healing, corneal epithelial toxicity, and crystalline keratopathy are reported with the use of topical administration of corticosteroids.

It is important that patients on topical corticosteroids be regularly monitored to assess the response to therapy as well as development *of side effects.*

PERIOCULAR STEROIDS

Indications. They are indicated in moderate to severe chronic or recurrent uveitis, cystoid macular oedema, and in cases with anterior chamber inflammation not responding adequately to topical corticosteroids.

Advantages. Periocular steroids offer the benefit of higher, local, and sustained drug to the eye with greater posterior segment penetration. The duration of effect is approximately 6–8 weeks.

Technique. Posterior injections are typically given via the posterior sub-Tenon approach using the Smith and Nozik technique (Fig. 5.4.2). Orbital floor injections provide an alternative to posterior sub-Tenon injection. Anterior injections are often given subconjunctivally on the

inferior or superior bulbar surface. Local injection of depot preparation of a long-acting triamcinolone acetonide (40 mg/0.5 ml) is given through the posterior sub-Tenon route and can be spaced 4–6 weeks apart.

Side effects of periocular steroids. Periocular administration may cause a variety of side effects, which include increased IOP and glaucoma, cataract, aponeurotic ptosis, enophthalmos and inadvertent globe perforation.

SYSTEMIC STEROIDS

Systemic corticosteroids play an important role in the management of intraocular inflammation.

Indications include inflammation; which is moderate to severe, bilateral, beyond anterior segment, resistant to local therapy, or associated with systemic disease.

Steroids available for oral administration include cortisone, hydrocortisone, prednisone, and fludrocortisone are the different. Prednisone is the most commonly used oral corticosteroid in the treatment of uveitis.

Relative potency of commonly available steroids is given in Table 5.4.4.

Initiation of therapy is typically 1 mg/kg daily followed by a slow taper once the inflammation is under control. Optimally, the dose should be

Table 5.4.4 *Potency of steroids with respect to their anti-inflammatory action and suppression of fibroplasia*

Drug	Relative anti-inflammatory activity	Systemic equivalent
Hydrocortisone	20	1.0
Cortisone	25	0.8
Prednisolone	5	4.0
Prednisone	5	4.0
Methylprednisone	4	5
Triamcinolone	4	5
Fludrocortisone	10	1.5
Dexamethasone	0.75	26
Betamethasone	0.6	33

less than 0.1 mg/kg daily within 3 months of initiating therapy. For immediate control of vision-threatening diseases (necrotizing scleritis, bilateral serous detachments), methyl-prednisolone sodium succinate can be given intravenously over a period of more than 30 min. The usual regimen consists of 250–1,000 mg/day (pulse dose) intravenously on 3 consecutive days. Table 5.4.5 outlines the guidelines for tapering and monitoring while on systemic corticosteroids.

Side effects. Systemic corticosteroids can cause a variety of systemic side effects, which have been summarised in Table 5.4.6.

Table 5.4.5 *Usual doses, tapering schedule, monitoring, and need of supplemental therapy with systemic corticosteroids*

Parameter	Suggested guidelines
Initial dose	1–1, 5 mg/kg/day
Maximum adult oral dose	60–80 mg/day
Maintenance dose (adult)	≤10 mg/day
Tapering schedule	Over 40 mg/day, decrease by 10 mg/day every 1–2 weeks
	40–20 mg/day, decrease by 5 mg/day every 1–2 weeks
	20–10 mg/day, decrease by 2. 5 mg/day every 1–2 weeks
	10–0 mg/day, decrease by 1 to 2.5 mg/day every 1–4 weeks
Monitor	Blood pressure, weight, glucose every 3 months
	Lipids (cholesterol and triglycerides) annually
	Bone density within first 3 months and annually thereafter
Supplemental therapy	Calcium 1500 mg daily and vitamin D 800 IU daily
	Oestrogens and antiresorptive agents as needed

Table 5.4.6 *Side effects of corticosteroids*

Fluid electrolytes	Sodium retention, potassium loss, fluid retention, hypokalemic alkalosis, hyperosmolar coma
Musculoskeletal	Muscle weakness, steroid myopathy, osteoporosis, aseptic necrosis of femoral and humeral heads, tendon rupture
Gastrointestinal	Nausea, increased appetite, peptic ulcer, perforation of small and large bowel, pancreatitis
Dermatologic	Poor wound healing, easy bruisability, increased sweating
Neurologic	Convulsions, headaches, hyperexcitability, moodiness, psychosis
Endocrine	Menstrual irregularities, Cushingoid state, suppression of adrenocortical pituitary axis, diabetes
Ophthalmic	Cataract, glaucoma, central serous retinopathy, activation of herpes
Others	Weight gain, thromboembolism

Intravenous methylprednisolone (IVMP)

IVMP is required when quick anti-inflammatory action is needed. The dose is 500 mg to 1 gram intravenous infusion with 0.9% normal saline or sodium lactate solution over 30 to 60 minutes daily for 3 consecutive days. It should be given in an intensive care unit set up to be able to manage any cardiopulmonary complication. IVMP should be followed by high dose oral steroid or immunosuppressive agent.[19] Figure 5.4.3A shows an active lesion of serpiginous choroiditis. This patient was subjected to a 3-day regimen of IVMP followed by high dose oral steroids and shows an early resolution (Fig. 5.4.3B).

INTRAVITREAL STEROIDS

Intravitreal corticosteroids, such as triamcinolone acetonide, are often used to manage non-infectious intermediate and posterior uveitis and

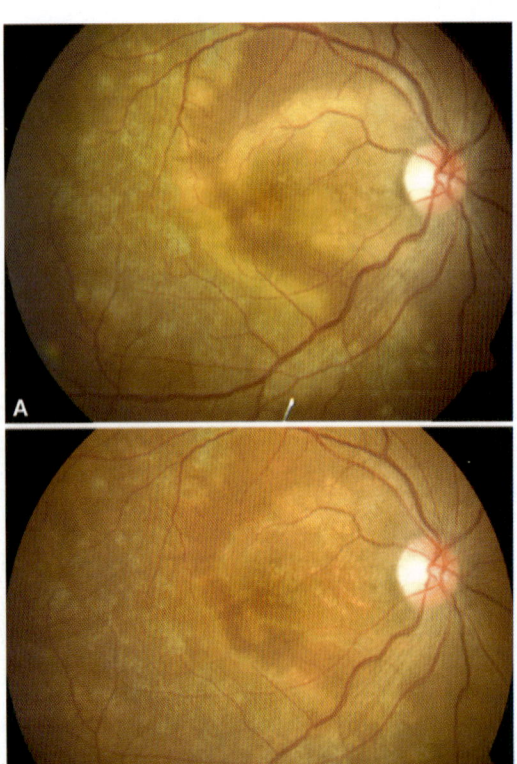

Fig. 5.4.3 *Fundus photograph of a patient with serpiginous choroiditis before (A) and after (B) intravenous methyl-prednisolone.*

its complications, such as cystoid macular oedema due to the direct action and hence greater efficacy.

Sustained release corticosteroid intraocular implants may be considered in place of repeated injections. Retisert contains fluocinolone acetonide that achieves sustained release of approximately 2.5 years. Another implant for treatment of non-infectious posterior uveitis is a dexamethasone intravitreal implant (Ozurdex).

Serious side effects include cataract, increased IOP, glaucoma, retinal detachment, vitreous haemorrhage, and endophthalmitis.

Intravitreal triamcinolone acetonide (IVTA)

Intravitreal injections of triamcinolone acetonide have increasingly been reported as a treatment of intraocular neovascular, oedematous or inflammatory disease. It can be used for chronic cystoid macular oedema (CME) due to uveitis. Complete resolution of CME has been reported in a significant proportion in majority of case series. Commonly used doses are 4 mg/0.1 ml and 2 mg/0.05 ml. One needs to monitor intraocular pressure following injection of triamcinolone. Rise of IOP is logically less in lesser doses. Endophthalmitis is also a major risk involved after intravitreal triamcinolone injections.

Intravitrial sustained release steroid implants

Fluocinolone acetonide sustained drug delivery device

It is a promising new therapy for the treatment of severe uveitis.

Retisert contains fluocinolone acetonide 0.59 mg (requires a surgical procedure to suture the implant to the scleral wall) that achieves sustained release of approximately 2.5 years. Fluocinolone acetonide devices release the drug at rate of approximately 2 microgram per day. Pure drug is compressed in a 1.5 mm tablet. Pellet is then coated in a polyvinyl alcohol and silicon laminated and affixed to a polyvinyl alcohol suture strut. The assembly is heat treated at 35° for 5 hours to change the PVA crystalline structure and to control drug delivery rate further and then gamma ray sterilised. Release occurs through a diffusion port in the coating. It is surgically implanted through the pars plana into the vitreous cavity of the patient (Fig. 5.4.4).

Favourable effects on inflammation, preservation or the improvement of visual acuity, reversal of CME, reduction or elimination of topical, periocular or systemic anti-inflammatory medications were observed. Raised intraocular pressure (IOP) and endophthalmitis are the major risks involved.

Multicentre uveitis steroid treatment (MUST) trial compared the efficacy and safety of local fluocinolone acetonide implant vs systemic treatments (systemic corticosteroids with or without adjuvant immunosuppressives for severe forms of uveitis including intermediate, posterior, and panuveitis over a 2-year time period). The study did not find any significant difference in efficacy, although there were increased ocular complications (cataract, raised IOP and glaucoma) when using the fluocinolone implant for non-infectious uveitis. Despite these safety concerns, the overall conclusion was that either approach is reasonable depending on the patient's individual situations and responses to therapy.

Iluvien implant is a non-erodable, injectable device consisting of fluocinolone acetonide by Alimera sciences. Its use in uveitis is under study.

Ozurdex

The Ozurdex 'bio-erodible' dexamethasone implant uses a solid polymer delivery system (Novadur delivery system), in which the biodegradable material is combined with dexamethasone to form a small rod-shaped implant which is injected into the vitreous using a specially designed injector.

Pharmacokinetics. Dexamethasone is released over about 6 months, the pharmacokinetics demonstrating a high initial concentration peak in the vitreous followed by a longer period of low-level release before the implant dissolves completely to H_2O and CO_2, leaving no residue.

Effects. It has shown favourable effects on visual acuity improvement and reduction of cystoid macular oedema. It may be needed to be repeated after 3 months.

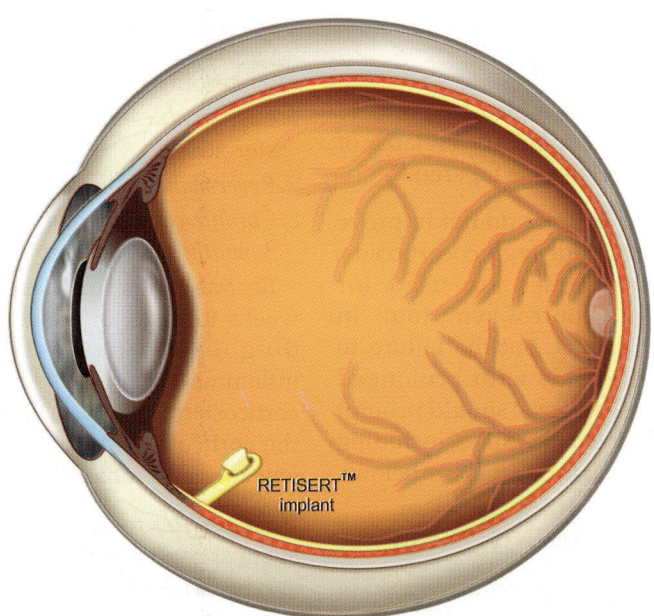

Fig. 5.4.4 *Intravitreal sustained release steroid implant (Retisert).*

Contraindications include ocular or periocular infections, advanced glaucoma, aphakic eyes with rupture of the posterior lens capsule, ACIOL with rupture of the posterior lens capsule and hypersensitivity.

Adverse effects include raised intraocular pressure, conjunctival haemorrhage, eye pain, cataract, vitreous haemorrhage, retinal detachment, and endophthalmitis.

HURON, a randomised controlled study, was undertaken to evaluate the role of intravitreal dexamethasone implant (Ozurdex) in the management of macular oedema associated with intermediate and posterior uveitis. Ozurdex was seen to have a favourable effect in the management of macular oedema, resolution of vitreous haze, improvement in visual acuity and subsequent improvement in the quality of life.

STEROID RESPONSIVENESS

The response to glucocorticoids in individual patients divides them into three general classes: steroid-responsive, steroid-dependent, and steroid-unresponsive.

Steroid-responsive patients improve clinically, generally within 1–2 weeks, and remain in remission as the steroids are tapered and then discontinued.

Steroid-dependent patients also respond to glucocorticoids but then experience a relapse of symptoms as the steroid dose is tapered.

Steroid-unresponsive patients do not improve even with prolonged high-dose glucocorticoids. Glucocorticoids sometimes are used for prolonged periods to control symptoms in steroid-dependent patients, but the failure to respond to glucocorticoids with prolonged remission (*i.e.* a disease relapse) should prompt consideration of alternative therapies, including immunosuppressives and infliximab (*see* below).

IMMUNOSUPPRESSIVE AGENTS

Immunomodulatory agents were introduced in the management of uveitis as an adjuvant of systemic corticosteroids.

INDICATIONS

The indications of use of these immuno-modulator agents are:

1. *Vision-threatening intraocular inflammation:*

Absolute indications
- Behcet's disease with retinal involvement
- Sympathetic ophthalmia
- Serpiginous choroiditis
- Systemic vasculitis
- Vogt-Koyanagi-Harada syndrome
- Necrotising scleritis
- Wegener's granulomatosis
- Polyarteritis nodosa
- Relapsing polychondritis with scleritis
- Juvenile idiopathic arthritis
- Ocular cicatricial pemphigoid

Relative indications
- Intermediate uveitis
- Retinal vasculitis with central vascular leakage
- Severe chronic iridocyclitis

2. *Inadequate response of corticosteroid treatment* with persistence of inflammation
3. *Failure of corticosteroid therapy* in controlling the inflammatory process
4. *Chronic corticosteroid dependency* or those requiring multiple injections
5. *Cases with unacceptable or intolerable side effects* of steroids
6. *Cases with contraindications to use* of corticosteroids
7. *Reversibility of disease process* with relapse
8. *Chronic corticosteroid treatment of greater than 3 months* and dose >10 mg/day.

Because most of these drugs take several weeks to have an effect, immunosuppressive drug regimens for initial therapy of ocular inflammation typically include high-dose oral corticosteroids as well. Once the disease is quiet, the corticosteroids are tapered either to a low level or, if possible, discontinued.

Prerequisites for the use of immunosuppressive agent are absence of infection, absence of hepatic and hematological contraindications facilities for follow up, informed consent, reversibility of the disease process.

Serious complications include renal and hepatic toxicity, bone marrow suppression, and increased susceptibility to infection. In addition, alkylating agents may cause sterility and increased risk of future malignancy. Although these agents may be associated with serious complications, they are extremely effective in treatment of ocular inflammatory disease in which patient is unresponsive to systemic corticosteroid or intolerant of it.

With recent advent of less toxic and more effective newer immunomodulators, many agents are now used as a first-line agent rather than an adjuvant drug.

Mechanism of action of various immuno-suppressive agents is summarised in Table 5.4.7 and Figure 5.4.5.

Salient features of action of various immuno-modulators along with their doses, side effects and indications have been outlined in Table 5.4.7.

Few specific points of each immunosuppressive agent are discussed below.

A. Antimetabolites

1. Azathioprine

Mechanism of action. It is a purine nucleoside analog (competitive inhibitor of purine synthesis), which interferes with adenine and guanine ribonucleotides by suppression of inosmic acid synthesis. This in turn interferes with DNA replication and RNA transcription. Azathioprine is a prodrug which is metabolized in liver and converted to its active form 6-

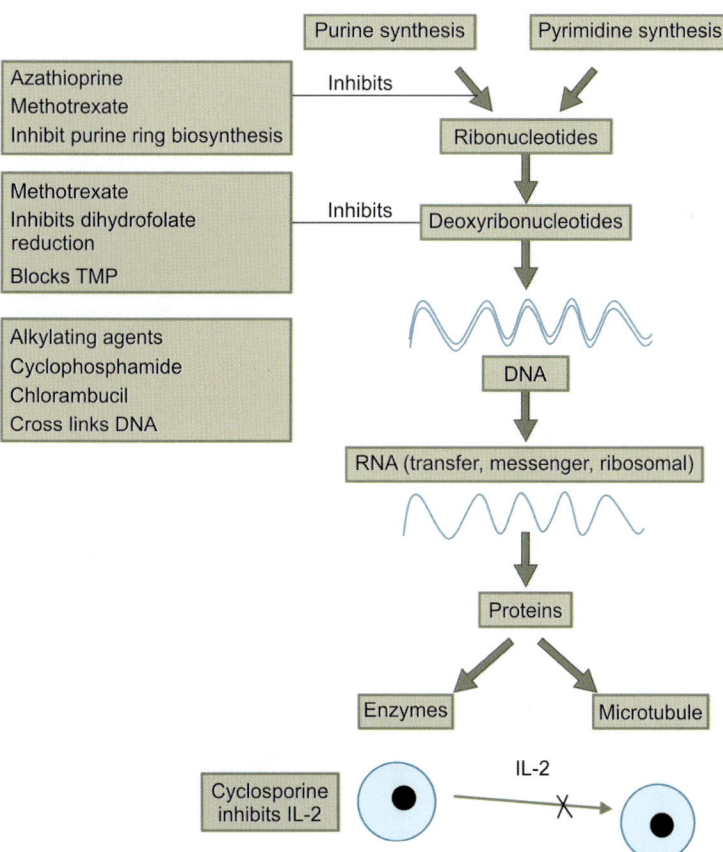

Fig. 5.4.5 *Mechanism of action of various immunosuppressive drugs.*

Table 5.4.7 *Immunosuppressants*

Class	Drugs	Mechanism of action	Dosage	Side effects	Specific indications
T cell signalling inhibitors	Cyclosporine	Inhibits nuclear factor of activated T lymphocytes (NF-AT) activation	2.5–5 mg/kg/d PO	Nephrotoxicity, hypertension, gingival hyperplasia, GI upset, paraesthesias	Behcet's disease, sarcoidosis, Vogt-Koyanagi-Harada syndrome, sympathetic ophthalmia, idiopathic posterior uveitis, pars planitis
	Tacrolimus	Inhibits NF-AT activation	0.1–0.2 mg/kg/d PO	Nephrotoxicity, hypertension, DM	Same as above
	Sirolimus	Inhibits T lymphocyte activation in G1Blunts T and B lymphocyte responses to lymphokines	6 mg loading dose IV and then 4 mg/day IV increasing by 2 mg increments	Gastrointestinal cutaneous at trough levels of > 25 ng/ml	Undergoing study. May benefit in various uveitis because of lower side effects
Anti-metabolites	Methotrexate	Folate analogue; dihydro-folate reductase inhibitor	7.5–25 µg/week PO	Hepatoxicity, ulcerative stomatitis, bone marrow suppression, diarrhoea	Sympathetic ophthalmia, scleritis, paediatric uveitis, JIA-associated iridocyclitis
	Azathioprine	Alters purine metabolism	100–200 mg/day PO	GI upset, hepatotoxicity, pneumonia, fatigue	Behcet's disease, Wegener's granulomatosis, systemic lupus erythematosus, scleritis, cicatricial pemphigoid, JIA-associated iridocyclitis
	Mycophenolate mofetil	Inhibits purine synthesis	1–3 gm/day PO	GI upset, hepatotoxicity	Sympathetic ophthalmia, scleritis, paediatric uveitis, JIA-associated iridocyclitis
Alkylating agent	Cyclophosphamide	Crosslinks DNA	1–2 mg/d PO	Sterile haemorrhagic cystitis, diarrhoea, nausea, GI ulceration	Wegener's granulomatosis, polyarteritis nodosa, necrotising scleritis, relapsing polychondritis, cicatricial pemphigoid, sympathetic ophthalmia, Behcet's disease

Contd..

Table 5.4.7 *Immunosuppressants (Contd...)*

Class	Drugs	Mechanism of action	Dosage	Side effects	Specific indications
	Chlorambucil	Cross- links DNA	2–12 mg/d PO	Haemorrhagic cystitis, sterility, increased risk of malignancy	Behcet's disease, sympathetic ophthalmia, JIA-associated iridocyclitis
Biologic response modifiers	Infliximab	TNF inhibition: –α TNF monoclonal-antibody	3 mg/kg IV weeks 0, 2, 6 and then q 6–8 weeks	Sterility, increased risk of malignancy Sepsis, lymphoma, autoantibodies, cost	Uveitis, JIA
	Adalimumab	TNF-inhibitor	40 mg q 1 week or q 2 weeks	Infusion reactions (TB reactivation for all TNF inhibitors) Malignancy/ lympho-proliferative diseases, lupus like syndrome, congestive heart failure	Along with other immunosuppressants
	Etanercept	TNF inhibition: soluble TNF receptor	25 mg bid/ week SC	Sepsis, lymphoma, autoantibodies, skin reactions, cost	Rheumatoid arthritis, JIA
	Daclizumab	Binds the α subunit of IL-2 receptor	1 mg/kg IV q 2 weeks × 5 doses	Headache, nausea, rash, stomach upset Granulomatous inflammation, infection, cost	
	Rituximab	Binds CD-20 positive lymphocytes (mainly B lymphocytes)	2 infusions 1 g IV given 2 weeks apart and repeated	Rare if any	
	Anakinra	IL-1 receptor antagonist	100 mg subcutaneous injection daily	Late onset neutropenia; few case reports	

mercaptopurine. It is more effective in preventing proliferation of T cells than B cells. Although, antibody production is unaffected.

Indications. Vogt-Koyanagi-Harada disease, sympathetic ophthalmia, Behcet's disease, Wegener's granulomatosis in remission, chronic iridocyclitis, scleritis, serpiginous choroiditis.

Dosage. 1.5–2.0 mg/kg/day; given as single dose or twice a day schedule.

Side effects. Bone marrow suppression with leucopenia and thrombocytopenia, hepatotoxicity.

Monitoring
- Total WBC count and platelet count—every 4 weeks
- Liver function test—every 3 months
  If total WBC count falls below 3,500 cells/mm^3 or platelet count falls below 1 lakh /mm^3, dosage of the drug should be adjusted or stopped.

2. Methotrexate

Mechanism of action. It is a folate analog. It inhibits the enzyme dihydrofolate reductase inhibiting the production of tetrahydrofolate which in turn inhibits formation of thymidylate, leading to inhibition of DNA replication and RNA transcription. It acts both on T and B cells. Methotrexate has little action on resting cells. It is mainly active against rapidly dividing immune cells.

Indications. Juvenile rheumatoid arthritis, children with pars planitis, sarcoidosis, and scleritis associated with connective tissue disorder.[11] Methotrexate is the first choice immunosuppressant in paediatric uveitis.

Dosage. 0.1–0.5 mg/kg/week; low dose therapy is started at a dose of 7.5 mg/week and it can be increased up to 25 mg/week. Generally given orally once a week.[12]

Side effects. Reversible hepatotoxicities, bone marrow suppression, dry cough and interstitial pneumonia.

Monitoring
- Complete blood count—monthly
- Liver function test (specially AST and ALT)— every 3–4 weeks

If parameters of the liver function tests are elevated to twice the normal, dosage of the drug should be adjusted or stopped.

3. Mycophenolate mofetil

Mycophenolate mofetil is derived from the fungus *Penicillium stoloniferum*.

Mechanism of action. It inhibits purine metabolism. It inhibits the enzyme inosine monophosphate dehydrogenase, which in turn inhibits the synthesis of guanosine thereby affecting the proliferation of B and T lymphocytes. Mycophenolate mofetil is a prodrug which is metabolised in liver and converted to its active form mycophenolic acid.

Indications. It is mainly used as alternative to azathioprine in Vogt-Koyanagi-Harada disease, sympathetic ophthalmia, Behcet's disease, Wegener's granulomatosis in remission, chronic iridocyclitis, scleritis, and serpiginous choroiditis.

Dosage. 1000 mg twice a day, available as 250 mg and 500 mg capsules.

Side effects. Weight loss, gastrointestinal upset and bone marrow suppression. Mycophenolate mofetil has lower side effects than other antimetabolites because it does not interfere with the salvage pathway of purine synthesis.

Monitoring
- Complete blood count—every month
- Liver function test (specially AST and ALT)— every month.

4. Leflunomide

Mechanism of action. It inhibits the enzyme dihydroorotate dehydrogenase, which in turn inhibits the synthesis of pyrimidine thereby affecting the repliction of DNA. Leflunomide is a prodrug which is metabolised in liver and converted to its active form teriflunomide.[15]

Dosage. Started with a loading dose of 100 mg/day for 3 days followed by 20 mg/day as maintenance.

Side effects. Reversible hepatotoxicity and leucopenia. Other reported side effects are gastrointestinal symptoms (including abdominal pain, diarrhoea, nausea with or without vomiting, gastritis and gastroenteritis), allergic reactions (e.g. rash, pruritus and rarely anaphylaxis), alopecia, infections and hypertension.

B. T cell inhibitors

1. Cyclosporine

It works on T cell by binding to an intracellular peptide know as cyclophylin which results in blockage of transcription and production of interleukins, activation of CD4 and CD8 T cells and production of other lymphokines such as interferon. Cyclosporine A is derived naturally from a fungus *Beauveria nivea*.

Cyclosporine is not a cytotoxic drug; it is a cytostatic drug, so inflammation may recur when the drug is stopped. For this rebound phenomenon, the drug is generally used for a long time.

Indications. Same as for azathioprine.

Dosage. 2–5 mg/kg/day in one or two divided doses.

Side effects. Renal toxicity, hypertension, hepatotoxicity, gingival hyperplasia, hypertrichosis.

Monitoring. Blood pressure and serum creatinine—initially every week until stable, then every 3–4 weeks.

2. Tacrolimus

The name tacrolimus is derived from "Tsukuba macrolide immunosuppressant" since it was the first macrolide immunosuppressant discovered. Its mechanism of action and indications of uses are similar to cyclosporine. Tacrolimus was first discovered in a soil fungus, but later it was revealed that the drug is actually produced by a bacterium *Streptomyces tsukubaensis*.

Dosage: 0.05 mg/kg/day

Side effects: Hypertension, cardiovascular toxicity, nephrotoxicity, hypercholesterolaemia, nephrotoxicity, myopathy and diabetes mellitus.

3. Sirolimus

Sirolimus inhibits activation of T and B cells by blocking the response to interleukin-2. Sirolimus is also known as Rapamycin as this macrolide immunosuppressant was first discovered in soil of an island "Rapa Nui".

Doasge: Starting dose is 4 mg daily.

Side effects: Gastrointestinal problems, dermatological, hyperlipidosis, leucopenia, thrombocytopenia.

Monitoring: Serum lipid profile and blood count.

c. Cytotoxic drugs

Some important examples are discussed below.

1. Cyclophosphamide

It is converted to an active metabolite which causes DNA crosslinking leading to DNA miscoding, breaks and defective repair of DNA, causing cell death. Cyclophosphamide inhibits both cellular and humoral immunity.

Indication. It is used when a rapid onset of action is needed, e.g. in case of severe ocular inflammation. It is also used in necrotising scleritis, Behcet's disease, Wegener's granulomatosis, systemic lupus erythematosus, refractory intermediate uveitis.

Dosage. Oral: 1–5 mg/kg/day; pulse doses of intravenous cyclophosphamide 500 mg/m² can be given once in 4 weeks.

Side effects. Haemorrhagic cystitis, carcinoma urinary bladder, bone marrow suppression, alopecia and sterility.

Monitoring. Complete blood count and routine urine analysis initially weekly at the initiation of therapy and then at least every 4 weeks once the dosage is stable. Cyclophosphamide therapy is discontinued/stopped, if WBC count is less than 3000/µl, platelet count is less than 75,000/ µl.

2. Chlorambucil

It substitutes an alkyl group for H⁺ in organic components causing crosslinking and thus interferes in DNA replication. Its main action is suppression of B cells.

Indications: Behcet's disease, sympathetic ophthalmia and serpiginous choroiditis.

Dosage: 0.1–0.2 mg/kg/day

Side effects: Bone marrow suppression, gastrointestinal upset, skin rash, azospermia and leucopenia.

Monitoring: Blood count—weekly at the initiation of therapy later monthly.

D. Biologicals

Biologicals are a group of biologically active proteins and monoclonal antibodies, which are directed mainly against specific cytokines or their receptors. These groups of drugs were introduced as an alternative therapy for refractory cases of uveitis about 15 years ago. They are also termed as *immunotherapy* or *biotherapy, biologic response modifiers,* etc.

Majority of the biologicals are either recombinant antibody or antagonist to particular cytokines or cell-surface receptors. However, they also include recombinant cytokines, like interferons too. Commonly available biologicals are summarised in Figure 5.4.1.

I. *TNF-α blockers*

TNF-α is a cytokine, produced in a soluble and membrane bound form by different cells of the immune system namely monocytes and macrophages. TNF-α act by binding to two types of receptors—the p55 or TNFR-1 and p75 or TNFR-2. TNF-α is one of the key components of the inflammatory response-increasing the transport of neutrophils, eosinophils to sites of inflammation, and through additional molecular mechanisms, like upregulations of vascular endothelial cell adhesion molecules, which initiate and amplify inflammation. They have been found in aqueous of eyes and in serum of patients with chronic uveitis.

Currently, there are three types of TNF-α blocker are available for the treatment of ocular inflmmation—infliximab, etanercept and adalimumab.

Infliximab

Infliximab is a genetically engineered monoclonal antibody (because the antibodies were produced from one cell that was grown into a clone of identical cells, it is called a monoclonal antibody) to TNF-α. As it is a combination of mouse and human antibody, it is called a chimeric monoclonal antibody. It reduces levels of interleukin-6 and chemokines, including macrophage chemoattractant protein-1, as well

as adhesion molecules, such as intercellular adhesion molecule-1. Infliximab is found to effective as a short-term immunosuppressive agent in non-infectious uveitis with relatively low side effects. However, repeated infusions are often needed to prevent recurrences. Infliximab has been found to be very effective in the treatmet of Behcet's disease, even in recalcitrant cases. The response to the infliximab therapy has been found to be rapid in onset and also found to be effective in controlling the extraocular manifestations of the disease. Reports suggest that infliximab therapy seemed to be well tolerated in children with chronic uveitis. However, in these paediatric cases, greter doses of the drug are needed.

The infliximab is administered as intravenous infusion in 5 to 10 mg/kg doses. The doses can be increased up to 20 mg/kg. The half-life of infliximab is about 10 days and biological effect of the drug persists for up to 60 days.

- *There is greater chance of reactivation of granulomatous infection* (e.g. tuberculosis) in patient taking infliximab. So, latent tuberculosis must be excluded before the administration of infliximab therapy using specific tests, such as interferon gamma assays.
- *Other serious side effects reported* are pulmonary embolism, congestive heart failure, lupus-like reaction and vitreous haemorrhage.
- *There are chances of development of antinuclear antibodies* in patients receiving multiple infusions.[3] For this reason, some advocates use of low-dose methotrexate or other immunosuppressive agent along with infliximab.

Etanercept

Etanercept is an engineered recombinant dimeric protein. It acts by competitively inhibiting the binding with TNF-α and TNF-β with their receptors. The drug was first approved for the treatment of rheumatoid arthritis. It has been tried for the treatment of chronic anterior uveitis in children, but the results are less encouraging than that of infliximab.[4] This may be due to the infliximab's dosage flexibility and its ability to bind both soluble and membrane-bound TNF. Infliximab forms stable bonds with both soluble and transmembrane forms of TNF-α, whereas etanercept forms a weak bond with trans-membrane forms. In a prospective study, Saurenmann et al reported better response to infliximab than to etanercept in reducing inflammatory activity of uveitis in children. In a retrospective study of 24 patients taking etanercept and 21 patients taking infliximab, Tynjala et al reported more effective improvement of inflammatory activity in the infliximab treated group. Also Smith et al in a randomized, placebo-controlled, double-masked study reported no significant differences in the anterior segment inflammation between patients treated with etanercept and placebo.

Administration and dose. Etanercept is injected subcutaneously. The dosage is 25 mg twice a week. Side effects of etanercept are similar to that of infliximab.

Adalimumab

It is an IgG monoclonal antibody to human necrosis factor. Adalimumab has an added advantage over infliximab as it is a fully humanised antibody. It has been found useful in chronic uveitis in children and Behcet's disease.

Route of administration and dose. The usual FDA approved dosage for treating rheumatoid arthritis is 40 mg injected subcutaneously every 2 weeks. However, it may be sufficient to treat intraocular inflammation in little lower doses.

Though initial reports are seems to be promising for the use of adalimumab and lower incidence of side effects, such as injection site reaction and the formation of neutralising antibodies, but prospective, randomised trials are needed to confirm the utility of the drug in the treatment of intraocular inflammation.

A comparison of the three TNF-α blockers has been summarised in the Table 5.4.8.

II. *Cytokine receptor antibodies*

Daclizumab

It is an IgG monoclonal antibody that binds to α-subunit (55kDa α chain of the IL-2 receptor complex is known as TAC /CD 25) of the IL-2 receptor blocking the effect of IL-2 and thus inhibits the proliferation of T cells. It is used for the prophylaxis of acute allograft rejection mainly in kidney transplant patients. In a non-randomized trial, daclizumab has been found to be beneficial in patients with uveitis, scleritis, or mucous membrane pemphigoid unrespon-sive to other drugs. In another nonrandomised, open label study, daclizumab was found to improve or stabilise best corrected visual acuity in 80% cases in patients with chronic, non-infectious, sight-threatening bilateral cases of uveitic conditions, like sarcoidosis,Vogt-Koyanagi-Harada disease, etc. The tretment protocol includes two induction dosage of 2 mg/kg every 2 weeks apart and maintenance dosage of 1 mg/kg every 2–4 weeks for next 22 weeks. Common side effects are skin rashes, lympha-denopathy and oppurtunistic infections.

Table 5.4.8 *Comparison of three TNF-α blockers*			
Properties	*Infliximab*	*Etanercept*	*Adalimumab*
Binding to TNF-α	Yes, both transmembrane and soluble form	Yes, but forms weak bond with transmembrane form	Yes, both transmembrane and soluble form
Binding to TNF-β	No	Yes	No
Preparation	Chimeric monoclonal antibody	Recombinant dimeric protein	Humanised monoclonal antibody
Half-life	10 days	4 days	14 days
Routes of administration	Intravenous	Subcutaneous	Subcutaneous
Dosage	5 to 10 mg/kg every 8 weeks	25 mg twice a week	40 mg every 2 weeks

III. Drugs acting against lymphocytes

Alemtuzumab

It is a recombinant DNA-derived humanized monoclonal antibody. It is directed against CD52-a marker present in the surface of lymphocytes. It remains on the surface, where it triggers the death of the target cells by initiating mainly two immune mechanisms— *complement cascade* and *natural killer cell* cytotoxicity.

There are case reports on the success of alemtuzumab in controlling severe posterior uveitis, refractory to conventional immunosuppression. In cohort study of 10 patients with refractory, non-infectious, ocular inflammatory disease with alemtuzumab, 8 out of 10 patients showed remission. But high incidence of infusion reaction and haematological toxicity has limited its use in intraocular inflammation.

Rituximab

It is a monoclonal antibody that acts against CD20-a marker expressed by B cells. CD20 is widely expressed on B cells, from early pre-B cells to later in differentiation, but it is absent on terminally differentiated plasma cells. Like alemtuzumab, rituximab causes a marked reduction of B cells. Rituximab has been shown to be effective in the treatment of chronic intraocular infections. Significant side effects are infusion reaction, neurological problems and infections.

IV. Interferons

Interferon-alpha

Interferon-alpha was the first cytokine that has been produced successfully with the help of recombinant technology. It is a low molecular glycoprotein produced by leucocytes. They are mainly involved in innate immune response against viral infection. It was first used in patients with Behcet's disease refractory to other immunosuppressive therapies. The usual dose is subcutaneous injection of 3 to 9 million units (IU) 3 times per week. Side effects are arthralgia, leucopenia, alopecia, and depression and injection site reaction.

TRIALS WITH IMMUNOSUPPRESSIVE AGENTS

There are various ongoing clinical trials related to immunosuppressive agents, which are:

Systemic Immunosuppressive Therapy for Eye Diseases (SITE) Cohort Study. To evaluate whether ocular immunosuppressive therapy is associated with a greater risk of death and of cancer.

Adalimumab in Uveitis Refractory to Conventional Therapy (ADUR Trial). To evaluate the efficacy and safety of the TNF-α inhibitor adalimumab in patients with active uveitis despite standard immunosuppressive therapy.

Interferon-α 2a Versus Cyclosporin A for Severe Ocular Behcet's Disease (INCYTOB) study

Choice of immunosuppressive agents should depend on familiarity with the drug, therapeutic action and adverse effects. One may use combination therapy of 2–3 immunosuppressive agents in vision-threatening, recalcitrant uveitis. Triple agent immunosuppressive has been used in serpiginous choroiditis.

ANTI-VASCULAR ENDOTHELIAL GROWTH FACTOR (ANTI-VEGF) AGENTS

Mechanism of action. VEGF is known to mediate its action in inflammation by mere fact of its induction in inflammation, its role in increasing vascular permeability and high level of VEGF in uveitic macular oedema eyes. Hence anti-VEGF agents can have an effective role in the management of uveitic macular oedema.

Intravitreal bevacizumab appears effective in reducing central macular thickness. Similar results have been achieved with ranibizumab.

Advantages. Anti-VEGF agents have the advantage over IVTA of being much less likely to cause cataract progression or a rise in IOP.

Disadvantages. However, they have less antiinflammatory effect, making them less suitable for the treatment of CME primarily driven by inflammation or if there is extensive breakdown of the blood–retina barrier.

CONCLUSION

The medical management forms the most important step in the effective treatment of uveitis and prevention of development of sequelae and complications. The need to individualise the therapy depends upon the type of uveitis and patient-related factors. Balance between all these factors will help us choose the best form of care needed for the patient. The continuous evolution of medical science with revolutionising discoveries adds to the armamentarium in the management of this enigmatic condition.

BIBLIOGRAPHY

1. Biswas J, Rao NA. Management of intraocular inflammation. In: Ryan SJ (Ed). Retina, Vol 2. St. Louis, CV Mosby, 1989; pp 139-46
2. Dodds EX. Toxoplasmosis. Curr. Opin. Ophthalmology 2006;17:557-61.
3. Foster CS, Vitale AT. Part II. Principles of Diagnosis and Therapy. Diagnosis and Treatment of Uveitis. Saunders, 2001; pp 141-214.
4. Goodman & Gilman's Manual of Pharmacology and Therapeutics, McGraw Hill, 2008;52:855-910.
5. Hemady RK, Chan AS, Nguyen ATQ. Immunosuppressive agents and nonsteroidal anti-inflammatory drugs for ocular immune and inflammatory disorders. Ophthalmol Clin N Am 2005;18:511-28.
6. Jabs DA, Rosenbaum JT, Foster S, et al. Guidelines for the use of immunosuppressive drugs in patients with ocular inflammatory disorders. Recommendations of an Expert Panel. Am J Ophthaalmology 2000;130:492-513.
7. Kaplan HJ. Intermediate uveitis (pars planitis, chronic cyclitis)-a four step approach to treatment. In: Saari KM (ed) Uveitis Update. Amsterdam: Excerpta Medica; 1984; pp 169-72.
8. Kuppermaann BD, Blumenkranz MS, Haller JA, Williams GA, Weinberg DV, Chou C, Whitcup SM. Randomized controlled study of an intravitreous dexamethasone drug delivery system in patients with persistent macular edema. Arch Ophthalmology 2007;125:309-17.
9. Lau.CH, Missotten T, Salzmann J, Lightman SL. Acute retinal necrosis features, management and outcomes. Ophthalmology 2007;114:756-76.
10. Lindstedt EW, Barsma GS et al. Anti- TNF-alpha therapy for site threatening uveitis. Br. J. Ophthalmology 2003;89:533-6.
11. Markomichelakis NN, Halkiadkakis I, Papciethymiou-orhcan S et al. Intravenous pulse methylpredisolone therapy for acute treatment of serpiginous choroiditis. Ocul Imm Inflamm 2006;14:29-33.
12. Medical management of Uveitis. Intraocular inflammation and Uveitis, Section 9. Basic and clinical sciences, American Academy of Ophthalmology, 2011-12; 98-135.
13. Nussenblatt RB. Philosophy, goals, and approaches to medical therapy. Uveitis Fundamentals and Clinical Practice, 4th edition, Mosby Elsevier, 2010; pp 76-113.
14. Paul AG. A review of evidence guiding the use of corticosteroids in the treatment of intraocular inflammation. Ocular Immunology and inflammation-2004;12:169-192.
15. Samson CM, Waheed N, Baltztziz S et al. Methotrexate therapy for chronic non-infectious uveitis: analysis of a case series of 160 patients Ophthalmology-2001;108:1134-39.
16. Stanbury RM, Graham EM. Systemic corticosteroid therapy-side effects and their management. Br J Ophthalmol. 1998;82:704-708.
17. Sugita S. Intravitreal anti-inflammatory treatment for uveitis. Br. J. Ophthalmology 2001; 91:135-136.
18. Tempest-Roe S, Joshi L, Dick AD, Taylor SR. Local therapies for inflammatory eye disease in translation: past, present and future. BMC Ophthalmology 2013;13(1):39.
19. Thorne JE, Jabs DA, Quazi FA et al. Mycophenolate mofetil therapy for inflammatory eye disease. Ophthalmology 2005;112:1472-77.
20. Young S, Larkin G, Branley M et al. Safety and efficacy of intravitreal triamcinolone for cystoid macular edema inuveitis. Clin. Exp Ophthalmology 2001;29:2-6.

5.5 SURGICAL MANAGEMENT AND INTERVENTIONS IN UVEITIS

Introduction

Diagnostic Surgical Interventions in Uveitis

• Indications

• Surgical procedures

Therapeutic Surgical Interventions in Uveitis

• Cataract surgery in uveitis

• Glaucoma filtration surgery

• Pars plana vitrectomy

INTRODUCTION

Surgical interventions in patients with uveitis may be associated with flare up of intraocular inflammation, increased risk of complications and needs a very meticulous pre- as well as post-operative follow-up and monitor for intraocular inflammation.

Surgical interventions in a patient with uveitis may be required for:

• Diagnostic purpose, as well as

• Therapeutic purposes.

DIAGNOSTIC SURGICAL INTERVENTIONS IN UVEITIS

Indications

• Atypical clinical presentations

• Non-responsive to empirical treatment with corticosteroids/immunosuppressant.

• Rapidly progressive disease with inconclusive non-invasive work-up.

• Strong suspicion of malignancy.

Surgical procedures

The diagnostic surgical intervention is indicated in patients with uveitis who present with atypical clinical picture, or show poor response to therapy and are strongly suspected of infectious or malignant etiology.

The main aim is to obtain the sample that can be subsequently subjected to histopathology, microbiology, immunology and molecular biologic tests so as to reach a specific diagnosis.

Diagnostic surgical interventions include:

• Aqueous and vitreous samples

• Iris and ciliary body biopsy

• Chorioretinal biopsy

Note. Surgical diagnostic interventions have been described in detail in Chapter 5.3: Pathological Diagnostic Tests in Uvetis.

THERAPEUTIC SURGICAL INTERVENTIONS IN UVEITIS

The therapeutic surgical interventions required in uveitis include:

• Intravitreal injections

• Intravitreal implants

• Cataract surgery in uveitis

• Glaucoma surgery in uveitis

• Pars plana vitrectomy in uveitis

• Surgical interventions for band keratopathy

CATARACT SURGERY IN UVEITIS

Indications

• *Phaco-antigenic uveitis.* Active inflammation as a result of leakage of lens proteins, and thus cataract surgery is mandatory.

• *Visually significant cataract* where cataract extraction is likely to improve the vision.

• Cataract impairing visualisation of the posterior segment

• Catarct extraction is likely to improve the visualisation of posterior segment.

• Cataract impairing visualisation of the posterior segment in a patient undergoing vitreoretinal surgery.

Causes of poor visual outcome following cataract extraction in uveitis patients

The primary goal of surgery is to improve vision. However, successful visual outcome depends not only on successful surgery but also on pre-existing irreversible structural damage. Factors which would adversely affect the visual out-come include:

• Presence of concurrent glaucoma

- Hypotony
- Band-shaped keratopathy
- Extensive posterior synechiae
- Retinal detachment
- Optic atrophy
- Cystoid macular oedema
- Macular atrophy or hole
- Epiretinal membranes
- Vitreous opacities

Important Points to consider

- Adequate preoperative control of inflammation. The most important step in cataract surgery in uveitis. Elimination of inflammation for at least three months (preferably 6 months) before surgery is desirable. It is important to remember to operate only when cells are absent (0 to 5) in the anterior chamber as assessed on slit-lamp examination.
- *In cases with vitritis*, though reduction of vitreous cells is desirable but the debris and few vitreous cells may persist even in the inactive stage and cannot be completely eliminated.
- *Preoperative medications* should include: Oral prednisone 1 mg/kg/day, along with topical prednisolone acetate 1% eyedrops, starting two days before the day of surgery along with oral and topical non-steroidal anti-inflammatory agents, depending on the type of uveitis and surgeon's discretion.
- Immunosuppressive agents, such as azathioprine 1 to 2 mg/kg, can be started at least four weeks or earlier. In patients with severe uveitis, corticosteroids are contraindicated.
- *Patients with Fuch's uveitis* do not require preoperative corticosteroids.

Procedure

Phacoemulsification with considerations

Phacoemulsification is the preferred technique in patients with cataract and uveitis. One should take care of the following to minimze postoperative inflammation:

- Smaller incision scleral/clear corneal is desirable.
- Minimize the iris trauma and iris prolapse during surgery.

- Reduction of iris stretch during nucleus expression in case extracapsular cataract extraction is being planned.
- In-the-bag placement of the IOL with an intact capsulorhexis.

Managing the small pupil during cataract surgery

- *Posterior synechia* can be separated with an iris hook under viscoelastic cushion that help in achieving pupillary dilation.
- *Fibrous, thick pupillary membranes* may be divided with Vannas scissors and stripped from the margins using forceps.
- *Mechanical stretching of the pupil* with dilators is possible and leads to pupillary dilation but is best avoided as this would lead to rupture of iris vessels and increased inflammation postoperatively.
- *Iris retractors* or hooks can be gently applied to hold the pupil.
- *Multiple small sphincterotomies* can be made with Vannas scissors to cause dilation of the pupil.
- *In cases with ring synechia or extensive anterior synechia*, a peripheral or a sector iridectomy may be required.

Intraocular lens implantation

A PCIOL can be safely implanted in cases of idiopathic non-granulomatous anterior uveitis, HLA-B27 associated uveitis, and Fuchs' heterochromic iridocyclitis. Others have also reported moderate success in VKH, sympathetic ophthalmia, Behçet's disease, pars planitis and any burnt out or inactive uveitis.

Prognosis following IOL implantation in uveitis

Good to excellent outcome is anticipated in:
- Fuchs' heterochromic iridocyclitis
- Burnt-out or inactive idiopathic anterior uveitis
- HLA-B27 associated uveitis
- Inactive toxoplasmosis

Moderate to good outcome is anticipated in:
- Pars planitis
- Behçet's disease
- Intermediate uveitis
- Sympathetic ophthalmia

- Birdshot retinochoroidopathy
- Vogt-Koyanagi-Harada syndrome
- Sarcoidosis, inactive infections, such as tuberculosis, syphilis and borreliosis

Poor outcome anticipated (IOL contraindicated)
- Juvenile rheumatoid arthritis
- Uveitis in less than 12 years of age
- Hypotony associated with uveitis
- Chronic granulomatous recurrent uveitis
- Advanced disease (VKH, sympathetic ophthalmia, Behçet's)

Note. While IOL implantation is the preferred practice in most cases of adult uveitic cataracts, most specialists consider IOL implantation contraindicated in children with JIA-associated uveitis, since the IOL is presumed to act as a scaffold for the formation of intraocular membranes further leading to cyclitic membranes, hypotony and eventual phthisis bulbi.

Complications

I. Intraoperative

1. *Complications and other commonly encountered intraoperative complications* of cataract surgery (posterior capsular tear, etc.) may occur during this surgery.

2. *Zonular dehiscence* may be more frequent due to weakening of zonules from long-standing inflammation.

3. *Amsler's sign* (bleeding from filiform iris vessels) can be seen in Fuch's heterochromic iridocyclitis.

4. *Hyphema* may result from trauma to iris vessels during mechanical stretching of pupils and synechiotomy, and due to bleed from iris new vessels. Hyphema can be managed on the operating table by tamponading with an air injection or intracameral adrenaline for vasoconstriction. Postoperative hyphema can either be lysed with tissue plasminogen activator (10 microgram in 0.1 ml of buffered saline) or intense anti-inflammatory therapy alone may suffice. In case of a large clot in the anterior chamber, surgical removal is advisable.

II. *Postoperative complications*

1. *Postoperative inflammation* is the most common complication incountered in three different entities which need consideration are as below:

i. *Severe postoperative inflammation.* This is likely to happen more if the preoperative inflammation is not adequately controlled or there is lot of iris manipulation intraoperatively. The management includes intense topical corticosteroids and cycloplegics; and oral steroids and immunosuppressives, if necessary. Recombinant tissue plasminogen activator injection into the anterior chamber may help disperse the fibrinous reaction. The sequelae of severe inflammation include cellular deposits on the IOL, posterior synechia and IOL capture, papillary block glaucoma, inflammatory membranes, hypotony and cystoid macular oedema; therefore, preoperative control of this inflammation is of utmost importance.

ii. *Recurrences of uveitis.* Recurrent episodes of the primary disease may continue to occur following cataract surgery. This may be precipitated by the inflammatory stimuli secondary to the surgical trauma or may be unrelated. Prompt institution of corticosteroids in full immunosuppressive doses (1 mg/kg body weight or more) is indicated.

iii. *Persistent postoperative inflammation.* In some patients, the postoperative inflammation (that is different from the recurrence of inflammation) may continue to persist long after the surgery. The causes include:

a. Excessive surgical manipulation results in severe and prolonged breakdown of the blood–aqueous barrier, resulting in accumulation of inflammatory cells, fibrin and debris on the IOL surface

b. Three-piece lenses with polypropylene haptics.

c. *Sulcus-fixated, anterior chamber-fixated lenses:* Mechanical irritation of the iris in ciliary or sulcus-fixated lenses may serve as a source of constant irritation with cytokine release and inflammatory cell migration at the site of inflammation.

d. Inadequate treatment.

2. *Cystoid macular oedema (CME).* CME is a major cause of reduced postoperative visual

acuity. The incidence of postoperative CME in these eyes ranges from 18 to 56%. The management of CME includes combination of corticosteroid drops, non-steroidal drops and acetazolamide, followed by injection of peri-ocular corticosteroids (40 mg triamcinolone acetonide in the sub-Tenon space). In refractory CME, oral prednisolone and other immuno-suppressive agents (as steroid-sparing) may be required. Intravitreal injection of triamcinolone (4 mg in 0.1 ml) or long-acting dexamethasone implants may be considered.

3. *Glaucoma.* A transient rise of postoperative IOP is common after surgery and is managed with antiglaucoma medications including beta-blockers and carbonic anhydrase inhibitors. Miotics and prostaglandin analogues should be avoided. Pre-existing glaucoma may get exacerbated in some cases. Secondary angle closure due to posterior synechia or pupillary block due to inflammatory membranes or IOL capture may too result in the development of secondary glaucoma. A planned peripheral iridectomy intraoperatively or Nd:YAG laser iridotomy postoperatively would help. However, the iridotomy may get closed due to fibrinous reaction. In cases of glaucoma not controlled medically or by laser, filtering surgery, usually trabeculectomy with anti-metabolite or valve implant may be performed.

4. *Posterior capsular opacification (PCO)* is a common occurrence after surgery for uveitic cataract and nearly one-third of the patients would require Nd:YAG laser capsulotomy. Recurrent and chronic uveitis can also cause the appearance of fibrous membranes and dense fibrosis in certain cases and many of these thick capsular opacifications especially in children may need surgical membrenectomy.

5. *Hypotony.* Hypotony may occur temporarily, as a result of ciliary body shutdown secondary to inflammation, and may respond to intensive anti-inflammatory treatment. Tractional ciliary body detachment may also cause hypotony, for which surgical excision of the membranes and IOL explantation combined with pars plana vitrectomy and silicon oil insertion may be necessary. UBM is a useful tool to detect ciliary body detachment.

GLAUCOMA FILTRATION SURGERY

Secondary glaucoma may occur in patients with chronic long-standing uveitis and is more commonly seen in patients with Fuch's uveitis and chronic anterior uveitis. Though the medical management remains the mainstay of therapy in these eyes, many of these patients may need surgical intervention.

Indications for Glaucoma surgery

- Progressive optic disc damage and un-controlled IOP despite maximum medical therapy.
- Pupillary block glaucoma
- Neovascular glaucoma

Preoperative considerations

- It is often not possible to wait for 3 months for the control of inflammation prior to per-forming surgery.
- Topical corticosteroids are needed pre-operatively in many of these patients as these help in reducing the conjunctival inflammatory cells as well.
- Oral corticosteroids in the dose of 0.5–0.75 mg/kg/day may be administered in the pre-operative period. In cases where the primary disease is not inactive.
- *In patients with co-existent cataract and glaucoma,* it is advisable to do glaucoma surgery first and catract surgery to be taken up later after a period of 6 months or so.

Procedures

A. Trabeculectomy

This is the most commonly performed and well-tolerated procedure in eyes with uveitic glaucoma, special considerations include:

- *Antimetabolites, like mitomycin C,* may be used intraoperatively. Since patients with uveitis show excessive inflammatory response and fibrous proliferation in the postoperative period, the risk of failure of procedure are high.
- *Monitoring* these patients closely for the post-operative inflammation.
- Topical corticosteroids for longer duration in the postoperative peroid are often required in these eyes.

B. Glaucoma drainage devices

Indications for these devices in uveitic glaucoma are as follows:

- Failed trabeculectomy with antimetabolites.
- Children with chronic anterior uveitis, like JIA.
- Eyes with neovascular glaucoma.
- Aphakic eyes.

C. Cyclodestructive procedures

These procedures have a risk of inducing inflammation and may result in hypotony progressing to phthisis bulbi. Thus, these procedures should preferably be avoided in eyes with uveitic glaucoma.

PARS PLANA VITRECTOMY

Pars plana vitreous (PPV) surgery is increasingly being performed both for diagnostic and therapeutic purposes in the management of patients with uveitis.

Types of PPV based on Indications

Based on indications, PPV can be broadly classified into the following categories:

- Diagnostic PPV,
- Therapeutic PPV, and
- Combined diagnostic and therapeutic PPV.

Diagnostic PPV

The diagnostic vitrectomy is indicated in patients with uveitis who present with atypical clinical picture, or show poor response to therapy and are strongly suspected of infectious or malignant etiology. The main aim is to obtain the vitreous humour sample that can be subsequently subjected to microbiology, immunology and molecular biologic tests so as to reach a specific diagnosis.

Diagnostic vitrectomy could involve any of the following:

- Vitreous tap/aspiration
- Vitreous biopsy
- Chorioretinal biopsy.

Indications

- Atypical clinical presentations

- Non-responsive to empirical treatment with corticosteroids/immunosuppressant.
- Rapidly progressive disease with inconclusive non-invasive work-up.
- Strong suspicion of malignancy.

Note. Diagnostic PPV is described in detail in Chapter 5.3 on Pathological Diagnostic Tests in Uveitis.

Therapeutic PPV

Therapeutic vitrectomy serves two purposes:
- *Physically removing the vitreous with resident inflammatory cells and the mediators of inflammation;*
- *Managing the secondary effects of uveitis*, i.e. non-resolving vitreous haemorrhage, cystoid macular oedema, epiretinal membranes, abnormal vitreoretinal tractions, choroidal neovascular membranes and retinal detachments. This is generally done in the chronic inactive stage of uveitis.

Indications

- Media opacities obscuring the visual axis.
- Tractional or combined retinal detachment
- Cystoid macular oedema
- Macular pucker
- Ciliary traction causing hypotony.

Diagnostic–therapeutic PPV

This involves taking the undiluted vitreous humour for laboratory tests and then performing the complete vitrectomy with removal of posterior hyaloid membrane to prevent/cure complications associated with severe uveitis. This also allows thorough intraocular distribution of drugs.

Preoperative considerations

- Unlike cataract surgery, the preoperative corticosteroids are not required in patients undergoing PPV for TRD, vitreous opacities, CME or macular pucker as these procedures are performed in the inactive stage of the disease.
- *Topical corticosteroid administration* in the preoperative period may be required, if there is any inflammation.

• *It is important to ascess the pupillary dilation* in the preoperative period as many of these eyes may require iris hooks to dilate pupil intra-operatively.

• *Preoperative ultrasound biomicroscopy* is required in eyes with cyclitic membrane and hypotony to ascess the structrual damage to ciliary body.

Procedure

• Standard three-port transconjunctival pars plana vitrecomy is done.

• Smaller gauges (25 G and 27G) are preferrable.

• In eyes with complicated cataract and hypotony, pars plana lensectomy, vitrectomy with posterior hyloid separartion is done. This is followed by insertion of fourth port for endoillumator to allow bimanual dissection and peeling of cyclitic membrane.

• Silicon oil tamponade is used in these eyes to maintain the IOP in the postoperative period.

• *Inferior iridectomy* is important to make in these eyes with silicon oil.

Postoperative care

The PPV is generally very well tolerated and majority would not require systemic steroids in the postoperative peroid. However, these eyes need to monitored closely for any signs of post-operative inflammation that may be managed with increased frequency of topical as well as systemic corticosteroids, if required.

BIBLIOGRAPHY

1. Androudi S, Ahmed M, Fiore T, et al. Combined pars plana vitrectomy and phacoemulsification to restore visual acuity in patients with chronic uveitis. J Cataract Refract Surg 2005;31:472-8.

2. deSmet MD, Gunning F, Feenstra R. The surgical management of chronic hypotony due to uveitis. Eye 2005;19:60-4.

3. Malinowski SM, Pulido JS, Folk JC. Long-term visual outcome and complications associated with pars planitis. Ophthalmology 1993;100:818-24.

4. O'Connell SR, Majji AB, Humayun MS, deJuan E Jr. The surgical management of hypotony. Ophthalmology 2000;107:318-23.

5. Tabbara KF, Chavis PS. Cataract extraction in patients with chronic posterior uveitis. Int Ophthalmol Clin 1995;35(2);121-31.

6. Yu EN, Paredes I, Foster CS. Surgery for hypotony in patients with juvenile idiopathic arthritis-associated uveitis. Ocular Immunol Inflamm 2007;15:11-7.

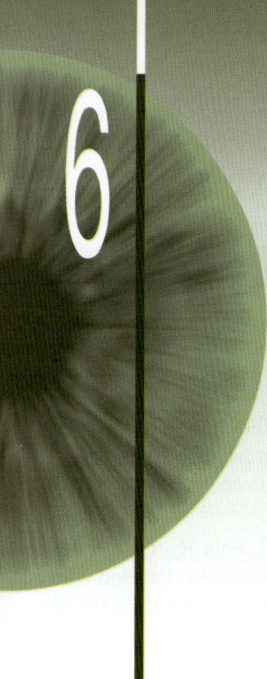

6   INFECTIOUS UVEITIS

6.1   BACTERIAL UVEITIS

6.1.1 TUBERCULAR UVEITIS

Introduction
• Tuberculosis
• Historical aspects of ocular tuberculosis
Etiopathogenesis
• Infective vs immunological etiology
• Stages of pathogenesis of ocular tuberculosis
Clinical Spectrum
Ocular surface tuberculosis
• Tuberculosis of eyelids
• Conjunctival tuberculosis
• Tubercular scleritis
Intraocular tuberculosis
• Tubercular anterior uveitis
• Tubercular intermediate uveitis
• Choroidal tubercles
• Tubercular retinal periphlebitis
• MSC or SLC
• Tubercular panuveitis

Tubercular optic neuropathy
Diagnostic Modalities
• Laboratory diagnosis of intraocular tuberculosis
• Ancillary diagnostic tests
Treatment: Considerations and Difficulties
• Treatment
• Difficulties in management

INTRODUCTION

Tuberculosis (TB) is a major health problem in developing nations, immigrant populations and immunocompromised patients. The 19th global report on TB by WHO in 2014, reports data from over 200 countries that accounts for 99% of world's TB cases. Nine million cases were reported to develop TB in 2013.[1] Of these 24% were in India alone. 1.1 million (13%) of these were HIV positive. The incidence of ocular TB has been reported variably from different countries. It varies from 0.4 to 10% in different reports across India.[2-4]

Historical aspect: Ocular TB can involve any structure in the eye

The earliest description of ocular TB was given by Maiti e-Jan for an iris lesion,[7] long before the bacillus was discovered by Koch in 1882.[8] Gueneau de Mussy first described choroidal tubercles in a patient of miliary tuberculosis in 1830 while in 1883 Julius von Michel identified the organism in the eye.[9]

ETIOPATHOGENESIS

Infective versus immunological etiology

Pathogenesis of ocular TB has been controversial, the debate being between an infective etiology vis-a-vis an immunological response to distant tubercular foci. The former is strongly supported by reports on histologically proven ocular tuberculosis showing acid-fast bacilli[10] or tubercular granuloma,[11] experimental animal studies of ocular tuberculosis,[12] detection of *M. tuberculosis* DNA in clinically suspected cases of ocular TB by molecular detection methods,[13, 14] and decrease in recurrence of disease on treatment with anti-tubercular medicines;[15] proof for latter is less convincing.

Stages of pathogenesis of ocular tuberculosis

Pathogenesis of any extrapulmonary TB infection can be divided into three stages:[16,17]

1. Stage of dissemination of bacteria from the site of primary infection, i.e. lungs, to the eye. After inhalation of the infected aerosol, the organism is ingested by the alveolar macrophages and from there it is transported to hilar lymph nodes. The macrophages present the antigen to T helper cells (T_H1) via major histocompatibility complex II (MHC II). Adaptive immunity, however, may take 5–7 days to develop and this is the time when macrophages, which have ingested *M. tuberculosis*, disseminate to various extrapulmonary sites including eye.

2. Localization of bacteria in different ocular tissues. In the eye, the retinal pigment epithelial (RPE) cells have properties similar to macrophages, such as phagocytosis and expression of Toll like receptors (TLRs). Recently, infected RPE cells have been shown to have greater survival rates than macrophages, thereby providing sanctuary for *M. tuberculosis* as dormant organisms.

3. Stages of bacterial reactivation and initiation of inflammation in those tissues. The factors contributing to reactivation of the bug, in apparently immunocompromised individuals remains unknown still. Certain proteins secreted by mycobacteria called 'resuscitation-promoting factors', have been associated with reactivation of chronic infection.[18]

CLINICAL SPECTRUM

Ocular tuberculosis shows variations in the disease spectrum and can affect any ocular tissue from the lids to the optic nerve.

Common presenting manifestations are a choroidal mass with or without inflammatory signs (34%), choroiditis or chorioretinitis (27%), vitritis (24%), iridocyclitis (13%), and panuveitis (11%).[5] The disease causes significant morbidity with moderate to severe visual impairment in nearly half the patients.[6]

This chapter highlights the:
• Clinical spectrum of intraocular TB,
• Definitive and ancillary diagnostic modalities, and
• Preferred practice pattern in its management.

A. OCULAR SURFACE TUBERCULOSIS

1. Tuberculosis of lids

Lid abscesses simulating chalazia have been reported due to tuberculosis.

2. Conjunctival tuberculosis

Conjunctival TB is primary in origin with the organism either visible on biopsy or isolated on culture. Eyre who had extensively worked on conjunctival TB, found that only 4.4% patients showed any evidence of pulmonary involvement[19] while many others believed that is it is almost always primary.

Clinically, it manifests as chronic conjunctivitis with a mass or superficial ulceration, usually with regional lymphadenopathy.

Treatment is with systemic and local anti-tubercular drugs, like amikacin and streptomycin.

3. Corneal lesions in tuberculosis

Phlyctenular conjunctivitis and interstitial keratitis have been associated with tuberculosis. However, many authors found very few patients of active pulmonary tuberculosis having these manifestations and hence hypothesis of immune-mediated reaction to tuberculoprotein was proposed.

Treatment revolves around the use of topical steroids.

4. Tubercular scleritis

Tubercular scleritis can be necrotizing or non-necrotizing and may also present as sclero-uveitis. Verhoeff, based on his experiments on rabbit postulated the pathogenesis of scleral TB. He proposed that the bacilli reached the ciliary body through blood, got secreted into the aqueous, infiltrated the trabecular meshwork and thereafter the sclera.[20] Bloomfield demonstrated acid-fast bacilli in the biopsy from sclera and also grew it in culture.[21]

Treatment of tubercular scleritis is prolonged. It includes the use of:
- *Systemic anti-TB and local therapy.*
- *Role of steroids* is controversial and there are groups both for and against its use.

B. INTRAOCULAR TUBERCULOSIS

Uveal involvement leads to a wide-spectrum of manifestations. Posterior uveitis is the most common (42%), followed by anterior uveitis (36%), intermediate uveitis (11%) and panuveitis (11%).[22]

1. Tubercular anterior uveitis

It presents as unilateral or bilateral iridocyclitis. Although a non-granulomatous inflammation does not rule out TB, it manifests classically with granulomatous inflammation characterized by (Fig. 6.1.1.1):
- *Mutton fat keratic precipitates.*
- *Koeppe and Busacca nodules*, on iris which are typically smaller than those in sarcoid.

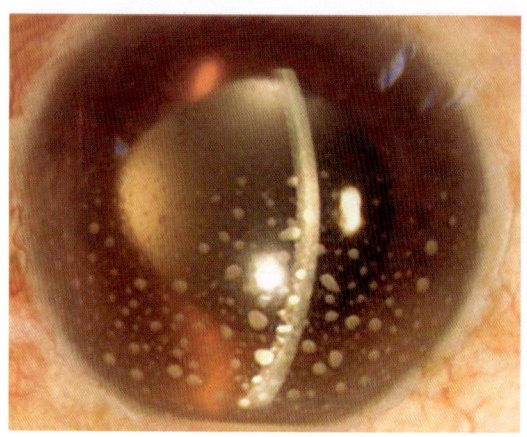

Fig. 6.1.1.1 *Tubercular anterior uveitis.*

- *Broad posterior synechiae* are noted as against sarcoidosis in which, peripheral anterior synechiae seem to dominate.

2. Tubercular intermediate uveitis

Features of tubercular infection are not very specific and include vitritis, vitreous snowballs, peripheral granulomas, vascular sheathing and cystoid macular oedema.

Treatment includes local or systemic steroids:
- *Topical medications* take care of spill over anterior uveitis.
- *Posterior sub-Tenon injection* may help resolve any associated cystoid macular oedema (CME).
- *Intravitreal dexamethasone implant* may be useful in non-responding vitritis/ CME cases.
- *Therapeutic vitrectomy* can be useful for eyes with persistent inflammation.

3. Choroidal tubercles

Choroidal tubercles or tuberculomas are the most frequent ocular manifestation seen in patients with active pulmonary tuberculosis. Illingworth and Wright found that 60% patients with miliary tuberculosis had choroidal tubercles[23] while in non-miliary active cases it varied between 5.5% and 30%.

Clinical features
- *Tuberculomas* appear as creamy yellow choroidal elevations with indistinct margins (Fig. 6.1.1.2).
- *Serous retinal detachment* may occur overlying the tuberculom.

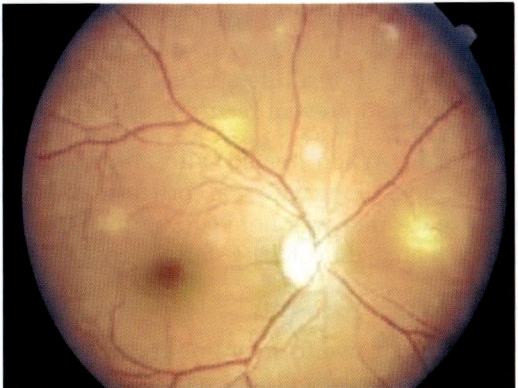

Fig. 6.1.1.2 *Choroidal tubercles.*

- *Subretinal abscess* formation may occur due to excessive tissue destruction.
- As the lesions heal, they tend to become hyper-pigmented and their margins become sharper.
- *Retinal involvement* is usually secondary to choroidal involvement.

Histologically, these tubercles have shown caseating granuloma with tubercle bacilli.[24]

Ancillary investigations show following features:
- *Fluorescein angiography* characteristically shows an early hypofluorescence followed by late hyperfluorescence.
- *Fundus autofluorescence* shows hyperauto-fluorescence during active phase and hypo-autofluorescence during the healed phase of the disease.

Differential diagnosis
Important differentials include sarcoid granu-loma and metastasis from distant primaries, like breast or lung.

4. Tubercular retinal periphlebitis
Commonly called as vasculitis, retinal peri-phlebitis represents the infiltration of lympho-cytes in the perivascular space.

Clinical features. Clinically visualized as:
- *Perivascular yellowish exudation* associated with intraretinal haemorrhages (Fig. 6.1.1.3). Being usually occlusive, it shows extensive capillary non-perfusion areas along with vessel staining and leakage on fluorescein angiography.

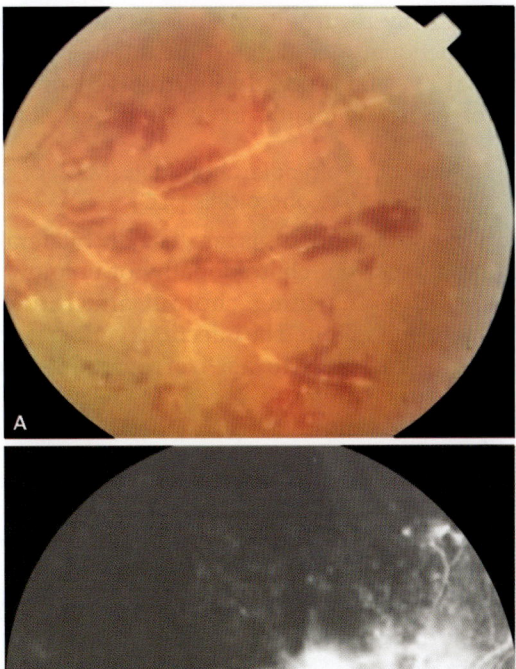

Fig. 6.1.1.3 *Tubercular retinal periphlebitis.*

- *Presence of healed or active choroiditis* patches usually overlying blood vessels are considered to be highly suggestive of tuberculosis.

Pathogenesis. Although Gilbert did demonstrate tubercle bacilli around the retinal vein in a patient with retinal periphlebitis,[25] it is infrequently seen in patients with active pulmonary tuberculosis. Donahue et al noted that only seven of 10,524 patients with systemic TB had retinal perivasculitis.[26] Polymerase chain reaction (PCR) based analysis of ocular samples have linked Eales disease to ocular TB, although it is considered to be immune-mediated rather than infectious.

Natural history of the disease includes an inflammatory vascular occlusion leading to ischaemia and hence neovascularisation, followed by recurrent vitreous haemorrhages and tractional retinal detachment. The contralateral eye may already be involved or get involved in few months in 90% of the cases.

5. Multifocal serpiginoid choroiditis (MSC) or serpiginous-like choroiditis (SLC)

Serpiginous choroiditis is rare, usually bilateral, chronic, recurrent choroidopathy of unknown cause, affecting inner choroid and retinal pigment epithelium. The infectious counterpart is being referred to as "serpiginous-like choroiditis" or more recently "multifocal serpiginoid choroiditis" (Fig. 6.1.1.4).[15]

Clinico-investigative profile. A typical lesion would show areas of healing in the centre with the outer border progressing in serpiginous fashion.

- *Fluorescein angiography* shows an early hypofluorescence followed by late hyperfluorescence.
- *Fundus autofluorescence* shows hyperautofluorescence at the active border and hypo-autofluorescence in healed areas.

Note. Monitoring the disease progression with serial fundus pictures, especially autofluorescence, helps in the assessment of disease course and treatment response.

Pathogenesis
- *Multifocal serpiginoid choroiditis*; besides being associated with tuberculosis, is also implicated to be associated with other infective etiologies, such as herpes virus, toxoplasmosis, fungus, etc.

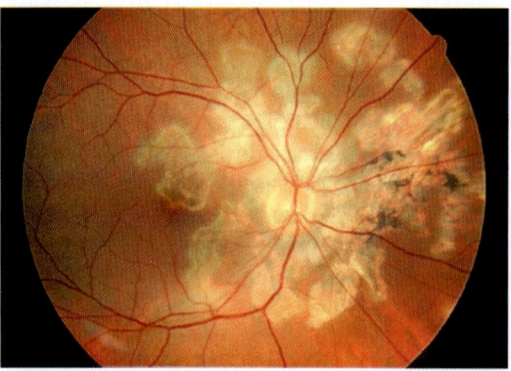

Fig. 6.1.1.4 *Serpiginous-like choroiditis in tuberculosis.*

- *Disease is typically recurrent*; and hence identification of the organism becomes important to institute specific antimicrobial therapy and prevent recurrences.

Treatment. When treated with antitubercular medications along with oral corticosteroids, the recurrence rate was noted to be much lower (9.7%) than that treated by steroids only (75%).[15]

6. Tubercular Panuveitis

- Tubercular uveitis may present with *generalized intraocular inflammation* involving both anterior and posterior segments of the eye.
- *Sometimes a mixed picture may also be noted*, like periphlebitis in one eye with MSC or panuveitis like picture in the other eye.
- Culture and microscopy proven cases of *endophthalmitis* and *panophthalmitis* have been reported.

C. TUBERCULAR OPTIC NEUROPATHY

The optic nerve may be involved either as an extension of the choroidal involvement or via hematogenous route. It can also be involved as a complication of meningitis presenting as optic disc oedema and a macular star.

Signs specific for tubercular uveitis

Gupta et al proposed four signs that were noted to be specific for tubercular uveitis. These were:
- *Broad-based posterior synechiae* (93%),
- *Retinal vasculitis without choroiditis* (97%),
- *Retinal vasculitis with choroiditis* (99%), and
- *Serpiginous-like choroiditis* (98%).[27]

Note. A history of contact must always be elicited while suspecting intraocular tuberculosis. The presence of any of the above warrant further investigation, especially in endemic area.

DIAGNOSTIC MODALITIES

A. LABORATORY DIAGNOSIS OF INTRAOCULAR TUBERCULOSIS

A definitive diagnosis can be made either by direct demonstration of the tubercular bacillus, by culture of the organism or by detection of bacillary DNA in the clinical sample by special molecular techniques, like PCR.

I. Aqueous humour and vitreous tap sample testing

Sample collection

Biopsy of ocular tissue is not only difficult but is also associated with significant comorbidity. Hence, samples used generally in intraocular TB are either aqueous or vitreous humour.

- *Presence of cells in aqueous humour* should be confirmed on slit-lamp before sampling as the organism is intracellular.
- *Aqueous tap* (100–200 µl) is done using 26G or a smaller needle under topical anaesthesia in an operating room. Vitreous biopsy is performed with a 23/25/27 G vitrectomy cutter.

Aqueous humour or vitreous sample testing

1. Microscopy

The sample obtained should preferably be centrifuged and then stained either with Ziehl-Neelsen stain or special immunofluorescent stains. Being a paucibacillary disease, the demonstration of tubercular bacilli under a microscope is usually a difficult task. While about 5000 to 10,000 bacilli per ml must be present to be detected on stained smears, 10–100 viable bacteria per ml may suffice to be grown in culture.

2. Culture

The fluid specimens should be inoculated as soon as possible with 1 part of specimen to 5 to 10 parts of liquid media including both agar base (Middlebrook 7H-10) and egg base (Lowenstein Jensen) media.[28] The generation time of *M. tuberculosis* is 12–18 h and colonies take 2–3 weeks to develop.[29] The culture must be kept for minimum 8 weeks and examined every week.

3. Molecular techniques (polymerase chain reaction)

Detection of DNA by nucleic acid amplification tests (NAATs) like polymerase chain reaction (PCR), provides another definitive diagnostic test modality. It uses simple principle of amplification of mycobacterial DNA, to detect it in the samples obtained.

PCR testing of three types:

i. *Qualitative PCR.* It detects the presence of DNA but does not quantify the load. The initial PCR studies for ocular TB were based on single target/uniplex PCR, with IS6110 as the gene target.[30] However, it was found that this gene was absent in about 11% of the population[31] and hence the use of multi-target PCR using three genes—protein b, MPB 64 and IS6110, as targets was advocated. It showed improved sensitivity (73.68%) and specificity (100%).[32]

ii. *Quantitative PCR (real-time or q-PCR).* It measures the number of DNA copies in the sample. This can potentially help in ruling out false positive results and besides verifying the result of treatment through serial monitoring of DNA load.

iii. *Nested PCR.* It is a modified conventional PCR to increase the sensitivity of PCR. It is a two-step PCR. In first step, DNA is amplified by outer primers and in second step internal/inner primers are used to further amplify the first step-amplified product.

Limitations of PCR. The test detects the presence of DNA in the patient's sample. But it cannot differentiate between viable and non-viable organisms. Detection of mycobacterial RNA in ocular fluid samples can indicate presence of viable bacteria in the eye.

II. Biopsy

In case an iris, retinal or choroidal lesion has been biopsied, histology may show signs of characteristic granuloma, with or without caseation. Close differentials simulating the histology include sarcoidosis, syphilis and leprosy.

B. ANCILLARY DIAGNOSTIC TESTS

1. Radiography

Chest X-ray is done to detect signs of active pulmonary tuberculosis, like consolidation, cavitation, satellite lesions or hilar lymphadenopathy or signs of old healed TB including fibrosis, calcified pulmonary nodules or hilar lymph nodes. Many studies by now have shown absence of any radiologic features in cases of ocular TB proven otherwise by definitive diagnostic tests. High resolution computed tomography (HRCT) may help in picking up lesions better than conventional radiography[33] while positron emission tomography (PET) scan may demonstrate metabolic activity in mediastinal lymph nodes which are not highlighted in HRCT.[34]

2. Tuberculin skin test/mantoux test

Basics. The old tuberculin (Koch;1890) consisted of filtered and evaporated heat stabilized culture of *M. tuberculosis*. It contained extracellular toxins that showed cross-reactivity with non-mycobacterial bacilli. Purified protein derivative (PPD) was made in 1940 by Siebert by auto-claving and extracting cultures of *M. tuberculosis*. It contains lesser exogenous substances. An intermediate strength of PPD, 5 TU, is used for the test.

Methodology. The solution must be injected within one hour of drawing the solution in the syringe. Using a 26 G or smaller gauge needle, 0.1 cc (5 TU) is injected intradermally into the dorsal aspect of left forearm. A wheal of 6–10 mm is usually produced. Results are interpreted 48–72 hours after injection and induration is measured transversely through point of injection.

Interpretation. Larger the reaction, more specific it becomes while smaller induration can be because of atypical mycobacterial infections. Induration of more than 5 mm in HIV patients or in individuals staying in areas where atypical mycobacterial infections are rare, is considered to be significant. According to CDC guidelines, the test is reported positive, if the size is ≥15 mm in non-endemic population, ≥10 mm in TB endemic population and ≥5 mm in immune deficient patients, those having chest radiographic signs of healed TB and those having recent contact with active TB.[35] After a recent infection, acquired immunity takes about 2–10 weeks to develop and this is signaled by a positive tuberculin test.

False negatives can be seen either due to erroneous testing or anergy conditions, like sarcoidosis, uraemia, Hodgkin's disease, etc. A false positive test is seen in a case of prior exposure to atypical mycobacteria or BCG vaccination, although the effect of BCG vaccine has been said to wane away by 3–5 years.

"Booster effect" is a phenomenon of increased reaction seen on sequential PPD testing and may occur either due to a remote tuberculosis infection or by sensitisation with atypical mycobacteria.[36] Hence while interpreting TST test, main considerations include the size of induration, history of contact, prevalence of atypical mycobacterial infections, age and immune status of the patient and concomitant clinical signs suggestive of active tuberculosis.

3. Interferon-gamma release assay (IGRA)

When the bacillus enters the body, it reacts against it and is engulfed by the macrophages. Interferon gamma (IFN-γ) is released by the peripheral blood cells on stimulation. There are specific DNA regions of difference (RD1) which are absent in BCG strains but present in all *M. tuberculosis* strains. These regions encode two proteins, early secreted antigen target 6 (ESAT-6) and culture filtrate protein 10 (CFP-10). Measurement of IFN-γ can be done either by ELISA (Quanti-FERON-TB Gold In-Tube Assay, Celestis) or Elispot (T-SPOT.TB assay, Oxford Immunotec) technique.[37] Although being highly specific, it does not differentiate between an active or latent infection.The sensitivity of IGRA is similar to TST but being more specific, it helps in evaluating a positive TST and to exclude a false-positive one.

TREATMENT: CONSIDERATIONS AND DIFFICULTIES

TREATMENT

Treatment of ocular TB is done with a combination of ATT and corticosteroids (topical, local or systemic).

Antitubercular treatment (ATT)

ATT is required for a minimum of 6 months in total—two months of four-drug therapy (isoniazid 5 mg/kg daily, rifampicin 450 mg daily, pyrazinamide 30 mg/kg daily and ethambutol 15 mg/kg daily) followed by a 4-month continuation phase of isoniazid and rifamipicin. Some advocate the use of ATT for 9 months as well, although no significant difference as compared to 6 months has been reported.

A phenomenon of "paradoxical worsening" has been reported to occur in 24.5% patients commencing ATT medication, which is generally managed well by escalating steroids.[38]

DIFFICULTIES IN MANAGEMENT

1. *Difficulty in definitive diagnosis.* There is a significant overlap in clinical presentation of ocular TB and other uveitic entities. Hence, diagnosis is usually based on clinical signs and ancillary testing after carefully excluding other infectious and non-infectious conditions. However, in 42 cases of histopathologically proven cases of ocular TB, 40% of tested patients had negative TST and 57% had normal chest radiograph.[39] In another series of 80 PCR positive patients, 44% patients had negative PPD skin test, and 83% had normal chest radiograms.[13] Hence the definitive diagnostics need to be improved to aid in management.

2. *Secondary complications,* like cataract, secondary angle closure glaucoma, vitreous haemorrhage, cystoid macular oedema, macular scars, choroidal neovascular membraneand tractional retinal detachment need simultaneous treatment to preserve best possible vision.

3. *Drug resistance.* The multi-dug resistance (MDR-TB) and extensively drug resistance TB (XDR-TB) has been a matter of concern and proven cases of resistant ocular TB have been shown in recent past which improved on alteration of conventional therapy.

4. *Drug toxicity.* Besides the systemic and liver toxicity of many antitubercular drugs, the ocular toxicity, especially of ethambutol must be kept in mind. Any decrease in vision without any obvious cause, must be dealt with caution.

To conclude, two special things that make intraocular tuberculosis interesting, are the wide range of clinical manifestations caused by the same organism and the overlap of disease spectrum with other infectious and non-infectious entities. Careful look out for clinical signs and confirmation of diagnosis with lab tests helps in clinching the diagnosis.

REFERENCES

1. WHO REPORT 2014 Global Tuberculosis Report (online). www.who.int/tb/publications/global_report/en/
2. Das D, Biswas J, Ganesh SK. Pattern of uveitis in a referral uveitis clinic in India. Indian J Ophthalmol 1995;43(3): 117–121.
3. Singh RGV, Gupta A. Patterns of uveitis in a Referral eye clinic in North India. Indian J Ophthalmol. 2004;52:121–5.
4. Biswas J, Madhavan HN, Gopal L, Badrinath SS. Intraocular tuberculosis: clinicopathologic study of five cases. Retina. 1995;15(6):461–8.
5. Demirci H, Shields CL, Shields JA, Eagle RC Jr. Ocular tuberculosis masquerading as ocular tumors. Surv Ophthalmol 2004;49(1):78–89.
6. Basu S, Monira S, Modi RR et al. Degree, duration, and causes of visual impairment in eyes affected with ocular tuberculosis. J Ophthalmic Inflamm Infect. 2014;4(1):3.
7. Maitre-Jan A. Traite des maladies des yeux, Troyes, 1711, p 456. Found in Duke-Elder S: System of Ophthalmology: Diseases of the Uveal Tract, Vol 9. St Louis, CV Mosby, 1966, p 248.
8. Koch R. Die Aetiologie der Tuberkulose. Berlin Klin Wochenschrif. 1882;19:221–30.
9. Friedberg DM, Lorenzo-Latkany M. Ocular complications. In: Rom WN, Garay SM, eds. Tuberculosis, 2nd Ed. Philadelphia: Lippincott Williams & Wilkins; 2004, pp 465–476.
10. Rao NA, Saraswathy S, Smith RE. Tuberculous uveitis: distribution of *Mycobacterium tuberculosis* in the retinal pigment epithelium. Arch Ophthalmol 2006;124:1777–9.
11. Basu S, Mittal R, Balne PK, Sharma S. Intra-retinal tuberculosis. Ophthalmology. 2012;119: 2192–3.e2.
12. Rao NA, Albini TA, Kumaradas M, et al. Experimental ocular tuberculosis in guinea pigs. Arch Ophthalmol 2009;127:1162–6.
13. Gupta V, Arora S, Gupta A, et al. Management of presumed intraocular tuberculosis: possible role of polymerase chain reaction. Acta Ophthalmol Scand 1998;76(6):679-82.
14. Mohan N, Balne PK, Panda KG, et al. Polymerase chain reaction evaluation of Multifocal Serpiginoid Choroiditis. Ocul Immunol Inflamm 2014; 22(5):384–90.
15. Bansal R, Gupta A, Gupta V, et al. Tubercular serpiginous-like choroiditis presenting as multifocal serpiginoid choroiditis. Ophthalmology 2012;119:2334–42.

16. Krishnan N, Robertson BD, Thwaites G. The mechanisms and consequences of the extra-pulmonary dissemination of Mycobacterium tuberculosis. Tuberculosis (Edinb) 2010;90:361–6.

17. Basu S, Wakefield D, Biswas J, Rao NA. Pathogenesis and pathology of intraocular tuberculosis. Ocul Immunol Inflam. 2015;23:4, 353–7.

18. Russell-Goldman E, Xu J, Wang X, Chan J, Tufariello JM. A *Mycobacterium tuberculosis* Rpf double-knockout strain exhibits profound defects in reactivation from chronic tuberculosis and innate immunity phenotypes. Infect. Immun 2008;76:4269–81.

19. Eyre JWH: 'Tuberculosis of the conjunctiva: its etiology, pathology, and diagnosis. Lancet 1912; 7:1319–1328.

20. Verhoeff FH. The experimental production of sclerokeratitis and chronic intraocular tuberculosis. Trans Am Ophthalmol Soc 1913; 13(Pt 2):469–85.

21. Bloomfield ST, Mondino B, Cray GK. Scleral tuberculosis. Arch Opthalmol W. 1976;954–956.

22. Gupta A, Gupta V. Tubercular posterior uveitis. Int Ophthalmol Clin 2005;45(2):71–88.

23. Illingworth RS., Wright T: Tubercles of choroid. Br Med J 1948;2(4572):365–8.

24. Barondes MJ, Sponsel WE, Stevens TS, Plotnik RD. Tuberculous choroiditis diagnosed by chorio-retinal endobiopsy. Am J Ophthalmol 1991; 112(4):460–1.

25. Gilbert W. Ueber Periphlebitis and Endovaskuli-tisder Nctzhautge fassenebslbemerkungenuber Sklcrolische. Tuberkulose und septische Ader-hauterkrankuiigen Klin Monnlshl Augenheilkd 1935;97:335–49.

26. Donahue HC. Ophthalmologic experience in a tuberculosis sanatorium. Am J Ophthalmol 1967; 64(4):742–8.

27. Gupta A, Bansal R, Gupta V, Sharma A, Bambery P. Ocular signs predictive of tubercular uveitis. Am J Ophthalmol 2010;149(4):562–70.

28. Helm CJ, Holland GN. Ocular Tuberculosis. Surv Ophthalmol 1993;38(3):229–56.

29. Tabbara KF. Tuberculosis. Curr Opin Ophthalmol 2007;18:493–501.

30. Kotake S, Kimura K, Yoshikawa K, et al. Polymerase chain reaction for the detection of Mycobacterium tuberculosis in ocular tuber-culosis. Am J Ophthalmol 1994;117:805–6.

31. Chauhan DS, Sharma VD, Prashar D, et al. Molecular typing of mycobacterial tuberculosis isolates from different parts of India based on IS6110 element polymorphism using RFLP analysis. Indian J Med Res 2007;125:577–81.

32. Sharma K, Gupta V, Bansal R, Sharma A, Sharma M, Gupta A. Novel multi-targeted polymerase chain reaction for diagnosis of presumed tubercular uveitis. J Ophthalmic Inflamm Infect 2013;3(1):25.

33. Sharma Ganesh SK, Roopleen, Biswas J, Veena N. Role of high-resolution computerized tomo-graphy (HRCT) of the chest in granulomatous uveitis: a tertiary uveitis clinic experience from India. Ocul Immunol Inflam. 2011;19(1):51–7.

34. Doycheva D, Pfannenberg C, Hetzel J, et al. Presumed tuberculosis-induced retinal vasculitis, diagnosed with positron emission tomography (18F-FDG-PET/CT), aspiration biopsy, and culture. Ocul Immunol Inflamm 2010;18(3):194–9.

35. American Thoracic Society. Targeted tuberculin testing and treatment of latent tuberculosis infection. MMWR Recomm Rep 2000;49:1e51 (A)

36. Reichman LB. Tuberculin skin testing. Chest 1979;76(6 suppl):764–70.

37. Mazurek GH, Jereb J, Lobue P, Iademarco MF, Metchock B, Vernon A. Guidelines for using the QuantiFERON-TB gold test for detecting *Myco-bacterium tuberculosis* infection, United States. MMWR Recomm Rep 2005;54(RR-15):49–55.

38. Basu S, Nayak S, Padhi TR, Das T. Progressive ocular inflammation following antitubercular therapy for presumed ocular tuberculosis in a high endemic setting. Eye (Lond) 2013;27(5): 657–62.

39. Wroblewski KJ, Hidayat AA, Neafie RC, et al. Ocular tuberculosis: A clinicopathologic and molecular study. Ophthalmology 2011;118:772–7.

6.1.2 UVEITIS IN LEPROSY

Pathogenesis and Types of Leprosy
Pathogenesis
Types of leprosy
Based on immunity
• Lepromatous lyprosy
• Tuberculoid leprosy
WHO classification
• Paucibacillary leprosy
• Multibacillary leprosy
Ridley-Jopling system
• Intermediate leprosy
• Tuberculoid leprosy
• Borderline tubculoid leprosy
• Mid-borderline leprosy
• Borderline lepromatous leprosy
• Lepromatous leprosy
Ocular Manifestations
Leprotic uveitis
• Autoimmune acute uveitis
• Neuroparalytic form of uveitis
• Iris and lepra pearls
Paralysis of ophthalmic division of 5th nerve and facial nerve
Diagnosis and Treatment
• Diagnosis
• Treatment

PATHOGENESIS AND TYPES OF LEPROSY

PATHOGENESIS

Leprosy is a chronic inflammatory disease caused by *Mycobacterium leprae*. *Mycobacterium laprae* is an acid-fast, pleomorphic, obligate intracellular bacillus that closely resembles *Mycobacterium tuberculosis*. The most likely route of infection is postulated to be through upper respiratory tract though exact mode of infection remains unknown.[1,2] *Mycobacterium leprae* affects skin, anterior segment of the eye as well as peripheral nerves. The organism cannot grow on culture but can be grown in the footpads of mice or nine-banded armadillos because they, like humans, are susceptible to leprosy.

TYPES OF LEPROSY

I. Based on immune response

Based on the immune response of the host, leprosy can be classified as lepromatous or tuberculoid.

1. *Lepromatous leprosy* form of disease develops in individuals with poor immune response. Thus the disease in this form of leprosy is widespread affecting skin, peripheral nerves, eyes, upper respiratory tract, testes, bones and reticuloendothelial systems. As a result, the patient may present with:
• *Leonine facies* (nasal widening, thickened ear lobules with thickening of skin)
• *Saadle-shaped nasal deformity*
• *Claw hand deformity* due to ulnar nerve palsy.
• *Loss of peripheral sensations* might result in the repeated trauma causing shortening and loss of digits.

2. *Tuberculoid leprosy* on the other hand is seen in patients with good immunity and is restricted to the involvement of skin and peripheral nerves resulting in development:
• Hypopigmented, annular cutaneous lesions that are hypoanaesthetic associated with
• Thickening of cutaneous sensory nerves.

II. WHO classification

WHO has classified the disease into:
Paucibacillary leprosy (5 or less skin lesions with no bacteria seen on skin smears)

Multibacillary leprosy (more than 5 lesions or bacteria detected on skin smears or both)

III. The Ridley-Jopling system

The Ridley-Jopling system of classfication is used commonly in clinical studies. It classifies leprosy as below:
1. *Intermediate leprosy.* Characterized by the presence of few flat lesions on the skin that may heal spontaneously or progress to a more severe variety.
2. *Tuberculoid leprosy.* Characterized by the presence of a few flat lesions that may heal spontaneously, persist or progress to a more severe variety. This form may have nerves involvement too.

3. Borderline tuberculoid leprosy. In this form of leprosy, the lesions are like tuberculoid but smaller and more numerous. These lesions may persist, revert to tuberculoid, or advance to another form. The enlargement of nerves is less common.

4. Mid-borderline leprosy. This is characterized by the presence of moderate numbness, reddish plaques with swollen lymph glands. The lesions may persist, regress, or progress to other forms of leprosy.

5. Borderline lepromatous leprosy. The skin lesions in this form of leprosy are flat, sometimes raised bumps, plaques, and nodules, sometimes numb; may regress, persist, or progress.

6. Lepromatous leprosy. This form of disease has many lesions with bacteria; hair loss; nerve involvement; limb weakness; disfigurement. There is no spontaneous regression in this form of leprosy. The ocular involvement is commonest in this form of leprosy.

OCULAR MANIFESTATIONS

Major ocular manifestation include chronic granulomatous uveitis due to infiltration of iris with bacilli while nerve damage may result in small undilating pupil. Leprosy can produce the following lesions in the eye.

I. Leprotic uveitis

The reported incidence of uveitis in leprosy is variable, ranging between 5.3 and 63%.[4-7] Leprosy can produce three different forms of uveitis:[1-3, 4-8]

1. Autoimmune acute uveitis. The first form of uveitis is typically acute and results from type II hypersensitivity reaction due to increased antigenic and antibodies load. The antibodies in this form of leprosy are not protective; instead they form antigen–antibody complexes that cause recurrent inflammations including erythema nodosum and uveitis. This produces acute granulomatous iridocyclitis with mutton fat keratic precipitates, hypopyon, posterior synechiae and rarely conjunctival leproma. The onset is acute and patient has to seek medical advice because of the acute onset.

2. Neuroparalytic form of uveitis. In this form of leprosy, during bacteremic phase, a large number of leprae bacilli get loaded in the uveitis tract. These bacilli lead to slow degeneration of the nerves leading to atrophy of the dilator muscle resulting in small-undilated pupil. In long-standing cases, the pupil becomes miotic associated with iris atrophy.

3. Iris and lepra pearls. This is the third form of uveitis characterised by the development of iris and lepra pearls; both of which are made up of dead as well as live bacilli. Clinically, these are seen as white sand grains on the surface of iris. These may enlarge slowly, become pedunculated, detach from the surface of iris and produce pseudohypopyon in the anterior chamber. The lepra pearls are pathogonomic of leprosy. *Mycobacterium leprae* tend to localise in the iris stroma early during the stage of bacterial dissemination throughout the body and may keep multiplying in the stromal mononuclear cells, which in turn take the appearance of 'foam cells'. These cells containing "globi" are made up of closely packed acid-fast bacilli that in turn coalesce and become clinically visible as 'iris lepromas' (Fig. 6.1.2.1).

II. Paralysis of ophthalmic division of 5th nerve and facial nerve

Paralysis of ophthalmic division of 5th nerve and facial nerve resulting in lid abnormalities and corneal hypoaesthesia that can cause secondary corneal infections.

DIAGNOSIS AND TREATMENT

DIAGNOSIS

1. Majority, of the patients are already diagnosed with systemic disease first and the ocular manifestations come later. That makes the diagnosis easier. If the patient does not have any systemic manifestation and presents to the ophthalmologist for the first time with the clinical manifestations described above and especially if the patient is from the geographic area that is endemic for leprosy, a thorough systemic investigation is required to rule out leprosy as a possible etiology of uveitis. The characteristic clinical signs are diagnostic of leprosy.

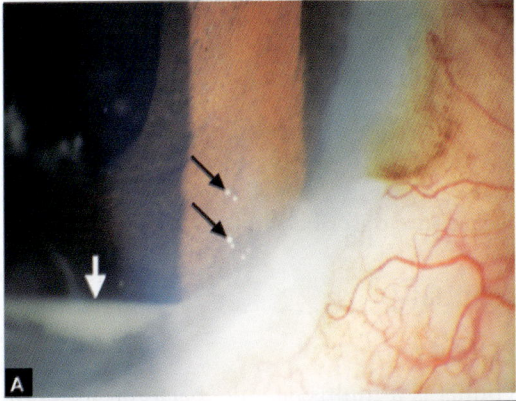

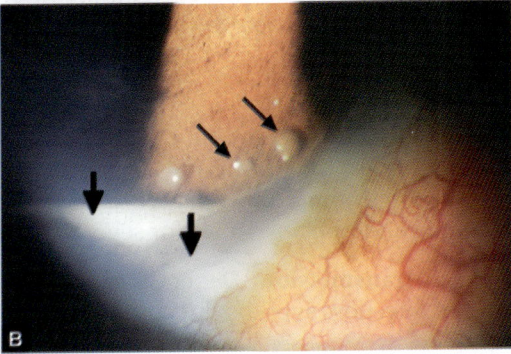

Fig. 6.1.2.1 *Anterior segment photograph in a patient with lepromatous leprosy: A, shows lepra pearls (thin arrows) with pseudohypoyon (thick arrow); B, Same eye, following treatment with topical corticosteroids and mydriatics shows hypopyon that has become organized and chronic with the appearance like a retrocorneal membrane (thick arrows) with iris lepromas (thin arrows). (Photograph courtesy of Dr Manohar Babu, Aravind Eye Hospital, Coimbatore).*

2. Lepramine test involves subcutaneous injection of inactivated *Mycobacterium leprae*. It is strongly positive in tuberculoid leprosy and negative in lepromatous disease.

3. Detection of Mycobacterium leprosy from eye. The eyes of patients with lepromatous leprosy may harbour live bacilli or antigen long after the skin has become bacteriologically negative. These acid-fast organisms can be detected from the aqueous humour or a scleral nodule for confirmation of the diagnosis. Since the eye disease is paucibacillary in nature, PCR of the aqueous humour is a more sensitive technique as it amplifies the organisms.

TREATMENT

Chemotherapy is quite effective and has improved the prognosis as well as reduced the risk of ocular complications in leprosy. The patients with type 2 reactions may require intensive topical and systemic corticosteroids, mydriatic agents as well as oral anti-leprosy treatment. *First-line multidrug treatment* includes three drugs for 6 months. These drugs include Rifampicin 600 mg administered first day of every month; clofazimine given as an oral dose of 300 mg first day of every month followed by 50 mg/day; and dapsone 100 mg per day. However, the patient may continue to have progressive ocular inflammation despite the completion of anti-leprosy treatment. Thus it is important to keep examining the eyes for any recurrences even after the completion of anti-leprosy treatment.

REFERENCES

1. Hogeweg M, Faber WR. Progression of eye lesions in leprosy: ten-year follow-up study in the Netherlands. Int J Leprosy 1991;59:392–7.
2. Lewallen S, Tungpakorn NC, Kim SH, et al. Progression of eye disease in "cured" leprosy patients: implications for understanding the pathophysiology of ocular disease and for addressing eye care needs. Br J Ophthalmol 2000;84:817–21.
3. Fe Eleanor FP, Tranquilino TF, Rodolfo MA, et al. Methods for the classification of leprosy for treatment. Clinical Infectious Diseases 2007; 44:1096–99.
4. Thompson K, Job CK. Silent iritis in treated bacillary negative leprosy Int J Lepr Other Mycobact Dis 1996;64:306–10. 21.
5. Desikan P, Desikan KV. Persistence of lepromatous granuloma in clinically cured cases of leprosy. Int J Lepr Other Mycobact Dis 1995; 63:417–21.
6. Ebenezer D, Gigi JE, Charles K. Job pathology of iris in leprosy. Br J Ophthalmol 1997;81:490–2.
7. Canizares O, Costello M, Gigli I. Erythema nodosum type of lepra reaction. Arch Ophthalmol 1962;85:29–40.
8. Hussein N, Ostler HB. Hansen disease. In: Pepose JS, Holland GN, Wilhelmus KR, (Eds). Ocular Infection and Immunity. St.Louis, Mosby, 1996; pp 1421–9.
9. Spaide R, Nattis R, Lipka A, Amico RD. Ocular findings in leprosy in the United States. Am J Ophthalmol 1985;100:411–6.

6.1.3 SYPHILITIC AND OTHER SPIROCHAETAL UVEITIS

General considerations
• Spirochaetes
Syphilis
Etiology
• Treponema pallidum
• Mode of transmission
Clinical spectrum
Congenital syphilis
• Systemic features
• Ocular menifestations
Acquired syphilis
• Primary syphilis
• Secondary syphilis
• Latent syphilis
• Tertiary syphilis
List of ocular lesions of syphilis
• Syphilitic uveitis
Diagnosis and treatment
• Diagnosis
• Treatment
Lyme Disease
• Etiology
• Clinical features
• Diagnosis and treatment
Leptospirosis
• Etiology
• Clinical features
• Diagnosis and treatment

GENERAL CONSIDERATIONS

SPIROCHAETES

Spirochaetes are motile, helicles flexible bacteria, which have gram-negative type cell wall. These are thin and twisted spirally along the long axis and hence the name spirochaetes (*speria* means coiled and *chaite* means hair). They have lengthwise fibrils called *endoflagella* that allow them to move.

Classification of spirochaetes and diseases produced by them is summarised in Table 6.1.3.1. Only a few common spirochaetal diseases are described in this chapter.

SYPHILIS

ETIOLOGY

Syphilis is a multisystemic, bacterial infection caused by the spirochaete *Treponema pallidum*.

Treponema pallidum is a spirochaete and possesses the gram-negative envelope. It cannot be stained by simple aniline dyes or Gram's method. It is a strict parasite and cannot survive long out of the human body. However, it can be cultivated and remains viable for several days.

Mode of transmission. Depending upon the mode of infection, syphilis can be congenital or acquired.

1. *Congenital syphilis* results from the transplacental transmission of *T. pallidum* from the infected mother to the fetus. Untreated primary or secondary syphilis is almost invariably transmitted to the fetus, whereas transmission in later stages of the disease occurs less frequently. Congenital syphilis is perventable with proper treatment of the mother; therefore, all expected mothers should have a VDRL test at the beginning and near the end of pregnancy.

2. *Acquired syphilis* occurs due to ability of *T. pallidum* to penetrate the intact mucous membranes or abraded skin. The modes of transmission include:

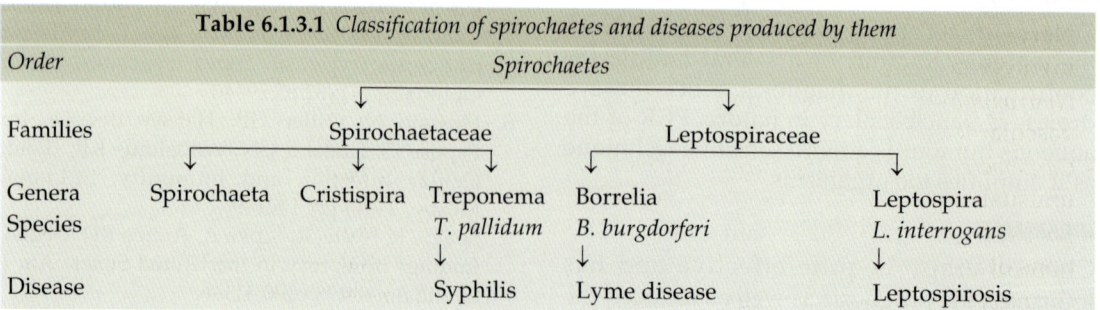

Table 6.1.3.1 *Classification of spirochaetes and diseases produced by them*

Order	Spirochaetes				
Families		Spirochaetaceae		Leptospiraceae	
Genera	Spirochaeta	Cristispira	Treponema	Borrelia	Leptospira
Species			*T. pallidum*	*B. burgdorferi*	*L. interrogans*
			↓	↓	↓
Disease			Syphilis	Lyme disease	Leptospirosis

- *Sexual transmission* is the most common mode of contracting acquired syphilis. The treponemas are present in the superficial genital lesions and pass from one partner to the other. During sexual intercourse including orogenital and anorectal contact.
- *Kissing* is also a mode of transmission, though less common.
- Blood transfusion from infected person is another rare mode of transmission.

Note. The disease is most infectious in patients with untreated primary and secondary syphilis. Disease can also be transmitted by patients with early latent syphilis, especially if they have mucocutaneous involvement. However, patients with late latent syphilis and tertiary syphilis are not infectious.

CLINICAL SPECTRUM

CONGENITAL SYPHILIS

Systemic features

Early congenital syphilis (up to 2 years of age) may not manifest until several days after birth.
Clinical features include:
- *Skin rash* may develop which have generalised distribution and resembling secondary syphilis, except that in the infant the rash may be vesicular or bullous.
- *Rhinitis*, also called the snuffles, may develop.
- *Other features* include hepatosplenomegaly, jaundice, osteochondritis, abdominal distress, low weight, pneumonia and severe anaemia.

Late congenital syphilis (older than 2 years of age) is characterised by:
- *Hutchinson teeth*, i.e. notched, thin, upper incisors with abnormal spacing.
- *Mulberry molars* and abnormal face
- *Nerve deafness* due to VIII cranial nerve involvement.
- *Neurosyphilitic features* due to meningo-vascular lesions.
- *Cardiovascular complications* are comparatively unusual.
- *Bony changes* include saber shins and perforations of the hard palate.
- *Cutaneous lesions* such as shagades.

- *Hutchinson's triad* refers to occurrence of Hutchinson teeth, nerve deafness and interstitial keratitis.

Ocular manifestations

Ocular manifestations of congenital syphilis include:
1. *Interstitial keratitis.* Interstitial keratitis (IK), usually associated with anterior uveitis, is a peculiar feature of congenital syphilis.

Pathogenesis. It is now generally accepted that the disease is a manifestation of local antigen–antibody reaction. It is presumed that *Treponema pallidum* invades the cornea and sensitises it during the period of its general diffusion throughout the body in the foetal stage. Later a small scale fresh invasion by *Treponema* or toxins excite the inflammation in the sensitised cornea. The inflammation is usually triggered by an injury or an operation on the eye.
2. *Uveitis.* Peculiar features are:
- *Uveitic manifestations* of congenital syphilis include multifocal chorioretinitis and less commonly retinal vasculitis.
- *Pigmentary retinitis* characterized by salt and pepper fundus appearance may result from ocular inflammatory disease. Such lesions may affect the peripheral retina, posterior pole, or a single quadrant. These changes are not progressive and may be associated with normal vision.
- *Bilateral secondary degeneration of RPE*, which may mimic retinitis pigmentosa, is less commonly described fundoscopic variation.
3. *Glaucoma.* Secondary glaucoma can also occur as a result of congenital syphilis keratouveitis.

AQUIRED SYPHILIS

Clinical features of acquired syphilis can be divided into four stages:
- Primary syphilis
- Secondary syphilis
- Latent syphilis, and
- Tertiary syphilis

Primary syphilis

Chancre is the predominant lesion of primary syphilis and appears about 4 weeks after infection.

- *Characteristic features*, the chancre is painless, relatively avascular, circumscribed, indented lesion of 1–2 cm in size, which later erodes in the centre to form a painless ulcer. Serous fluid from these lesions is teeming with spirochaetes. Chancre heals in 3–6 months.
- *Common sites of chancre* in males are penis, anus, and rectum, and in females cervix, vulva, and perineum. Small lesions may also occur on the lips, tongue, buccal, mucosa and skin. Chancres of eyelids and conjunctiva are also reported.

Lymphadenitis of inguinal lymph nodes in male and pelvic lymph nodes in female may occur due to spread of *Treponema* from primary site of infection. The involved lymph nodes are swollen, discrete, rubbery and non-tender. From lymph nodes, the *Treponema* enter the blood-stream in large number.

Secondary syphilis

Primary syphilis heals, even if untreated, within 3–6 weeks. However, the untreated cases develop secondary syphilis due to general dissemination of *Treponema* within 2–6 months after the primary lesions heal.

Characteristic features include:
- *Constitutional symptoms* are fever, malaise, nausea, anorexia, headache and joint pain.
- *Diffuse erythematous cutaneous lesions,* i.e. papulomacular rashes particularly on the trunk and extremity.
- *Mucous patches* in the nasopharynx, and mucosa of genitalia. These lesions discharge large number of *Treponema*.
- *Condylomata* at mucocutaneous junctions in vulva, anus.
- *Generalized lymphadenopathy* is a common features of both primary and secondary syphilis.
- *Other organs,* like joints, kidneys, liver and gastrointestinal tract, can also be involved.
- *Ocular involvement* as anterior uveitis may occur is about 10–15% of cases.

Latent syphilis

Once the lesions of secondary syphilis heal, the disease become latent and can be detected only by serological test.

Early latent syphilis is the first year after healing of secondary lesions. In this stage, a few patients may have recurrences of infectious muco-cutaneous lesions.

Late latent phase of syphilis occurs after 1 year of disappearance of secondary lesions, many cases remain disease free for a larger period and may undergo even natural cure. However, about 40% cases develop manifestation of tertiary syphilis.

Tertiary syphilis

Tertiary syphilis, also called the late syphilis, develops decades after the primary infection. It is a slowly progressive destructive inflammatory disease that may affect any organ. Its lesions can be arranged in three groups:

1. *Benign lesions of tertiary syphilis* are called gummas, the chronic granulomatous lesion that heal with scaring and fibrosis. Gummas are known to involve skin, mucous membrane, bones, but can occur in almost any tissue and have also been reported to involve choroid of the eye.

2. *Cardiovascular syphilis* may involve heart and aorta. Aortitis, aortic aneurysm and aortic valvular insufficiency may occur.

3. *Neurosyphilis* is characterised by wide-spectrum of manifestations:
- *Asymptomatic neurosyphilis* in some patients who have a CSF positive for CDRL test.
- *Meningovascular syphilis* presents as an aseptic meningitis causing palsies of many cranial nerves.
  Argyll Robertson pupil, characterised by a smll, irregular pupil that is unreactive to light but normally reactive to accommodation can occur due to involvement of base of brain.
- *Parenchymatous neurosyphilis* or *meningo-encephalitis* may occur with progressive lobs of cortical functions. Patients may experience altered mental status, irritability, reduced memory, poor judgment, delusions, syphilitic psychosis and seizures.
- *Tabes dorsalis* refers to involvement of posterior columns and posterior roots of spinal cord

resulting in severe nabbing pain in lower limbs, ataxia, hyperaesthesia, paraesthesia, reduced tendon reflexes, Charcot arthropathy and Argyll Robertson pupil.

LIST OF OCULAR LESIONS OF SYPHILIS

Ocular manifestations occurring in different stages of syphilis are summarised below.

Congenital syphilis
- Bilateral interstitial keratitis
- Pigmentary retinitis (salt and pepper)
- Keratouveitis
- Inflammatory glaucoma

Acquired syphilis
Primary syphilis
- Chancres of eyelid
- Chancres of conjunctiva

Secondary syphilis
- *Eyelids:* Blepharitis, madarosis
- *Lacrimal apparatus:* Dacryocystitis, dacryo-adenitis
- *Conjunctiva:* Conjunctivism
- *Sclera:* Episcleritis, scleritis
- *Cornea:* Keratitis
- *Uvea:* Iris nodules, iridocyclitis, chorioretinitis
- *Vitreous:* Vitritis
- *Retina:* Neuroretinitis, perivasculitis, disc oedema, exudative retinal detachment

Tertiary syphilis
- *Orbit:* Periostitis of orbital bones
- *Eyelids:* Gummas
- *Sclera:* Episcleritis, scleritis
- *Cornea:* Unilateral interstitial keratitis, punctate stromal keratitis
- *Uvea:* Anterior and posterior uveitis, chorio-retinitis
- *Lever:* Dislocation
- *Posterior segment:* Vitritis, chorioretinitis, neuro-retinitis, retinal vasculitis, venous and arterial occlusive disease, macular oedema, pseudo-retinitis pigmentosa, CNVM
- *Neuro-ophthalmic manifestation:* Argyll Robertson pupil, oculomotor palsies, neuropathy, retro-bulbar neuritis.

Syphilitic uveitis

Syphilitic anterior uveitis

Acute plastic anterior uveitis typically occurs in the secondary syphilis and also as Herxheimer reaction seen after 24–48 hours of therapeutic dose of penicillin.

Gummatous anterior uveitis occurs late in the secondary syphilis and rarely during the tertiary stage of syphilis. It is characterized by formation of yellowish red highly vascularised multiple nodules arranged near the papillary border or ciliary of iris.

Syphilitic posterior uveitis

Syphilitic posterior uveitis may occur in following forms:
- *Multifocal choroiditis*, which is usually bilateral.
- *Acute posterior placoid chorioretinitis*, which is characterized by bilateral, large, solitary, placoid, pale-yellowish subretinal lesions
- *Neuroretinitis*, which can end in secondary optic atrophy.
- *Retinal vasculitis*, both venous and arterial, and may be of occlusive type also.

DIAGNOSIS AND TREATMENT

DIAGNOSIS

Once suspected, the clinical diagnosis of syphilitic lesions, is confirmed by following laboratory tests:

A. *Demonstration of Treponema in exudates and fluid* from genital and rectal lesions by:
- Dark ground microscopy, and
- Direct fluorescent antibody staining for *Treponema pallidum* (DFA-Tp)

B. *Demonstration of Treponema in tissues* by:
- Immunofluorescence or
- Silver staining

C. *Demonstration of treponemal antigen* in lesions by:
- Enzyme immunoassay, and
- Polymerase chain reaction (PCR) test

D. *Serological tests*

i. *Non-treponemal test* also called as *standard tests for syphilis* (STS): These tests, in which cardiolipin or lipoidal antigen is used, include the following:

1. Rapid plasma reagin (RPR) test
2. Venereal disease research lab (VDRL) test
3. Kahn test
4. Wassermann reaction

ii. *Treponemal tests*, in which treponemes are used as antigen, are of two types:

a. Tests using cultivable treponemes:
  • *Treponema pallidum* immobilization, i.e. TPI test

b. Tests using killed *Treponema*:
  • *Treponema pallidum* agglutination (TPA) test
  • *Treponema pallidum* immune adherence (TPIA) test
  • Fluorescent treponemal antibody (FTA) test
  • Fluorescent treponemal antibody absorption (FTA-ABS) test
  • IgM (FTA-ABS) test

iii. *Tests using T. pallidum extract*
  • *Treponema pallidum* haemagglutination (TPHA) tests.
  • Enzyme immunoassay (EIA)

TREATMENT

Syphilitic uveitis is treated as recommended for neurosyphilis by CDC (Center for Disease Control and Prevention) as below:

Primary treatment regimen consists of *Aqueous penicillin*, G 18–24 million units (MU) given intravenously (IV) as 3–40 MU every 4 hours for 10–14 days.

Alternative treatment regimen consists of:
• *Procaine penicillin* 2.4 MU intramuscularly (1MU) daily for 10–14 days, and
• *Probenecid* 500 mg orally 9.0 for 10–14 days.

LYME DISEASE

ETIOLOGY

Causative bacteria; Lyme disease (borreliosis) caused by the spirochaete *Borrelia burgdorferi*, is widespread in USA, where it is the most common vector-borne infection. It has been reported from other parts of the world also.

Natural hosts for *B. burgdorferi* are wild and domestic animals, such as mice and other rodents, deer, sheep, cattle, horses and dogs.

Transmitting vector is *Ixodes* tick that becomes infected whilst feeding on the infected animals. The organisms grow in the midgut of the tick and are transmitted to humans by regurgitation of the gut contents during the blood meal.

Age and sex predisposition. The disease affects men (53%) slightly more than women and has a bimodal distribution with incidence peaks in children ages 5–14 years and in adults 50–59 years.

Season. Disease is more common between months of May to August.

CLINICAL FEATURES

General features

General features can be divided into three stages:
Stage 1: Immediate stage or local disease. This is characterised by:
• *Erythema migrans*, a small red macule that develops at the site of bite within 2 to 20 days. The lesion enlarges and becomes a papule and the paracentral area may clear forming *Bull eye appearance*.

Stage 2: Early stage or disseminated disease. This stage occurs several weeks to 4 months after the initial bite and is characterised by:
• *Erythema chronicum migrans* (ECM), i.e. multiple skin rashes involving the sites remote from the site of bite.
• *Monoarthritis* or *oligoarthritis* involving large joints, particularly knee joint.
• *Constitutional symptoms* (fever, malaise, headache, stiff neck) and lymphadenopathy.
• *Neurological involvement*; in the form of meningitis, encephalitis, painful rediculitis and Bell's palsy may occur in 30–40% patients.

Stage 3: Late stage or persistent disease. This stage occurs 5 months or more after the initial bite and is characterised by:
• *Chronic arthritis* of large joints.
• *Chronic neurological syndrome* with polyneuropathy, encephalopathy, radiculopathy, memory loss and neuropsychiatric disease.
• *Acrodermatitis, chronic atrophic,* i.e. skin discolouration which is most evident in limbs, and may eventually result in shiny atrophy.
• *Myocarditis* may also occur in few patients.

Ocular features

Variable ocular involvement may occur in different stages of the disease. In general, reported ocular features include:

- *Follicular conjunctivitis.* It is a common manifestation seen in stage 1 of the disease.
- *Episcleritis.* It is a comparatively less commonly seen manifestation of stage 1 and stage 3 of the disease.
- *Keratitis.* It is the most common manifestation of stage 3 of disease. Keratitis typically occurs as bilateral, patchy, focal, stromal and subepithelial infiltrates. However, peripheral infiltrates may also be seen. Keratitis is considered an immune phenomenon rather than infection.
- *Intraocular inflammatory disease, i.e. uveitis.* It may occur as anterior uveitis, intermediate uveitis, peripheral multifocal choroiditis, retinal periphlebitis and neuroretinitis associated with vitritis.
- *Orbital myositis* may occur rarely.
- *Neuro-ophthalmic manifestations* include ocular motor nerve palsies, optic neuritis, reversible Horner's syndrome and 7th nerve palsy.

DIAGNOSIS AND TREATMENT

Diagnosis

Clinical diagnosis of lyme disease is mode from the typically features including ECM.

Serological testes include ELISA, indirect immunofluorescence and haemagglutination tests. However, these tests lack specificity and may give positive results in cases of relapsing fever, syphilis, yawn, pinta, leptospira infection and collagen disease.

Lyme disease patients may give a positive FTA-ABS test, though VDRL test is negative.

CDC 2-step protocol recommendation for diagnosis of active disease or previous infections includes:
1. IFA or ELISA for IgM and IgG, followed by
2. Western Immunoblot testing

Treatment

Antibiotics, like doxycycline, amoxicillin, cefuroxime are useful for the treatment of Lyme disease. Jarisch-Herxheimer reaction occurs in 15% patients following antibiotic therapy.

Intraocular inflammatory disease in Lyme disease needs to be treated with intravenous ceftriaxone 2 g daily for 14–28 days.

LEPTOSPIROSIS

ETIOLOGY

Causative bacteria. Leptospirosis is caused by a gram-negative spirochaete.

Leptospira interrogans: This species had over 200 pathologic strains.

Natural reservoirs. Leptospira is primarily a parasite of vertibrates other than human, such as rodents, dogs, pigs and cattle. The organisms localize in the kidneys, colonie in the convoluted tubules and continuously shed in the urine of reservoir animals, thereby contaminating the environment.

Mode of transmission. Humans acquire infection through contact with water, soil or vegetation contaminated with animal urine. The pathogenic Leptospira enter the body through cuts or abrasions of the skin. They may also enter through the mucous membrane of nose, mouth or eye. The organisms enter the blood of human and invade various tissues and organs, particularly the kidneys, liver, meninges and conjunctiva.

CLINICAL FEATURES

Clinical features of leptospirosis include two phases:

Leptospiremic phase occurs after an incubation period of 1 to 4 weeks (average 13 days) and lasts for 4 to 9 days. It is characterised by:
- *Constitutional symptoms* which have abrupt onset include fever, chills, severe headache (frontal, bitemporal or retro-orbital) severe muscular pain, vomiting and diarrhoea.
- *Conjunctival hyperaemia* is a characteristic finding that usually appears on third or fourth day of disease.

Immune phase of leptospirosis occurs due to appearance of the antibodies in the serum beginning on 6th to 12th day of the illness. Its clinical course is variable and is characterised by:

- *High fever with meningismus* occurs in 50% of the patients. CSF examination in such patients shows pleocytosis with mildly elevated protein levels.
- *Neurological features* include encephalitis, peripheral neuropathies, and optic neuritis, palsy of 6th, 7th and 8th cranial nerves.
- *Spontaneous abortion* is reported in patients with leptospirosis during pregnancy.
- *Uveitis*, both anterior and posterior, may occur during immune phase.

Weil's disease

Weil's disease refers to a severe form of leptospirosis, characterised by following features:

- *Renal and hepatocellular dysfunction* occurs on 3rd to 6th day after infection and manifestating as jaundice, azotaemia, anaemia and persistent fever.
- *Neurological features* may include optic neuritis, facial nerve paralysis and altered mental status.
- *Subconjunctival and retinal haemorrhages* may occur in severe form of disease.
- *Anterior uveitis* of moderate to severe degree, is of consistent occurrence. Therefore, leptospirosis must be ruled out in patients with uveitis of unknown cause.

List of ocular manifestations in leptospirosis

Leptospiraemic phase
- Conjunctival hyperaemia

Immune phase
- Palpebral herpes
- Facial nerve palsy
- Subconjunctival haemorrhages
- Scleral icterus
- Iridocyclitis
- Posterior segment lesions: Optic neuritis, posterior uveitis with retinal exudates, and retinal haemorrhage

DIAGNOSIS AND TREATMENT

Diagnosis

Clinical diagnosis

Clinically, leptospirosis must be considered a possible cause of pyrexia of uncertain origin (PUO), particularly in those patients who may have been exposed to various animal hosts or have been swimming in water contaminated with animal urine.

Leptospiral uveitis needs to be differentiated from other causes of uveitis. High prevalence of bilaterality and vitreous inflammation, the frequency of CME, and the absence of occlusive retinal vasculitis and peripheral retinal neo-vascularisation differentiate this entity from HLA-B27 associated uveitis, idiopathic pars planitis, Behcet's disease and Eales disease, respectively.

Investigations

Diagnosis of leptospirosis may be established by:
- Demonstration of leptospirosis in body fluids, and
- Serological tests

Demonstration of the leptospirosis in blood, CSF and urine can be done by dark ground microscopy of the centrifugal samples.
- *Blood examination* is useful in early stages of the disease, as leptospirosis disappears from the blood after 8 days.
- *Urine examination* may show leptospirosis in the second week and intermittently thereafter for 4–6 weeks.

However, practically, it is not possible, because the process is very resource demanding.

Serological tests

Genus-specific tests are:
- Complement fixation test
- Sensitised erythrocyte lysis and haemagglutination test
- Enzyme-linked immunosorbent assay (ELISA), which is capable of detecting IgM and IgG leptospiral antibodies.

Serogroup and serovar specific tests are:
- Macroscopic agglutination test (MAT), and
- Microscopic agglutination test

Treatment

Mild infection
- Doxycycline 100 mg PO, BID × 7 days, or
- Amoxicillin 500 mg PO, QID × 7 days, or
- Ampicillin 550–750 mg PO QID × 7 days

Moderate to severe infection
- Penicillin G 1.5 MU IV QID × 10 days, or
- Ampicillin 0.5–1g IV QID × 10 days, or
- Ceftriaxone 1 gm IV QID × 10 days

Severe uveitis or neurological abnormalities or arthritis
- Ceftriaxone 2 g/days IV × 14–21 days.

BIBLIOGRAPHY

1. Becerra LI, Ksiazek SM, Savino PJ, et al. Syphilitic uveitis in human immunodeficiency virus infected and noninfected patients. Ophthalmology 1989;96:1727–30.
2. McLeish WM, Pulido JS, Holland S, et al. The ocular manifestations of syphilis in the human immunodeficiency virus type 1-infected host. Ophthalmology 1990;97:196–203.
3. Neetens A, Smets RM. Ocular complications of neuro-syphilis. Bull Soc Belge Ophtalmol 1986; 213:83–6.
4. Ormerod LD, Puklin JE, Sobel JD. Syphilitic posterior uveitis: correlative findings and significance. Clin Infect Dis 2001;32:1661–73.
5. Rajapure V, Tirwa R, Poudyal H, Thakur N. Prevalence and risk factors associated with sexually transmitted diseases (STDs) in Sikkim. J Community Health 2013;38:156–62.
6. Rathinam SR. Ocular leptospirosis. Curr Opin Ophthalmol 2002;13:381–6.
7. Shalaby IA, Dunn JP, Semba RD, Jabs DA. Syphilitic uveitis in human immunodeficiency virus-infected patients. Arch Ophthalmol 1997;115:469–73.
8. Shukla D, Rathinam SR, Cunningham ET. JrLeptospiral uveitis in the developing world. Int Ophthalmol Clin 2010;50:113–24.
9. Spoor TC, Wynn P, Hartel WC, Bryan CS. Ocular syphilis: acute and chronic. J Clin Neuro-ophthalmol 1983;3:197–203.
10. Uglietti A, Antoniazzi E, Pezzotta S, Maserati R. Syphilitic uveitis as presenting feature of HIV infection in elderly patients. AIDS 2007; 21:535–7.

6.1.4 OCULAR NOCARDIOSIS

- Etiology
- Clinical features
- Diagnosis and treatment

ETIOLOGY

Nocardiosis is a potentially lethal systemic disease caused by the bacterium *Nocardia asteroides*. *Nocardia* is found in the soil and initial infection occurs by ingestion or inhalation of the organism. Ocular involvement occurs by haematogenous spread of the bacteria.

CLINICAL FEATURES

Systemic features include:
- Pneumonia
- Disseminated abscess

Ocular lesions include any of the following:
- Diffuse iridocyclitis with anterior chamber cells and flare,
- Marked vitritis, and multiple choroidal abscesses with overlying retinal detachment.
- Isolated, unilateral chorioretinal mass with minimal vitritis to retinal detachment.

DIAGNOSIS AND TREATMENT

Diagnosis is made from:
- Clinical features of the disease, and
- Microbiological investigations in the form of Gram staining and culture of aqueous and/or vitreous taps.

Treatment consists of systemic sulphonamide for 6 weeks in immunologically competent patients and up to 1 year in immunomodulated patients.

BIBLIOGRAPHY

1. Bozbeyoglu S, Yilmaz G, Akova YA, et al. Choroidal abscess due to nocardial infection in a renal allograft recipient. Retina 2004; 24:164–6.
2. Climenhaga DB, Tokarewicz AC, Willis NR. Nocardia keratitis. Can J Ophthalmol 1984;19: 284–6.

3. Korkmaz C, Aydinli A, Erol N, et al. Widespread nocardiosis in two patients with Behcet's disease. Clin Exp Rheumatol 2001;19:459–62.
4. Ng EW, Zimmer-Galler IE, Green WR. Endogenous nocardia asteroides endophthalmitis. Arch Ophthalmol 2002;120:210–3.
5. Ng EW, Zimmer-GallerIE, GreenWR. Endogenous Nocardia asteroides endophthalmitis. Arch Ophthalmol 2002;120(2):210–3.
6. Phillips WB, Shields CL, Shields JA, et al. Nocardiachoroidal abscess. Br J Ophthalmol 1992;76:694–6.
7. Rogers SJ, Johnson BL. Endogenous nocardia-endophthalmitis: report of a case in a patient treated for lymphocytic lymphoma. Ann Ophthalmol 1977;9:1123–31.
8. Sridhar MS, Gopinathan U, Garg P, et al. Ocular nocardia infections with special emphasis on the cornea. Surv Ophthalmol 2001;45:361–78.
9. Suppiah R, Abraham G, Sekhar U, et al. Nocardial endophthalmitis leading to blindness in a renal transplant recipient. Nephrol Dial Transplant 1999;14:1576–7.
10. Yap EY, Fam HB, Leong KP, Buettner H. Nocardiachoroidal abscess in a patient with systemic lupus erythematosus. Aust N Z J Ophthalmol 1998;26:337–8.

6.1.5 UVEITIS IN CAT-SCRATCH DISEASE

- Etiology
- Clinical features
- Diagnosis
- Treatment

ETIOLOGY

Cat-scratch disease (CSD) is a systemic bacterial infection caused by *Bartonella henselae*.

Primary reservoirs of Bartonella henselae are cats and the disease is transmitted to human by scratches, licks, and bites of domestic cats, particularly kitten and hence the name 'cat-scratch disease'.

Vector for transmission of organisms from cat to cat is *Cat flea*.

CLINICAL FEATURES

Systemic manifestations of CSD include:
- *Flue-like illness* of mild to moderate severity.

- *Cutaneous lesions* at the site of cat-scratch may occur in the form of an erythematous papule, vesicle or pustule.
- *Lymphadenopathy* of draining lymph nodes is from primary site of lesion may occur.
- *Disseminated disease*, though rare, may occur as encephalopathy, aseptic meningitis, hepatosplenic disease, pneumonia and pleural or pericardial effusion.

Ocular involvement in 5–10% cases may occur as:

Parinaud oculoglandular syndrome, i.e. unilateral granulomatous conjunctivitis with regional lymphadenitis.

Posterior segment involvement occurs as:
- *Neuroretinitis* which earlier has been labelled as: Leber's idiopathic stellate neuroretinitis; is characterised by optic disc oedema and macular star formation.
- *Recurrent idiopathic neuroretinitis*
- Discrete, focal or multifocal retinal and/or choroidal lesions.
- Arterial and venous occlusions are also reported.
- Other posterior segment complications include epiretinal membrane. Peripapillary angiomatosis, white-dot-syndrome, intermediate uveitis.

Anterior chamber inflammation and vitritis of some degree is usually associated with posterior segment lesions. Some patients may have penuveitis.

DIAGNOSIS

Diagnosis of CSD suspected from the characteristic clinical features is substantiated by following tests:
- *Indirect fluorescent antibody (IFB) assay* for the detection of serum *anti-B. henselae* antibodies
- *Enzyme immunoassay (EIA)* with an IgG together with Western blot analysis.
- *PCR-based tests* that target the *B. henselae* DNA or bacterial 165 rRNA gene.
- *Skin testing* can also be done.
- *Bacterial cultures* can be made from the cutaneous lesions.

TREATMENT

- *Systemic antibiotics.* Oral doxycycline 100 mg BD, for 2–4 weeks, or other antibiotics, such as erythromycin, rifampin, ciprofloxacin and gentamicin, are effective.
- *Oral corticosteroids* along with antibiotics may hasten the recovery of ocular posterior segment lesions.
- *Immunomodulatory treatment*, for a long-term is recommended for the subset of patients with recurrent idiopathic neuroretinitis.

BIBLIOGRAPHY

1. Cunningham ET, Koehler JE. Ocular bartonellosis. Am J Ophthalmol 2000;130(3):340–9.
2. Curi AL, Machado D, Heringer G, et al. Cat-scratch disease: ocular manifestations and visual outcome. Int Ophthalmol 2010;30(5):553–8.
3. Khurana RN, Albini T, Green RL, Rao NA, Lim JI. Bartonellahenselae infection presenting as a unilateral panuveitis simulating Vogt-Koyanagi-Harada syndrome. Am J Ophthalmol 2004; 138(6):1063–5.
4. Ormerod LD, Dailey JP. Ocular manifestations of cat-scratch disease. Curr Opin Ophthalmol 1999;10(3):209–16.
5. Ormerod LD, Skolnick KA, Menosky MM, Pavan PR, Pon DM. Retinal and choroidal manifestations of cat-scratch disease. Ophthalmology 1998;105(6):1024–31.
6. Roe RH, Michael Jumper J, Fu AD, Johnson RN, Richard McDonald H, Cunningham ET. Ocular bartonella infections. Int Ophthalmol Clin. 2008;48(3):93–105.

6.1.6 UVEITIS IN WHIPPLE'S DISEASE

- Etiology
- Clinical features
- Diagnosis and differential diagnosis
- Treatment

ETIOLOGY

Whipple's disease is a chronic multisystem disease caused by a small gram-positive bacillus, *Tropheryma whipplei*. The bacillus is an actinobacterium, has low virulence but high infectivity. Disease occurs more commonly in aged Caucasian men.

CLINICAL FEATURES

1. *Gastrointestinal features* are the primary manifestation of disease and include:
- Diarrhoea
- Steatorrhoea
- Malabsorption
- Abdominal pain associated with
- Weight loss.
2. *Migrating arthritis* usually involving large joints.
3. *CNS symptoms* may occur is 10% cases and include seizures, dementia and coma.
4. *Neuro-ophthalmic features* include cranial nerve palsies, Nystagmus ophthalmoplegia.
5. *Intraocular involvement* is seen is 5% cases in the form of:
- *Panuveitis*, characterised by anterior uveitis, moderate vitreous and diffuse chorioretinal inflammation.
- *Retinal vasculitis* may occur in the perifoveal and midperipheral region; and retinal vascular occlusions, retinal haemorrhages and cotton wool spots.
- *Optic disc oedema* and later, optic atrophy may also occur.

DIAGNOSIS AND DIFFERENTIAL DIAGNOSIS

Differential diagnosis of uveitis with retinal vasculitis and multisystem involvement include:
- SLE disease
- PAN, and
- Behcet's disease.

Diagnosis of Whipple's disease is made from:
- *Clinical features* of multiple system involvement
- *PCR analysis* of blood, aqueous humour and vitreous may show *T. whipplei* DNA.
- *Duodenal biopsy*, that show PAS positive bacillus in macrophages in the intestinal villi, is the gold standard for diagnosis in suspected patients.

TREATMENT

Systemic antibiotic of choice is double-strength trimethoprim sulfamethoxazole for a long period (approximately one year). In patients allergic to sulfamethoxazole other antibiotics, such as ceftriaxone, tetracycline or chloramphenicol, may be given. Retinal vasculitis, usually respond to systemic antibiotics but neurological deficit may become permanent.

BIBLIOGRAPHY

1. Avila MP, Jalkh AE, Feldman E, Trempe CL, Schepens CL. Manifestations of Whipple's disease in the posterior segment of the eye. Arch Ophthalmol 1984;102:384–90.
2. Leland TM, Chambers JK. Ocular findings in Whipple's disease. South Med J 1978;71:335–7.
3. Rickman LS, Freeman WR, Relman DA, et al. Uveitis caused by Tropherymawhippelii. N Engl J Med 1995;332:363–6.
4. Wechsler B, Fior R, Reux I, et al. Uveitis: late complication of undiagnosed Whipple disease. Rev Med Interne 1995;16:687–90.

6.1.7 RICKETTSIAL DISEASES AND THE EYE

General Considerations
Systemic Features of Rickettsioses
• Pathogenesis
Ocular Manifestations
• Clinical features
• Symptoms
• Anterior segment lesion
• Posterior segment lesion
• Neuro-ophthalmic manifestations
Diagnosis and differential diagnosis
• Diagnosis
• Differential diagnosis
Treatment

GENERAL CONSIDERATIONS

Rickettsioses are zoonoses due to obligate intracellular gram-negative bacteria. Most of them are transmitted to humans by the bite of infected ticks. Ricketsial agents are classified into three major categories: the spotted fever group, the scrub typhus, and the typhus group.

Systemic Features of Rickettsioses

The presence of high fever, headache, general malaise and skin rash in a patient living in or travelling back from a region endemic for rickettsioses. A local skin lesion, called "tache noire" (black spot) may develop at the site of arthropod bite.

Pathogenesis

Invasion of the vascular endothelial cells by the organism causes endothelial injury and tissue necrosis, and stimulation of coagulation process with subsequent development of occlusive vasculitis.

OCULAR MANIFESTATIONS
Clinical features

Symptoms. Most often asymptomatic or present with complaints, such as:
• Decreased vision
• Redness
• Scotoma and
• Floaters.

Anterior segment lesions include:
• *Conjunctivitis* (can be unilateral or bilateral)
• *Conjunctival petechiae* and subconjunctival haemorrahges
• *Non-granulomatous anterior uveitis*

Psterior segment lesions include (Fig. 6.1.7.1):
• *Vitritis with retinitis* (white retinal lesions)
• *Retinitis and retinal vascular changes* are the most common and typical manifestations of rickettsial infecfion.
• *Macular star, cystoid macular oedema* and *serous retinal detachment*
• *Subclinical retinal and choroidal vascular involvement* visible on FFA or ICG

Neuro-ophthalmic manifestations, such as optic disc oedema, optic disc staining, optic neuritis, neuroretinitis, and ischaemic optic neuropathy, third and six cranial nerve palsies can occur following rickettsial infections.

DIAGNOSIS AND DIFFERENTIAL DIAGNOSIS

Diagnosis is confirmed by:
• Weil-Felix test
• Immunofluorescence assay (IFA)

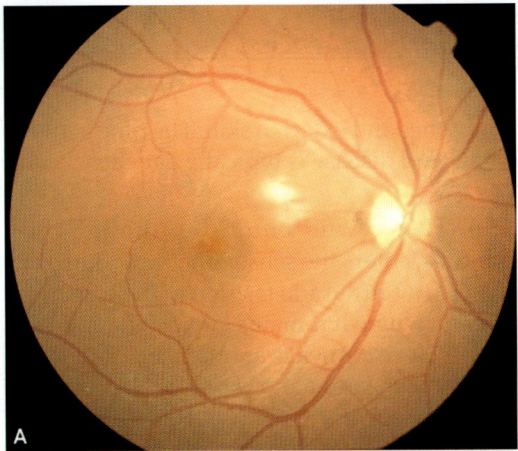

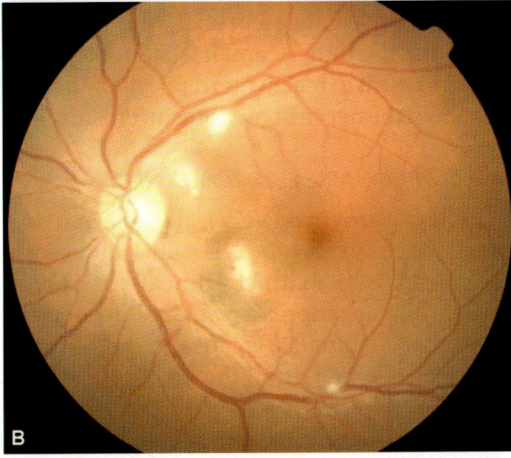

Fig. 6.1.7.1 *Fundus photograph of a patient with rickettsial retinitis and macular oedema in both eyes.*

- Polymerase chain reaction (PCR), and
- Rapid immunochromatographic test (RICT) for rickettsia.

Differential diagnosis includes
- Toxoplasmosis,
- Cat-scratch disease, and
- Chikungunya retinitis

TREATMENT

Antibiotic therapy is a below:
- *Doxycycline* is the drug of choice in the treatment of rickettsioses.
- *Fluoroquinolones*, because of their good ocular penetration, might be a better therapeutic option for the treatment of intraocular involvement.

Corticosteroid therapy may be required in addition to antibiotic treatment

BIBLIOGRAPHY

1. Alio J, Ruiz-Beltran R, Herrero-Herrero JI, Hernandez E. Retinal manifestations of Mediterranean spotted fever. Ophthalmologica 1987;195:31–7.
2. Fontaine M, Saraux H, Ganen J. Rickettsioses et uvéites. Bull Mém Soc Fr Ophthalmol 1960;73:491–9.
3. Helmick CG, Bernard KW, D'Angelo LJ. Rocky Mountain spotted fever: clinical, laboratory, and epidemiological features of 262 cases. J Infect Dis 1984;150:480–8.
4. Khairallah M, Ladjimi A, Chakroun M, Messaoud R, Ben Yahia S, Zaouali S, Ben Romdhane F, Bouzouaia N. Posterior segment manifestations of Rickettsia conorii infection. Ophthalmology 2004;111(3):529–34.
5. Khairallah M, Zaouali S, Ben Yahia S, Ladjimi A, Messaoud R, Jenzeri S, Attia S. Anterior ischemic opticneuropathy associated with Rickettsia conorii infection. J Neuro-ophthalmol 2005;25:212–4.
5. Lebas M, Bernaerts-Lebas M. Rickettsioses et affections oculaires. Bull Soc Belge Ophthalmol 1963;135:437–41.
6. Pinna A, Sechi LA, Serru A, et al. Endogenous panuveitis in a patient with Rickettsia conorii infection. Acta Ophthalmol Scand 2000;78:608–9.

6.2 VIRAL UVEITIS

6.2.1 HERPETIC UVEITIS

• Herpes viruses
• Herpes zoster ophthalmicus
• Herpetic anterior uveitis
• Viral scleritis
• Necrotizing herpetic retinopathy

HERPES VIRUSES

Herpetic eye disease is among the most common causes for infectious uveitis. It may affect healthy as well as immunocompromised hosts, although its clinical presentation varies accordingly.

VIROLOGY OF HERPES SIMPLEX VIRUS

The herpes simplex virus (HSV) is a ubiquitous, large double-stranded DNA virus that has an icosahedral capsid. Human herpes viruses can remain dormant in cells and can periodically reactivate. As these viruses have an affinity for the sensory ganglion cells, they are called neurotrophic viruses. Based on virus-specific antigens, HSV can be differentiated into two types: type 1 (HSV-1) and type 2 (HSV-2). HSV-1 infections are found more commonly in the orolabial area and HSV-2 in the genital area. Ocular disease is usually caused by HSV-1 rather than HSV-2, one exception is neonatal herpetic keratitis, 75% of which is caused by HSV-2.

Herpes simplex virus 1 (HSV-1) causes oral, facial, and ocular lesions.

Herpes simplex virus 2 (HSV-2) causes mainly genital lesions in adults, very rarely ocular diseases in adults, neonatal herpes simplex keratitis.

Humans are the only natural host or reservoir of HSV. So only source of infection is human being infected with HSV. Close personal contact is thought to be necessary for the spread of HSV. Major portals of entry are the mucous membranes and external skin. The time between contact and disease is typically between 3 and 9 days.

The HSV virus enters epithelial cells, replicates, enters the sensory nerve endings and travels in a retrograde fashion to the trigeminal ganglion where it remains latent and replicates. Many believe cornea is another such site where HSV remains latent and replicates. After initial replication in the trigeminal ganglion, HSV usually travels back down the nerve in an ante grade fashion to cause a primary infection in 1–6% of patients. It then remains latent till certain triggers cause it to reactivate, replicate, and travel back down the nerve to cause recurrent infection.

VIROLOGY OF VARICELLA-ZOSTER VIRUS

Varicella-zoster virus (VZV), also referred to as human herpes virus type 3, is a ubiquitous virus that causes two distinct clinical conditions, varicella or chickenpox, a primary infection and herpes zoster (shingles) is caused by reactivation of the latent VZV within the sensory ganglia. The term "Herpes zoster" derives from the Greek words *herpein*, meaning "to spread" or "to creep" and *zoster*, meaning "girdle" or "zone."

Varicella-zoster is a DNA virus belonging to the herpes virus family and it is the smallest (150 to 200 nm in diameter) of the viral genomes within the herpes virus family. Its viral structure includes a core of double-stranded DNA surrounded by an icosahedral nucleocapsid, with an outer cell membrane.

Human beings are the only known natural host of VZV. VZV is a heat-labile virus, which spreads from cell to cell by direct contact. After primary infection, VZV is transported to the various dorsal roots or trigeminal ganglia and neural cell bodies where it enters a state of latency in either the ganglion satellite cells or within the neurons. Any sensory ganglion may be involved with herpes zoster. In the order of frequency, the dermatomes most commonly affected are thoracic, cranial, cervical, lumbar, and sacral. The mechanism of reactivation is not known. However, it has been established that impairment of the host's cellular immunity plays an important role in reactivation of HZV.

Once reactivated, the virus replicates within cells of the dorsal root ganglion and the resultant virions via axonal transport travel to the skin or mucous membrane. Virion transport produces associated abnormal skin sensations, pain, and tenderness followed by the characteristic unilateral dermatomal eruption of herpes zoster.

HERPES ZOSTER OPHTHALMICUS

Primary infection by VZV presents as varicella or chickenpox, a contagious and usually benign childhood illness occurring in annual spring epidemics.

- *Incubation period* of classical varicella or chickenpox is about 2 weeks.
- *Prodromal symptoms,* like fever, malaise anorexia, headache, sore throat, etc.
- *Skin lesions* can be described as maculopapulovesicular rash, which appears one after another, so lesions in various stages are present simultaneously.
- *Infectious period* is ~1 week after the appearance of each crop of lesions or until they crust and shed.

Herpes zoster ophthalmicus (HZO) can be defined as HZV involvement of the ophthalmic division of the fifth cranial nerve. The ophthalmic division of the fifth cranial nerve further divides into the nasociliary, frontal, and lacrimal branches, of which the frontal nerve is most commonly involved with HZO and lacrimal branch is least commonly involved in HZO. The nasociliary nerve innervates the anterior and posterior ethmoidal sinuses, skin of both eyelids and the tip of the nose, conjunctiva, sclera, cornea, iris, and choroid. Hutchinson was the first to describe the signs and symptoms of herpes zoster ophthalmicus in 1865. The classical Hutchinson's sign is defined as skin lesions at the tip, side, or root of the nose is strong predictor of ocular inflammation and corneal denervation in HZO.

CLINICAL FEATURES

The classical herpes zoster infection starts with prodromal symptoms, like fever, malaise, etc.

- *Lid oedema* is usually the first sign of HZO which can present with pruritus, hypoesthesia, or pain.
- *Skin lesions* start with maculopapular rash and progress to a vesicular skin eruption. New skin lesions continue to appear for 3 to 5 days. VZV infection involves deep dermis in contrast to herpes simplex, which is limited to the epidermis. In most patients, the vesicles heal within 2 to 3 weeks, leaving some scar.

Clinical spectrum of HZO is summarised in Table 6.2.1.

Table 6.2.1 *Clinical spectrum of herpes zoster ophthalmicus*	
Structures involved	*Clinical manifestations*
Skin, eyelid	Trichiasis, ectropion, entropion, madarosis, or poliosis, contraction scars, entropion, cicatricial ectropion, trichiasis, permanent loss of lashes, epicanthoid lesions, and paralytic ptosis
Conjunctiva	Follicular conjunctivitis, petechial haemorrhages, pseudomembranes
Lacrimal system	Epiphora as a result of scarring and obstruction of nasolacrimal duct.
Sclera	Diffuse or nodular scleritis
Cornea	Punctate epithelial keratitis, pseudodendritic keratitis, disciform keratitis, neurotrophic corneal ulcers
Uvea	Anterior uveitis, haemorrhagic iritis, secondary glaucoma
Optic nerve	Argyll Robertson pupil, Ischemic optic neuritis
Retina	Vasculitis, occlusion of the central retinal vein with haemorrhage, central retinal artery occlusion, and ischaemic retinitis, acute retinal necrosis syndrome
Cranial nerves	The third, fourth, and sixth cranial nerves may be involved separately or simultaneously.

TREATMENT

Supportive treatment. Treatment of varicella is primarily supportive and includes maintenance of adequate hydration with fluid intake; nonaspirin antipyretics, cool baths, and careful hygiene and antiseptic dressings to the skin lesions to prevent secondary bacterial infection from pruritic skin lesions.

Intravenous acyclovir is sometimes required to treat varicella in immunocompromised individuals. Acyclovir, valacyclovir, and famciclovir are currently FDA-approved for treatment of herpes zoster in the United States. These agents are guanosine analogs and interfere with viral thymidine kinase and DNA polymerase, leading to viral DNA chain termination. Intravenous acyclovir is the treatment of choice for severely immunocompromised individuals, like post-organ transplantation, patients with acquired immune deficiency syndrome, leucopenia, and patients with disseminated zoster.

Zoster immune globulin is often recommended for the susceptible individuals at risk for severe infection, like premature infants, neonates, the immunocompromised, and adults.

HERPETIC ANTERIOR UVEITIS

Iridocyclitis is the most common presentation of herpetic uveitis. In herpetic eye disease, iritis may accompany inflammation of other surrounding structures (keratitis, endotheliitis, or trabeculitis). Also, patients with HSV keratitis may develop a concomitant or subsequent iridocyclitis.

Approximately 40% of patients with herpes zoster ophthalmicus may develop iritis and most of them usually presents within the first week of acute disease, but VZV associated anterior uveitis can occur months after acute herpes zoster. As mentioned before, cutaneous involvement at the side of the tip of the nose indicate nasociliary nerve involvement (Hutchinson's sign) with increased risk of eye involvement. The diagnosis of VZV associated anterior uveitis can be very difficult in absence of previous skin eruption or zoster dermatitis ("*zoster sine herpete*").

CLINICAL PRESENTATION OF HSV AND VZV ASSOCIATED ANTERIOR UVEITIS

- *Patients present with signs and symptoms typical of iridocyclitis* including photophobia, pain, and ciliary flush.
- *Unilateral iridocyclitis with recurrences* is very common presentation.
- *Corneal ghost scarring* indicative of a previous infectious epithelial keratitis associated with iritis should arouse suspecsion of HSV iritis.
- *Herpetic anterior uveitis may be granulomatous*, but more commonly is *non-granulomatous* characterised by fine keratic precipitates.
- *Anterior chamber cellular reaction* that can range from mild to severe is seen on slit-lamp examination. Posterior synechiae may develop. Haemorrhages or hyphema, though rare, can occur.
- *Focal areas of iris atrophy* may be seen in HSV uveitis and may be seen into transilluminating areas of iris on retroillumination. Iris atrophy results from ischaemic necrosis of the iris stroma.
- *Ischaemic occlusive vasculitis* of iris with ciliary body inflammation and segmental iris distortion and sectoral iris atrophy may be associated with zoster iritis.
- *HSV associated endotheliitis* can present as one of the three morphological forms: disciform, diffuse and linear. The affected endothelium may take many months to recover. It may be very difficult to distinguish between viral stromal inflammation and stromal oedema secondary to an endotheliitis.
- *Endothelial decompensation* can be seen in cases with chronic infection leading to persistent corneal oedema.
- *Trabeculitis* may occur, which usually results in acute severe elevation of intraocular pressure.
- *Inflammatory secondary glaucoma* accompanying viral uveitis can also be due to the following mechanisms:
  - Trabecular meshwork blockage by cellular debris, iris pigment, or blood
  - Peripheral anterior synechiae
  - Pupillary block glaucoma from posterior synechiae; or

– Structural changes through the trabecular meshwork.

- *Posterior subcapsular cataract* formation develops from prolonged chronic uveitis or chronic steroid administration for uveitis treatment.

TREATMENT

Topical corticosteroids and cycloplegics are the mainstay of treatment of viral anterior uveitis. Proper control of anterior chamber inflammation with topical corticosteroids and cycloplegic agents, to prevent formation of synechiae, is essential part of the therapy. Patients with herpetic anterior uveitis may require prolonged corticosteroid therapy with very gradual tapering.

- *Oral corticosteroids* may be necessary at times.
- *Topical antiviral therapy* is usually ineffective, but oral antivirals are often beneficial. Topical antivirals are used in cases with significant corneal involvement, like keratouveitis or endotheliitis.
- *Systemic antivirals* form a crucial part in management of herpetic uveitis. The oral antiviral dosages are acyclovir 400 mg five times daily or valacyclovir 500 mg two times daily for patients with HSV and acyclovir 800 mg five times daily or valacyclovir 1000 mg three times daily for VZV disease. Oral antiviral therapy has been shown to diminish the number of recurrences and reduce the incidence and severity of the inflammation in patients with herpetic anterior uveitis when given on a long-term basis.
- *Topical and oral antiglaucoma medications* are often necessary to control the ocular hypertension, especially during the first days of treatment.

VIRAL SCLERITIS

Viral involvement of scleral and episcleral tissues is very rare and most commonly associated with herpes group of viruses.

Herpes zoster ophthalmicus can cause an episcleritis, anterior scleritis, or rarely posterior scleritis. Both episclera and sclera can become affected during the acute stages of HZO or later.

Scleritis can be diffuse anterior or nodular in nature and has a tendency to progress toward the perilimbal area which can lead to peripheral limbal vasculitis and peripheral ulcerative keratitis.

Scleral thinning and staphyloma formation can occur in cases of long-standing scleritis.

Herpes simplex-related scleritis is relatively rare. Scleritis in such cases is usually accompanied by keratitis and uveitis. Ischaemia with occlusion of conjunctival and scleral vessels is typical.

NECROTIZING HERPETIC RETINOPATHY

Necrotizing herpetic retinopathy is a clinical spectrum of posterior uveitis and retinitis and is subdivided into acute retinal necrosis (ARN) and progressive outer retinal necrosis (PORN).

ACUTE RETINAL NECROSIS

Age and sex. Acute retinal necrosis generally affects healthy, immunocompetent individuals regard less of sex or race. The disease affects typically young adults. A *bimodal age* distribution has been described by various authors with peaks at 20 and 50 years of age. However, ARN has been reported in children also.

Laterality. Acute retinal necrosis generally begins with unilateral disease. Second eye becomes involved in one-third cases usually within 1 to 6 weeks. The longest interval reported between the involvements of two eyes is 34 years.

Etiology

Acute retinal necrosis is caused by multiple members of the herpes virus family.

- *Varicella-zoster virus* (VZV) accounts for the majority of cases.
- *Other viruses* include herpes simplex type 1 (HSV-1) and type 2 (HSV-2), and rarely cytomegalovirus (CMV) and Epstein-Barr virus (EPV).
- *It has been reported* that varicella-zoster virus or herpes simplex virus type 1 causes acute retinal necrosis syndrome in patients older than 25 years, whereas herpes simplex virus

type 2 causes acute retinal necrosis in patients younger than 25 years.

Clinical picture

Symptoms. Early symptoms are usually very minimal and patients may complain of irritation, redness, photophobia and floaters. Some patients complain of mild-to-moderate ocular pain, which may be worse with eye movements.

Anterior segment examination reveals mild to moderate anterior uveitis. In some patients, there may be increased intraocular pressure due to secondary glaucoma.

Posterior segment involvement occurs within 1 to 2 days. *Characteristic triad* of lesions encountered in acute retinal necrosis consists of moderate to severe vitritis, confluent necrotizing retinitis and vasculitis.

- *Ophthalmoscopically, the retinal necrosis appears* as well-demarcated, multifocal patches of yellowish-white infiltrates in the periphery at the level of deep retina and retinal pigment epithelium.
- *Lesions usually start in midperiphery* and do not follow the architecture of retinal vessels.
- *Border between the necrosis and normal retina appears* well defined, smooth, and geographic; and retinal haemorrhages, although present, are not a prominent feature.
- *Active vasculitis* is characterised by vascular sheathing and perivascular small intraretinal haemorrhages. Characteristically arteries are more affected than veins.
- *Over the few weeks, retinal necrosis becomes confluent* and progresses rapidly and circumferentially toward the posterior pole.
- *Macular involvement.* It should be kept in mind that although the involvement of macula is not a characteristic feature of acute retinal necrosis, its involvement does not preclude the diagnosis.
- *As the retinal necrosis and sloughing progresses,* resultant debris accumulation and inflammation of vitreous ensues often giving rise to a dense vitreous haze.

Course of the disease. With treatment, resolution of acute retinal necrosis begins approximately

in 3 weeks. In untreated patients, inflammation starts resolving 6 to 12 weeks after the onset of symptoms. Retinal thinning and atrophy starts at the peripheral margins and gradually moves centrally. Meanwhile, retinal pigment epithelium perturbation develops with areas of clearing they form a characteristics "Swiss-cheese appearance". Vitreous organization and traction continue to develop during this phase. The thin atrophic retina often contributes to the development of retinal holes or tears, which typically appear at the junction of normal and affected retina. Retinal holes, combined with vitreous traction, lead to retinal detachment in up to 75% of cases. Thus retinal detachments in acute retinal necrosis patients have both a rhegmatogenous and tractional component.

Stages of acute retinal necrosis are:
- *Stage 1:* Necrotizing retinitis
  A: Discrete areas of peripheral retinitis
  B: Confluent areas of peripheral retinitis, papillitis, macular oedema
- *Stage 2:* Vitreous opacification/organisation
- *Stage 3:* Regression of retinal necrosis and secondary pigmentation of the lesions with contraction and condensation of the vitreous base.
- *Stage 4:* Retinal detachment
  A: Acute retinal tears or detachment with traction, or proliferative vitreoretinopathy
  B: Chronic retinal detachment

Diagnosis

Diagnosis of acute retinal necrosis is usually based on the clinical appearance and course. However, patients with atypical presentation should be investigated as a delay in initiation of treatment may significantly affect the visual prognosis. Conventional methods of viral isolation, like viral culture, are cumbersome and time consuming. The best option for investigating such challenging cases with diagnostic dilemma is polymerase chain reaction. PCR has been proved more than 90% sensitive for detection of VZV, HSV and CMV. With the advent of newer technique, like real-time PCR, which helps quantitative estimation of the pathogen, aqueous or vitreous specimen can be analysed in conditions where the cause of a severe uveitis may not be obvious.

Diagnostic criteria for acute retinal necrosis by American Uveitis Society

In 1994, the Executive Committee of the American Uveitis Society published some diagnostic criteria for acute retinal necrosis. These includes:

- One or more discrete foci of retinal necrosis in the periphery
- Rapid disease progression in the absence of therapy
- Circumferential spread of the lesions
- Occlusive arteriolar vasculopathy, and
- A prominent vitreous or anterior chamber inflammatory reaction.

Other characteristics that support, but are not required for, the diagnosis of acute retinal necrosis include optic neuropathy, scleritis and pain.

Treatment

A. Medical therapy

1. *Antiviral agents.* The aim of medical therapy in acute retinal necrosis is rapid recovery of the disease and prevention of fellow eye involvement. As majority of cases of ARN are due to either HSV or VZV infections, intravenous acyclovir is the current medical treatment of choice for acute retinal necrosis.

Acyclovir is a guanine analogue with activity against VZV, HSV-1, HSV-2, and Epstein-Barr virus, although most strains of CMV are resistant to it. Recommended therapeutic regimen consists of induction with 15 mg/kg/d intravenous acyclovir in 3 divided doses for 7 to 10 days and oral antiviral medication is then with either acyclovir (800 mg 5 times a day), valacyclovir (1 g 3 times a day), or famciclovir (500 mg 3 times a day) is continued up to six weeks or more.

Effects of acyclovir therapy in acute retinal necrosis cases are:

- Regression of the retinal necrosis is usually seen within four days.
- Forty-eight hours after treatment initiation, progression of new and existing lesions usually occurs.

- Complete regression occurs on average 32.5 days after treatment.
- Reduce the short-term incidence of bilateral involvement, but do not prevent it.
- The risk of fellow eye involvement reduces from 65 (in cases of untreated cases) to 25% at 2 years follow-up.

Often few patients, mainly the immunosuppressed patients do not respond to treatment with acyclovir. It should be kept in mind that as discussed earlier in differential diagnosis section of this article, CMV retinitis mimicking the acute retinal necrosis may not respond to treatment with acyclovir. In such cases or in cases with acyclovir stains of HSV and VZV, ganciclovir or valacyclovir can be used. Though ganciclovir is highly effective against HSV and VZV, but for its greater risks of systemic toxicity, it should be used cautiously. Valacyclovir, the L-valyl ester of acyclovir, is a prodrug which is rapidly and nearly completely converted to acyclovir after oral administration. It has an excellent bioavailability which yields serum acyclovir levels comparable to intravenous acyclovir and requiring less frequent dosing than oral acyclovir. So, the drug has the same antiviral indications with the advantage of simpler dosing and it is as safe as oral acyclovir. Huynh et al reported that the oral administration of valacyclovir quickly leads to substantial vitreous acyclovir concentrations demonstrating the successful use of valacyclovir in the primary treatment of acute retinal necrosis. However, it is not recommended in immunocompromised or HIV-seropositive patients.

2. *Corticosteroids.* Corticosteroid has been used to inflammatory component of acute retinal necrosis because vitritis and vitreous organisation progress in spite of effective antiviral treatment. Corticosteroid helps in reducing intraocular inflammation and clearing vitreous haze in acute retinal necrosis, however, they do not have any beneficial effect in reducing severity of the clinical entity and its lesions. It should be kept in mind that corticosteroid therapy in acute retinal necrosis should be started only after initiation of antiviral therapy as it can promote viral replication. Recommended dosage is 1 to 2 mg/kg for 1 week and

224 | **Disorders of Uvea and Sclera**

the drug is tapered over 2 to 6 weeks. Topical corticosteroid can be used to treat anterior segment inflammation, if present.

3. *Antithrombotic therapy.* Some authors suggest the antithrombotic therapy to combat vascular obstructive complications of the acute retinal necrosis. However, till now, there is no clinical trial that has proven efficacy of anti-thrombotic agents in acute retinal necrosis.

B. Laser photocoagulation

The major devastating sequela of acute retinal necrosis is retinal detachment which occurs in up to 75% of patients. Prophylactic confluent laser photocoagulation posterior to the areas of active retinitis likely to create a "new artificial ora serrata" posterior to the affected zones in which retinal holes are likely to develop. A reduction in occurrence of retinal detachment to 17% in patients with laser photocoagulation compared with 67 % in non-laser treated patients has been reported by Sternberg and its associates.

C. Surgical management of retinal detachment

Surgical management of retinal detachment in acute retinal necrosis patients is often frustrating. The reasons for difficulty in repairing retinal detachment in acute retinal necrosis patients have been described by Blumenkranz et al, who explained three reasons:

- Multiplicity and posterior location of retinal breaks, for which selection of an appropriate scleral buckle becomes very difficult,
- Presence of vitreous traction and proliferative vitreoretinopathy, and
- Higher rate of postoperative complications due to the inflammatory nature of the disease.

However, with the help of techniques, like pars plana vitrectomy, air–fluid exchange, endolaser, and gas or silicone oil tamponade, varying reports of success rate, even up to 100%, have been published.

PROGRESSIVE OUTER RETINAL NECROSIS (PORN)

PORN is a variant of a necrotizing herpetic retinopathy, usually seen in immunocompro-mised patients. This clinical entity was first described by Forster and colleagues in 1990 in two human immunodeficiency virus (HIV) patients.

Etiology

Varicella-zoster virus and herpes simplex virus have been implicated in the cause of PORN.

Clinical picture

- *Mild non-granulomatous anterior uveitis* is seen.
- *Early disease* is characterised by multifocal deep retinal opacification.
- *Fulminant, rapidly progressive necrotising retino-pathy* which starts at the posterior pole and spreads toward the peripheral retina is typical of PORN. These lesions coalesce quickly and progress to total full-thickness retinal necrosis leading to early retinal detachment in majority of patients.
- *Occlusive vasculitis and vitritis* are uncommon unlike ARN.

Therapy

Treatment of PORN is very frustrating and visual prognosis is very poor because of the resistance to antiviral and occurrence of retinal detachment.

High-dose intravenous acyclovir has been used with inconsistent success.

BIBLIOGRAPHY

1. Cunningham Jr. ET Diagnosing and treating herpetic anterior uveitis. Ophthalmology 2000; 107:2129–30.
2. Falcon MG, Williams HP. Herpes simplex kerato-uveitis and glaucoma. Trans Opthalmol Soc UK 1978;98:101–4.
3. Gaynor BD, Margolis TP, Cunningham Jr. ET Advances in diagnosis and management of herpetic uveitis. Int Ophthalmol Clin 2000; 40(2): 85–109.
4. Goldstein DA, Mis AA, Deschenes JG. Iris atrophy in herpes simplex uveitis. Invest Ophthalmol Vis Sci 1995;36:S150.
5. Harding SP, Lipton JR, Wells JC. Natural history of herpes zoster ophthalmicus: predictors of postherpetic neuralgia and ocular involvement. Br J Ophthalmol 1987;71:353–8.
6. Kimura SJ. Herpes simplex uveitis: a clinical and experimental study. Trans Am Ophthalmol Soc 1062;60:441–70.

7. Schacher S, Garweg JG, et al. Diagnosis of herpetic uveitis and keratouveitis. Klin Monatsbl Augenheilkd 1998;212:359–62.
8. Tabbara KF, Chavis PS. Herpes simplex anterior uveitis. Int Ophthalmol Clin 1998;38 (4):137–47.
9. Wilhelmus KR, Falcon MG, Jones BR. Herpetic iridocyclitis. Int Ophthalmol 1981;4:143–50.
10. Womak LW, Liesegang TJ. Complications of herpes zoster opthalmicus. Arch Ophthalmol 1983;101:42–5.

6.2.2 OCULAR INVOLVEMENT IN ACQUIRED IMMUNODEFICIENCY SYNDROME (AIDS)

General considerations
Ocular manifestations of HIV/AIDS
- Ocular adnexal and anterior segment lesions
- Posterior segment lesions
- Orbital lesions
- Neuro-ophthalmic lesions
- Immune recovery uveitis
Pre-HAART era and present scenario

GENERAL CONSIDERATIONS

In 1981, acquired immunodeficiency syndrome (AIDS) was originally described by the United States Centers for Disease Control and Prevention (CDC); when few cases of carinii pneumonia (PCP) and Kaposi's sarcoma occurred in homosexuals and IV drug abusers.[1] In 1983, human immunodeficiency virus (HIV), a retrovirus similar to human T-lymphotrophic virus (HTLVs) was described the cause for this HIV/AIDS spectrum.[2] Two types of HIV have been described: HIV-1 and HIV-2. HIV-1 accounts for the most number of cases, globally and it is much more infective and virulent than HIV-2. HIV-2 is mainly confined to western Africa.

ORIGIN

HIV is believed to have originated in non-human primates in west-central Africa and was transmitted to humans in the early 20th century. Chimpanzees and sooty mangabey have been believed to be the source of HIV 1 and HIV 2, respectively.

AIDS is the end stage of the clinical infection by HIV. Following infection, a person may experience a flu-like illness. This is followed by prolonged asymptomatic phase and as the disease progresses; a person may contract common infections, like tuberculosis and other opportunistic infections. This is followed by AIDS, the last stage characterised by AIDS defining illnesses, like *Pneumocystis carinii* pneumonia (PCP), oral candidiasis, CMV retinitis, Kaposi's sarcoma and many others.

GLOBAL SCENARIO OF HIV/AIDS

According to the World Health Organization (WHO), there were approximately 35 million people worldwide living with HIV/AIDS in 2013.[3] Of these, 3.2 million were children (<15 years old). An estimated 2.1 million individuals worldwide became newly infected with HIV in 2013; this includes over 240,000 children (<15 years).[3]

CONTRIBUTION OF HIV/AIDS TO GLOBAL BLINDNESS

It is difficult to assess the contribution of HIV/AIDS towards global blindness; as most studies have been done in developed nations while a huge population of the HIV/AIDS patients lives in developing and underdeveloped nations. Ocular complications affect 50–75% of HIV/AIDS patients in some point of their life. CMV retinitis is the most common cause of ocular blindness related to AIDS-related complications.[4] Other causes include HSV and HZV retinitis, HIV ischaemic microvasculopathy, ocular tuberculosis, ocular syphilis and cryptococcal infections. With the advent of HAART, life expectancy has increased in HIV/AIDS patients and hence the prevalence of blindness related to HIV/AIDS is expected to increase further.

OCULAR MANIFESTATIONS OF HIV/AIDS

Ocular manifestations in AIDS were first described by Dr Holland and his team, way back in 1982; before the causative agent could be identified as HIV in 1983.[5]

HIV can affect every tissue of the eye and can be the presenting feature of the disease too. The most common manifestations are dry eyes, retinal microvasculopathy and CMV retinitis.

CMV retinitis is the commonest ocular opportunistic infection in India, even in the HAART era.[6] In developing countries, like India, opportunistic infections in HIV/AIDS have significant variations as compared to developed countries. Newer manifestations of known opportunistic diseases and newer diseases are commonly seen especially in post-HAART era. Ocluar TB should be kept in mind especially in Indian scenario.[7-9]

The various manifestations of the disease are given in Table 6.2.2.1.

A. OCULAR ADNEXAL AND ANTERIOR SEGMENT LESIONS

Adnexal manifestations of HIV/AIDS include molluscum contagiosum, herpes zoster ophthalmicus, Kaposi's sarcoma, various other viral, bacterial and protozoal infections of the eyelid and adnexa, Stevens-Johnson syndrome and other microvascular abnormalities.[10]

KAPOSI'S SARCOMA

Kaposi's sarcoma (KS) is a tumour caused by human herpes virus type 8 (HHV8). It was originally described in 1872, by Dr Moritz Kaposi, a Hungarian dermatologist.[11]

Four clinical subtypes have been described:
- Classic KS
- African endemic KS
- KS in iatrogenically immunosuppressed patients, and
- AIDS-related KS. It is more widely known as an AIDS-defining illness.

Sites of lesions. It commonly causes skin lesions but can affect the oral cavity, gastrointestinal tract, respiratory tract and other viscera.
- *Cutaneous lesion* can be solitary, localised or disseminated and usually appear as a reddish, violaceous or bluish-black macules, papules, nodules or plaques (Fig. 6.2.2.1).

Treatment options include excision, cryosurgery, radiotherapy, chemotherapy or a combination therapy.

In about 40–50% AIDS-related KS, HAART treatment can cause regression of lesions.

Table 6.2.2.1 *Various ocular manifestations of HIV/AIDS*

A. *Ocular adnexal lesions*
  1. Molluscum contagiosum.
  2. Herpes zoster ophthalmicus.
  3. Kaposi's sarcoma.
  4. Herpes simplex virus cutaneous infection.
  5. Pyogenic infection of the eyelid and adnexa.
  6. Stevens-Johnson syndrome.

B. *Conjunctiva and sclera lesions*
  1. Dry eyes.
  2. Kaposi's sarcoma.
  3. Conjunctival microvasculopathy.
  4. Microsporidial conjunctivitis.
  5. Herpes virus conjunctivitis.
  6. Squamous cell carcinoma of the conjunctiva.
  7. Scleritis.

C. *Cornea lesions*
  1. Dry eyes and corneal complications.
  2. Infective keratitis (herpes simplex, varicella zoster, microsporidia).
  3. Herpes zoster ophthalmicus.
  4. Syphilitic keratitis.

D. *Anterior uveitis*
  1. Rifabutin induced.
  2. Cidofivir induced.
  3. Spillover from CMV retinitis and other lesion.

E. *Posterior segment lesions*
  1. HIV retinopathy
  2. CMV retinitis
  3. Acute retinal necrosis (ARN)
  4. Progressive outer retinal necrosis (PORN)
  5. Herpes zoster retinopathy
  6. Ocular tuberculosis
  7. Ocular syphilis
  8. Toxoplasma retinochoroiditis
  9. Pneumocystis choroidopathy
  10. *Mycobacterium avium intracellulare* infections
  11. Fungal endophthalmitis (Cryptococcus, Candida)
  12. Histoplasmosis
  13. Intraocular lymphoma

F. *Orbital lesions*
  1. Burkit's lymphoma
  2. Orbital cellulitis (esp. Aspergillus).

G. *Neuro-ophthalmic lesions*
  1. Optic neuropathy.
  2. Cranial nerve palsies.
  3. Lagophthalmos.

H. *Immune recovery uveitis* (IRU)

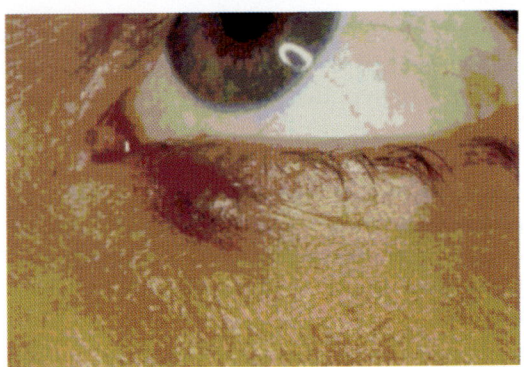

Fig. 6.2.2.1 *Kaposi's sarcoma in a patient with AIDS.*

- In general, KS responds to combination chemotherapy, like conventional adriamycin, bleomycin sulfate and vinblastine sulphate (ABV) combination therapy.
- Other agents include liposomal daunorubicin, doxorubicin, paclitaxel, etoposide, cisplatin, interferon alpha-n3 and alpha-2a.

MOLLUSCUM CONTAGIOSUM

Molluscum contagiosum (MC), also known as *water warts*, is a viral infection of the skin and mucous membrane caused by a double-stranded DNA pox virus by the name of molluscum contagiosum virus (MCV). It occurs in 5–18% of HIV-infected patients. Characteristic skin lesion is a single small elevation with central umbilication. However, in AIDS patients (Fig. 6.2.2.2),

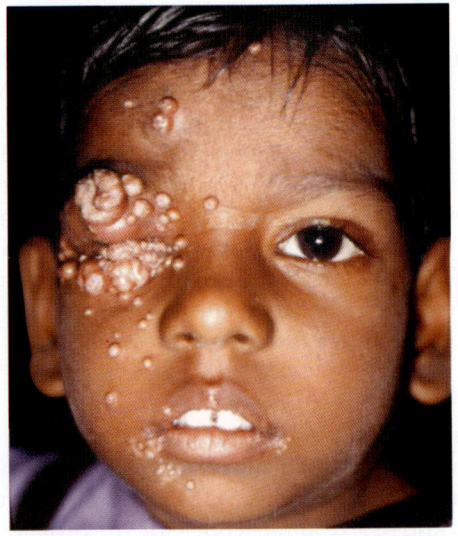

Fig. 6.2.2.2 *Molluscum contagiosum in an HIV infected patient.*

lesions are multiple, bilateral and involve trunk, axillae, antecubital and popliteal fossae, face, or genital/crural area apart from face and neck. In HIV infected patients, lesions are difficult to eradicate and recurs. However; HAART therapy causes early regression and may cause resolution of lesions. Apart from HAART therapy, other treatment options include local excision, medical management and laser therapy. Medical management includes 5% imiquimod, podophyllotoxin, cantharidin, retinoin, trichloroacetic acid, combination of salicylic acid and lactic acid and cidofovir cream.

HERPES ZOSTER OPHTHALMICUS

Herpes zoster ophthalmicus is caused by reactivation of chickenpox virus, also known as human herpes virus 3. Younger non-diabetic patients without any other medical or surgical history should raise a suspicion of HIV/AIDS.

Lesions. It causes vesicles and gradual crusting in a well-defined dermatomal region. It can lead to other eye lesions, like conjunctivitis, corneal ulcers and scarring, uveitis, glaucoma, retinitis, cytoid macular oedema, optic neuritis, nerve palsies, post-herpetic neuralgia and post-herpetic itch.

Treatment. It is usually treated with antivirals like acyclovir, valacyclovir and famciclovir.

- Conventional treatment includes 800 mg of oral acyclovir five times daily for a period of 7 to 10 days.
- Topical antibiotics, steroids and lubricants are added according to the coexisting conditions and complications.

CONJUNCTIVAL MICROVASCULOPATHY

These changes occur in 70–80% of HIV/AIDS patients. These changes are multifactorial, like direct injury by the HIV itself, immune complex deposition, blood viscosity changes and vessel wall changes. These changes include vascular contour changes, like narrowing, dilatation, comma-shaped vessels and aneurysms formation. Treatment is usually not needed.

DRY EYES

Dry eyes are usually seen as a long-term sequela of various other corneal and adnexal manifestations. It is seen in about 10–20% patients. Direct injury to the lacrimal glands by the HIV itself has also been postulated as a cause for it.

Treatment is as for other cases of dry eyes along with HAART.

INFECTIOUS KERATITIS AND SCLERITIS

Viral keratitis is the most common cause of infectious keratitis in HIV/AIDS patients. HSV and HZV viral keratitis in these patients tend to recur frequently and are at times resistant to treatment.

Bacterial and fungal keratitis is not as common as viral keratitis in HIV/AIDS patients. Candida, microsporidial and *Fusarium solani* keratitis should raise a suspicion of HIV/AIDS.

Granulomatous conjunctivitis of Cryptococcus, fungal or tubercular origin can also be seen.

Scleritis can also be seen in HIV/AIDS, but rarely. Syphilis can cause scleritis in these patients.

SQUAMOUS CELL CARCINOMA OF THE CONJUNCTIVA

Squamous cell carcinoma (SCC) of conjunctiva is usually seen in old male HIV/AIDS patients. But, its incidence has been increasing with many younger people affected; especially women. The incidence of HIV positivity in SCC of conjunctiva can be as high as 75% especially in African nations. Many causative theories, like HIV infection, HPV infection, sunlight exposure, and trauma, have been known. Many treatment modalities are present but the tumour is known for recurrences and the end stage result is poor.

ANTERIOR UVEITIS

Anterior uveitis is seen in HIV/AIDS patients in association with retinitis, retinochoroiditis or drug toxicity.

- CMV, HSV and VZV retinitis are usually associated with mild anterior segment reaction too.
- Severe anterior segment reaction should arouse a suspicion of toxoplasmosis, tuberculosis or syphilis.

Rifabutin-associated uveitis

This drug is used in treating *Mycobacterium avium complex* (MAC) infections. MAC infections are commonly seen in HIV/AIDS patients. It can present as anterior, intermediate or posterior uveitis.

Treatment includes discontinuing the drug along with topical steroids and cycloplegics.

Cidofovir-associated uveitis

Cidofovir is a DNA polymerase inhibitor used in the treatment of CMV infections. Anterior uveitis has been seen after intravitreal as well as intravenous administration of cidofovir. Anterior uveitis has also been reported after treatment with cidofovir for ocular as well non ocular CMV retinitis. It has been associated with immune recovery uveitis.

Treatment involves discontinuation of cidofovir, aggressive topical steroids and cycloplegics. Although, outcomes are good but complications, like posterior synechiae, cataract and hypotony, can occur.

B. POSTERIOR SEGMENT LESIONS

HIV RETINOPATHY

HIV retinopathy is a non-infectious involvement of the retina in HIV/AIDS patients characterised by retinal haemorrhages, cotton wool spots, microaneurysms, telangiectatic vessels and capillary non-perfusion areas (Fig. 6.2.2.3). It occurs in around 70% of HIV/AIDS patients. Cotton wool spots are the earliest and most consistent finding, seen in about 60–70% HIV/AIDS patients. Though it is not a vision-threatening condition but its presence can be considered as a disease progressing sign.

CMV RETINITIS

Human CMV is a double-stranded DNA virus belonging to the b subgroup of herpes viruses (human herpes virus 5). The CMV genome is 230 kbp in size and encodes for 162 proteins, 45 of which are essential for replication in human

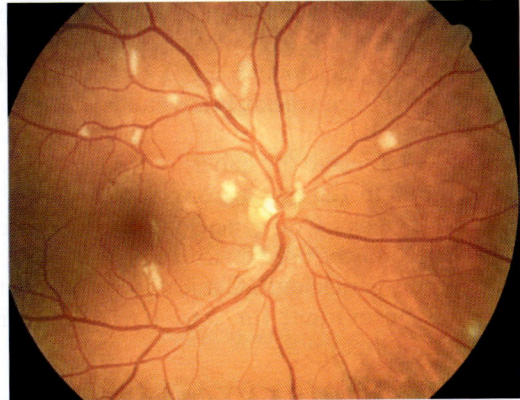

Fig. 6.2.2.3 *HIV retinopathy.*

fibroblasts. CMV is a ubiquitous human virus. CMV is transmitted through placental transfer, breastfeeding, saliva, sexual contact, blood transfusions, and organ or bone marrow transplants.

Pathogenesis of CMV infection

Pathogenesis of CMV retinitis is summarised in Fig. 6.2.2.4. Cytomegalovirus retinitis is the most common opportunistic ocular infection in patients with AIDS, affecting 30–40% of them. HIV-induced retinal microvasculopathy may contribute to facilitated access of CMV to retinal glial tissue. CMV infection progresses from the retinal vasculature horizontally through glial cells and vertically through Mueller cells, to result in full-thickness necrosis. CMV-infected cells contain eosinophilic cytoplasmic and nuclear viral inclusion bodies that result in the typical owl's eye appearance on hematoxylin and eosin stain.

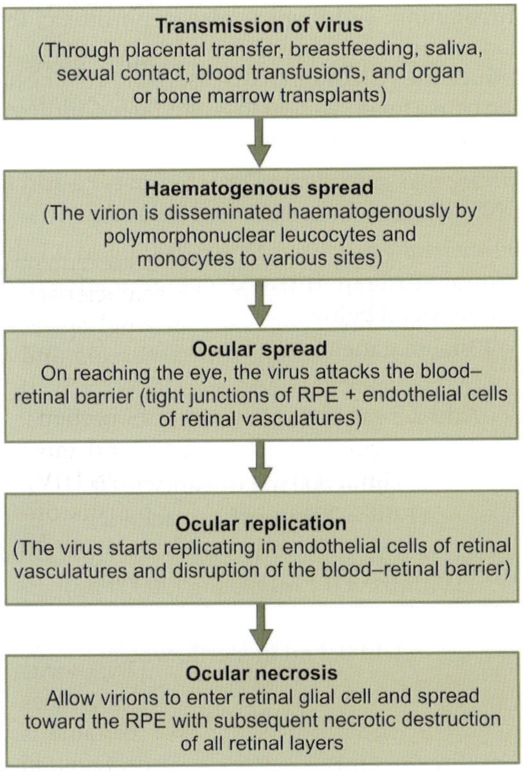

Clinical pictures

Patterns of CMV retinitis: Classically, three patterns of active lesions have been described:

1. *Haemorrhagic CMV retinitis* is characterised by—with a predominance of retinal haemorrhage interspersed with retinal necrosis (Fig. 6.2.2.5).
2. *Brush fire CMV retinitis* is characterised by—a progressively expanding yellow-white margin surrounding necrotic retina (Fig. 6.2.2.6).
3. *Granular CMV retinitis* is characterised by—with a central atrophic area surrounded by punctate white granular satellite lesions without retinal haemorrhage.

Zone grading system.

- *Zone 1:* Area within 1500 mm of the optic nerve or 3000 mm of the fovea.
- *Zone 2:* Zone 1 to the equator defined by the ampullae of the vortex veins.

Transmission of virus
(Through placental transfer, breastfeeding, saliva, sexual contact, blood transfusions, and organ or bone marrow transplants)

↓

Haematogenous spread
(The virion is disseminated haematogenously by polymorphonuclear leucocytes and monocytes to various sites)

↓

Ocular spread
On reaching the eye, the virus attacks the blood–retinal barrier (tight junctions of RPE + endothelial cells of retinal vasculatures)

↓

Ocular replication
(The virus starts replicating in endothelial cells of retinal vasculatures and disruption of the blood–retinal barrier)

↓

Ocular necrosis
Allow virions to enter retinal glial cell and spread toward the RPE with subsequent necrotic destruction of all retinal layers

Fig. 6.2.2.4 *Pathogenesis of CMV retinitis.*

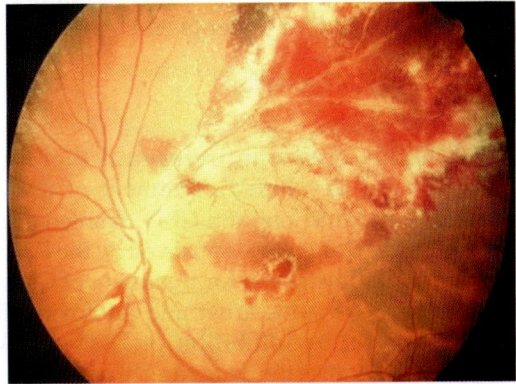

Fig. 6.2.2.5 *Haemorrhagic CMV retinitis in a patient with AIDS.*

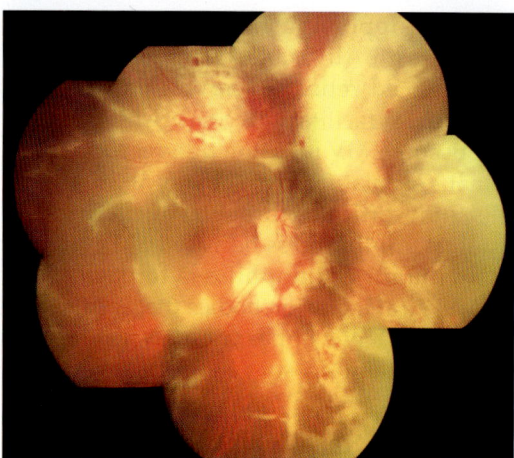

Fig. 6.2.2.6 *CMV retinitis fulminant.*

- *Zone 3:* Remaining anterior retina, up to ora serrata.

Note. Zone 1 lesions are considered most sight-threatening.

Progression of CMV retinitis. There is distinction between the affected area and normal retina, which allows us to measure the progression rate of CMV retinitis. The lesions in CMV retinitis spread much more slowly than HSV or varicella-zoster retinitis. If untreated, progression of CMV retinitis is, on average, 24 mm/d but can be as fast as 160 mm/d. Choroid remains largely unaffected

Rate of progression of CMV retinitis defined as extension of existing retinal lesions or observation of new lesions in patients with AIDS has drastically decreased from 3.0 events per patient per year (PY) in the pre-HAART era to the current level of 0.1/PY. Even in patients with low CD4+ T cell counts, the progression does not exceed 0.6/PY for patients on HAART.

Treatment of CMV retinitis

Pre-HAART era

Before highly active antiretroviral therapy (HAART) was developed, treatment of CMV retinitis required life-long anti-CMV maintenance therapy. Three drugs were approved by the Food and Drug Administration for treatment of CMV retinitis: ganciclovir, foscarnet, and cidofovir. All three drugs act by inhibition of CMV DNA polymerase. Because the drugs are virostatic, not virocidal, they must be continued indefinitely in patients with persistent immunosuppression.

Systemic therapy is initiated with induction therapy consisting of 2 weeks of twice-daily intravenous ganciclovir 5 mg/kg or foscarnet 90 mg/kg, or once-weekly intravenous cidofovir 5 mg/kg, followed by maintenance therapy consisting of once-daily ganciclovir 5 mg/kg or foscarnet 90 to 120 mg/kg, or cidofovir 5 mg/kg every 2 weeks. Oral ganciclovir 1 to 2 g three times daily may be used instead of maintenance intravenous ganciclovir. Clinical improvement may not be evident for 2 to 4 weeks after initiation of therapy.

Side effects with anti-CMV drugs: The patients with systemic anti-CMV medications should be carefully monitored. Dose adjustments are necessary for all three drugs, depending on renal function. Ganciclovir is marrow-suppressive and can cause leucopenia, anaemia and thrombocytopenia. Foscarnet is nephrotoxic and can cause painful genital ulcerations. In addition, the use of intravenous ganciclovir or foscarnet requires the use of a central venous catheter because the drugs must be given daily, and catheter-related infections can be life-threatening. Cidofovir is also nephrotoxic; the concurrent use of probenecid is necessary to reduce the risk of renal disease, but probenecid can cause fever, weight loss and rash. Cidofovir can also cause iritis and ocular hypotony.

Intravenous ganciclovir: Dose: 5–7 mg/kg add to DNS/RL for 1 hour infusion; twice daily.

Intravitreal ganciclovir: Dose: 2000 μg in 0.1 ml. Preparation of intravitreal ganciclovir is summarized below:

1 vial of ganciclovir (cymevene) = 500 mg
↓

Add 2.5 ml of sterile water for injection
↓

2.5 ml = 500 mg of ganciclovir
(1 ml = 200 mg of ganciclovir)
↓

Withdraw 0.1 ml {20 mg (20000 μg)}
↓

Add 0.9 ml of sterile water
↓

1 ml = 20000 μg
↓

Withdraw 0.1 ml (0.1 ml= 2000 μg of ganciclovir)

HAART era

Natural history of CMV retinitis has dramatically changed since the introduction of HAART. HAART is a combination of nucleoside reverse transcriptase inhibitors and protease inhibitors. These antiretroviral drugs disrupt two critical viral functions:

- Reverse transcription of viral RNA into DNA
- Proteolytic processing of viral proteins

The HIV protease enzyme is responsible for the processing of polyprotein precursors and its inhibition by protease inhibitors results in the production of non-infectious virions. HAART is highly efficient in reducing HIV viral replication and increasing CD4+ T cell count. In patients on intravenous ganciclovir, the risk of retinal detachments is 14-fold higher compared with those receiving intravitreal ganciclovir injections.

ACUTE RETINAL NECROSIS AND PROGRESSIVE OUTER RETINAL NECROSIS

Acute retinal necrosis (ARN) (Fig. 6.2.2.7) and progressive outer retinal necrosis (PORN) (Fig. 6.2.2.8) are the two recognizable clinical patterns of necrotising herpetic retinopathy (NHR), most commonly caused by VZV. Both are a very severe retinitis and the severity depends upon the level of immune compromise.

Differential diagnosis. Early lesions are difficult to distinguish from CMV retinitis. Table 6.2.2.2 helps to distinguish ARN, PORN and CMV retinitis.

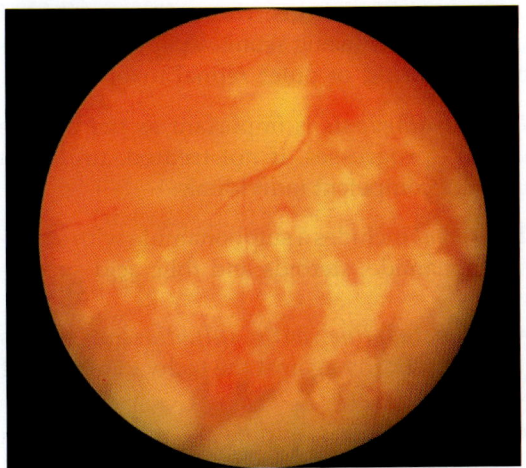

Fig. 6.2.2.7 *Acute retinal necrosis (ARN).*

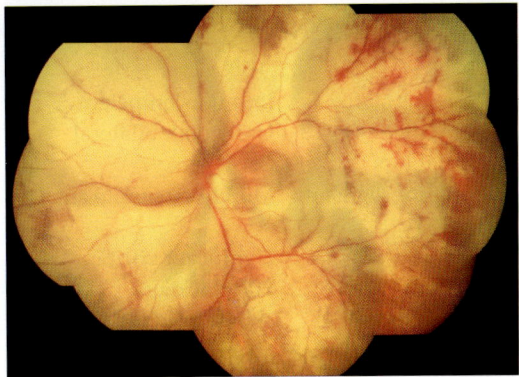

Fig. 6.2.2.8 *Progressive outer retinal necrosis (PORN) in an HIV-infected patient.*

Treatment includes:

- *IV acyclovir* 500 mg, eighth hourly for 1–2 weeks followed by oral aciclovir 800 mg five times daily is usually the mainstay therapy.
- *Additional low-dose systemic steroids* are necessary, at times.
- *Oral valacyclovir,* which has better bio-availability, can be given in a dose of 1 g three times daily as an efficient alternative. Treatment with antivirals may be required for up to 6–8 months in some cases.
- *Prophylactic laser barrage* can be done, whenever necessary.

OCULAR TUBERCULOSIS

Tuberculosis is the most common opportunistic systemic infection, although ocular tuberculosis is not that common.

Ocular tuberculosis can affect any part of the ocular tissue and adnexa. It can affect the eyelids, orbit, lacrimal glands, conjunctiva, keratitis, sclerokeratitis, scleritis, anterior uveitis, iris nodules.

Posterior segment manifestations include choroiditis, choroidal granulomas, endophthalmitis, subretinal abscess and panophthalmitis.

Diagnosis. Polymerase chain reaction (PCR) and histopathologic examination are very helpful in the diagnosis of ocular TB.

Treatment. Ocular TB can have an aggressive presentation and may not resolve with ATT, in patients with AIDS. The newly emerging trend

Table 6.2.2.2 *Differentiating features of ARN, PORN and CMV retinitis*

Characters	ARN	PORN	CMV retinitis
1. Immune status	Immunocompetent	Immunocompromised	Immunocompromised
2. Laterality	Unilateral/bilateral	Bilateral	Unilateral/bilateral
3. Visual loss	Gross	Early loss of vision	Variable
4. Anterior segment uveitis	Mild to moderate anterior	Mild anterior uveitis	Usually normal
5. Vitritis	Significant vitritis	No/minimal vitritis	No/minimal vitritis
6. Retinal involvement	Full thickness	Deep retinal involvement	Full thickness with granular border
7. Pattern	Multifocal, peripheral	Multifocal, early macular	Unifocal, mid-periphery
8. Vasculitis	Common	Uncommon	Seen
9. Retinal haemorrhages	Common	Uncommon	Common
10. Retinal detachment	Common	Common	Less common
11. Optic nerve	Common	Uncommon involvement	Uncommon
12. Progression	Rapid	Rapid	Slow

of immune reconstitution inflammatory syndrome, can lead to paradoxical worsening of TB; if HAART is initiated before ATT. Patients with AIDS should have regular ophthalmic screening.

OCULAR SYPHILIS

Characteristic features. Ocular syphilis tends to be aggressive, severe and relapsing in HIV/AIDS patients. All patients with ocular syphilis should be screened for HIV/AIDS.

- *Anterior segment involvement* includes conjunctival chancre, conjunctivitis, gummata, scleritis and anterior uveitis.
- *Posterior segment lesions* include chorioretinitis, optic neuritis, papilloedema or optic perineuritis. But in the era of HAART, syphilis can present with vitritis or panuveitis.

Diagnosis. Up to 38% of HIV-positive patients can be seronegative despite active syphilitic disease, making the diagnosis more difficult. Diagnostic tests include serologic screening and confirmatory tests, such as the rapid plasma reagin or fluorescent treponemal antibody absorbent tests, respectively. Direct examination using darkfield microscopy or biopsy of suspicious lesions can be performed, if results are uncertain.

Treatment of ocular syphilis consists of high-dose IV penicillin G 12–24 million units/day for 14 days.

TOXOPLASMA RETINOCHOROIDITIS

Toxoplasma gondii, a protozoon, affects about 10% of AIDS patients while toxoplasmic retino-choroiditis is relatively rare.

Clinical features. Its presentation in HIV/AIDS patients differs from immunocompetent patients. Lesions can be larger, multiple, bilateral, with minimal vitritis and resolves without scars. It can cause iritis, vitritis, choroiditis, multifocal or diffuse necrotizing retinitis, papillitis or retrobulbar neuritis, or outer retinal toxoplasmosis.

Prompt diagnosis is important as the disease usually progresses, if not treated, unlike in immunocompetent individuals.

Treatment includes a sulphonamide with a non-sulphonamide, steroids and folic acid supplements.

- *Pyrimethamine with sulfadiazine* works synergistically against the tachyzoite form of *T. gondii*.
- *In patients allergic to sulfa drugs*, combination of clindamycin and azithromycin gives god results.

- *Spiramycin* is the drug of choice in pregnant females.
- *Topical steroids* and *cycloplegics* can be used based on the severity of anterior uveitis.
- *Treatment continues* till all lesions resolve.
- *Long-term prophylaxis* continues till patient's CD4 counts raise above 200 cells/ml for six or more months and then can be discontinued.

PNEUMOCYSTIS CHOROIDOPATHY

Pneumocystis carinii, a unicellular protozoon, usually presents as pneumocystis pneumonia (PCP). It spreads to choroidal layers through a haematogenous route and is more common in patients treated with aerosolised pentamidine.

Characteristic features. Disseminated life-threatening *P. carinii* infection should be suspected, if *P. carinii* choroidopathy is seen. It has decreased in recent times due to the avoidance of aerosolised pentamidine use and with systemic cotrimoxazole prophylaxis.

Treatment. IV pentamidine is very effective and given daily for 3 weeks followed by maintenance therapy.

FUNGAL ENDOPHTHALMITIS

The most common intraocular fungal infections are Candida and Cryptococcus in immuno-compromised individuals.

Candida endophthalmitis is uncommon and occurs in patients with a history of indwelling venous catheters or in patients who are IV drug abusers.

- *Disseminated candidal infection* can involve multiple area including oral cavity (Fig. 6.2.2.9) and eye.
- *Candida endophthalmitis* is characterised by multiple fluffy-creamy-white chorioretinal lesions with overlying vitreous inflammation and snowballs (Fig. 6.2.2.10).

Cryptococcus neoformans is also a common fungal infective agent in AIDS.

- It manifests as meningitis, resulting in papilloedema, and optic neuropathy.
- Chorioretinitis and cranial nerve palsies are also seen, which indicate a poor prognosis.

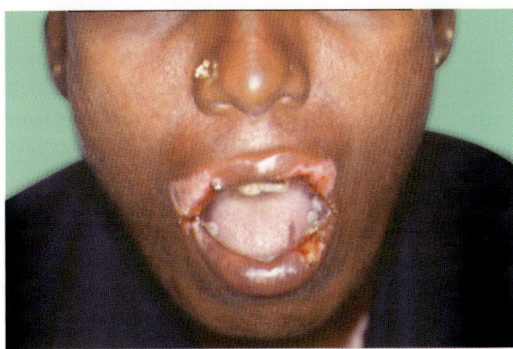

Fig. 6.2.2.9 Oral candidiasis in an HIV-infected patient.

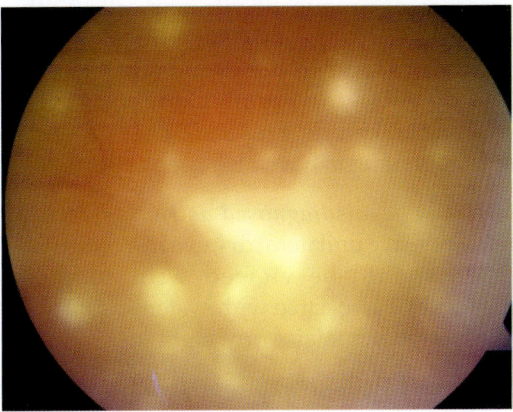

Fig. 6.2.2.10 Candida endophthalmitis.

Treatment. Systemic and intravitreal antifungal agents may be effective.

HISTOPLASMOSIS

H. capsulatum is a small, gram-positive, dimorphic fungus. The organism is endemic in the central and eastern United States.

Organism enters the body via the respiratory tract by inhalation of spores.

HIV/AIDS infection is an important risk factor for disseminated histoplasmosis which may involve liver, spleen, lymph nodes, and bone marrow.

Disseminated histoplasmosis has a fulminant course and high mortality in HIV/AIDS patients.

CRYPTOCOCCAL CHORIORETINITIS

C. neoformans is budding yeast-like fungus. Infection is usually acquired from pigeon and other bird dropping and through inhalation. It primarily affects the lungs, brain and meninges. Most intraocular infection occurs in association with cryptococcal septicaemia, seen in immuno-compromised patients, like HIV/AIDS patients.

LYMPHOMAS

3.5–5% of AIDS-defining illnesses are contributed by Non-Hodgkin's lymphoma (NHL). NHL can be seen in HIV patients of any age and a CD4 cell count of <50 cells/ml.

Characteristic features. It is characterised by the presence of prominent vitreous cells, with or without subretinal exudation. Primary NHL has also been found in the eyelids of patients as rapidly enlarging erythematous lesions, lid swelling and ptosis. Proptosis, gaze palsies and ophthalmoplegia have also been reported.

NHL can be misdiagnosed as KCS. Hence, any unresponsive unilateral dry eye in a patient with AIDS should be viewed with suspicion, especially if associated with systemic symptoms, such as fever, malaise or weight loss.

Treatment. Radiotherapy and/or chemotherapy are helpful. Interferon alpha has also been used as a part of the treatment modality.

C. ORBITAL LESIONS

Orbital lesions are uncommon in HIV/AIDS.

Most common orbital manifestations include orbital lymphoma and orbital cellulitis by *Aspergillus* fungus infection. They are usually seen in patients with CD4 counts less than 100 cells/ml.

Lymphoma is treated with chemotherapy and radiation. Orbital cellulitis responds well to systemic antibiotics and antifungals.

D. NEURO-OPHTHALMIC LESIONS

Neuro-ophthalmic complications are seen in approximately 10–15% of patients who are infected with HIV.

Common lesions include optic neuropathy, cranial nerve palsies, papilloedema and optic atrophy.

Commonly caused by toxoplasmosis, crypto-coccosis, VZV, CMV, progressive multifocal leucoencephalopathy, CNS and orbital lymphoma.

E. IMMUNE RECOVERY UVEITIS

Immune recovery uveitis (IRU) is part of the immune reconstitution inflammatory syndrome (IRIS), which has been described in other organs and with other opportunistic infections.[12] IRU was first described in 1998 to be a consequence of rapid immune reconstitution after the use of HAART among patients with HIV infection.

AIDS Clinical Trial Group defined IRU as a 'decrease in vision and at least two of the following signs in the absence of active CMVR:

- Presence of >2+ inflammatory cells in vitreous by slit-lamp examination
- Cystoid macular edema (CME) or
- Epiretinal membrane formation in patients receiving potent antiretroviral therapy with evidence of immune reconstitution'.[13]

Risk factors for IRU. A low CD4 count, HLA A8-18, extent of retinitis and history of treatment with cidofovir are significant risk factors for IRU at the time of starting HAART.[14]

Clinical features. IRU can present as cataract, vitritis, cystoid macular oedema, disc oedema and epiretinal membrane.

PRE-HAART ERA AND PRESENT SCENARIO (HAART ERA)

Highly active antiretroviral therapy (HAART) is a combination therapy of two or more nucleoside reverse transcriptase inhibitors along with either a protease inhibitor or a non-nucleoside reverse transcriptase inhibitor. It is the current accepted protocol for managing patients with HIV/AIDS infections. HAART is typically commenced when the patient demonstrates a low CD4 count (200–350 cells/mm^3) and may be susceptible to opportunistic infections.[15]

It leads to a decrease in the viral loads and return of CD4 counts to normal; indicating restoring of natural immune response. This HAART-mediated improvement of the immune function in patients with AIDS has changed the clinical presentation of many opportunistic infections, especially CMV and also to treatment. Newer ocular diseases in patients on HAART have been reported. HAART-led immune recovery has also allowed some patients with ocular infections, such as CMV retinitis to discontinue specific anti-CMV therapy without the reactivation of eye disease.

CONCLUSION

Ocular manifestations of HIV/AIDS are many and can present in many forms and at various stages of the disease; especially in HAART era. Thus, regular comprehensive ocular examination is very important along with regular monitoring of CD4 counts, general health and other opportunistic infections. Since large majority of HIV/AIDS patients are visually asymptomatic; comprehensive examination in adherence to universal precautions are utmost importance, especially in country like ours.

REFERENCES

1. Gottlieb MS, Schroff R, Schanker HM, et al. 'Pneumocystis carinii pneumonia and mucosal candidiasis in previously healthy homosexual men: evidence of a new acquired cellular immunodeficiency'. The New England Journal of Medicine 1981;305:1425–31.
2. Barre-Sinoussi F, Chermann J-C, Rey F, Nugeyre MT, Chamaret S, Gruest J, et al. 'Isolation of a T lymphotropic retrovirus from a patient at risk for acquired immune deficiency syndrome (AIDS)'. Science, May 20, 1983.
3. Source: UNAIDS website; www.unaids.org.
4. Shukla DS, Rathinam SR, Cunningham ET. Contribution of HIV/AIDS Global Blindness. Int Ophthalmol Clin 2007;47:27–43.
5. Holland GN, Gottlieb MS, Yee RD, et al. Ocular disorders associated with a new severe acquired cellular immunodeficiency syndrome. Am J Ophthalmol 1982;93:393–402.
6. Sudharshan S, Kaleemunnisha S, Banu AA, et al. "Ocular lesions in 1,000 consecutive HIV-positive patients in India: a long-term study". Journal of Ophthalmic Inflammation and Infection, vol. 3, article 2, 2013.
7. Biswas J, Madhavan HN, George AE, Kumarasamy N, and Solomon S. "Ocular lesions associated with HIV infection in India: a series of 100 consecutive patients evaluated at a referral center." American Journal of Ophthalmology, vol. 129, no. 1, 2000; pp. 9–15.
8. Ocular lesions in AIDS in India. In: Biswas J, editor. Practical Guidelines for Diagnosis and Management. Chennai: Gnanodaya Press, 2001.
9. Biswas J, Sudharshan S. Ophthalmic manifestations of HIV/AIDS. In: Brian J Hall, editor, A Textbook on HIV/AIDS in the Post-HAART Era, Connecticut, PmPH, 2011; pp.293–318.
10. Biswas J, Sudharshan S. Anterior segment manifestations of human immunodeficiency virus/acquired immune deficiency syndrome. Ind J Ophthalmol 2008;56:363–75.
11. Kaposi M. "Idiopathisches multiples Pigmentsarkom der Haut". Arch. Dermatol. Syph. 1872;4 (2): 265–273.
12. Jabs DA. Cytomegalovirus retinitis and the acquired immunodeficiency syndrome –bench to bedside: LXVII Edward Jackson Memorial Lecture. Am J Ophthalmol 2011;151(2):198–216.e1.
13. Holland GN, Vaudaux JD, Shiramizu KM, et al; Southern California HIV/Eye Consortium. Characteristics of untreated AIDS-related cytomegalovirus retinitis. II. Findings in the era of highly active antiretroviral therapy (1997 to 2000). Am J Ophthalmol 2008;145(1):12–22.
14. Otiti-Sengeri J, Meenken C, van den Horn GJ, Kempen JH. Ocular immune reconstitution inflammatory syndromes: Immune restoration disease. Curr Opin HIV & AIDS 2008;3:432–437.
15. Jabs DA, Van Natta ML, Holbrook JT, Kempen JH, Meinert CL, Davis MD. Studies of the Ocular Complications of AIDS Research Group. Longitudinal study of the ocular complications of AIDS: 1. Ocular diagnoses at enrollment. Ophthalmology 2007;114(4):780–786.

6.2.3 CHIKUNGUNYA AND EYE

General considerations
• Chikungunya virus
• General features of chikungunya
• Pathogenesis
Ocular manifestations
• Ocular lesions
• Uveitis in chikungunya
Management
• Differential diagnosis
• Diagnosis
• Treatment

GENERAL CONSIDERATIONS

Chikunguny virus

Chikungunya virus is a single-stranded RNA virus of the genus Alphavirus in the family Togaviridae.

It is transmitted to humans by the bite of infected mosquitoes, primarily *Aedes aegypti*,[1] and sometimes by *Aedes albopictus*. Chikungunya fever is a debilitating viral infection caused by chikungunya virus, first described by Robinson[2] and Lumsden[3] in 1955. Its name is derived from Makonade word meaning "that which bends up," in reference to the stooped posture developed as a result of arthritis.

Epidemic of chikungunya fever has been reported in the past from different parts of the world.[4] Although the virus had been passive for quite sometime, recent reports of outbreaks of chikungunya fever in several parts of southern India have confirmed the re-emergence of the virus.[5]

General features of chikungunya

• *Chikungunya virus* was recognized to cause illness that was self-limiting and characterized by sudden onset of fever with chills, headache, malaise, arthralgia or arthritis, vomiting, myalgia, skin rash and low back pain.
• *Incubation period* is about 2–4 days. Although chikungunya fever typically lasts for 3–7 days and recovery was usually the outcome, yet certain patients experienced persistent joint symptoms for weeks or months and occasionally years after the initial onset of illness.

• *Neurological complications*, such as meningo-encephalitis, have been reported during the first Indian outbreak as well as the recent French Reunion island's outbreak.[7] Other neurological signs include bilateral external ophthalmoplegia, upper motor neuron facial palsy, hemiparesis, incongruous homonymous hemianopias suggestive of optic tract lesions.[8]
• *Complications* including death have been reported in the current outbreak. The increased virulence has been attributed to absence of the herd immunity as well as the possible emergence of a new strain.[6,7]

Pathogenesis

The systemic manifestation of the fever may be related to viraemia, and in the case of joints involvement, it is believed to be immune-mediated from the viral antigen and antibody reactions.

• *Exact mechanism of ocular involvement* following chikungunya infection remains unknown. Simultaneous occurrence of systemic and ocular disease suggests the possibility of direct viral involvement of ocular structure.
• *Late involvement of ocular tissue suggests* a delayed immune response. Antigenic mimicry between the stimulating virus-derived antigens and normal or altered host tissue proteins, immediate hypersensitivity reactions and stimulations of a pathogenic lymphocytic reaction may be responsible for this delayed immune response.[15]

OCULAR MANIFESTATIONS

Ocular manifestations can be present at the time of systemic illness or after the systemic illness. It can be unilateral or bilateral presentation.

Ocular symptoms are redness, blurred vision, floaters, pain, watering, photophobia, irritation and diplopia.

Ocular lesions

Ocular lesions reported include: Conjunctivitis,[9] iridocylitis,[10,12,13] Fuchs' heterochromic irido-cyclitis,[19] episcleritis,[10] scleritis, keratitis,[12] retinitis,[10,20] choroiditis,[11] neuroretinitis,[12,21] panuveitis,[12] optic neuritis,[12,13] central retinal artery occlusion,[12] exudative retinal detachment,[12] secondary glaucoma,[9, 14] cranial nerve palsies,[12] bilateral external ophthalmoplegia,[8] upper motor neuron facial palsy,[8] and incongruous homonymous hemianopias.[8]

Uveitis in chikungunya

Ocular manifestations of chikungunya virus infection are likely to be encountered during an epidemic. Iridocyclitis is the commonest, other vision-threatening presentations, such as retinitis and optic neuritis, can also be seen in chikungunya fever. Ophthalmologists need to be aware of the chikungunya uveitis, which can result in visual impairment.

Two distinct presentations are seen in this infectious uveitis including anterior and posterior uveitis.

Anterior uveitis

Among the ocular features, anterior uveitis is the commonest manifestation. It can be unilateral or bilateral. It can have non-granulomatous or granulomatous presentation which can be associated with increased intraocular pressure with open angles. Posterior synechiae is not common.

Posterior uveitis

Symptoms. Patients may present with history of loss of vision, colour vision defect, central or centrocaecal scotoma and peripheral field defects.

Signs are as below:
- *Anterior segment* may be quiet with normal intraocular pressure.
- *Posterior segment* lesions include posterior pole retinitis, neuroretinitis, optic neuritis,[13] (Figs 6.2.3.1A and B) and retrobulbar neuritis.
- *Chikungunya retinitis* occurs several weeks after the primary illness which is similar to herpetic retinitis in immunoincompetent individuals, the former is characterized by minimal vitritis, retinitis and retinal oedema. The retinal vessel involvement in the posterior pole may be associated with haemorrhages (Figs 6.2.3.1A and B). Whereas in acute retinal necrosis, severe vitritis with multifocal

retinitis lesions is seen primarily in the retinal periphery. Although chikungunya retinitis may morphologically mimic the herpetic viral retinitis, the history of fever, joint pains and skin rash prior to the onset of the visual symptoms are helpful in the clinical diagnosis, particularly in the endemic regions.

Fluorescein angiography (Figs 6.2.3.1C to F) and OCT (Figs 6.2.3.1G and H) are useful in detecting retinal changes.

MANAGEMENT

Differential diagnosis

Chikungunya clinically resembles dengue, and hence should be differentiated from dengue fever, by absence of dengue IgM and IgG antibodies in the serum and also by platelet count. Syphilis, tuberculosis, sarcoidosis, dengue, herpes, cytomegalovirus and human immunodeficiency virus infections are to be ruled out.

Diagnosis

- Virus isolation, serological tests and molecular techniques are used to diagnose chikungunya infections.
- *Confirmation of chikungunya virus* infection can be performed by real-time polymerase chain reaction[19] or by virus isolation.[16] These are rapid confirmatory tests of choice, if the illness is of less than seven days duration.
- *Beyond seven days, diagnosis* is possible only with the detection of chikungunya-specific IgM in the serum.[17]
- *The temporal association between the systemic mani festations*, the ocular changes and the positive IgM serology will help us to make a diagnosis of chikungunya associated ocular changes.

Treatment

- *Topical steroids* and *cycloplegic agents* in case of anterior uveitis.
- *Topical beta blockers* and oral or topical carbonic anhydrase inhibitors for associated increase in intraocular pressure.
- *Systemic steroids* are used to control the inflammation in posterior uveitis, panuveitis and optic neuritis.

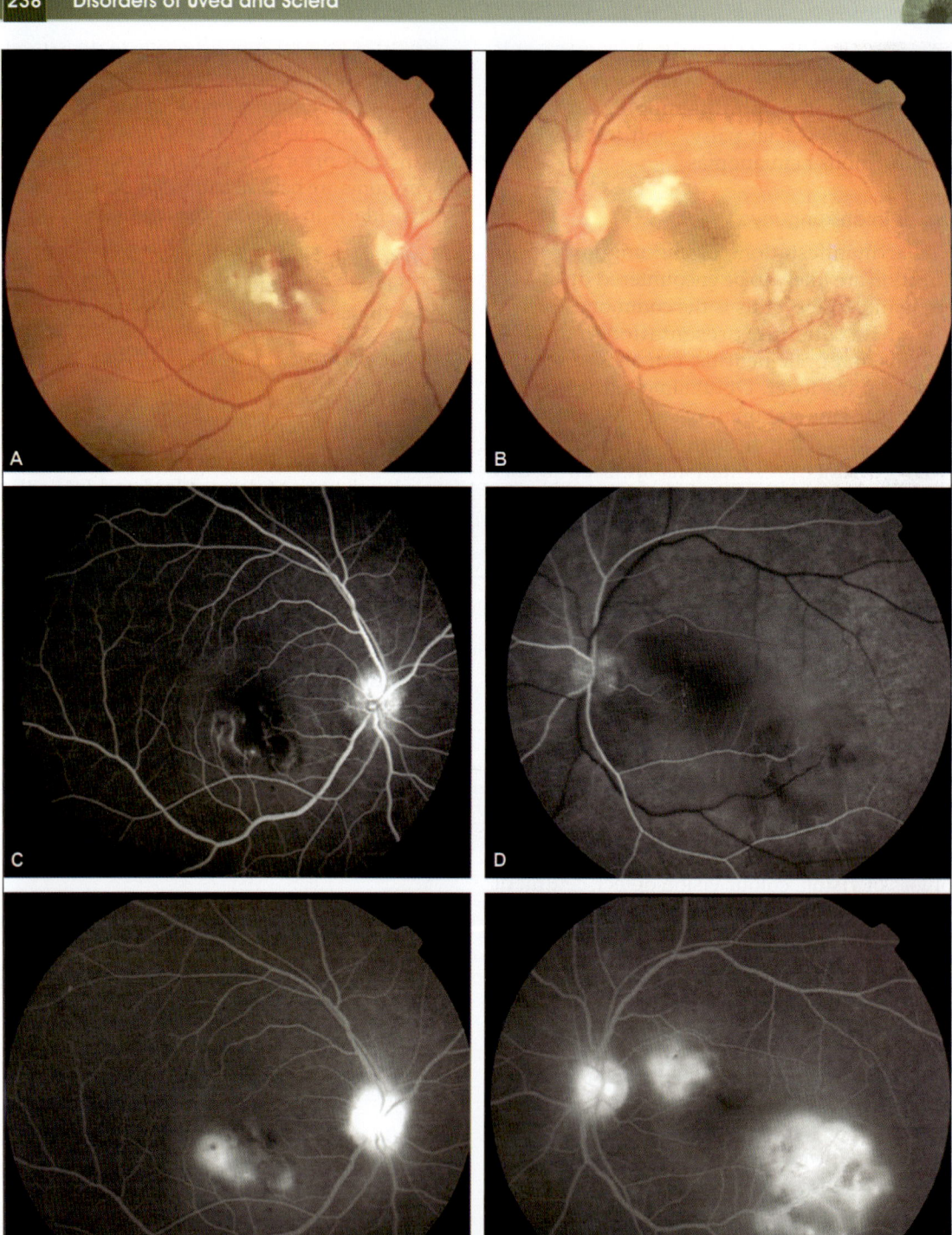

Fig. 6.2.3.1 *Chikungunya retinitis: A, Fundus photograph shows hyperaemic disc with retinitis with haemorrhages in the right eye; B, Multifocal retinitis, left eye; C, Early hypofluorescence with disc leakage; D, Early hypofluorescence in the posterior pole; E and F, Late hyperfluorescence with disc leakage.*

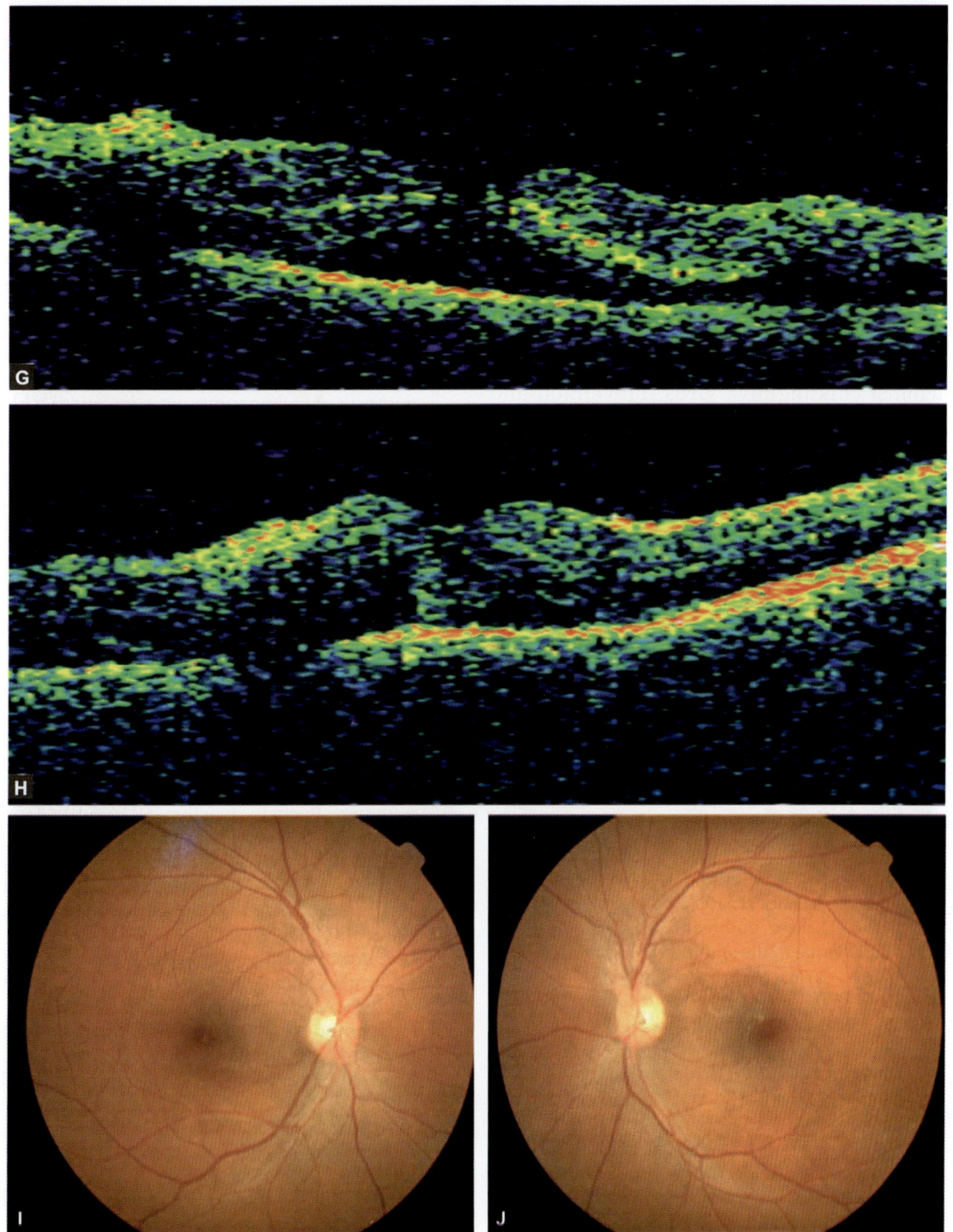

Fig. 6.2.3.1 *Chikungunya retinitis (contd.):* G, *Optical coherence tomography shows increased reflectivity in the nerve fibre layer zone corresponding to the areas of retinitis with after shadowing in the right eye; H, ECT left eye reveals fluid-filled spaces in the outer retina with subfoveal serous detachment; I and J, Resolved retinitis with visual acuity improving to 6/6, N6 in right eye and left eye, respectively.*

- *Non-aspirin analgesics and antipyretics* are used to manage fever and associated joint pains are treated with chloroquine phosphate.[18]
- *Antiviral therapy.* No specific antiviral therapy is available for chikungunya, however, few cases have been treated with acyclovir (empirically) along with systemic steroids.[10] The efficacy of acyclovir against chikungunya is doubtful, further studies are needed to address this issue.

Note. After resolution, full recovery can occur (Figs 6.2.3.1 I and J).

Prevention. There is no vaccine that protects one against chikungunya virus. Prevention and control depend on surveillance, early identification of outbreak, vector control and by use of protective measures to prevent being bitten by an infected mosquito.

REFERENCES

1. Calisher CH, Shope RE, Brandt W, et al. Proposed antigenic classification of registered arboviruses I (Togaviridae, Alphavirus). Intervirology 1980; 14:229–232.
2. Robinson MC. An epidemic of virus disease in Southern Province, Tanganyika Territory, in 1952–53. I. Clinical features. Trans R Soc Trop Med Hyg 1955; 49:28–32.
3. Lumsden WH. "An epidemic of virus disease in Southern Province, Tanganyika Territory, in 1952-53; II. General description and epidemiology". Trans Royal Society Trop Med Hyg 1955;49:33–57.
4. WHO. Disease outbreak news: Chikungunya and Dengue in the south west Indian Ocean. 17 March, 2006: http://www.who.int/csr/don/2006_03_17/en. (Accessed 10 January 2008).
5. WHO. Disease outbreak news: Chikungunya in India. 17 October, 2006: www.who.int/csr/don/2006_10_17/en.(accessed 10 January 2008)
6. Mourya DT, Mishra AC. Chikungunya fever. Lancet 2006;368:186–7.
7. Schuffenecker I, Iteman I, Michault A, Murri S, Frangeul L, Vaney MC, et al. Genome micro-evolution of chikungunya viruses causing the Indian Ocean outbreak. PLoS Med 2006; 3:e263.
8. WHO Disease outbreak news. Chikungunya and Dengue in the South West Indian ocean. 2006 Available from: http://www.who.int/csr/don/2006_03_17/en. [cited on 2006 Mar 17]
9. Parola P, Lamballerie X, Jourdan J, et al. Novel chikungunya virus variant in travelers returning from Indian Ocean islands. Emerg Infect Dis Volume 12, Number 10 2006 Oct. http://www.cdc.gov/ncidod/EID/vol12no10/06-0610.htm Accessed December 15th 2006
10. Mahendradas P, Ranganna SK, Shetty R, Balu R, Narayana KM, Babu RB, Shetty BK. Ocular manifestations associated with chikungunya. Ophthalmology 2007 Jul 11;
11. Chanana B, Azad RV, Nair S. Bilateral macular choroiditis following Chikungunya virus infection. Eye 2007;21(7):1020–1.
12. Lalitha P, Rathinam S, Banushree K, Maheshkumar S, Vijayakumar R, Sathe P. Ocular involvement associated with an epidemic outbreak of chikungunya virus infection. Am J Ophthalmol 2007;144(4): 552–6.
13. Mittal A, Mittal S, Bharati MJ, Ramakrishnan R, Saravanan S, Sathe PS. Optic neuritis associated with chikungunya virus infection in South India. Arch Ophthalmol 2007;125(10): 1381–6.
14. Mittal A, Mittal S, Bharathi JM, Ramakrishnan R, Sathe PS. Uveitis during outbreak of Chikungunya fever. Ophthalmology. 2007;114(9):1798.
15. Mahalingam S, Meanger J, Foster PS, Lidbury BA. The viral manipulation of the host cellular and immune environments to enhance propagation and survival: a focus on RNA viruses. J Leukoc Biol 2002;72:429–39
16. Rohani A, Yulfi H, Zamree I, Lee HL. Rapid detection of chikungunya virus in laboratory infected Aedes aegypti by reverse-transcriptase-polymerase chain reaction (RT-PCR). Trop Biomed 2005;22(2):149–54.
17. Kumarasamy V, Prathapa S, Zuridah H, Chem YK, Norizah I, Chua KB. Re-emergence of chikungunya virus in Malaysia. Med J Malaysia 2006;61(2): 221–5.
18. Brighton SW. Chloroquine phosphate treatment of chronic chikungunya arthritis. An open pilot study. S Afr Med J 1984;66:217–8.
19. Mahendradas P, Shetty R, Malathi J, Madhavan HN. Chikungunya virus iridocyclitis in Fuchs' heterochromic iridocyclitis. Indian J Ophthalmol 2010;58(6):545–7.
20. Murthy KR, Venkataraman N, Satish V et al. Bilateral retinitis following chikun- gunya fever. Indian J Ophthalmol 2008;56(4):329–31.
21. Mahesh G, Giridhar A, Shedbele A. A case of bilateral presumed chikungunya neuroretinitis. Indian J Ophthalmol 2009;57(2):148–50.
22. Mahendradas P, Avadhani K, Shetty R. Chikungunya and the eye: a review. J Ophthalmic Inflamm Infect 2013;3(1):35. doi: 10.1186/1869-5760-3-35.

6.2.4 DENGUE UVEITIS

General considerations
• Dengue fever
• Systemic features
Ocular manifestations
• Pathogenesis
• Clinical features
Diagnosis and treatment
• Diagnosis
• Treatment

GENERAL CONSIDERATIONS

Dengue fever is the most common mosquito-borne viral disease in humans. It is caused by the dengue virus, a flavivirus. It is transmitted by the *Aedes aegypti* mosquito. This arthropod-borne disease is endemic in more than 100 countries and commonly seen in tropical and subtropical regions.[1]

Systemic features. In addition to fever, dengue infection can also cause headaches, myalgia and thrombocytopenia, resulting in bleeding manifestations, such as a purpuric rash. Hypotension may also occur in the dengue shock syndrome which carries a high mortality rate.[1] Visual loss has been reported in cases of eyes affected with dengue fever.[2–7]

OCULAR MANIFESTATIONS

Pathogenesis

The exact *mechanism of the ocular involvement* in dengue infection is unclear.

The average onset of ocular symptoms from the onset of illness is about 7 days.[6,8–10] This delay as well as the lower the serum complement C3 levels in patients with maculopathy supports an immune-mediated mechanism rather than direct viral infection of the eye.[9,10]

Clinical features

Subconjunctival haemorrhage of petechial type which was associated with a platelet count of less than 50,000 in an East Indian population was the commonest ocular involvement.[8]

Symptoms. Patients can present with floaters, central scotoma and sudden decrease in vision in the eyes. The involvement is bilateral and asymmetrical.

Signs include:
• *Anterior segment involvement* is mild and associated with the presence of cells in the anterior chamber and the vitreous.[6]
• *Fundus findings* (Figs 6.2.4.1A and B) can be disc hyperaemia, disc oedema, retinal haemorrhages,[6] sheathing of the veins,[6] yellow subretinal dots, retinal pigment epithelium mottling, round foveal swelling [foveolitis][12]

DIAGNOSIS AND TREATMENT

Diagnosis

Diagnosis of dengue fever

Diagnosis of dengue fever is based on:
• Typical clinical presentation
• Positive dengue IgM serology, real-time automated reverse transcriptase (RT-PCR), or both.
• Serial serum platelet measurements tracked the thrombocytopenic pattern.[9]

Diagnosis of dengue retinitis

Diagnosis of dengue maculopathy is based on:
• *Clinical features* as well as the imaging studies,
• In dengue, maculopathy involves both the retinal as well as the choroidal circulations, hence fluorescein and indocyanine green angiography are important modalities in the assessment of extent of involvement in the retina.[7,11]

Imaging studies
• *Fundus fluorescein angiography* (FFA) shows the presence of blocked fluorescence corresponding to the areas of retinal haemorrhages (Figs 6.2.4.1C and D) and staining of the lesions with vascular leakages (Figs 6.2.4.1E and F) in both eyes.
• *Indocyanine green angiography* (ICG) in the mid to late phases may manifest hypofluorescent dark dots corresponding to the yellow subretinal lesions, suggesting involvement of the choriocapillaris with large choroidalvasculopathy.[12]
• *Optical coherence tomography (OCT)* is indispensable in detecting and monitoring the progress of foveolitis and exudative retinal detachment (Figs 6.2.4.1G and H).

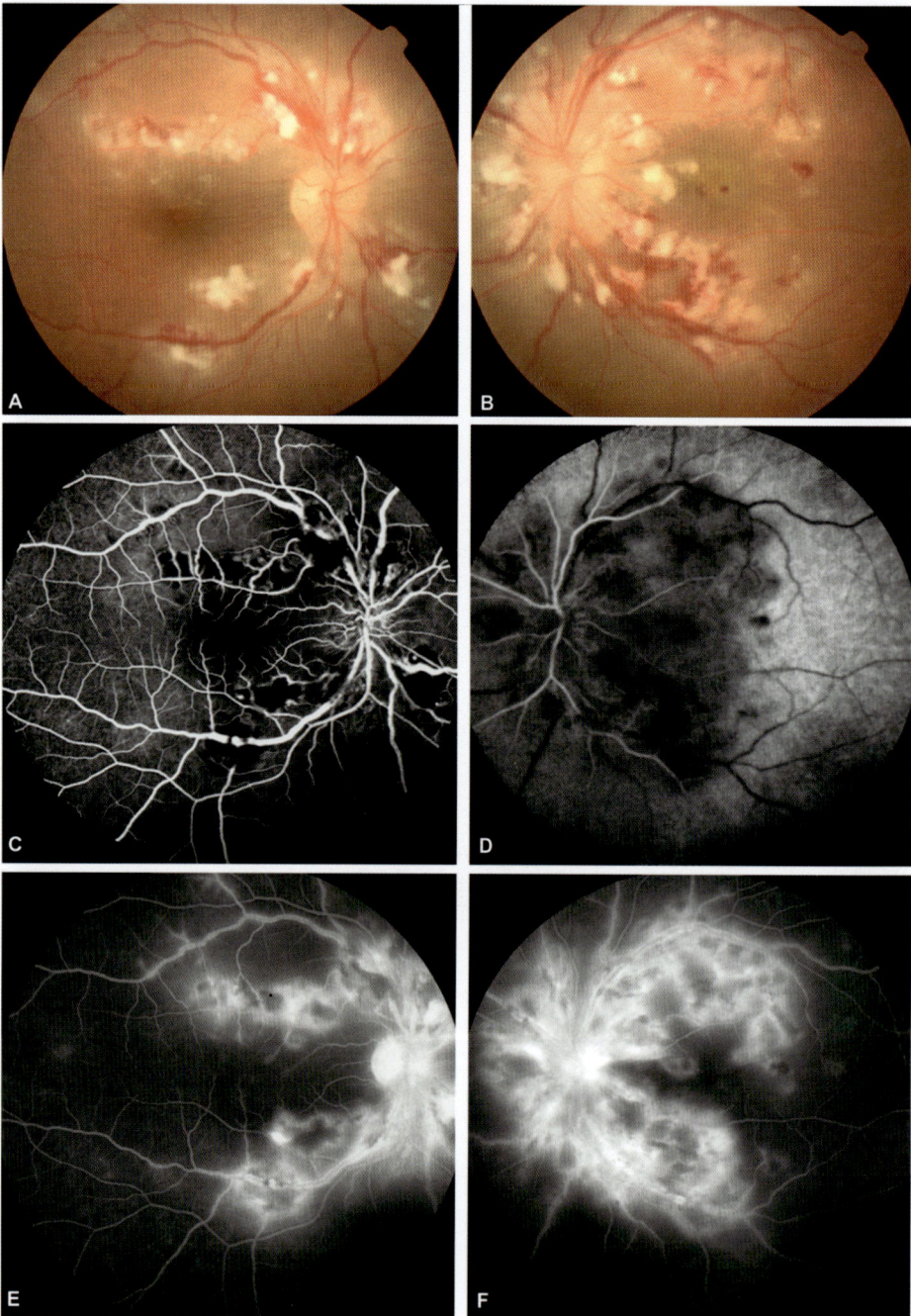

Fig. 6.2.4.1 *Dengue uveitis:* *A, Fundus examination of the right eye revealed mild hyperaemic disc, full thickness retinal opacification, retinal haemorrhages along the arcade of vessels, macular oedema with internal limiting membrane folds; B, Left eye showed hyperaemic disc, multiple cotton wool spots, superficial retinal haemorrhages with macular oedema; C, Early phase fluorescein angiogram showing multiple areas of hypofluorescence with staining of the veins in the right eye; D, Early phase fluorescein angiogram showing areas of hypofluorescence in the posterior pole with absent filling of the retinal veins in the left eye; E, Late phase showing disc leak, staining of the lesions and the veins with diffuse vascular leakage in the right eye; F, Late phase showing disc leak, staining of the lesions with leakage from the lesions and vessels in the posterior pole in the left eye.*

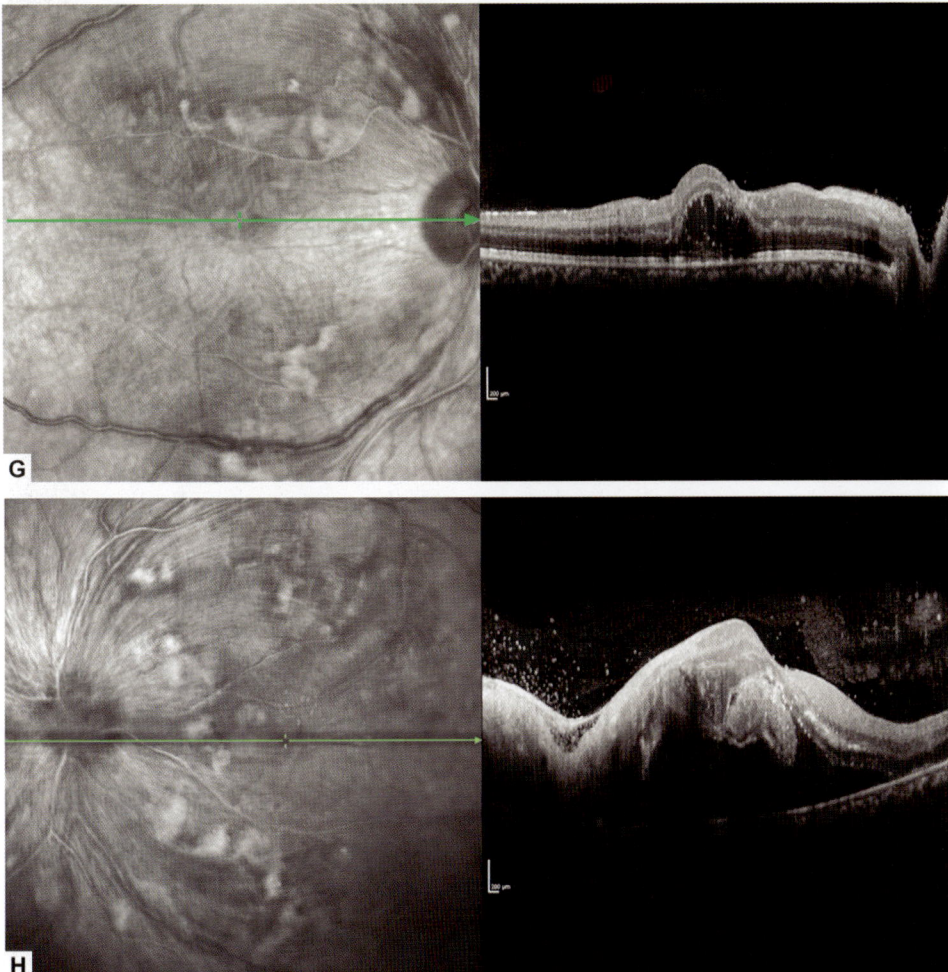

Fig. 6.2.4.1 *Dengue uveitis (contd.):* G, High definition spectral domain optical coherence tomography shows hyperreflective dots in the posterior vitreous cavity suggestive of posterior vitreous cells, hyporeflective cystic space in the outer retina with inflammatory infiltrate in the retinal layers in the right eye; H, High definition spectral domain optical coherence tomography shows hyperreflective dots in the vitreous cavity, with the presence of severe neurosensory retinal detachment accounting for the poor vision in the left eye.

Treatment

Ocular manifestations of dengue infection can be self-limiting illness. However, immuno-suppression with topical, periocular, oral, intra-venous steroids and immune globulins has been used with variable success. [7, 11]

REFERENCES

1. World Health Organization. Dengue Hemorr-hagic Fever: Diagnosis, Treatment and Control (2nd edn), Geneva, Switzerland: WHO; 1997.

2. Wen KH, Sheu MM, Chung CB, Wang HZ, Chen CW. [In Chinese] The ocular fundus findings in dengue fever. Gaoxiong Yi Xue Ke Xue Za Zhi 1989;5:24–30.

3. Haritoglou C, Scholz F, Bialaslewicz A, Klauss V. Ocular manifestations in dengue fever. [In German] Ophthalmologe 2000;97:433–6.

4. Haritoglou C, Dotse SD, Rudolph G, Stephan CM, Thurau SR, Klauss V. A tourist with dengue fever and visual loss. Lancet 2002;360:1070.

5. Haritoglou C, Dotse SD, Rudolph G, Stephan CM, Thurau SR, Klauss V. A tourist with dengue fever and visual loss. Lancet 2002;360:1070.

6. Chlebicki MP, Ang B, Barkham T, Laude A. Retinal haemorrhages in 4 patients with dengue fever. Emerg Infect Dis [serial on the Internet] 2005 May Available at http://www.cdc.gov/ncidod/EID/vol11/n005/04- 0992.htm

7. The Eye Institute Dengue-related Ophthalmic Complications Workgroup. Ophthalmic complications of dengue. Emerg Infect Dis [serial on the Internet]. 2006 Feb Available at http://www.cdc.gov.ncidod/EID/vol12no02/05-0274.htm

8. Bacsal K, Chee SP, Cheng CL, Flores JVPG. Dengue-associated maculopathy. Arch Ophthalmol 2007;125:501–10.

9. Kapoor HK, Bhai S, John M, Xavier J. Ocular manifestations of dengue fever in an East Indian epidemic. Can J Ophthalmol 2006;41:741–6.

10. Mehta S. Ocular lesions in severe dengue hemorrhagic fever (DHF). J Assoc Physicians India 2005;53:656–7.

11. Su DHW, Bacsal K, Chee SP, et al. Prevalence of dengue maculopathy in patients hospitalized for dengue fever. Ophthalmology 2007;114:1743–7.

12. Soon-Phaik Chee. Ocular manifestations of dengue fever. In: Amod Gupta, Vishali Gupta, Carl P Herbort, Moncef Khairallah, editors. Uveitis Text and Imaging. Jaypee brothers medical Publishers (P) Ltd; 2009, pp. 699–705.

6.2.5 WEST NILE DISEASE

- Systemic features
- Ocular manifestations

SYSTEMIC FEATURES

West Nile virus (WNV), first isolated in 1937 in the West Nile district of Uganda, is an enveloped single-stranded RNA flavivirus. It is transmitted to humans by infected Culex mosquito vector with wild birds serving as its reservoir.

Incubation period of WNV ranges from 3 to 14 days.

Asymptomatic. About 80% of human infections are apparently.

Symptoms are seen in approximately 20% of persons infected become symptomatic. These include high-grade fever, headache, myalgia, malaise, nausea, vomiting, skin rash, arthralgia, weakness, and pharyngitis. The acute illness is self-limiting, typically lasting less than a week. Severe neurologic disease (meningoencephalitis), frequently associated with advanced age and diabetes.

OCULAR MANIFESTATIONS

Symptoms

- Decreased vision
- Floaters

Signs

- *Bilateral multifocal chorioretinitis*, with typical clinical (Figs 6.2.5.1A and B) and fluorescein angiographic features (Figs 6.2.5.1C and D), is the most common finding, but numerous other ocular manifestations can occur.
- *Diabetes mellitus appears to be a potential risk factor* for developing severe neurologic disease and also severe chorioretinitis.
- *Numerous retinal changes can occur*, including retinal haemorrhages, focal or diffuse vascular sheathing, vascular leakage, and occlusive vasculitis.
- Recently, Rathinam et al have reported a different spectrum of West Nile retinitis in South India in a non-diabetic, non-linear pattern of retinitis in a younger indivisuals.

DIAGNOSIS AND TREATMENT

Diagnosis

- ELISA IgM antibody >1:30; sensitivity 100%
- Real-time polymerase chain reaction (RT-PCR) and re-time loop-mediated isothermal amplification (RT-LAMP) assays.
- Genotyping of RT-PCR amplified product
- Antigen capture ELISA

Differential diagnosis

- Chikungunya retinitis
- Dengue retinitis
- Cat-scratch disease

Treatment

- *Antivirals drugs,* such as ribavirin and newer drugs, like interferon α, β and intravenous immunoglobulins, can be used to treat the systemic infection. However, there is no

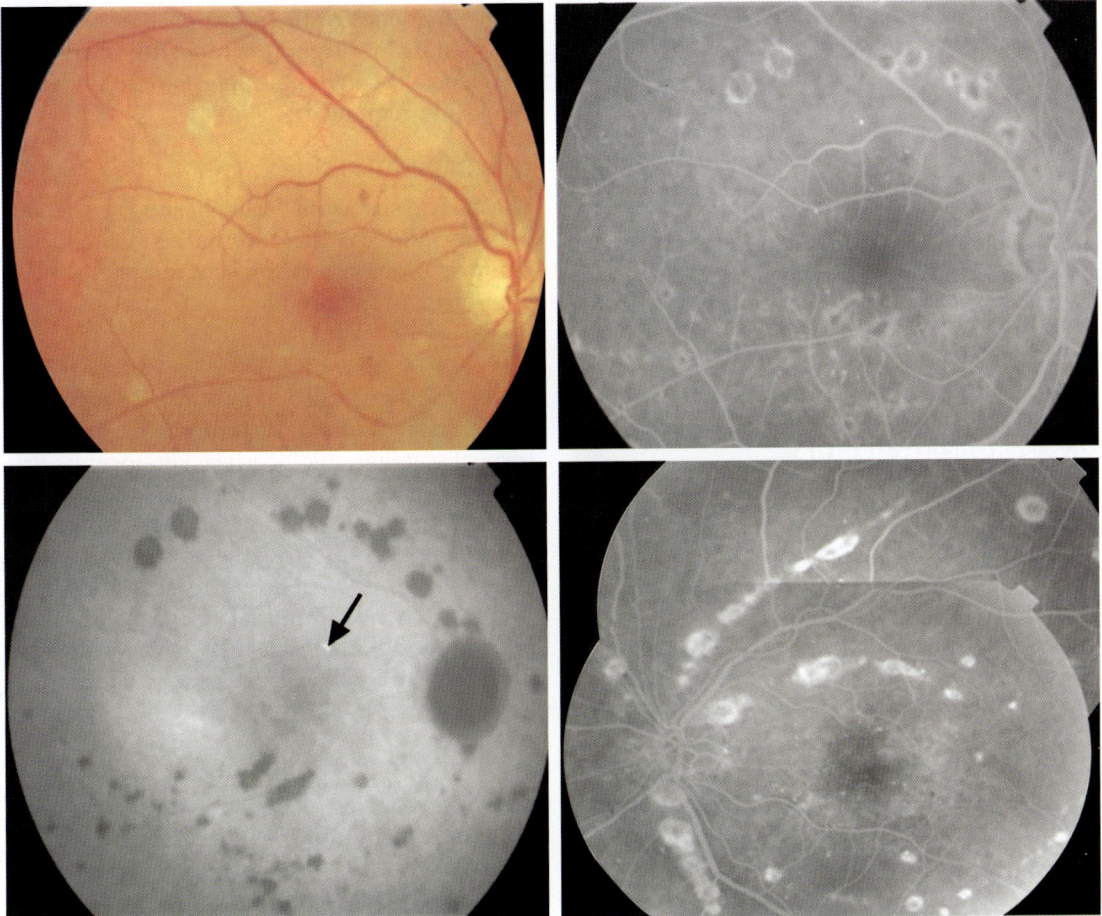

Fig. 6.2.5.1A to D *West Nile virus infection with multiple partial atrophic, pigmented chorioretinal lesions in the right eye and multiple linear streaks of chorioretinitis, which follow the course of retinal nerve fibres in another case of West Nile infection. (Courtesy: Moncef Khairallah).*

specific proven systemic treatment for West Nile virus infection.

• *Symptomatic therapy* with topical and systemic steroids is used to control the eye inflammation.

BIBLIOGRAPHY

1. Chan CK, Limstrom SA, Tarasewicz DG, Lin SG. Ocular features of West Nile virus infection in North America: a study of 14 eyes. Ophthalmology 2006;113:1539–46.
2. Eidsness RB, Stockl F, Colleaux KM. West Nile chorioretinitis. Can J Ophthalmol 2005;40:721–4.
3. Kaiser PK, Lee MS, Martin DA. Occlusive vasculitis in a patient with concomitant West Nile virus infection. Am J Ophthalmol 2003;136:928–30.
4. Khairallah M, Ben Yahia S, Attia S, et al. Severe ischemic maculopathy in a patient with West Nile virus infection. Ophthalmic Surg Lasers Imaging 2006;37:240–2.
5. Khairallah M, Ben Yahia S, Ladjimi A, et al. Chorioretinal involvement in patients with West Nile virus infection. Ophthalmology 2004;111:2065–70.
6. Kuchtey RW, Kosmorsky G, Martin D, Lee MS. Uveitis associated with West Nile virus infection. Arch Ophthalmol 2003;121:1648–9.
7. Myers JP, Leveque TK, Johnson MW. Extensive chorioretinitis and severe vision loss associated with West Nile virus meningoencephalitis. Arch Ophthalmol 2005;123:1754–6.
8. Seth RK, Stoessel KM, Adelman RA. Choroidal neovascularization associated with West Nile virus chorioretinitis. Semin Ophthalmol 2007; 22:81–4.

9. Shaikh S, Trese MT. West Nile virus chorio-retinitis. Br J Ophthalmol 2004;88:1599–60.
10. Shukla J, Saxena D, Rathinam S, Lalitha P, Joseph CR, Sharma S, Soni M, Rao PV, Parida M. Molecular detection and characterization of West Nile virus associated with multifocal retinitis in patients from southern India. Int J Infect Dis 2012;16(1):e53–9.
11. Sivakumar RR, Prajna L, Arya LK, Muraly P, Shukla J, Saxena D, Parida M. Molecular diagnosis and ocular imaging of West Nile virus retinitis and neuroretinitis. Ophthalmology. 2013;120(9):1820–6.

6.2.6 RUBELLA UVEITIS

Introduction
Congenital Rubella Syndrome
- Epidemiology
- Clinical features
- Ocular features
- Systemic features
- Etiopathogenesis
- Diagnosis
- Treatment
Acquired Rubella
- Epidemiology
- Clinical features
- Etiopathogenesis
- Diagnosis
- Treatment

INTRODUCTION

Rubella virus (German Measles) is a single-stranded RNA virus with a lipid envelope belonging to the family of Togaviridae.[1] It causes acute, contagious and exanthematous disease.[2] It can present as congenital rubella syndrome (CRS) or acquired rubella.

CONGENITAL RUBELLA SYNDROME

EPIDEMIOLOGY

Rubella was considered one of the most important causes of blindness before the development of vaccination programmes. However, even today, 5–20% of women of child bearing age who lack antibodies to rubella are suspectible to the infection.

The incidence of the occurrence depends on the gestational age at which the mother is infected. No congenital defects noted after 20 weeks of pregnancy.[3]

CLINICAL FEATURES

The clinical spectrum of rubella involves ocular, hearing and cardiac anomalies. Congenital malformations can be present at birth, shortly after birth, or later in life.[4,5]

Ocular features

It has an incidence of 30–78% among the population. Ocular findings include microphthalmia, corneal scarring, microcornea, keratoconus, iris hypoplasia, cataracts, glaucoma, and "salt and pepper" retinopathy (Fig. 6.2.6.1).[6] The retinopathy can remain non-progressive or can progress to cause tissue destruction and scarring.[7] It is complicated by subretinal neovascularisation presenting as a sudden loss of vision or as a disciform scar at macula presenting with gradual loss of vision.[8–11]

Systemic features

- *Hearing* features, i.e. sensorineural deafness is the most common systemic finding noted in rubella.
- *Cardiac* features include patent ductus arteriosus, intraventricular septal defect and pulmonic stenosis.
- *CNS features* are mental retardation, and encephalitis.
- GIT features include hepatosplenomegaly.

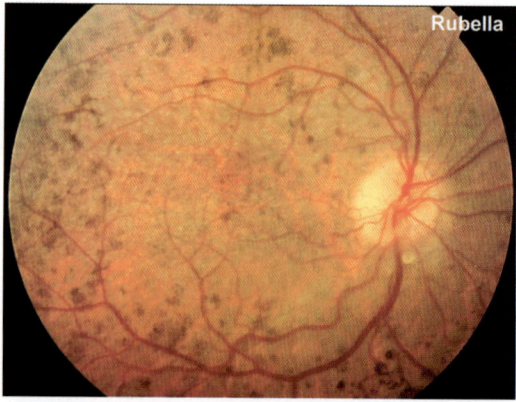

Fig. 6.2.6.1 *Salt and pepper retinopathy in congential rubella.*

- *Pulmonary features* include interstitial pneumonitis.

ETIOPATHOGENESIS

The infection in the fetus can occur either as a primary placental infection or through the ascending routed from cervix.[12,13] The virus causes inhibition of cellular multiplication during organogenesis leading to tissue destruction and scarring. Moreover, focal necrosis of the ciliary epithelium, pars plicata and pars plana is characteristic of the rubella infection in eye.[14]

DIAGNOSIS AND TREATMENT

Diagnosis

The diagnosis of rubella can be made by:
- *History* of any maternal infection during the pregnancy especially in the first trimester.
- *Clinical examination* for ocular and systemic congenital anomalies.
- Serology
- *Isolation of virus from nose*, throat, urine, blood, and cerebrospinal fluid.
- *Molecular diagnostic* tests such as polymerase chain reaction from the ocular fluids.
- *Fundus fluorescein angiography*. Revealing hyperfluoresence and hypofluorescence due to diffuse retinal pigment epithelium mottling.

Treatment

The treatment for congenital rubella syndrome is symptomatic.
- *In active cases of rubella*, isolation of the child till cultures become negative should be advocated.
- *In case of subretinal neovascularisation*, photo-coagulation is advised.

Preventive measures by giving immuno-globulins to mothers susceptible to infection can prevent maternal as well as congenital anomalies.[2]

ACQUIRED RUBELLA

EPIDEMIOLOGY

Since the vaccination programmes, acquired rubella is more commonly in the age group above 19 years. The vaccination programmes focus on children to prevent epidemics and on young women of childbearing age to prevent maternal and congenital rubella.[15,16] It is reportedly more common in winters and springs, although it is seen to have sporadic pattern in large cities.[17]

CLINICAL FEATURES

Acquired rubella presents as:
1. *Prodromal stage of fever and malaise.* It occurs within 1–5 days before the onset of rash.[18]
2. *Rubella exanthema.* An erythematous and maculopapular rash first appears on face and then spreads towards hand and feet. It eventually involves the entire body within 24 hours and disappears on 3rd day.
3. *Lymphadenopathy* is invariably present
4. *Ocular complications* for acquired rubella includes:
- *Conjunctivitis*, which is seen in almost 70% patients.
- *Epithelial keratitis* in 7.6%, and
- Retinitis in rare cases.[19-22]
- *Systemic complications*, like encephalitis, arthritis and thrombocytic purpura, are also seen.

Note. Further, the rubella virus is associated with the pathogenesis of Fuchs' heterochromic iridocyclitis.[23]

ETIOPATHOGENESIS

Rubella infection is acquired through respiratory tract.[24,25] It travels to the regional lymph nodes. The virus undergoes replication thereafter and causes viraemia. The infection is identified by the presence of IgG,IgM,IgA antibodies in the serum.

DIAGNOSIS AND TREATMENT

Diagnosis

Due to lack of pathognomonic evidence, the diagnosis can be difficult. However, virus isolation is important and can be done through:
- *Serology* of the virus from nose, throat, urine, etc.
- *Molecular diagnostic tests,* like real-time PCR from ocular fluids can help.

- *Ig and IM levels.* An increase in the IgG antibodies to four times or presence of newly detected IgM rubella-specific antibodies are seen.

Treatment

- The treatment for acquired rubella is aimed symptomatic.
- In cases of retinitis, systemic steroids should be given.[26,27]

REFERENCES

1. Basic and Clinical Science Course, American Academy of Ophthalmology. Section 9. San Francisco; LEO; 2011; Chapter 7, Intraocular Inflammation and Uveitis; 197–268.
2. Letko E, Foster S. Rubella. In: Foster S, Vitale AT, editors. Diagnosis and Treatment of Uveitis; 2nd ed. New Delhi: Jaypee Brothers Medical Publishers (P) Ltd; 2013.
3. Sallomi SJ. Rubella in pregnancy. A review of prospective studies (from the literature. Obstet Gynecol 1966;27:252–6.
4. Hancock MT, Huntley CC, Sever JL. Congenital rubella syndrome with immunoglobulin disorder. J Pediatr 1968;72:636–45.
5. Murphy AM, Reid RR, Pollard I, et al. Rubella cataracts. Further clinical and virologic observations. Am J Ophthalmol 1967;64:1109–19.
6. Albert and Jackobiec's Principles and Practice of Opthalmology; vol1; 3rd edition; Chapter 95; Infectious causes of Posterior Uveitis; p 1173–1193; Saunder Elseveir.
7. Collis WJ, Cohen DN. Rubella retinopathy: a progressive disorder. Arch Ophthalmol 1970; 84:33–5.
8. Deutman AF, Grizzard WS. Rubella retinopathy and subretinal neovascularization. Am J Ophthalmol 1978;85(1):82–7.
9. Frank KE, Purnell EW. Subretinal neovascularization following rubella retinopathy. Am J Ophthalmol 1978;86(4):462–6.
10. Orth DH, Fishman GA, Segall M, et al. Rubella maculopathy. Br J Ophthalmol 1980;64:201–5.
11. Slusher MM, Tyler ME. Rubella retinopathy and subretinal neovascularization. Ann Ophthalmol 1982;14:292–4.

12. Sever JL, South MA, Shaver KA. Delayed manifestations of congenital rubella. Rev Infect Dis 1985;7(Suppl 1):S164–9.
13. Vaheri A, Vesikari T, Oker-Blom N, et al. Isolation of attenuated (rubella-vaccine virus from human products of conception and (uterine cervix. N Engl J Med 1972;286:1071–4.
14. Boniuk M, Zimmerman LE. Ocular pathology in the rubella syndrome. Arch Ophthalmol 1967; 77(4):455–73.
15. Communicable Disease Center. Rubella Surveillance. Atlanta GA: Centers for Disease Control, 1969.
16. Hambling MH. Effect of a vaccination program on the distribution of rubella antibodies in women of childbearing age. Lancet 1975;1:1130–8.
17. Communicable Disease Center. Provisional Information in Selected Notifiable Diseases in the United States and on Deaths in Selected Cities for Week Ended September 3, 1964. MMWR 1964;13:349–60.
18. Gross PA, Portnoy B, Mathies AW Jr, et al. A rubella outbreak among adolescent boys. Am J Dis Child 1970;119(4):326–31.
19. Zimmerman LE. Histopathologic basis for ocular manifestations of congenital rubella syndrome. Am J Ophthalmol 1968;65(6):837–62.
20. Matoba A. Ocular viral infections. Pediatr Infect Dis. 1984;3: 358–68.
21. Gerstle C, Zim KM. Rubella-associated retinitis in adult. Report of a case. Mt Sinai J Med 1976; 43(3):303–8.
22. Hayashi M, Yoshimura N, Kondo T. Acute rubella retinal pigment epithelitis in an adult. Am J Ophthalmol 1982;93:285–8.
23. De Groot Mijnes JD, De Visser L. Rubella virus is associated with Fuchs' heterochromia iridocyclitis. Am J Ophthalmol 2006;141(1); 212–4.
24. Johnson BL, Cheng KP. Congenital aphakia: a clinicopathologic report of three cases. J Pediatr Ophthalmol Strabismus 1997;34(1):35–9.
25. O'Neill JF. Strabismus in congenital rubella. Arch Ophthalmol 1967;77(4):450–4.
26. Hayashi M, Yoshimura N, Kondo T. Acute rubella retinal pigment epithelitis in an adult. Am J Ophthalmol 1982;93:285–8.
27. Kazarian EL, Gager WE. Optic neuritis complicating measles, mumps, and rubella vaccination. Am J Ophthalmol 1978;86:544–7.

6.3 FUNGAL UVEITIS

General Considerations
- Definition

Etiology and Clinical Profile of known Fungal Uveitis Entities
Candida uveitis
- Etiology
- Clinical features
Aspergillus uveitis
- Etiology
- Clinical features
- Histology
Fusarium uveitis
- Etiology
- Clinical features
Cryptococcus uveitis
- Etiology
- Ocular manifestation
Coccidioidomycosis uveitis
- Etiology
- Ocular manifestations
Histoplasma uveitis
- Etiology
- Ocular manifestations

Management of Fungal Endophthalmitis
- Differential diagnosis
- Investigations
- Treatment

GENERAL CONSIDERATIONS

DEFINITION

Fungal uveitis is an intraocular inflammation caused by fungi, such as *Candida, Aspergillus, Fusarium, Histoplasma,* etc.

Fungi can enter the eye either exogenously, endogenously or locally from the extension from periocular tissues. The two main types of fungal infections are exogenous and endogenous endophthalmitis.

Exogenous endophthalmitis is caused by inoculation of the eye by microorganisms from the external environment and most commonly occurs as a complication of ocular surgery, trauma, or intravitreal injections. This form has a characteristic history and signs typical of endophthalmitis and is unlikely to be confused with endogenous variety of uveitis.

Endogenous endophthalmitis is caused by haematogenous spread of infectious organisms from distant sites of the body. It has been estimated that endogenous endophthalmitis accounts for 2 to 15% of all cases of endophthalmitis.

ETIOLOGY AND CLINICAL PROFILE OF KNOWN FUNGAL UVEITIS ENTITIES

CANDIDA UVEITIS

Etiology

Candida albicans (a yeast) is a common nasocomial pathogen that can spread to the eye through haematogenous spread, resulting in the development of Candida endophthalmitis.

Predisposing risk factors. Patients with Candida fungal endophthalmitis usually have one or more of the following predisposing systemic conditions:
- Diabetes mellitus
- Intravenous drug use
- Liver diseases
- Renal failure
- History of recent hospitalization, surgical intervention especially abdominal surgery.
- Cancer
- Indwelling intravenous lines
- Immunosuppression secondary to organ transplantation
- HIV/AIDS
- Hyperalimentation
- Immunosuppressive therapy
- Bacterial sepsis requiring broad-spectrum systemic antibiotics

Clinical features

Presenting symptoms are ocular pain, decreased vision and floaters.

Clinical signs include:
- *Fluffy white exudates* in the vitreous cavity often called 'puff balls' along with presence of white vitreous opacities forming a 'string of pearls' appearance is a very typical feature.

- *Whitish chorioretinitis lesions* may be associated which may progress with the development of satellite lesions. The chorioretinitis lesions may be bilateral and multiple. Often, extensive lesions may be present in the retinal periphery without causing symptoms.
- *Severe anterior uveitis* without any retinitis lesions may rarely be the presenting feature.
- *Scleritis* may also be a lesion in some cases.
- *Endophthalmitis and event panophthalmitis* usually develop soon in untreated cases.
- *Multiple creamy white lesions* with minimal or no vitritis may be the presenting feature in severely immunocompromised patients.

Figures 6.3.1 to 6.3.4 are clinical photographs of a patient with Candida endophthalmitis.

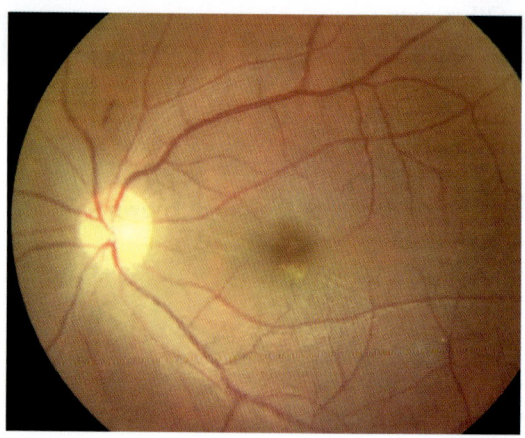

Fig. 6.3.3 *Fundus photograph left eye 2 weeks following pars plana vitrectomy showing improved media clarity of the posterior pole.*

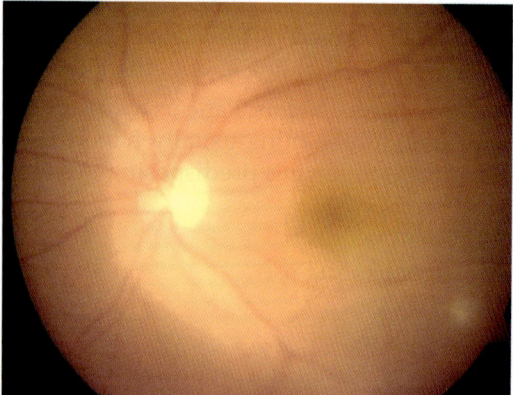

Fig. 6.3.1 *Fundus photograph left eye of a patient with suspected endogenous Candida endophthalmitis showing normal looking posterior pole.*

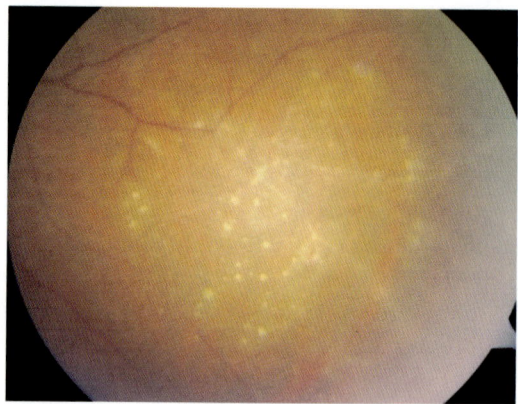

Fig. 6.3.4 *Fundus photograph left eye inferior retina showing vitreous debris with occluded vessels seen typically in endophthalmitis.*

Histopathology

- *Progressive inflammation in the vitreous cavity.* Vitreous is the main site of localisation of yeast, resulting in formation of vitreous abscess.
- *Involvement of retina and uveal tract* is minimal. Retinal vessels are also spared.

ASPERGILLUS UVEITIS

Etiology

Aspergillus species are ubiquitous saprophytic spore-forming moulds commonly present in soil and decaying vegetable matter.

- *Aspergillus fumigatus* is the most common causative agent of human aspergillosis.

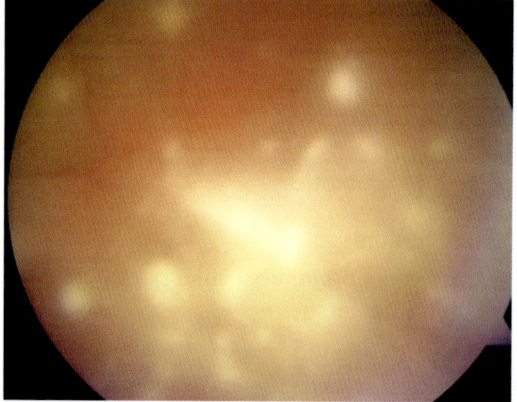

Fig. 6.3.2 *Fundus photograph left eye inferior retina showing puff-balls in the vitreous cavity. The culture was positive for Candida albicans.*

- *Other common species* include A. flavus, A. niger, A. terreus, etc.
- *Ocular involvement* occurs through haemato-genous dissemination of organisms from the lungs.

Risk factors include:

- Severe chronic pulmonary diseases
- Severe immunosuppression, e.g. orthotopic liver transplantation
- Intravenous drug abuse or drug-induced immune suppression.
- Valvular cardiac surgery

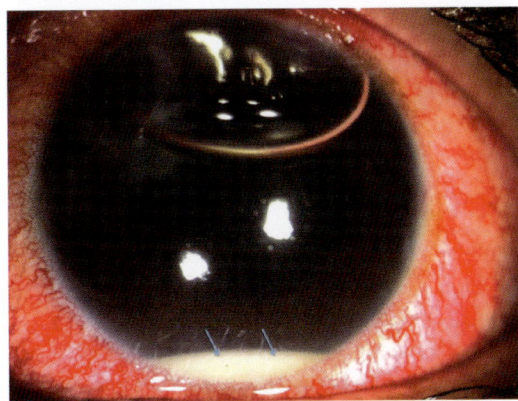

Fig. 6.3.5 *Convex hypopyon (arrows) following cataract surgery.*

Clinical features

Presenting symptoms are characterised by a more rapid onset of pain and decreased vision with more fulminant course.

Clinical signs include:

- *Yellowish infiltrative subretinal or choroidal lesions* which often develop in the macular region and have indistinct margins.
- *Vascular occlusions* may also develop.
- *Subhyloid hypopyon* may develop due to the inferior gravitational layering of inflammatory exudates in either or both the subhyaloid and subretinal space.
- *Full thickness retinal involvement* may occur with abscess formation that may soon break into the vitreous cavity.
- *Vitreous is invaded*, eventually after the breaking of retinal or sublyoid abscess giving a picutre of fungal endophthalmitis.
- *Anterior segment* also involved finally.

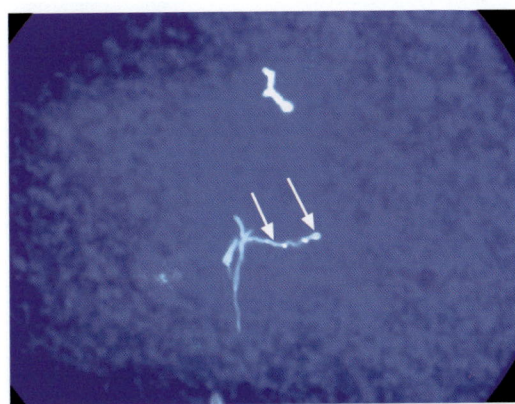

Fig. 6.3.6 *Calcofluor smear from the hypopyon aspirate shows septate hyphae (arrows).*

Figures 6.3.5 to 6.3.10 show clinical presentation, smear pictures, and effect of treatment in two patients with Aspergillus uveitis.

Histology

- *Acute inflammatory response* is seen in the choroid, subretinal space, retina and vitreous.
- *Vessel wall invasion* is common in retinal and choroidal vessels.
- *Vitreous involvement* is relatively less as compared to Candida uveitis.

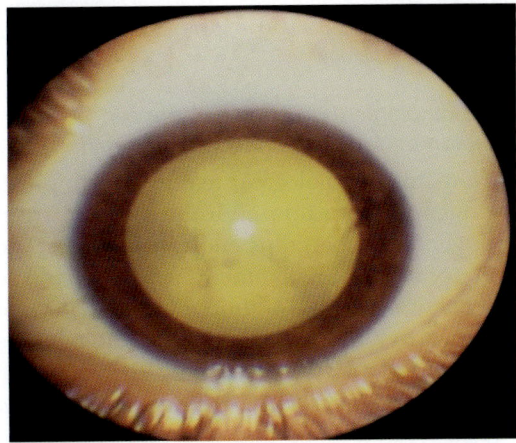

Fig. 6.3.7 *Left eye of a 32-year-old woman shows loss of red reflex following a single infusion of dextrose 5%.*

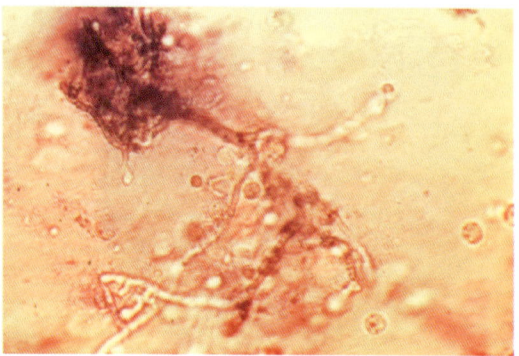

Fig. 6.3.8 *Vitreous tap was done and KOH smear of same eye as in Fig. 6.3.7 shows septate hyphae suggestive of Aspergillus. Culture was positive for Aspergillus fumigatus. Patient underwent pars plana vitrectomy.*

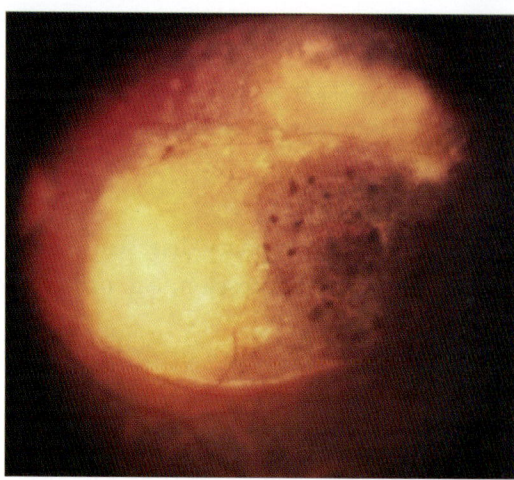

Fig. **6.3.10** *Fundus photograph left eye taken 6 months later shows a large scar.*

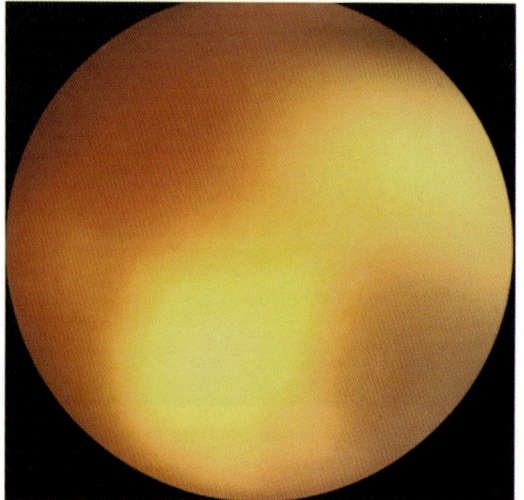

Fig. 6.3.9 *Fundus picture taken 3 days later shows residual abscess on the posterior pole. Patient continued to receive oral antifungal therapy.*

Histopathological differences between Candida and Aspergillus endophthalmitis

Various histopathological features distinguish endogenous Candida endophthalmitis from endogenous Aspergillus endophthalmitis. The primary site of involvement is usually in the inner choroid in both, although rarely it may be confined to the retina. The histopathology has some important differences:

1. *Aspergillus tends to invade the choroidal and retinal vessel walls* and growths along the choriocapillaris; preferentially along sub-retinal pigment epithelium and subretinal space. The vascular invasion is associated with retinal necrosis and haemorrhages and the tendency for horizontal spread results in the development of large scars.

2. *Eyes with Candida show small foci of retinal damage* from invasion of the organisms. Unlike the extensive retinal necrosis and choroidal damage noted histopathologically in eyes with Aspergillus infection. In Candida endophthalmitis, most of the inflammatory response has been found to be in the vitreous in the form of multiple microabscesses surrounding the organisms.

3. *Abscesses* in cases with Candida are multiple and small, while eyes with aspergillosis usually have larger abscesses and macular involvement is more common.

4. *Heavy infiltration of acute inflammatory cells* in the retina, subretinal space and choroid is seen in eyes with Aspergillus endophthalmitis, unlike Candida infection.

FUSARIUM UVEITIS

Etiology

Fusarium is a filamentous mould found commonly in the plants and soil.

• *Endogenous endophthalmitis* due to Fusarium is very rare and has been reported in leukaemia or other severe immunosuppressive states.

• *Exogenous infection* has been reported after cataract surgery.

Clinical features

Clinical features include:

- Fibrinous reaction in anterior chamber,
- Progressive vitritis,
- Retinal ischaemia, and
- Retinal necrosis.

CRYPTOCOCCUS UVEITIS

Etiology

Cryptococcus neoformans (yeast) is found in the pigeon droppings that can be inhaled via respiratory droplets resulting in the development of ocular infection in immunocompromised host.

Ocular Manifestations

Ocular lesions include:

- Multifocal choroiditis,
- Exudative retinal detachment,
- Vasculitis/sheathing,
- Optic disc swelling, and
- Rarely endophthalmitis.

COCCIDIOIDOMYCOSIS

Etiology

Coccidioidomycosis (dimorphic fungus) too is found in the soil and the infection is acquired via respiratory route.

Ocular manifestations

Ocular lesions include:

- Multifocal choroiditis,
- Exudative retinal detachment,
- Vasculitis/sheathing, and
- Retinal haemorrhages.

HISTOPLASMA UVEITIS

Etiology

Histoplasma capsulatum is a diphasic fungus found in the soil. The infection is acquired via respiratory tract due to inhalation of aerosolised bird droppings that contain this fungus. These organisms first enter the lungs and then disseminate through haematogenous route to other organs including liver, spleen, kidney, eye, etc.

Presumed ocular histoplasmosis syndrome (POHS) is thought to be caused by the fungus *Histoplasma capsulatum* (though the fungus has not been isolated from the affected eyes); as the disease is more common in areas where histoplasmosis is endemic (e.g. Mississippi-Ohio-Missouri river vally) and 90% of patients with POHS show positive histoplasmin skin test. POHS has also been reported from United Kingdom, suggesting that perhaps some other etiological agents are also capable of producing the disease.

Ocular manifestations

I. Endophthalmitis: This is seen in generalised systemic disease and shows involvement of retina and uveal tract.

II. Choroidal granuloma that is solitary.

III. Presumed ocular histoplasmosis syndrome (POHS): This syndrome is characterised by the following:

- *Absence of anterior segment and vitreous inflammation* is typical of POHS.
- *Histo spots.* These are atrophic spots scattered in the mid-retinal periphery. They are roundish, yellowish-white lesions measuring 0.2 to 0.7 disc diameter in size. These begin to appear in early childhood and represent the scars of disseminated histoplasma choroiditis.
- *Macular lesion.* It starts as atrophic macular scar (macular histo spot); followed by a hole in the Bruch's membrane, which then allows ingrowth of capillaries leading to subretinal choroidal neovascularisation. Leakage of fluid from the neovascular membrane causes serous detachement, which when complicated by repeated haemorrhages constitutes haemorrhagic detachemnt. Ultimately, there develops fibrous disciform scar, which is associated with a marked permanent visual loss.

Differential diagnosis

Differential diagnosis for POHS includes sarcoidosis, Vogt-Koyanagi-Harada syndrome, sympathetic ophthalmia, punctate inner choroiditis. Majority of the patients with OHS are asymptomatic and may become symptomatic only when they develop CNV in the macular or peripapillary regions. These CNVs need to be managed with anti-VEGF injections with monoclonal antibodies (bevacizumab, ranibizumab, aflibercept). The thermal laser for extrafoveal and juxtafoveal CNVs and subfoveal surgery for subfoveal CNVs is not currently practiced.

MANAGEMENT OF FUNGAL ENDOPHTHALMITIS

Management of fungal endophthalmitis includes:
- Differential diagnosis,
- Investigations,
- Treatment,
- Outcome, and prognosis.

DIFFERENTIAL DIAGNOSIS

Endogenous fungal endophthalmitis may be the first manifestation of an underlying systemic disorder in an apparently healthy individual.

Other conditions that may produce a similar clinical picture are:
- Bacterial endogenous endophthalmitis
- Toxoplasma retinochoroiditis
- Acute retinal necrosis
- CMV retinitis
- Progressive outer retinal necrosis
- Non-infective causes, like sypilitic chorioretinitis, Behcet's disease , primary intraocular lymphoma and other masquerade syndromes.

INVESTIGATIONS

1. *Systemic workup.* A thorough history taking for any predisposing factors, such as intravenous drug abuse, long-standing corticosteroid treatment, organ transplantation, diabetes, etc. should be done. Blood and urine cultures should be sent to establish a disseminated fungal infection although poor sensitivity has been reported even in patients with a proven systemic focus of fungal infection.

2. *Ultrasonography.* In cases with significant vitreous inflammation, it helps in elucidating posterior segment details, such as the extent of vitreous and scleral involvement, presence of any subretinal or choroidal abscess, retinochoroidal thickening and retinal detachment.

3. *Microbiological evaluation.* The vitreous fluid obtained either by doing a vitreous tap or during a diagnostic/therapeutic vitrectomy should be sent for microbiological evaluation, such as KOH, Calcoflour white stain, Gomori Methenamine stain, Gram and Giemsa stain, etc. along with culture sensitivity.

4. *Polymerase chain reaction (PCR).* Since the sensitivity of conventional fungal cultures is not high, and the culture growth rates are slow, longer times are required before final results can be obtained. Thus, an early diagnosis can be important in ensuring prompt and effective management of the endophthalmitis. PCR is well suited for the detection of fungal moieties due to its specificity and applicability for use with small samples, such as ocular specimens.

TREATMENT

I. Medical treatment

Medical management includes oral administration of antifungal drugs for 4–6 weeks to all the patients with endogenous fungal endophthalmitis.

- *Amphotericin B* use has reduced significantly in the recent times due to problem of nephrotoxicity.
- *Newer drugs,* including fluconazole and voriconazole have good ocular bioavailability and can be used more safely.
- *Voriconazole* is effective against both Candida and Aspergillus. Voriconazole dose is 6 mg/kg × 2 doses followed by 4 mg/kg two times a day.
- *Fluconazole* dose is 12 mg/kg loading dose followed by a daily dose of 6–12 mg/kg/day.
- Total duration of therapy is 4–6 weeks and can be extended depending on the patient response.
- *Medical therapy may be given in combination with* pars plana vitrectomy in severe cases and intravitreal antifungal agents in moderate cases. Voriconazole 100 µg/0.1 ml or Amphotericin 5 µg/0.1 ml may be used for intravitreal injections.

II. Surgical treatment: Pars plana vitrectomy

- *Early pars plana vitrectomy* (PPV) is recommended for sight-threatening endogenous endophthalmitis with vitritis.

- *Vitreous sample* obtained at the time of surgery can provide useful information about the diagnosis from smears, cultures and PCR. It also allows removal of loculated areas of infection that would not respond to systemic antifungal agents and decreases the overall burden of organisms.
- *PPV* is usually combined with the administration of intravitreal antifungal agents (discussed above in medical treatment).
- *Half-life of antifungal agents* administered directly into the vitreous after or at the time of vitrectomy is shortened and that repeated administration may be necessary.

OUTCOME AND PROGNOSIS

Key to successful outcome is early diagnosis and management.

Candida endophthalmitis has a relatively better prognosis than Aspergillus.

Factors associated with poor outcome include:
- Poor baseline visual acuity
- Retinal detachments
- Posterior pole involvement resulting in scar at the posterior pole that compromises the visual gain.

BIBLIOGRAPHY

1. Essman TF, Flynn HW Jr, Smiddy WE, et al. Treatment outcomes in a 10-year study of endogenous fungal endophthalmitis. Ophthalmic Surg Lasers 1997;28(3):185–94.
2. Graham DA, Kinyoun JL, George DP. Endogenous Aspergillus endophthalmitis after lung transplantation. Am J Ophthalmol 1995;119:107–9.
3. Gupta A, Gupta V, Dogra MR, Chakrabarti A, Ray P, Ram J, Patnaik B. Fungal endophthalmitis after a single intravenous administration of presumably contaminated Dextrose infusion fluid. Retina 2000;20:262–8.
4. Rao NA, Hidayat A. A comparative clinicopathologic study of endogenous mycotic endophthalmitis: variations in clinical and histopathologic changes in candidiasis compared to aspergillosis. Transactions of the American Ophthalmological Society 2000; 98:183–94.
5. Samiy N, D'Amico DJ. Endogenous fungal endophthalmitis. Int Ophthalmol Clin 1996;36: 147–62.
6. Shen X, Xu G. Vitrectomy for endogenous fungal endophthalmitis. Ocul Immunol Inflamm 2009; 3(3):148–52.
7. Tanaka M, Kobayashi Y, Takebayashi H, et al. Analysis of predisposing clinical and laboratory findings for the development of endogenous fungal endophthalmitis. A retrospective 12-year study of 79 eyes of 46 patients. Retina 2001; 21(3):203–9.

6.4. PARASITIC UVEITIS

6.4.1 OCULAR TOXOPLASMOSIS

Etiopathogenesis
• Toxoplasma gondi
• Hosts
• Life cycle of *T. gondii*
• Transmission of infection
• Pathogenesis of ocular lesions
Clinical Types
Congenital toxoplasmosis
• Clinical feature
Acquired toxoplasmosis
Clinical feature plasmic
Recurrent retinochoroiditis
• Clinical features
Diagnosis
• Clinical diagnosis
• Laboratory diagnosis
Treatment
• Clinical treatment regimen
• Alternative other treatment regimens
• Prophylactic treatment in recurrent cases
• Prophylactic treatment during intraocular surgery

ETIOPATHOGENESIS

Ocular toxoplasmosis is caused by the protozoan parasite *Toxoplasma gondii*. The parasite has been reported to infect approximately 13 to 50% of the world's population. Ocular toxoplasmosis is the most important cause of infectious posterior uveitis worldwide.

Toxoplasma gondii

An obligatory parasite is one that is completely dependent on its host and cannot survive without it, e.g. hookworms.

A facultative parasite is one that can change its lifestyle between free-living in the environment and parasitic according to the surrounding conditions, e.g. *Strongyloides stercoralis*.

Toxoplasma gondii is an intracellular ubiquitous-parasite and exists in three forms:

• *Tachyzoite*, which can infect any nucleated cells,
• *Tissue cysts containing many bradyzoite*, which is formed during chronic phase of infection, and
• *Oocyst* (eggs of the parasite, contains sporozoites), which is formed in intestine of infected cats.

Strains. There are primarily three strains of *Toxoplasma gondii*—namely type I, II and III. Many atypical strains of the organism are also reported.

Hosts

T. gondii has a broad range of hosts. Life cycle of parasite is completed or require following hosts:

Definitive host (DH) that harbours the adult or sexually mature stages of the parasite (or in whom sexual reproduction occurs). Members of cat family are definitive host. This means sexual part of life cycle of the parasite takes place in this hosts.

Intermediate host (IH) that harbours larval or sexually immature stages of the parasite (or in whom asexual reproduction occurs).

Human and other animals (cattle, sheep and pig) are knows intermediate hosts.

Life cycle of Toxoplasma gondii

Replication of *T. gondii* occurs independently by one of the two mechanisms of life cycle (Fig. 6.4.1.1.):
• Sexual cycle
• Asexual cycle

Sexual cycle. Members of the cat family are the definitive hosts and sexual reproduction of the parasite occurs only in the epithelial cells of the feline intestinal tract.

The products of the sexual reproduction, *oocysts* contain *sporozoites*. Once oocysts are shed from cats, they can remain viable in the environment for long periods of time.

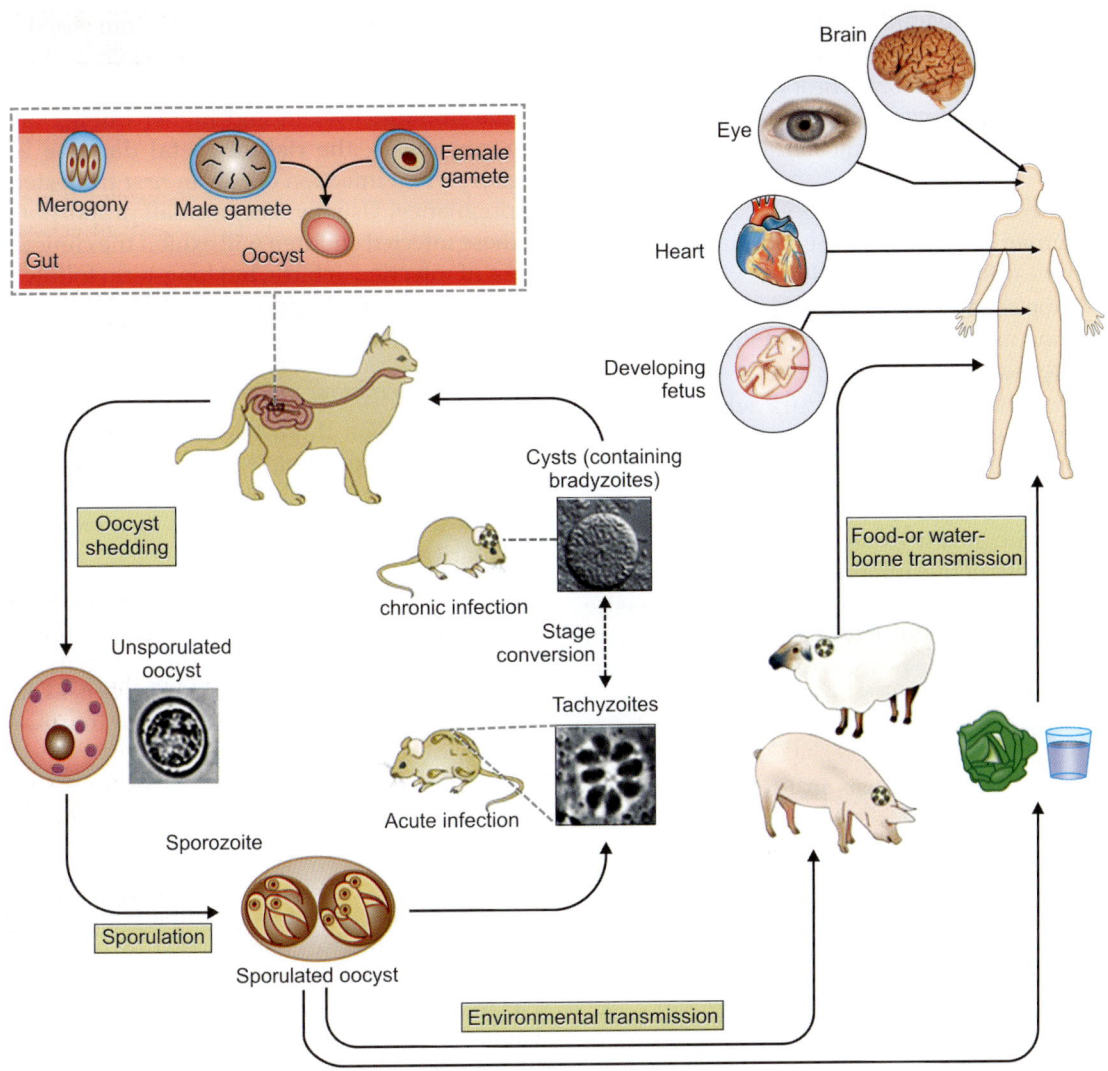

Fig. 6.4.1.1 *Life cycle of Toxoplasma gondii.*

Asexual cycle occurs in any nucleated cell sub-population of any intermediate host. Following ingestion, oocysts develop into the tachyzoites. Tachyzoites eventually undergo asexual reproduction and produce bradyzoites, which persist in the tissues in a viable cyst form. This asexual reproduction can occur in either cats or in intermediate hosts, like pigs, cows, and human beings. The cysts contain hundreds to thousands of bradyzoites, and have a propensity for cardiac tissue, muscle, and neural tissue, including the retina.

Transmission of infection

Human infection with *T. gondii* human, i.e. transmission of the parasite to human being can occur in following ways:

By ingestion of undercooked or raw meat of an intermediate host (lamb, pork, and beef) containing cysts bradyzoites.

By consumption of unwashed vegetables contaminated with oocysts.

- *By inadvertent contamination of hands* when disposing of cat litter trays and then subsequent transfer on to food. Infants can be infected by eating dirt (pica) containing cysts.

• *By transplacental or vertical transmission* of the parasite (tachyzoite) to foetus from mother (congenital toxoplasmosis).

Pathogenesis of ocular lesions

In human being, two forms of the parasite are found—cysts and tachyzoites.

• *Toxoplasma gondii* believed to invade human retina and can transform into cystic form in inner sensory retina.

• *Necrotising retinitis* occurs when the cyst ruptures and tachyzoites replicate in retinal cells with inflammatory reaction to surrounding retina and choroid.

Note. In contrast to tachyzoites, which cause tissue destructive inflammatory disease as they proliferate, cysts do not stimulate tissue inflammation. Cysts have been found to remain viable outside the host in soil for at least 1 year.

CLINICAL TYPES

Systemic toxoplasmosis in humans occurs in three forms:
• Congenital,
• Acquired, and
• Recurrent.

CONGENITAL TOXOPLASMOSIS

Congenital toxoplasmosis is much more common than the acquired form. Fetus gets infestation through transplacental route from the mother.

Scenario of toxoplasmosis in mother

Severity of congenital toxoplasmosis is dependent on the duration of gestation at the time of maternal infection. Maternal infection during early pregnancy may result in stillbirth, whereas infection occurring during late pregnancy may result in convulsions, paralysis, hydrocephalus and visceral involvement.

1. *Infection in mother before pregnancy or in very early pregnancy*

It is to be understood that if mother had contracted the infection earlier or before pregnancy, the maternal antibody developed during the infection, will prevent foetus from *T. gondii*. However, because of the immaturity of the immune system and higher impact on organogenesis, the risk of foetal damage is highest when infection occurs in first trimester of pregnancy. Usually, only a small proportion of these infected children will exhibit the clinical signs of infection at birth, but long-term follow-up has shown that approximately 80% of the infected children will develop sequelae.

2. *Infection in mother in late pregnancy*

Pregnant women those who are not infected with parasite before pregnancy are at the highest risk of transmission of infection to the foetus in the last trimester, possibly due to increased vascularity of the placenta.

Clinical feature

Common clinical features of congenital toxoplasmosis are summarised in Figure 6.4.1.2. An infants may be born with active or inactive disease.

Active disease consisits of retinochoroiditis and is of very-very rare occurrence in congenital toxoplasmosis.

Inactive disease. Most of the infants are born with inactive disease characterised by bilateral punched out heavily pigmented chorioretinal scar in the macular area (Fig. 6.4.1.3), which is usually discovered when the child is brought for defective vision or squint checkup.

ACQUIRED TOXOPLASMOSIS

In the past, acquired toxoplasmosis was considered of doubtful existence and most toxoplasmosis was thought to be congenital but acquired disease is increasingly recognized. The infestation is acquired by eating the undercooked meat of intermediate host containing cyst form of the parasite. Most of the patients are subclinical (asymptomatic); and the typical chorioretinal lesion similar to congenital toxoplasmosis is discovered by chance. Other lesions include punctate outer retinal toxoplasmosis (PORT). More common in HIV + patients.

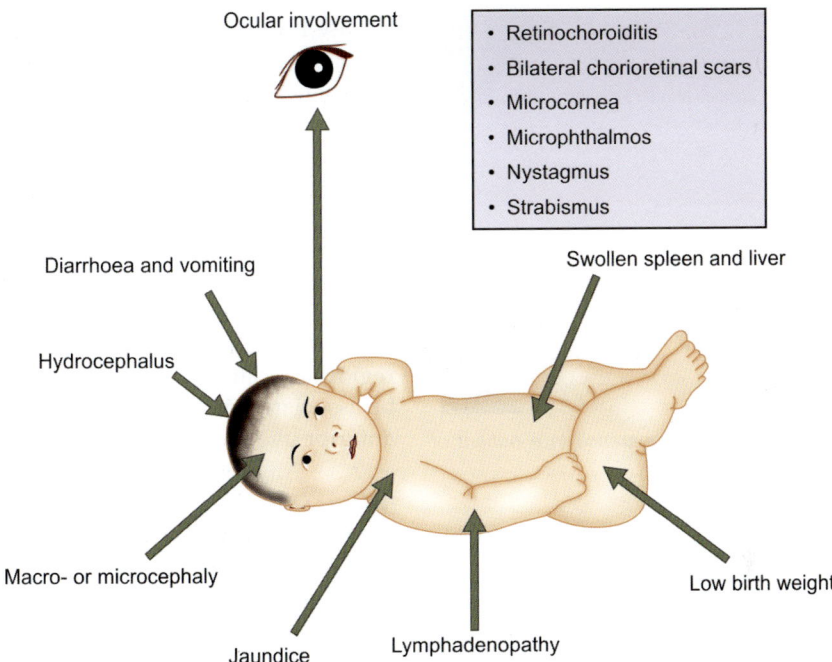

Ocular involvement

- Retinochoroiditis
- Bilateral chorioretinal scars
- Microcornea
- Microphthalmos
- Nystagmus
- Strabismus

Diarrhoea and vomiting

Swollen spleen and liver

Hydrocephalus

Macro- or microcephaly

Low birth weight

Jaundice   Lymphadenopathy

Fig. 6.4.1.2 *Clinical features of congenital toxoplasmosis.*

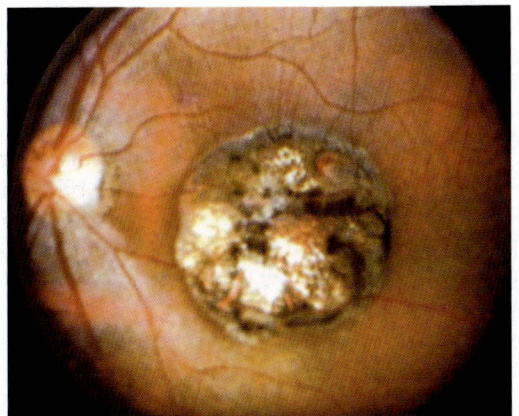

Fig. 6.4.1.3 *Healed central toxoplasma chorioretinits.*

Clinical features

Symptoms

Floaters with or without blurred vision are most common symptoms of ocular toxoplasmosis patients.

- *Severe reduction of vision*, if macula is involved.
- *Ocular pain and redness* are usually uncommon and can occur in case of severe anterior segment inflammation.

Signs

1. *Focal necrotising retinitis:* Ocular toxoplasmosis typically manifests as a localized necrotising retinitis. Characteristic lesion can be seen as a grey-white focus of retinal necrosis at the edge of a pre-existing pigmented chorioretinal scar (satellite lesion).

2. *Dense vitritis:* Vitritis can be severe and sometimes so dense that it can hinder an adequate view of the posterior segment. Visualisation of white retinal lesion hazily through a dense vitritis, has given the dictum *"headlight in the fog"* for ocular toxoplasmosis (Fig. 6.4.1.4).

3. *Granulomatous anterior uveitis:* The associated iritis can be mild to severe with granulomatous features.

4. *Increased intraocular pressure:* Ocular toxoplasmosis may be associated with increased intraocular pressure.

5. *Punctate outer retinal toxoplasmosis (PORT):* PORT is characterised by small multifocal lesions at the level of the deep retina that are associated with scant overlying vitreal inflammation.

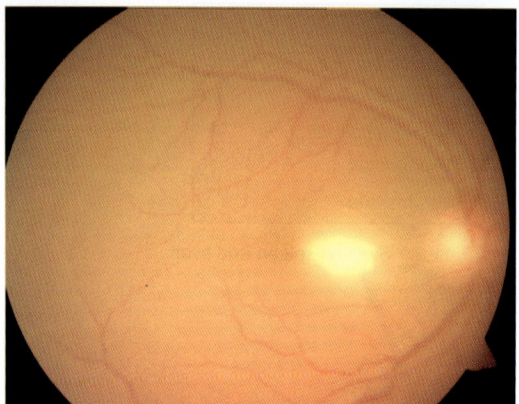

Fig. 6.4.1.4 *Headlight in fog appearance in a patient of ocular toxoplasmosis.*

6. Atypical presentation of ocular toxoplasmosis: Atypical presentation, like retinal vasculitis, neuroretinitis, vitritis, iritis, and papillitis, may also be seen. Recurrences are often seen and may occur years after the original lesion resolved.

7. Ocular toxoplasmosis in immunocompromised individuals: Ocular toxoplasmosis in immunocompromised patients especially in AIDS patients can cause a severe, fulminant disease often with central nervous system involvement, which carries a poor prognosis and may be rapidly fatal, if untreated.

8. Healed lesion of ocular toxoplasmosis: Ocular toxoplasmosis is usually self-limiting disease in immunocompetent patients. The inflammatory response in the eye gradually subsides and the lesions usually heal in 6 to 8 weeks of time. The healing is characterised by sharper border of the retinitis lesions and increased pigmentations. The typical healed lesion of ocular toxoplasmosis is a punched out scar with increased hyperpigmentation at the border of the lesion often mimicking a coloboma.

RECURRENT TOXOPLASMIC RETINOCHOROIDITIS

Pathogenesis. The parasites reaching the foetus through placenta involve its brain and retina, and also excite antibodies formation. After healing of the active retinal lesion (with which the infant is born), the parasites remain encysted therein inactive form. After about 10–40 years (average 25 years), the retinal cysts rupture and release hundreds of parasites, which by direct invasion cause a fresh lesion of focal necrotising retinochoroidits, adjacent to the edge of old inactive pigmented scar. In addition to this lesion, an inflammation in the iris, choroid and retinal vessels is excited due to antigen–antibody reaction.

Characteristic features. Recurrent toxoplasmic retinochoroiditis is a very common disease. It is characterised by a whitish-yellow, slightly rasied area of infiltration located near the margin of old punched out scarred lesion in the macular region associated with severe vitritis. There may be associated non-granulomatous type of mild anterior uveitis.

Clinical diagnosis

Diagnosis of ocular toxoplasmosis is almost always clinical. Laboratory diagnosis of this clinical entity is of paramount importance in cases of atypical presentations, subclinical infections, etc. Also it must be remembered that many of the serological tests used for diagnosis of toxoplasma infection are often positive in general populations and do not necessitate any active treatment.

Serological diagnosis

Serological diagnosis of ocular toxoplasmosis is confirmed by measurement of intraocular parasite-specific antibody production, which is an indirect proof of the presence of the parasite within the eye.

• **An acute T. gondii infection** can be demonstrated by detection of specific IgM or IgA antibodies, or both, in the blood. Immunoglobulin M usually appears in the first week after infection, peaks at 1 month, and disappears after 9 months.

• **For the detection of congenital toxoplasmosis,** IgA antibodies are often used, because the IgM production is still weak in newborns and IgG antibodies can be of maternal origin. Though the presence of anti-*T. gondii* IgG antibodies does not confirm the diagnosis, a negative IgG usually discards the possibility. Anti-*T. gondii* IgG antibodies can persist at high titres for years after the acute infection and there is a high prevalence of such antibodies in the general population.

Thus the presence of specific antibodies in the form of cell-mediated immunity in the blood of patients is not discriminatory for ocular disease and may not even be related to the ocular lesion.

- *Demonstration of local synthesis of specific antibodies* is a valuable diagnostic tool in ocular toxoplasmosis. Intraocular antibody production is considered to be significant, if the relative amount of specific antibodies (compared to the total immunoglobulin level found in the aqueous) exceeds the relative amount of these antibodies in the serum. This intraocular production of antibody can be calculated by the Goldmann-Witmer (GW) coefficient according to the following formula.

GW coefficient = (Intraocular anti-Toxoplasma IgG/intraocular IgG)/(Serum anti-Toxoplasma IgG/serum IgG)

- *Polymerase chain reaction (PCR)* has also been tried for detection of ocular toxoplasmosis. The use of intraocular antibody titre along with PCR yields higher sensitivity. Recently, real-time PCR has been utilised as a rapid and sensitive technique for quantitatively evaluating ocular samples for the presence of *Toxoplasma gondii*.

TREATMENT

As discussed earlier, ocular toxoplasmosis in immunocompetent patient is a self-limiting disease. Small peripheral lesion generally does not require any treatment. However, prompt treatment is warranted for lesions within the temporal arcade, closer proximity to the disc or macula and in cases of severe vitritis.

Various drugs and combination of drugs have been used to treat ocular toxoplasmosis.
Triple therapy. Classicial treatment regiments. The most common treatment for ocular toxoplasmosis consists of pyrimethamine-sulfadiazine combination and corticosteroids.

- *Pyrimethamine.* This therapy consists of an initial dose of 75 to 100 mg of pyrimethamine daily for two days followed by a 25 to 50 mg dose daily.
- *Sulfadiazine* 2 to 4 g daily for two days, followed by a 500 mg to 1 g dose every six hours as well as 5 mg of folinic acid daily for four to six weeks.

- *Oral prednisolone* (1 mg/kg daily) is given from the third day of therapy and tapered over two to six weeks.

Other treatment regimens include:
- *Quadruple drug therapy* (classic regimen plus clindamycin)
- *Single or combined use of clindamycin,* trimethoprim-sulfamethoxazole, spiramycin, minocycline, azithromycin, atovaquone and clarithromycin.
- *Recent regimen.* As the first drug combination for the treatment of ocular toxoplasmosis, the recent choice is trimethoprim (80 mg)/ sulfamethoxazole (400 mg) every 12 hours and oral clindamycin 300 mg four times a day along with oral prednisone (1 mg/kg started after three days). Systemic corticosteroids are used as an adjunct to minimize collateral damage from the inflammatory response.

Treatment during pregnancy, include spiramycin and sulfadiazine (2–4 g PO single dose, loading dose, followed by 1 g PO QID) can be used in the first trimester. Throughout the second trimester, spiramycin, sulfadiazine, pyrimethamine, and folinic acid are recommended. Spiramycin, pyrimethamine, and folinic acid may be used during the third trimester.

Treatment in patients with HIV/AIDS. These patients require extended systemic treatment due to frequent cerebral involvement and high frequency of recurrent ocular disease.

Prophylactic treatment in recurrent cases. Recently, the use of long-term intermittent trimethoprim/sulfamethoxazole (1 tablet taken every 3 day) has recommended to decrease the risk of reaction among patients with recurrent toxoplasmic retinochoroiditis. A similar strategy may be useful as prophylaxis in patients with ocular toxoplasmosis and HIV/AIDS.

Prophylactic treatment during intraocular surgery, e.g. cataract surgery in patient with inactive toxoplasmosis may be considered with anti-toxoplasmic agents, particularly in those with threat to optic disc or fovea. However, still there is no consensus with respect to this treatment approach.

BIBLIOGRAPHY

1. Atmaca LS, Simsek T, Batioglu F. Clinical features and prognosis in ocular toxoplasmosis. Jpn J Ophthalmol 2004;48:386–91.
2. de-la-Torre A, Stanford M, Curi A, Jaffe GJ, Gomez-Marin JE. Therapy for ocular toxoplasmosis. Ocul Immunol Inflamm 2011;19:314–20.
3. Dodds EM. Toxoplasmosis. Cur Opin Ophthalmol 2006;17:557–61.
4. G, Rabiah P, McLeod R, Brézin A. Clinical manifestations of ocular toxoplasmosis. Ocul Immunol Inflamm 2011;19:91–102.
5. Garweg JG. Determinants of immunodiagnostic success in human ocular toxoplasmosis. Parasite Immunol 2005;27:61–68.
6. Glasner PD, Silveira C, Kruszon-Moran D, Martins MC, Júnior MB, Silveira S, Camargo ME, Nussenblatt RB, Kaslow RA, Júnior RB. An unusually high prevalence of ocular toxoplasmosis in southern Brazil. Am J Ophthalmol 1992;114:136–44.
7. Holland GN, Lewis KG. An update on current practices in the management of ocular toxoplasmosis. Am J Ophthalmol 2002;134:102–14.
8. Holland GN. Ocular toxoplasmosis: a global reassessment. Part I: Epidemiology and course of disease. Am J Ophthalmol 2003;136:973–88.
9. Noble A. Cataracts in congenital toxoplasmosis. J AAPOS. 2007;11:551–4.
10. Park YH. Toxoplasma gondii in the peripheral blood of patients with ocular toxoplasmosis. Br J Ophthalmol 2012;96:766.
11. Perkins ES. Ocular toxoplasmosis. Br J Ophthalmol 1973;57:1–17.
12. Schuman JS, Weinberg RS, Ferry AP, Guerry RK. Toxoplasmic scleritis. Ophthalmology 1988; 95:1399–1403.

6.4.2 TOXOCARIASIS

• Etiology
• Clinical features
• Differential diagnosis and diagnosis
• Prognosis and treatment

ETIOLOGY

Causative nematode. Toxocariasis is an infestation caused by an intestinal ascaris (roundworm) of dogs (*Toxocara canis*) and cats (*Toxocara cati*).

Pathogenesis. The eggs produced by the worms are released in the faeces of their natural hosts, i.e. dogs and cats. The humans, more commonly the young children (average age 7.5 years) who play with dogs and cats or eat dirt, are infested by ova of toxocara. After humans ingest Toxocara eggs, the larvae hatch. In humans, the nematodes larvae do not develop into adult worm but instead penetrate the intestinal mucosa, from which they are carried by the circulation to a wide variety of organs and may cause severe systemic infection labelled as visceral larva migrans (VLM) and ocular toxocariasis.

Visceral larva migrans (VLM) versus ocular toxocariasis is depicted in Table 6.4.2.1.

CLINICAL FEATURES OF OCULAR TOXOCARIASIS

Ocular toxocariasis is the ocular infestation by the larvae of toxocara. The condition is almost always unilatereal.

Presenting symptoms include:
• *Defective vision* in one eye.
• *Pain and photophobia* may be associated.

Table 6.4.2.1 *Visceral larva migrans versus ocular toxocariasis*

Features	VLM	Ocular toxocariasis
• Average age of onset	• 2 years	• 7.5 years
• History of pica	• Positive	• Less common
• General condition	• Child sick with history of fever, hepatosplenomegaly pneumonitis and even convulsions	• Healthy child
• White cell count	• Leucocytosis	• Normal
• Eosinophil count	• Eosinophilia	• Normal

- *Leucocoria* may be present in 25% of cases.
- *Strabismus* may be a presenting complaint in few patients.

Presenting signs include:

Anterior segment signs. The eye is typically white and quiet. However, non-granulomatous anterior inflammation and posterior synechiae may be present with severe disease.

Posterior segment signs

Common presentations are three distinct entities:
- Toxocara chronic endophthalmitis (in 25% of cases)
- Posterior pole granuloma (in 25% of cases)
- Peripheral granuloma (in 25% of cases)

Uncommon presentations include:
- Optic nerve granuloma
- Unilateral pars planitis with diffuse inflammatory exudates.

Chronic toxocara endophthalmitis

Age of onset is 2–10 years, seen in 25% of cases.

Characteristic lessons include:
- *Anterior uveitis* unilateral and chronic.
- *Leukocoria* due to marked vitreous clouding. Thus the condition may mimic retinoblastoma.
- *Vitreous clouding* is a common feature (Fig. 6.4.2.1).
- *Cyclictic membrane* may also be formed.

Posterior pole granuloma

Age of onset is 6–14 years with unilateral visual impairment. Seen in 25% of cases.

Characteristic lesions include:
- *Granuloma* is seen as a yellowish-white round, solitary, raised nodule, about 1–2 disc diameter in size located either at the macula or in the centrocaecal area.
- *Signs of inflammations.* Cells and flare in the anterior segment as well as posterior segment are either absent or minimal.
- *Associated features* include vitreoretinal traction bands with or without localized tractional retinal detachment (TRD).

Peripheral granuloma

Age of onset varies from 6–40 years.

Characteristic features include:
- *Presenting symptoms.* May present with defective vision or peripheral granuloma may be asymptomatic and remain undetected throughout the life.
- *Incidence.* It is seen in about 50% of cases.
- *Peripheral granuloma* is seen as hemispheric mass, usually situated anterior to the equator (Fig. 6.4.2.2).
- *Associated features* include dense connective tissue strands in the vitreous cavity that may connect to disc and may even cause its dragging.
- *Signs of inflammation,* i.e. cells and flare, in the anterior as well as posterior segment are either absent or minimal.

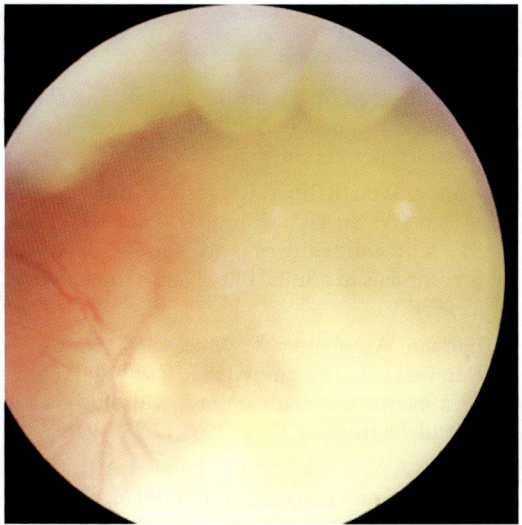

Fig. 6.4.2.1 *Toxocara endophthalmitis.*

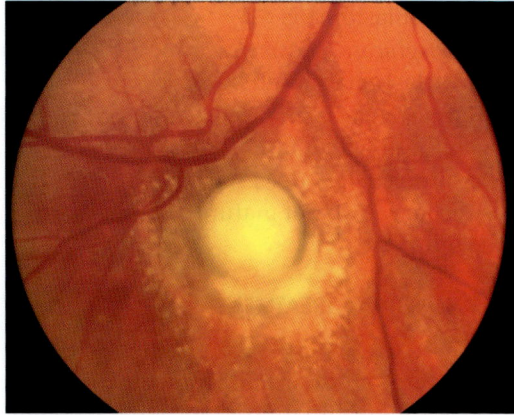

Fig. 6.4.2.2 *Peripheral granuloma in toxocariasis.*

DIFFERENTIAL DIAGNOSIS AND DIAGNOSIS

Differential diagnosis

Leukocoria due to toxocariasis needs to be differentiated from:

- *Retinoblastoma*, and
- *Other causes of leukocoria* in children, such as toxoplasmosis, persistent hyperplastic primary vitreous (PHPV), Coat's disease, advanced stage of retinopathy of prematurity (ROP), focal choroiditis in sarcoidosis or some other cause, and massive pars planitis.

Diagnosis

Clinical diagnosis is suspected from the characteristic features in children.

Investigations useful in arriving at diagnosis includes:

- *ELISA.* It is the most reliable and readily available test for evaluation of antibodies directed against toxocara. However, a positive test is consistent with but not necessarily diagnostic.
- *Ultrasound and CT scan* are useful in ruling out retinoblastoma due to absence of calcification in patients presenting with leukocoria. Also help in detecting vitreous bands and tractional retinal detachment.
- *OCT* can demonstrate larva which may produce a highly reflective signature, moving in the nerve fibre layer.
- *Fundus fluorescent angiography* may demonstrate signs of inflammatory disease.
- *Lactate dehydrogenase* aqueous to serum ratio in retinoblastoma is >1.
- *Phosphoglucose to isomerase* ratio in eyes with retinoblastoma should be >2.
- *Eosinophilia and hyperglobulinaemia* may be seen in children with VLM.
- *Stool examination* does not demonstrate ova, as the larvae do not mature to adult worm in the human.

PROGNOSIS AND TREATMENT

Prognosis

Prognosis is poor in children with chronic toxocara endophthalmitis. In general, determinants of the visual prognosis are:

- Degree of intraocular inflammation,
- Location of the inflammatory foci with respect to fovia,
- Presence or absence of CME, and
- Tractional membranes involving the optic nerve, macula and ciliary body.

Treatment

Treatment of toxocariasis still remains unclear and unsatisfactory. Suggested measures include:

Steroids, either periocular or systemic, may be used to reduce inflammation and prevent structural complications of the disease.

Antihelminthic drugs, such as thiabendazole or diethylcarbamazine should not be used alone, as the larvae per se may not induce that much inflammation as the killed one may. Therefore, these drugs, if at all to be given should be after the start of systemic steroids.

Vitrectomy, especially in chronic toxocara endophthalmitis, has been suggested as method to manage secondary effects of toxocariasis. Reports on successful removal of toxocara granuloma by vitrectomy are also available.

Enucleation with intraorbital implant may be required in children with irreversible visual loss, with hypotony and phthisis bulbi.

BIBLIOGRAPHY

1. Ahn SJ, Woo SJ, Hyon JY, Park KH. Cataract formation associated with ocular toxocariasis. J Cataract Refract Surg 2013;39:830–5.
2. Ahn SJ, Woo SJ, Jin Y, Chang YS, Kim TW, Ahn J, Heo JW, Yu HG, Chung H, Park KH, Hong ST. Clinical features and course of ocular toxocariasis in adults. PLoSNegl Trop Dis 2014; 8:e2938.
3. Barisani-Asenbauer T, Maca SM, Hauff W, Kaminski SL, Domanovits H, Theyer I, Auer H. Treatment of ocular toxocariasis with albendazole. J Ocul Pharmacol Ther. 2001;17:287–94.
4. Biglan AW, Glickman LT, Lobes LA Jr. Serum and vitreous Toxocara antibody in nematode endophthalmitis. Am J Ophthalmol 1979; 88:898–901.

5. Despommier D. Toxocariasis: clinical aspects, epidemiology, medical ecology, and molecular aspects. Clin Microbiol Rev 2003;16:265–72.

6. Gillespie SH, Dinning WJ, Voller A, Crowcroft NS. The spectrum of ocular toxocariasis. Eye (Lond)1993;7(Pt 3):415–8.

7. Good B, Holland CV, Taylor MR, Larragy J, Moriarty P, O'Regan M. Ocular toxocariasis in school children. Clin Infect Dis 2004;39:173–8.

8. Maetz HM, Kleinstein RN, Federico D, Wayne J. Estimated prevalence of ocular toxoplasmosis and toxocariasis in Alabama. J Infect Dis 1987; 156:414.

9. Maguire AM, Green WR, Michels RG, Erozan YS. Recovery of intraocular Toxocara canis by pars plana vitrectomy. Ophthalmology 1990; 97:675–80.

10. Mirdha BR, Khokar SK. Ocular toxocariasis in a North Indian population. J Trop Pediatr 2002;48:328–30.

11. Rubinsky-Elefant G, Hirata CE, Yamamoto JH, Ferreira MU. Human toxocariasis: diagnosis, worldwide seroprevalences and clinical expression of the systemic and ocular forms. Ann Trop Med Parasitol 2010;104:3–23.

12. Shields JA. Ocular toxocariasis. A review. Surv Ophthalmol 1984;28:361–81.

13. Stewart JM, Cubillan LD, Cunningham ET Jr. Prevalence, clinical features, and causes of vision loss among patients with ocular toxocariasis. Retina 2005;25:1005–13.

14. Suzuki T, Joko T, Akao N, Ohashi Y. Following the migration of a Toxocara larva in the retina by optical coherence tomography and fluorescein angiography. Jpn J Ophthalmol 2005;49:159–61.

15. Wilkinson CP, Welch RB. Intraocular toxocara. Am J Ophthalmol 1971;71:921–30.

16. Woodhall D, Starr MC, Montgomery SP, Jones JL, Lum F, Read RW, Moorthy RS. Ocular toxocariasis: epidemiologic, anatomic, and therapeutic variations based on a survey of ophthalmic subspecialists. Ophthalmology 2012;119:1211–7.

17. Yokoi K, Goto H, Sakai J, Usui M. Clinical features of ocular toxocariasis in Japan. Ocul Immunol Inflamm 2003;11:269–75.

18. Zygulska-Machowa H, Ziobrowski S. A case of ocular toxocariasis treated by xenon photo-coagulation. Klin Oczna 1987;89:213–4.

6.4.3 CYSTICERCOSIS

Etiopathogenesis
• Causative tapeworm
- Life cycle of taenia solium
• Transmission to human
Clinical Features
• Systemic cysticercosis
• Ocular cysticercosis
Diagnosis
• Clinical diagnosis
• B-san ultrasonography
• Diagnostic criteria for human cysticercosis
Treatment
• Medical treatment
• Destruction of larvae in situ
• Surgical remove of larvae

ETIOPATHOGENESIS

Causative tapeworm

Taeniasis in humans is a parasitic infection caused by the tapeworm species *Taenia saginata* (beef tapeworm), *Taenia solium* (pork tapeworm), and *Taenia asiatica* (Asian tapeworm). Taeniasis is commonly seen in Latin America, Eastern Europe, China and Southeast Asia.

Cysticercosis is caused by *Cysticercus cellulose*, the larval form of pork tapeworm, *Taenia solium* and occasionally by the larvae of beef tapeworm, *T. saginata*.

Life cycle of Taenia Solium

Hosts. The complete life-cycle of *Taenia solium* involves two hosts the pig and the human and life cycle of *Taenia saginata* involves the cow and the human. Humans act as the *definitive host* and pigs and cattle act as *intermediate hosts* for these parasites. Human beings harbour the adult tapeworm in their small intestines (Fig. 6.4.3.1).

Adult tapeworm consists of a scolex and a strobila.
• *Scolex* is the organ of attachment and consists of four suckers.
• *Strobila* consists of several segments known as proglottids. The mature proglottids are hermephroditic and produce eggs. The gravid or egg-carrying proglottids may contain 40,000–100,000 eggs depending on the species

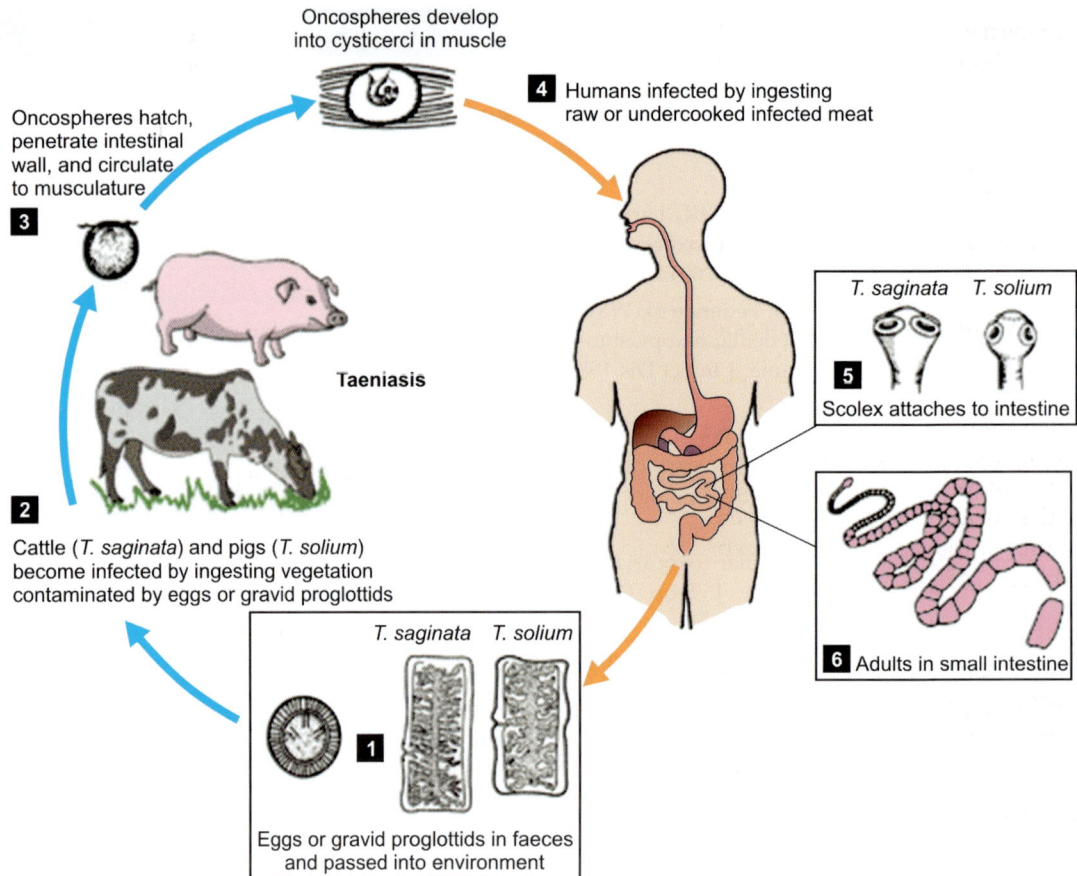

Fig. 6.4.3.1 *Life cycle of Taenia solium and Taenia saginata.*

of Taenia. These proglottids and the eggs are released with the faeces of infected individuals, which serve as a source of infection for pigs and cattle. After the ingestion of eggs, mature larvae or oncospheres are released in the gut of pigs and cattle and enter the bloodstream by penetrating the small intestine and migrate to skeletal and cardiac muscles where they develop into cysticerci. Cysticerci can survive in the host tissues for several years causing cysticercosis. The consumption of raw or undercooked meat containing cysticerci facilitates the spread of infection from pigs and cattle to humans.

Transmission to human

- *Human taeniasis*, i.e. intestinal tapeworm infestation in humans occurs by eating contaminated raw pork or beef.

- *Cysticerci transform into adult tapeworms* in humans which persist in the small intestines for years causing taeniasis.

- *Human cysticercosis*, i.e. infestations of body tissue by *Cyticercus cellulose* the larvae form of *Taenia solium* (pork tapeworm) occurs by drinking contaminated water or eating food contaminated with eggs of Taenia. The eggs are usually derived from faeces of contact with a taperworm carrier.

- *Autoinfection* may occur, if an individual with egg-producing taperworm ingests eggs derived from his or her own faeces.

CLINICAL FEATURES

Systemic cysticercosis

Systemic cysticercosis can occur any where in the body, but more commonly include:

Neurocysticercosis that can be detected in brain and cerebrospinal fluid (CSF) and can manifest as:

- Seizures
- Hydrocephalous, and
- Signs of raised intracranial pressure

Skeletal muscle cysticercosis anywhere in the body.

Subcutaneous tissue cysticercosis.

Ocular cysticercosis

Ocular cysticercosis can involve any part of the ocular system from orbit to the visual cortex. Symptoms of ocular cysticercosis largely depend on the location of the involvement and the severity of the inflammatory response induced at the site of involvement.

Types of ocular cysticercosis

Orbital cysticercosis can present as periocular swelling, proptosis and ptosis associated restriction of ocular motility. Superior rectus is the most commonly involved muscle.

Adnexal cysticercosis can involve eyelids, conjunctiva and rarely lacrimal gland.

Cysticercosis of the eyelid presents as a painless nodule.

Subconjunctival cysticercosis presents as painful epibulbar masses with congestion that move under the conjunctiva (Fig. 6.4.3.2).

Intraocular cysticercosis. Live cysticercus usually induces a mild to moderate inflammatory reaction in the anterior chamber or vitreous. Severe inflammatory response occurs when the parasite dies inside the eye. Death of a large cysticercus inside the eye usually results in blindness and phthisis, probably resulting from the release of chemical toxins from the parasite and subsequent intraocular inflammation.

- *Anterior chamber cysticercosis* has been reported to occur as free-floating cyst producing minimal inflammation. However, a dead parasite can produce severe iritis. The anterior segment signs are variable and range from a quiet eye without congestion to keratic precipitates with severe anterior chamber cellular reaction with or without a hypopyon.
- *Posterior segment* is the most commonly involved and anterior localisation of the cysts is less common. Cysticercus has been found more frequently in the subretinal space than in the vitreous cavity. Usually, in the early larval stage, the parasite enters the eye by the posterior ciliary arteries and rests in the subretinal space, often in the macular area. It may occasionally perforate the retina and reach the vitreous cavity.
- *Vitreous inflammation*, retinal detachment and proliferative vitreoretinopathy can occur. Vitritis is the most common posterior segment finding.
- *Intravitreal cysticerci* (Fig. 6.4.3.3) appear as translucent fluid-filled whitish cysts which measure approximately 3–6 disc diameters in size. Inside the cyst, a dense, white spot

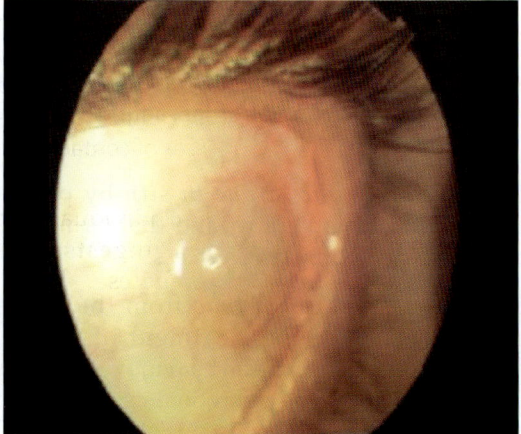

Fig. 6.4.3.2 *Subconjunctival cysticercosis.*

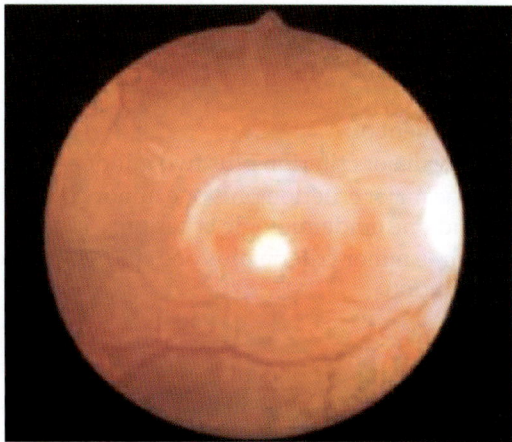

Fig. 6.4.3.3 *Intravitreal cysticercosis.*

corresponding to scolex can be seen. Sometimes movement of the cyst wall can be seen with indirect ophthalmoscopic examination.

- *Subretinal cysticercosis* can appear as acute retinitis with retinal oedema, haemorrhages and subretinal exudates retinal vessel sheathing, serous or exudative retinal detachment. If macula is involved, patients with subretinal cysticercosis may present with the complaints of a sudden central visual loss.

Optic nerve or CNS involvement may present with gradual painless diminution of vision, seizures or symptoms related to increased intracranial pressure.

Diagnosis

Clinical diagnosis of ocular cysticercosis is made from typical features described above.

- Often a part of large intravitreal cysticercus can be seen through the clear lens in careful slit-lamp examination.

B-scan ultrasonography is useful, particularly in the presence of opaque media. It shows well outlined round to oval echoluscent cyst with an echo dense nodule near inner wall of the cyst, which represents the scolex. In kinetic ultrasonography, spontaneous movement of the scolex can be seen. It is of paramount importance to rule out neurocysticercosis by neuroimaging studies in cases of diagnosed ocular cysticercosis.

Diagnostic criteria for human cysticercosis summarised in Table 6.4.3.1 is as below:

- *Diagnosis is confirmed by* either one absolute criterion or a combination of two major criteria, one minor criterion, and one epidemiologic criterion.
- Probable diagnosis is supported by the fulfillment of:
  1. One major criterion plus two minor criteria;
  2. One major criterion plus one minor criterion and one epidemiologic criterion;
  3. Three minor criteria plus one epidemiologic criterion.

Treatment

Medical treatment of ocular cysticercosis:

- *Antihelminthic drugs,* such as praziquantel is not helpful. The dead parasite also can cause severe inflammation.

Table 6.4.3.1 *Diagnostic criteria for human cysticercosis*

I. *Absolute criteria*
1. Demonstration of cysticerci by histologic or microscopic examination of biopsy material
2. Visualization of the parasite in the eye by funduscopy
3. Neuroradiologic demonstration of cystic lesions containing a characteristic scolex

II. *Major criteria*
1. Neuroradiologic lesions suggestive of neurocysticercosis
2. Demonstration of antibodies to cysticerci in serum by enzyme-linked immunoelectrotransfer blot
3. Resolution of intracranial cystic lesions spontaneously or after therapy with albendazole or praziquantel alone

III. *Minor criteria*
1. Lesions compatible with neurocysticercosis detected by neuroimaging studies
2. Clinical manifestations suggestive of neurocysticercosis
3. Demonstration of antibodies to cysticerci or cysticercal antigen in cerebrospinal fluid by ELISA (enzyme-linked immunosorbent assay)
4. Evidence of cysticercosis outside the central nervous system (e.g. cigar-shaped soft tissue calcifications)

IV. *Epidemiologic criteria*
1. Residence in a cysticercosis-endemic area
2. Frequent travel to a cysticercosis-endemic area
3. Household contact with an individual infected with *Taenia solium*

Source: Modified froms Del Brutto et al.

- *Systemic steroids* control inflammation together with surgical removal of larvae in preferred treatment.

Destruction of the larvae in situ by photocoagulation, cryotherapy, and diathermy has been reported with some success.

Surgical removal of larvae from the eye is considered to be the treatment of choice. Intravitreous cysticerci can be removed by pars plana vitrectomy and subretinal cysticerci can be removed by the transvitreous or trans-scleral route.

BIBLIOGRAPHY

1. Adegbehingbe BO, Soetan EO, Adeoye AO. Case report: intraocular cysticercosis. West Afr J Med 2003; 22(4):354–5.
2. Bartholomew RS. Subretinal cysticercosis. Am J Ophthalmol 1975; 79:670–3.
3. Chandra A, Singh MK, Singh VP, et al. A live cysticercosis in anterior chamber leading to glaucoma secondary to pupilary block. J Glaucoma 2007; 16(2):271–3.
4. Jain IS, Dhir SP, Chattopadhaya PR, Kumar P. Ocular cysticercosis in North India. Indian J Ophthalmol 1979; 27(2):54–8.
5. Kapoor S, Kapoor MS. Ocular cysticercosis. J Pediatr Ophthalmol Strabismus 1978; 15(3):170–3.
6. Labh RK, Sharma AK. Ptosis: a rare presentation of ocular cysticercosis. Nepal J Ophthalmol 2013; 5(9):133–5.
7. Li JJ, Zhang LW, Li H, Hu ZL. Clinical and pathological characteristics of intraocular cysticercosis. Korean J Parasitol 2013;51(2):223–9.
8. Messner KH, Kammerer WS. Intraocular cysticercosis. Arch Ophthalmol 1979; 97(6):1103–5.
9. Murthy GR, Rao AV. Sub-conjunctival cysticercosis. Indian J Ophthalmol 1980 28(2):77–8.
10. Natarajan S, Malpani A, Kumar Nirmalan P, Dutta B. Management of intraocular cysticercosis. Graefes Arch Clin Exp Ophthalmol 1999; 237(10):812–4.
11. Pushker N, Bajaj MS, Chandra M, et al. Ocular and orbital cysticercosis. Acta Ophthalmol Scand 2001; 79(4):408–13.
12. Rath S, Honavar SG, Naik M, Anand R, Agarwal B, Krishnaiah S, et al. Orbital cysticercosis: clinical manifestations, diagnosis, management, and outcome. Ophthalmology 2010; 117(3):600–5, 605.e1.
13. Sachdeva RS, Manchanda SK, Abrol S, et al. Freely mobile cysticercus in the anterior chamber. Indian J Ophthalmol 1995; 43(3):135–6.
14. Seo MS, Woo JM, Park YG. Intravitreal cysticercosis. Korean J Ophthalmol 1996; 10(1):55–9.
15. Sharma T, Sinha S, Shah N, et al. Intraocular cysticercosis: clinical characteristics and visual outcome after vitreoretinal surgery. Ophthalmology 2003; 110(5):996–1004.
16. Topilow HW, Yimoyines DJ, Freeman HM, et al. Bilateral multifocal intraocular cysticercosis. Ophthalmology 1981; 88(11):1166–72.
17. Wood TR, Binder PS. Intravitreal and intracameral cysticercosis. Ann Ophthalmol 1979; 11(7):1033–6.
18. Ziaei M, Elgohary M, Bremner FD. Orbital cysticercosis, case report and review. Orbit 2011; 30(5):230–5.

6.4.4 DIFFUSE UNILATERAL SUBACUTE NEURORETINITIS

- Etiology
- Clinical features
- Diagnosis and differential diagnosis

Diffuse unilateral subacute neuroretinitis (DUSN) is the term coined by Gas in 1978 to denote a typical set of presence of neuroretinitis associated within an otherwise normal young healthy individual subretinal mobile nematodes causing unilateral blindness.

ETIOLOGY

Causative nematodes over the year it has been reported that probably yet not confirmed, DUS or is caused by following two types of members:

1. *Ancylostoma caninum* (dog roundworm) or *Toxocara canis*, a small nematode measuring 400–1000 μm in length, over seen in most patients who lived in southeastern United States and was also reported in Caribbean and South America (Brazil).
2. *Baylisascaris procyonis* (the raccoon roundworm), a large worm that measles about 1500–2000 μm in length, has been seen in patients residing in northern and midwestern states and in Germany, China and Brazil.

Pathogenesis. The human gets infested after ingesting the eggs of nematodes. From these eggs, the larvae hatch and penetrate the intestinal mucosa from which they are carried by circulation to a wide variety of organ and tissues. Ocular form of larva migrans syndrome occurs when the larvae invade the eye and produce intraocular information.

CLINICAL FEATURES

Clinical features of DUSN can be described in two stages:

Early stage of DUSN

The young, otherwise healthy, patients present with an insidious onset of unilateral loss of central vision associated with transient visual obscuration.

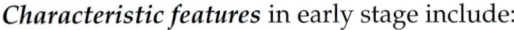

Characteristic features in early stage include:

- Vitritis, moderate to severe
- Optic disc, swelling (popillitis)
- Post equatorial fundus lesions, which are multiple, focal, evancscent, grey – white outer retinal lesions that vary in size from 1200 to 1500 μm. These may be associated with overlying serious retinal detachment. Subretinal mobile worms of small and large size have been reported to be visible in this stage.

Late stage of DUSN

Characteristic features of this stage reported include:

- Retinal arteriolar narrowing
- Optic atrophy
- Diffuse pigment epithelial degeneration, and
- Subretinal scarring.

DIAGNOSIS AND DIFFERENTIAL DIAGNOSIS

Differential diagnosis

Differential diagnosis of early stage of DUSN need to be made from:

- Sarcoid-associated uveitis
- Multifocal choroiditis and panuveitis (MCP) syndrome
- Acute posterior multifocal placoid pigment epitheliopathy (APMPPE)
- Multiple evanescent white dot syndrome (MEWDS)
- Serpiginous choroidopathy
- Behcet's disease
- Ocular toxoplasmosis
- Ocular histoplasmosis syndrome (OHP)
- Non-specific optic neuritis, and papillitis

Differential diagnosis in late stage of DUSN includes:

- Post-traumatic chorioretinopathy,
- Retinal vascular occlusion,
- Toxic retinopathy, and
- Retinitis pigmentosa.

Investigations

1. *Electroretinogram* (ERG) is subnormal even in early stage.

2. *Fluorescein angiography* demonstrates fluorescence of the gray-white lesions in the early angiogram stages. Perivascular staining and motted RPE window defects are also seen.
3. *ICG* demonstrates choroidal areas of hypofluorescence suggesting involvement of choroid in addition to subretinal space.

Definitive diagnosis

Definitive diagnosis is made when the careful examination with a contact lens or 90D/78D fundus examination demonstrates a mobile worm moving in the subretinal space. It may not be possible in every case because of marked vitritis.

TREATMENT

1. *Systemic corticosteroids* may help in transiently controlling inflammation, soon followed by recurrence.
2. *Antihelminthic drugs*, oral thiabendazole or albendazole may be helpful by killing the worm.
3. *Direct laser photocoagulation* of the worm, when localized in the early stage of disease, may be highly effective in halting progression of the disease and improving the vision. Laser should be applied first surrounding the nematode with a ring of burn, which restrict its movement, and then apply heavy burn to the entire area.

BIBLIOGRAPHY

1. Arevalo JF, Arevalo FA, Garcia RA, de Amorim Garcia Filho CA, de Amorim Garcia CA. Diffuse unilateral subacuteneuroretinitis. J Pediatr Ophthalmol Strabismus 2013;50(4):204–12.
2. Cai J, Wei R, Zhu L, Cao M, Yu S. Diffuse unilateral subacute neuroretinitis in China. Arch Ophthalmol 2000;118(5):721–2.
3. Cialdini AP, de Souza EC, Avila MP. The first South American case of diffuse unilateral subacute neuroretinitis caused by a large nematode. Arch Ophthalmol 1999;117(10):1431–2.
4. de Souza EC, Abujamra S, Nakashima Y, Gass JD. Diffuse bilateral subacute neuroretinitis: first patient with documented nematodes in both eyes. Arch Ophthalmol 1999;117(10):1349–51.
5. de Souza EC, Nakashima Y. Diffuse unilateral subacuteneuroretinitis. Report of transvitreal surgical removal of a subretinal nematode. Ophthalmology 1995;102(8):1183–6.

6. deAmorim Garcia Filho CA, Gomes AH, de A Garcia Soares AC, de Amorim Garcia CA. Clinical features of 121 patients with diffuse unilateral subacute neuroretinitis. Am J Ophthalmol 2012; 153(4):743–9.

7. Garcia CA, Gomes AH, Garcia Filho CA, Vianna RN. Early-stage diffuse unilateral subacute neuroretinitis: improvement of vision after photo-coagulation of the worm. Eye 2004;18(6):624–7.

8. Gass JD, Callanan DG, Bowman CB. Oral therapy in diffuse unilateral subacute neuroretinitis. Arch Ophthalmol 1992;110(5):675–80.

9. Gass JD, Scelfo R. Diffuse unilateral subacute-neuroretinitis. J R Soc Med 1978;71(2):95–111.

10. Gass JDM. Diffuse unilateral subacute neuro-retinitis. Stereoscopic Atlas of Macular Disease: Diagnosis and Treatment, 4th ed. 1997;622–8.

11. Harto MA, Rodriguez-Salvador V, Aviñó JA, Duch-Samper AM, Menezo JL. Diffuse unilateral subacute neuroretinitis in Europe. Eur J Ophthalmol 1999;9(1):58–62.

12. Martidis A, Greenberg PB, Rogers AH, Velázquez-Estades LJ, Baumal CR. Multifocal electro-retinography response after laser photo-coagulation of a subretinal nematode. Am J Ophthalmol 2002;133(3):417–9.

13. Mets MB, Noble AG, Basti S, Gavin P, Davis AT, Shulman ST, et al. Eye findings of diffuse unilateral subacute neuroretinitis and multiple choroidal infiltrates associated with neural larva migrans due to baylisascaris procyonis. Am J Ophthalmol 2003;135(6):888–90.

14. Meyer-Riemann W, Petersen J, Vogel M. [An attempt to extract an intraretinal nematode located in the papillomacular bundle]. Klin Monatsbl Augenheilkd 1999;214(2):116–9.

15. Moraes LR, Cialdini AP, Avila MP, Elsner AE. Identifying live nematodes in diffuse unilateral subacute neuroretinitis by using the scanning laser ophthalmoscope. Arch Ophthalmol 2002; 120(2):135–8.

16. Myint K, Sahay R, Mon S, Saravanan VR, Narendran V, Dhillon B. "Worm in the eye": the rationale for treatment of DUSN in south India. Br J Ophthalmol 2006;90(9):1125–7.

17. Myint K, Sahay R, Mon S, Saravanan VR, Narendran V, Dhillon B. The Indian case of live worm in diffuse unilateral subacute neuro-retinitis. Eye 2006;20(5):612–3.

18. Slakter JS, Ciardella AP. Diffuse unilateral subacute neuroretinitis. Retina Vitreous Macula 1998;806–812.

19. Souza EC, Casella AM, Nakashima Y, Monteiro ML. Clinical features and outcomes of patients with diffuse unilateral subacute neuroretinitis treated with oral albendazole. Am J Ophthalmol 2005;140(3):437–445.

6.4.5 ONCHOCERCIASIS

- Etiology
- Clinical features
- Diagnosis and treatment

Onchocerciasis (river blindness) is a common cause of blindness in African countries. It is known to be endemic in 37 countries and an estimated 18 million people are infected with onchocerciasis and an approximately 1–2 million are blind due to this disease worldwide. About 95% of infected persons reside in Africa, where the disease is most severe along the major rivers in 30 countries. Outside Africa, the disease occurs in Mexico, Guatemala, Ecuador, Columbia, Venezuella and Brazil in the America, and Yemen in Asia.

ETIOLOGY

Causative organism, the *Onchocerca volvulus*, is a filarial nematode parasite.

Natural hosts of this parasite are humans only.

Vector transmitting the disease from one human being to another is bite of female black flies the *Simulium genus*. These flies breed in fast-flowing streams of river; hence the name of disease—the river blindness.

Pathogenesis

- Infection is transmitted to other persons when a female black fly ingests microfilariae from the host's skin and these microfilariae then develop into irrespective larvae.
- The infective larvae are then deposited in the skin of other persons by the site of infected black fly. The larvae develop into mature adult worms that forms subcutaneous nodules.
- About 7 months to 3 years after infection, the gravid female worm releases microfilariae that migrate out of the nodules and spread throughout the body concentrating in the skin.

Ocular transmission of microfilariae probably occurs by multiple routes:

- *Direct invasion of cornea* from the conjunctival tissue.
- *Invasion of sclera* both directly from the conjunctiva and also through vascular bundles.
- *Haematogenous spread* is also a possible route.

CLINICAL FEATURES

General features

1. *Skin lesion* include:
- *Subcutaneous nodules* onchocercomata scattered throughout the body.
- *Pruritis and papular rashes* are generalized and mild to severe, sometimes even incapacitating.
- *Long-term changes in skin* include premature wrinkling, epidermal atrophy, hypo- or hyper-pigmentation, hyperkeratosis and scaling.

2. *Lymphadenopathy*, mild to moderate, is common, particularly in the inguinal and femoral area, where the enlarged nodes may hand down due to gravity (handing grain).

3. *Constitutional features*, some heavily infected individuals develop cachexia with loss of adipose tissue and muscle man.

Ocular features

In the endemic area, onchocerciasis is a common cause of corneal and posterior segment blindness. Ocular lesions include:

1. *Conjunctivitis* with photophobia is the most common early finding.

2. *Keratitis* in onchocerciasis occurs in two forms:
   - Microfilariae in corneal tissue
   - Punctate keratitis occurring due to acute inflammatory reactions surrounding dying microfilariae and manifesting as snowflake opacities, is common among younger patients. It resolves without apparent complication.
   - *Sclerosing keratitis* occurs in 1 to 5% of infected persons and is a common cause of corneal blindness in Africa.

3. *Anterior segment* signs are:
   - *Live microfilariae* can be seen swimming freely in the anterior chamber.

- *Anterior uveitis* may occur in about 5% of infected persons. Severely may vary from mild to severe.
- *Secondary glaucoma and complicated cataract* are common complications of anterior uveitis in onchocerciasis

4. *Posterior segment lesions* include:
   - *Chorioretinal lesions* develop as a result of atrophy and hyperpigmentation of RPE.
   - *Optic neuritis* invariably ending in optic atrophy is a posterior segment cause of blindness in onchocerciasis.

DIAGNOSIS AND TREATMENT

Diagnosis

Clinical diagnosis is based on the typical signs and a history of exposure is an endemic area.

Definitive diagnosis is made from:
- *Biopsy exciside subcutaneous nodule*, which may demonstrate adult worm.
- *Skinship biopsy*, which may demonstrate micro-filariae.

Serological tests include:
- *Eosinophilia* and elevated serum include IgG levels are common, but may occur in many parasitic infections.
- *Arrays to detect antibodies* to Onchocerca.
- *PCR and to detect Onchocerca DNA* are specialized laboratory tests, used for research purposes.
- *Mazzotti test* is reserved for cases not diagnosed with above tests. It is a provocative test based on *Mazzotti reaction* which is caused by massive worm killing by the drug *diethyl-carbamazine* (used earlier for treatment).

Treatment

Medical treatment with the drug ivermectin is presently first choice and maintaining of treatment. A single dose of 150 µg/kg body weight to be repeated annually for 10 years has been recommended. Recently, some studies recommend a single dose every 3 months to ameliorate pruritus and skin disease.

Note. Under Vision 2020: Global initiative for prevention of blindness yearly dose of ivermectin is recommended in endemic area.

Surgical excision of the nodules is recommended when located on the head (because of proximity of microfilariae-producing adult worms to the eye).

Topical treatment of uveitis with corticosteroid and cycloplegic eyedrops is an usual lines secondary glaucoma, when develops, need to be managed medically with betablodeen and carbonic anhydrase inhibitors.

BIBLIOGRAPHY

1. Ament CS, Young LH. Ocular manifestations of helminthic infections: onchocersiasis, cysticercosis, toxocariasis, and diffuse unilateral subacute neuro-retinitis. Int Ophthalmol Clin 2006; 46(2):1–10.
2. CDC. Parasites - Onchocerciasis (also known as River Blindness). CDC. Available at http://www.cdc.gov/parasites/onchocerciasis/disease.html.
3. Cooper PJ, Proaño R, Beltran C, Anselmi M, Guderian RH. Onchocerciasis in Ecuador: ocular findings in Onchocerca volvulus infected individuals. Br J Ophthalmol 1995;79(2):157–62.
4. Ejere HO, Schwartz E, Wormald R, Evans JR. Ivermectin for onchocercal eye disease (river blindness). Cochrane Database Syst Rev 2012; 8:CD002219.
5. Etya'ale D, Taylor HR. Onchocerciasis. Duane's Ophthalmology. Lippincott Williams & Wilkins; 2006. 5: Chapter 62.
6. Greene BM, Gbakima AA, Albiez EJ, Taylor HR. Humoral and cellular immune responses to Onchocerca volvulus infection in humans. Rev Infect Dis 1985;7(6):789–95.
7. Little MP, Breitling LP, Basáñez MG, Alley ES, Boatin BA. Association between microfilarial load and excess mortality in onchocerciasis: an epidemiological study. Lancet 2004; 363(9420): 1514–21.
8. Rowe SG, Durand M. Blackflies and whitewater: onchocerciasis and the eye. Int Ophthalmol Clin 1998;38(1):231–40.
9. The Carter Center. River Blindness Elimination Program. The Carter Center. Available at http://www.cartercenter.org/health/river_blindness/index.html.
10. World Health Organization. African Programme for Onchocerciacis Control (APOC). Available at http://www.who.int/apoc/onchocerciasis/ocp/en/.
11. World Health Organization. Prevention of Blindness and Visual Impairment. Onchocerciasis Control Programme (OCP). World Health Organization. Available at http://www.who. int/blindness/partnerships/onchocerciasis_OCP/en/.
12. Yaya G, Kobangué L, Kémata B, Gallé D, Grésenguet G. [Elimination or control of the onchocerciasis in Africa? Case of Gami village in Central African Republic]. Bull Soc Pathol Exot. 2014;107(3):188–93.

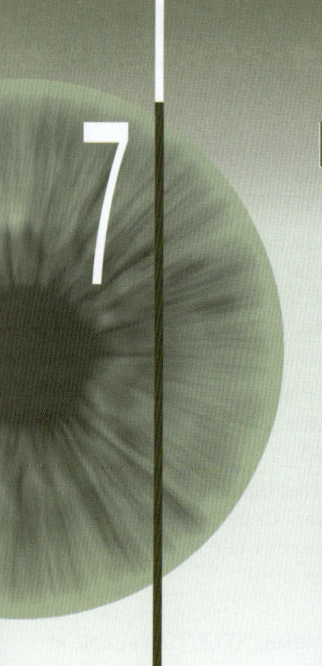

NON-INFECTIOUS UVEITIS

7

7.1 UVEITIS IN JUVENILE IDIOPATHIC ARTHRITIS AND SYSTEMIC RHEUMATIC DISEASE

7.1.1 UVEITIS IN JUVENILE IDIOPATHIC ARTHRITIS (JIA)

- General considerations
- Classification and features of JIA
- Uveitis in JIA
- Screening schedule for JIA

GENERAL CONSIDERATIONS

Juvenile idiopathic arthritis (JIA) is a chronic inflammatory arthritis involving multiple joints (knee, elbow, ankle and interphalangeal joints) in children below the age of 16 years. The disease is also referred as *juvenile rheumatoid arthritis,* though the patients are seronegative for rheumatoid factor. In 30% cases, polyarthritis is associated with hepatosplenomegaly and other systemic features, and the condition is labelled as *Still's disease.*

The diagnosis of juvenile idiopathic arthritis is based on the presence of arthritis in a child under 16 years which usually has at least 6 weeks duration and is usually with a negative rheumatoid factor test result and no other known cause for the joint disease.

CLASSIFICATION AND FEATURES OF JIA

It is classified as:

- Oligoarticular JIA
- Polyarticular JIA
- Systemic JIA

I. Oligoarticular JIA (40–60%)

- This is common in girls (5:1).
- Peak age of onset is around 2 years.
- Four or fewer joints are involved (often asymmetric) during first 6 months.
- Approximately 70% patients tested positive for antinuclear antibody.
- High risk of uveitis exists.

II. Polyarticular JIA (20–40%)

- It is common in girls (3:1).
- Peak age of onset is around 3 years.
- It involves 5 or more joints during first 6 months.
- Approximately 40% of these patients are tested positive for antinuclear antibody.
- Intermediate risk for uveitis exists.

III. Systemic JIA (Still's disease) (10–20%)

- The disease is of equal frequency in girls and boys, can occur at any age.
- A systemic form of JIA is characterised by a symmetric polyarthritis with an associated fever, rash, hepatosplenomegaly, and leucocytosis.
- Antinuclear antibody is positive in only 10% of patients.
- Has lower risk of uveitis.

UVEITIS IN JIA

Clinical profile

Laterally. Anterior uveitis associated with JIA is a bilateral (70%), chronic non-granulomatous disease affecting female children more than the male (4:1). It usually develops before the age of 6 years.

HLA association. Nearly half of the patients are positive for HLA-DW5 and 75% are positive for antinuclear antibodies (ANA).

Onset of uveitis is asymptomatic and the eye is white even in the presence of severe uveitis.

Therefore, slit-lamp examination is mandatory in children suffering from JIA.

Characteristic features. Characterised by anterior chamber cells and flare. Usually, patients only have 1 to 2+ cells, and once the uveitis has developed, chronic flare is typical. Anterior chamber cells and not flare should be used to determine the severity of disease and the need for therapy. The number of cells will fluctuate with the severity of inflammation and diminish with corticosteroid therapy. Similar to the uveitis associated with other arthropathies, the severity of the uveitis is unrelated to the severity of the underlying joint disease. Although the joint disease often diminishes with age, ocular disease frequently persists into adulthood.

Complications like posterior synechiae, complicated cataract and band-shaped keratopathy are fairly common (Fig. 7.1.1.1).

Management

Screening schedule for JIA

The American Academy of Pediatrics recommends a schedule for screening patients with JRA/JIA for uveitis. According to this schedule:

Pauci/polyarticular subtype at onset

+*ANA:* Every 3–4 months, if within the first 7 years of onset of arthritis; every 6 months, if beyond that.

−*ANA:* Every 6 months, if within the first 7 years of onset of arthritis; every 6 months thereafter.

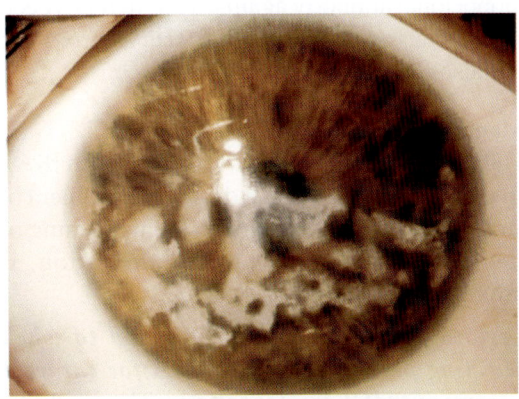

Fig. 7.1.1.1 *Complications of uveitis in juvenile idiopathic arthritis: Posterior synechiae, complicated cataract and band-shaped keratopathy.*

Systemic subtype at onset

Every 12 months irrespective of the onset of arthritis.

So screening of patients with JIA for early detection is must. Once uveitis is developed, it should be treated energetically.

Treatment

Steroids. Management of JRA/JIA includes treatment with topical corticosteroids. More severe cases may require systemic or periocular corticosteroids. In patients with chronic aqueous flare, in the absence of active cellular reaction, corticosteroids are not indicated. In this group of patients, however, mydriatics may be useful to keep the pupil mobile and prevent the formation of posterior synechiae.

Methotrexate. Complications such as growth retardation among others, seen with the chronic use of systemic corticosteroids in children are common. The presence of low-grade inflammation for a prolonged period can result in unacceptable ocular morbidity and visual loss. The use of weekly low-dose methotrexate may be considered in such patients as this can control uveitis, is well tolerated and eliminates the complications of chronic corticosteroid use.

Tumour necrosis factor. Another modality of treatment that may be tried in patients with JRA/JIA includes tumour necrosis factor inhibitors, such as *infliximab*, a chimeral monoclonal antibody against TNF-α. It has been seen to decrease not only the corticosteroid use but also the number of recurrences.[11]

Management of complicated cataract

The implantation of IOLs in patients with JRA/JIA remains controversial due to the problem of amblyopia, if left aphakic and the worsening of the aggressive nature of inflammation, if implanted.

Certain guidelines may be adhered to when selecting patients with JRA/JIA for cataract surgery with IOL implantation.[12] They include:
- *Good control of inflammation for at least 3 months* prior to surgery with systemic immunomodulatory therapy and without frequent instillation of topical medication.
- *Use of acrylic lenses* only.
- *Frequent follow-up* to detect any inflammation which must then be aggressively treated.
- *Use of long-term immunomodulatory therapy* pre- and postoperatively, not only perioperatively.
- *Feasibility of long-term follow-up* to detect late complications that may lead to loss of the eye.
- *A lack of hesitation to explant the IOL* in case of persistent postoperative inflammation and recurrent cyclitic membranes may result in less of eye.

BIBLIOGRAPHY

1. Acevedo S, Quinones K, Rao V, et al. Cataract surgery in children with juvenile idiopathic arthritis associated uveitis. Int Ophthalmol Clin 2008;48(2):1–7.
2. Anesi SD, Foster CS. The importance of recognizing juvenile idiopathic arthritis-associated uveitis and preventing blindness from it. Arthritis Care Res (Hoboken). 2012 Jan 9.
3. Boone MI, Moore TL, Cruz OA. Screening for uveitis in juvenile rheumatoid arthritis. J Pediatr Ophthalmol Strabismus 1998;35(1):41–3.
4. Ceisler EJ, Foster CS. Juvenile rheumatoid arthritis and uveitis: minimizing the blinding complications. Int Ophthalmol Clin 1996; 36(1):91–107.
5. Gallagher KT, Bernstein B. Juvenile rheumatoid arthritis. Curr Opin Rheumatol 1999;11(5):372–6.
6. Heiligenhaus A, Mingels A, Heinz C, et al. Methotrexate for uveitis associated with juvenile idiopathic arthritis: value and requirement for additional anti-inflammatory medication. Eur J Ophthalmol 2007;17(5):743–8.
7. Hemady RK, Baer JC, Foster CS. Immuno-suppressive drugs in the management of progressive, corticosteroid-resistant uveitis associated with juvenile rheumatoid arthritis. Int Ophthalmol Clin 1992;32(1):241–52.
8. Holland GN. Intraocular lens implantation in patients with juvenile rheumatoid arthritis-associated uveitis: an unresolved management issue. Am J Ophthalmol 1996;122(2):255–7.
9. Ilowite NT. Update on biologics in juvenile idiopathic arthritis. Curr Opin Rheumatol 2008; 20(5):613–8.

10. Imrie FR, Dick AD. Biologics in the treatment of uveitis. Curr Opin Ophthalmol 2007;18(6): 481–6.

11. Kanski JJ. Anterior uveitis in juvenile rheumatoid arthritis. Arch Ophthalmol; 95(10):1794–7.

12. Kesen MR, Setlur V, Goldstein DA. Juvenile idiopathic arthritis-related uveitis. Int Ophthalmol Clin 2008;48(3):21–38.

13. Kotaniemi K, Kaipiainen-Seppanen O, Savolainen A, et al. A population-based study on uveitis in juvenile rheumatoid arthritis. Clin Exp Rheumatol 1999;17(1):119–22.

14. Kotaniemi K. Late onset uveitis in juvenile-type chronic polyarthritis controlled with prednisolone, cyclosporin A and methotrexate. Clin Exp Rheumatol 1998;16(4):469–71.

15. Malleson P. Prevalence and outcome of uveitis in a regional cohort of patients with juvenile rheumatoid arthritis. J Rheumatol 1998;25(6):1242.

16. Nguyen QD, Foster CS. Saving the vision of children with juvenile rheumatoid arthritis-associated uveitis. JAMA 1998;280(13):1133–4.

17. Päivönsalo-Hietanen T, Tuominen J, Saari KM. Uveitis in children: population-based study in Finland. Acta Ophthalmol Scand 2000; 78(1):84–8.

18. Rabinovich CE. Treatment of juvenile idiopathic arthritis-associated uveitis: challenges and update. Curr Opin Rheumatol 2011; 23(5):432–6.

19. Tynjala P, Kotaniemi K, Lindahl P, et al. Adalimumab in juvenile idiopathic arthritis-associated chronic anterior uveitis. Rheumatology (Oxford) 2008;47(3):339–44.

20. Weiss AH, Wallace CA, Sherry DD. Methotrexate for resistant chronic uveitis in children with juvenile rheumatoid arthritis. J Pediatr 1998;133(2):266–8.

21. Wright T, Cron RQ. Pediatric rheumatology for the adult rheumatologist II: uveitis in juvenile idiopathic arthritis. J Clin Rheumatol 2007; 13(4):205–10.

22. Yu EN, Meniconi ME, Tufail F, et al. Outcomes of treatment with immunomodulatory therapy in patients with corticosteroid-resistant juvenile idiopathic arthritis-associated chronic iridocyclitis. Ocul Immunol Inflamm 2005;13(5): 353–60.

7.1.2 SYSTEMIC RHEUMATIC DISEASES AND EYE

Introduction
Rheumatoid arthritis
• General considerations
• Ocular manifestations
Systemic lupus erythematosus
• Systemic menifestations
• Ocular manifestations
• Antinuclear antibodies in SLE
Granulomatosis with polyangiitis
• Systemic menifestations
• Ocular manifestations
• Diagnostic tests
Scleroderma or systemic sclerosis
• General features
• Systemic manifestations
• Ocular manifestations
Polyarteritis nodsa
• General considerations
• Ocular manifestations
Relapsing polychondritis
• General considerations
• Ocular manifestations
Ankylosing spondylitis and the seronegative spondyloarthopathies
• Ankylosing spondylitis
• Reiter's syndrome (reactive arthritis)
• Acute anterior uveitis in seronegative spondyloathropathy

INTRODUCTION

Systemic rheumatic disease can be defined as a group of autoimmune disorders that have in common diffuse immunologic and inflammatory changes in small blood vessels and connective tissue. Ocular involvement is usually seen as a complication of systemic rheumatic disease. Often ophthalmic manifestations can be the first manifestations of a systemic rheumatic disease and present to an ophthalmologist. Thus it is very important to diagnose these spectrum of diseases, refer promptly to a rheumatologist as many of these conditions are lethal and timely intervention can save the life of patients. Ocular complications, associated with these disorders, can range from the very mild to the devastating. Common such systemic rheumatic diseases are:
• Rheumatoid arthritis (RA)

- Systemic lupus erythematosus (SLE)
- Granulomatosis with polyangiitis (GPA), formerly known as Wegener's granulomatosis
- Systemic sclerosis (SS)
- Polyarteritis nodosa (PAN)
- Relapsing polychondritis
- Ankylosing spondylitis (AS).

RHEUMATOID ARTHRITIS

Rheumatoid arthritis (RA) is the most common inflammatory arthritis, affecting about 1% of the population worldwide. RA has a wide-spectrum of disease manifestations and extra-articular involvement involving most organ systems.

GENERAL CONSIDERATIONS

Females are affected three times more than males, mostly aged 40 to 60.

Morning stiffness of the joints is the hallmark of the disease.

Rheumatoid factor is an autoantibody directed against the Fc region of IgG. Rheumatoid factor and IgG join to form immune complexes that contribute to the disease process.

Various immunoassays are available for detection of rheumatoid factor. The classic *Rose-Waaler test* is haemagglutination test, which depends on the ability of rheumatoid factor to agglutinate sheep erythrocytes coated with anti-sheep immunoglobulin. This test identifies only the IgM isotype of rheumatoid factor and not used routinely nowadays.

Enzyme-linked immunosorbent assay (ELISA) can measure IgG, IgA, and IgM rheumatoid factors. Some forms of rheumatoid arthritis, like oligoarticular rheumatoid arthritis, may be associated with a negative test for IgM rheumatoid factor but a positive test for IgG rheumatoid factor.

OCULAR MANIFESTATIONS

Ocular manifestations include (Fig. 7.1.2.1):
Dry eye is the most common ocular involvement in RA. One-third of patients with RA suffer with dry eyes and sometimes combined with a dry mouth (**Sjögren's syndrome**).

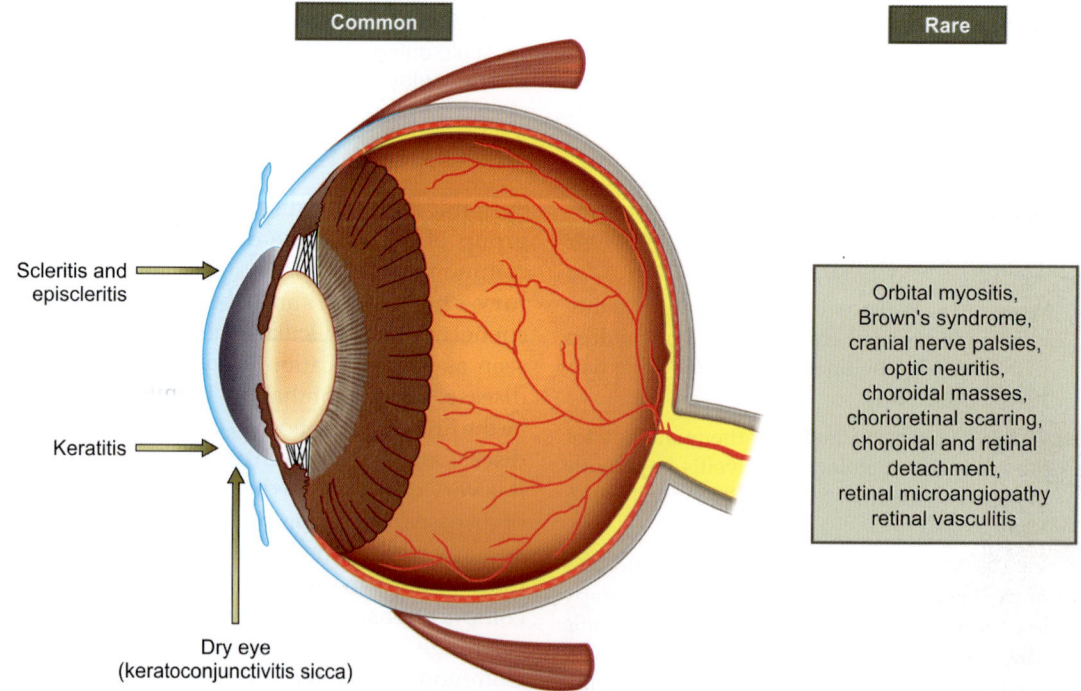

Common

Rare

Scleritis and episcleritis

Keratitis

Orbital myositis, Brown's syndrome, cranial nerve palsies, optic neuritis, choroidal masses, chorioretinal scarring, choroidal and retinal detachment, retinal microangiopathy retinal vasculitis

Dry eye (keratoconjunctivitis sicca)

Fig. 7.1.2.1 *Ocular manifestations of rheumatoid arthritis.*

Peripheral ulcerative keratitis (Fig. 7.1.2.2) occurring in patients with rheumatoid arthritis usually involves one sector, is rapidly progressive. It may be associated with peripheral corneal guttering or peripheral corneal melting.

Episcleritis can be seen in patients of RA.

Scleritis. RA is the most common systemic association of scleritis. Patients with RA more commonly have bilateral scleritis than patients with scleritis due to other systemic rheumatic diseases.

Scleromalacia perforans is a rare variant of necrotising scleritis and believed to occur due to obliterative endarteritis of the scleral vessels. It is seen most commonly in patients with long-standing rheumatoid arthritis, is clinically silent and painless.

SYSTEMIC LUPUS ERYTHEMATOSUS

Systemic lupus erythematosus (SLE) is a chronic multi-system autoimmune disorder which is characterised by production of self-directed antibodies. These antibodies cause widespread tissue and cell destruction by formation of immune complexes and misdirected inflammatory responses.

SYSTEMIC MANIFESTATIONS

Systemic manifestations of SLE include (Fig. 1.2.3.1):

• *Females*, mostly in the childbearing years, are four times more commonly affected than males.

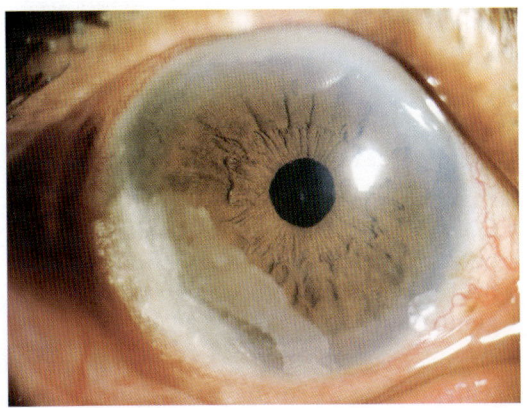

Fig. 7.1.2.2 *Peripheral ulcerative keratitis in rheumatoid arthritis.*

• *Skin* is one of the frequently involved organs in SLE and examination of skin can help one to clinch the diagnosis and progression of disease activity.

• *Malar rash (Butterfly rash)* on the bridge of the nose and cheeks is the commonest skin lesion seen in SLE. Photosensitivity when the skin is exposed to UV light is an important feature in SLE. Raynaud's phenomenon, acral cyanosis, periungual erythema and maculopapular rashes of the trunk or extremity can also be seen in these patients.

• *Alopecia*, associated with inflammatory involvement of scalp can be seen in SLE.

• *Arthropathy* seen in SLE is also known as Jaccoud's arthropathy. This arthropathy is generally non-erosive in nature and involves migratory arthralgia of multiple joints. This arthropathy has the same distribution of joints as rheumatoid arthritis, including the metacarpophalangeal joints, wrists, and metatarsophalangeal joints.

OCULAR MANIFESTATIONS

Ocular manifestations are as below:

Scleritis, though relatively rare, can be the initial presentation of SLE.

Episcleritis and dry eye are also seen in patients with SLE.

Optic nerve involvement, though rare, can be seen in the form of papillitis, retrobulbar neuritis, acute ischaemic optic neuropathy. Optic neuropathy in SLE believed to occur due to ischaemia, which may produce demyelination.

Retinal involvement in SLE is often termed as **lupus retinopathy** and may occur in the form of cotton-wool spots with or without retinal haemorrhages, and additional microvascular changes, including microaneurysms and capillary telangiectasia. *Occlusive vasculitis* is a hallmark of lupus retinopathy and results due to deposition of immune complexes. The hallmark of occlusive vasculopathy is cotton-wool spot. Occlusions of central and branch retinal arteries may occur.

Fundus fluorescein angiography is very important, if retinal involvement is suspected

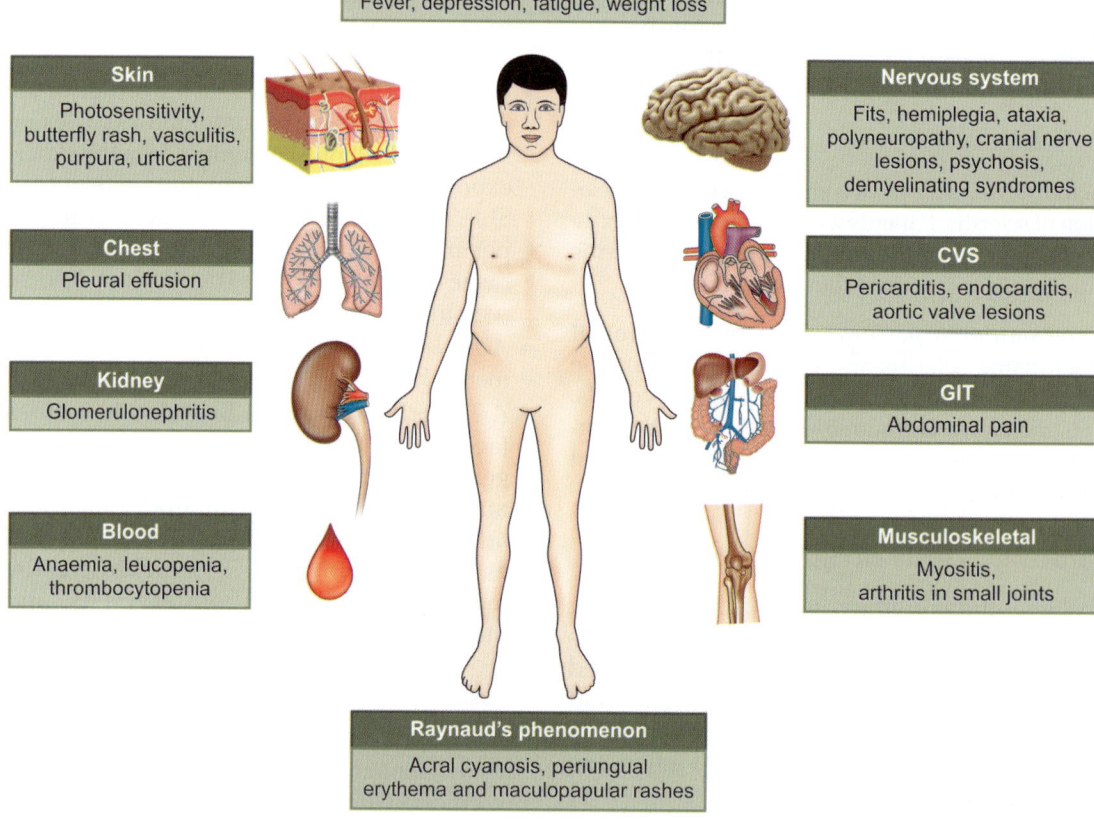

General
Fever, depression, fatigue, weight loss

Skin
Photosensitivity, butterfly rash, vasculitis, purpura, urticaria

Nervous system
Fits, hemiplegia, ataxia, polyneuropathy, cranial nerve lesions, psychosis, demyelinating syndromes

Chest
Pleural effusion

CVS
Pericarditis, endocarditis, aortic valve lesions

Kidney
Glomerulonephritis

GIT
Abdominal pain

Blood
Anaemia, leucopenia, thrombocytopenia

Musculoskeletal
Myositis, arthritis in small joints

Raynaud's phenomenon
Acral cyanosis, periungual erythema and maculopapular rashes

Fig. 7.1.2.3 *Systemic manifestations in SLE.*

in SLE. FFA helps to identify the areas of ischaemia, shunt vessels and neovascularisation.

Lupus choroidopathy, choroidal involvement in SLE, is less common than lupus retinopathy. It is usually associated with systemic hypertension. It is characterised by serous detachment of the retina and choroidal infarcts.

ANTINUCLEAR ANTIBODIES IN SLE

A variety of autoantibodies have been associated with SLE. Autoantibodies to a number of nuclear and cytoplasmic constituents may be present and may be the result of a generalized polyclonal B cell hyperactivity. Antinuclear antibodies (ANAs) are elevated in about 95% of patients with SLE. However, their absence does not rule out the diagnosis. In addition, ANAs can be seen in other systemic diseases.

GRANULOMATOSIS WITH POLYANGIITIS

Granulomatosis with polyangiitis (GPA) or *Wegener's granulomatosis* (WG) is characterised by formation of necrotising granulomas within small- to medium-sized vessels.

SYSTEMIC MENIFESTATIONS

- *Age and sex.* There is no age or gender predilection.
- *Classic triad* of the disease is characterised by necrotising granulomas of the respiratory tract, systemic vasculitis, and focal necrotising glomerulonephritis (Fig. 7.1.2.4).
- *Organs most often affected* in granulomatosis with polyangiitis, in decreasing order, are the upper respiratory tract, lung, kidney, skin, and orbit and eye.

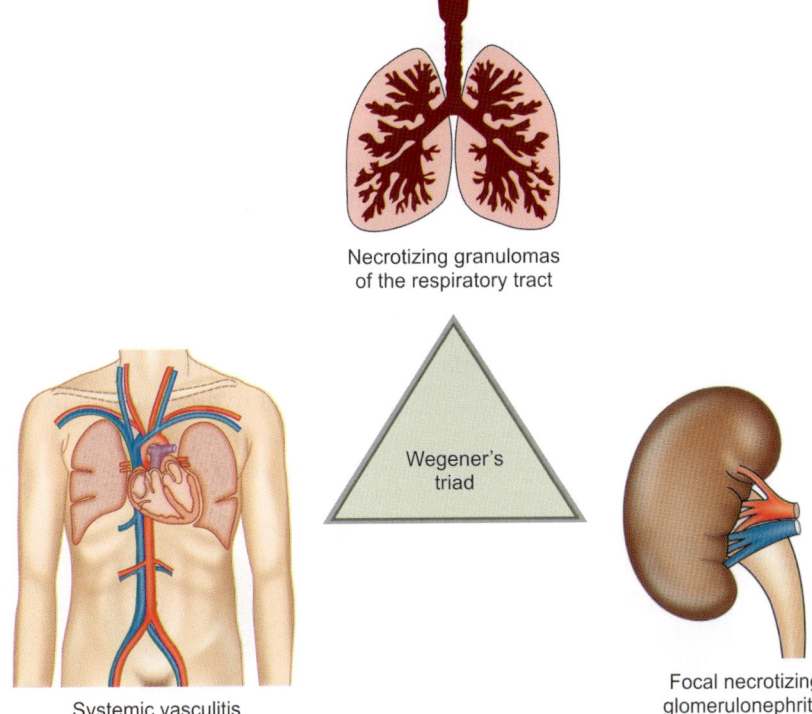

Fig. 7.1.2.4 *Classical triad of Wegener's granulomatosis.*

OCULAR MANIFESTATIONS

Ocular involvement can occur in approximately 50% patients with granulomatosis with poly-angiitis. In few of them, ocular involvement may be the initial presentation of the disease. Ocular manifestations include:

Scleritis is common in patients with granulo-matosis with polyangiitis and is of necrotising variety (Fig. 7.1.2.5), often associated with peripheral corneal changes and indicates severe systemic involvement and the need for more aggressive immunosuppressive therapy.

Proptosis can occur due to infiltration of the orbit with granulomatous tissue. In fact granulomatosis with polyangiitis is the only systemic inflammatory disease that may present with proptosis. Orbital inflammation or cellulitis can occur from extensive sinus involvement or purulent sinusitis and can lead to bony erosion of the ethmoid and nasal bones.

Compressive optic neuropathy and ophthalmo-plegia can occur from orbital involvement.

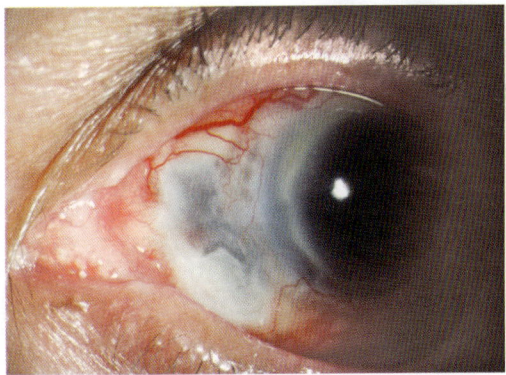

Fig. 7.1.2.5 *Necrotising scleritis in a case of WG.*

DIAGNOSTIC TESTS

Cytoplasmic antineutrophil cytoplasmic antibody (cANCA) is found to be more specific for granulomatosis with polyangiitis with reported sensitivity as high as 85–96%.

SCLERODERMA OR SYSTEMIC SCLEROSIS

Scleroderma or systemic sclerosis (SS) is a chronic multi-system disorder of unknown etiology.

GENERAL FEATURES

Sex. Females are affected three times more often than males.

Age. Relatively more common between 30 and 50 years of age.

Race. Black patients are affected twice as frequently as white patients.

SYSTEMIC MANIFESTATIONS

Systemic involvement of SS can be best described with the help of **ABCDCREST** criteria (Fig. 7.1.2.6):

• *Autoantibodies* to various body proteins.

• *Basilar pulmonary fibrosis* detected by chest radiograph as linear shadows or "honeycomb" reticular appearance.

• *Contracture of the joints* defined as permanent limitation of joint motion. The prayer sign is detected when a patient opposed the palmar surfaces of both hands with extended wrists. The sign is positive when the patient is unable to oppose the palms.

• *Dermal thickening* is often present.

• *Calcinosis cutis*, most often located on the fingers, is intra- and/or subcutaneous deposits of hydroxyapatite that can ulcerate the skin.

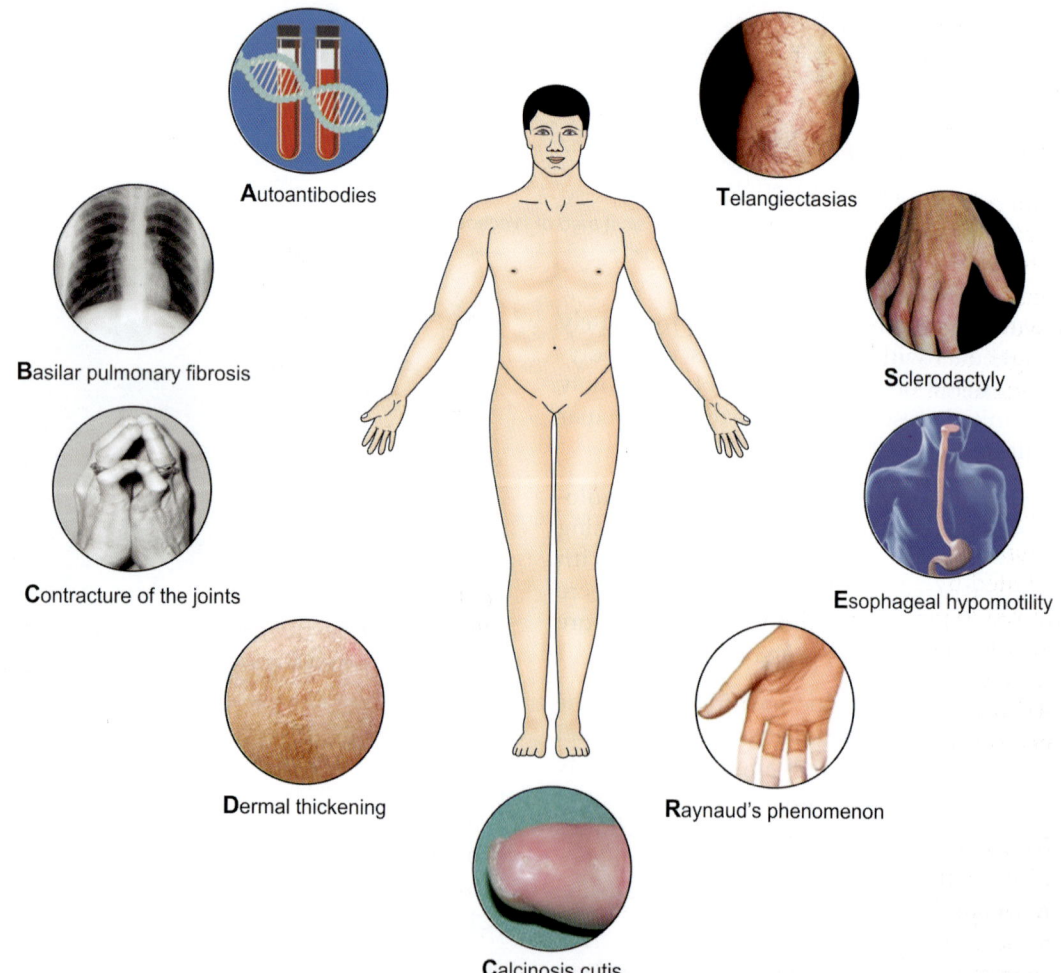

Autoantibodies

Telangiectasias

Basilar pulmonary fibrosis

Sclerodactyly

Contracture of the joints

Esophageal hypomotility

Dermal thickening

Raynaud's phenomenon

Calcinosis cutis

Fig. 7.1.2.6 *Systemic manifestations of systemic sclerosis (ABCDCREST criteria).*

- *Raynaud's phenomenon* is a sudden pallor of an acral structure (e.g. fingers, whole hand, toes, tip of nose, earlobe, or tongue). Raynaud's phenomenon is observed in 90–98% of SSc patients.
- *Esophageal distal hypomotility* is present.
- *Sclerodactyly* is symmetric thickening and tightening of the skin on the digits.
- *Telangiectasias* are seen in digits, face, lips, and tongue.

OCULAR MANIFESTATIONS

"Woody" texture of the eyelids or lid stiffness can be seen in these patients. Telangiectasia can be found on either upper or lower lids and is very small, rarely exceeds 1 mm in diameter.

Keratoconjunctivitis sicca (KCS) the most common ocular manifestation of SS KCS can sometimes be associated with secondary Sjogren syndrome (keratoconjunctivitis sicca in association with xerostomia or dry mouth).

Retinopathy in SS is similar to that seen in the other systemic vasculitides, with cotton-wool spots, exudates, neuroretinal oedema, intra-retinal haemorrhages and lipid degeneration. However, retinal involvements in SS is primarily thought to be due to renal involvement and hypertension.

POLYARTERITIS NODOSA

GENERAL CONSIDERATIONS

Necrotising vasculitis of medium-sized arteries, mediated by circulating immune complexes is referred to polyarteritis nodosa (PAN).

- *Sex.* Males are almost twice as affected as females, usually in the fourth to sixth decades.
- *All organs can be affected* in this systemic necrotising vasculitis.

OCULAR MANIFESTATIONS

- *Necrotising scleritis* with peripheral corneal ulceration is common in PAN patients.
- *Retinopathy* seen in PAN is usually secondary to accelerated hypertension and, therefore, characterised by arteriovenous nipping, cotton-wool spots, and flame-shaped haemorrhages.

RELAPSING POLYCHONDRITIS

Relapsing polychondritis is a rare but potentially life-threatening disorder characterised by recurrent inflammation and destruction of cartilaginous structures of the external ears, nose, larynx, and tracheobronchial tree, sometimes leading to their destruction.

GENERAL CONSIDERATIONS

- *Age and sex.* Relapsing polychondritis can occur in any age group with slight female preponderance.
- *Auricular chondritis* is a key manifestation of the disease and characterised by pain, tenderness, swelling of cartilaginous parts of the external ear, sparing the soft earlobe, which lacks cartilage.
- *"Cauliflower" deformity* of the pinna may occur due to recurrent inflammation.
- *Nasal chondritis* is less common than auricular chondritis. A *saddle-nose deformity* can sometimes result from cartilage collapse.
- *Laryngeal, tracheal, or bronchial chondritis* is relatively uncommon but can be life-threatening.

OCULAR MANIFESTATIONS

- *Episcleritis and scleritis* are the most common ocular involvement seen in relapsing polychondritis. Diffuse anterior scleritis is the most common subtype associated with, but other subtypes can also occur.
- *Anterior uveitis* can occur.
- *Peripheral ulcerative keratitis* can occur in 10% of the patients.
- *Proptosis* or *extraocular muscle palsy* can be seen.
- *Posterior segment involvement* is very common.

ANKYLOSING SPONDYLITIS AND THE SERONEGATIVE SPONDYLOARTHROPATHIES

Seronegative spondyloarthropathies are a group of disorders characterised by an absence of serum rheumatoid factor.

Clinical entities commonly included in this group are:
- Ankylosing spondylitis

- Reiter's syndrome
- Psoriatic arthritis
- Arthritis associated with inflammatory bowel disease (Crohn's, Whipple or idiopathic), and
- Juvenile-onset spondyloarthropathy

Characteristics of seronegative spondyloarthropathies are:

- Asymmetric peripheral arthritis involving predominantly lower limb
- Radiographic evidence of sacroiliitis
- Absence of rheumatoid factor
- Absence of subcutaneous nodules and other extra-articular features of rheumatoid arthritis
- Overlapping extra-articular features characteristic of the group (e.g. anterior uveitis)

Association with HLA-B27. HLA-B27 is a human leucocyte antigen (HLA) and a class I major histocompatibility complex (MHC). It has been estimated that approximately 50% of all cases of acute anterior uveitis are associated with the presence of HLA-B27.

ANKYLOSING SPONDYLITIS

Ankylosing spondylitis (AS) is an HLA-B27-associated chronic inflammatory disease of unknown etiology. It is characterised by inflammation, calcification and finally ossification of ligaments and joint capsules. The term ankylosing spondylitis is derived from the Greek words which means "bent vertebral disk".

- *Age and sex.* The condition typically affects young males in third or fourth decades.
- *Presenting symptoms.* Backache and stiffness of lower back is most common presenting symptoms.
- *Primarily affects the sacroiliac joints and the axial skeleton,* but peripheral joint involvement may also be seen.
- *Spine may become flexed* in flexion in AS, leading to severe limitation of spinal movement. Calcification of spinal ligaments may appear as *"bamboo spine"* radiologically.
- *Extra-articular manifestations* of AS are not rare and include acute anterior uveitis, aortic incompetence, cardiac conduction defects, fibrosis of the upper lobes of the lungs, neurologic involvement, or renal (secondary) amyloidosis.
- *Acute anterior uveitis* can be seen in one-fourth patients with AS. Though simultaneous involvement of both eyes is uncommon, the anterior chamber inflammation is usually severe, often with plastic fibrin, hypopyon and severe congestion and warrants rapid treatment with topical steroids and cycloplegics. Primarily, it is actue recurrent non-granulomatous type of iridocyclitis.

REACTIVE ARTHRITIS

Reactive arthritis (earlier known as *Reiter's syndrome*) was first described as a clinical triad of arthritis, nongonococcal urethritis, and conjunctivitis.

Reactive arthritis differs from infectious arthritis in that the infectious pathogens cannot be cultured from the joint fluid or synovium.

Reactive arthritis is characterised by:
- *Arthritis.* Acute, asymmetrical, migratory peripheral arthritis involving 3 to 4 joints, most commonly lower extremities.
- *Enthesopathy*
- *Mucocutaneous lesions* like painless mouth ulceration, circinate balanitis, etc.
- *Genitourinary involvement* including cystitis, cervicitis, prostatitis and epididymoorchitis.
- *Conjunctivitis* is usually bilateral, with follicular or papillary with mucopurulent discharge. It usually occurs after urethritis and precedes the arthritis.

ACUTE ANTERIOR UVEITIS IN SERONEGATIVE SPONDYLOARTHROPATHY

- *Anterior uveitis is the most important ocular disease in patients with spondyloarthropathies.* In fact, HLA-B27 is the strongest known genetic risk factor for acute anterior uveitis.
- *Acute anterior uveitis* is relatively more common in patients with ankylosing spondylitis than in other causes of seronegative arthropathy.
- *Uveitis is usually unilateral* but both eyes become affected during the course of the disease.

- *Age and sex.* Males are affected about 2.5 times more frequently with HLA-B27 acute anterior uveitis than females and first attack of uveitis usually occurs between 20 and 40 years of age.
- *Presenting symptoms.* Patient usually presents with complaints of severe pain, photophobia, and watering.
- *Signs.* Acute anterior uveitis is characterised by severe circumcorneal congestion (ciliary flush), sticky, fibrinoid aqueous in the anterior chamber with or without hypopyon, posterior synechiae formation.
- *Posterior segment* is relatively rare to get involved.
- *Secondary glaucoma is common* in these patients. During acute phase of inflammation, intra-ocular pressure is usually reduced due to ciliary body shutdown. Subsequently intra-ocular pressure is increased due to iris bombé or synechial angle closure.

BIBLIOGRAPHY

1. Barisani-Asenbauer T, Maca SM, Mejdoubi L, Emminger W, Machold K, et al. Uveitis – a rare disease often associated with systemic diseases and infections – a systematic review of 2619 patients. Orphanet J Rare Dis 2002; 7:57.
2. Reddy CV, Foster CS. Systemic lupus erythe-matosus. In: Albert DM, Jakobiec FA, (eds). Principles and Practice of Ophthalmology, vol 5. Philadelphia: Saunders, 1994:2894–2901.
3. de Andrade FA, Foeldvari I, Levy RA. Auto-immune uveitis. In: Shoenfeld Y, Cervera R, Gershwin ME (eds) Diagnostic criteria in auto-immune diseases. 1st edition, Humana Press, New Jersey, USA, 2008;461–5.
4. Díaz-Valle D, Méndez R, Arriola P, Cuiña R, Ariño M. Noninfectious systemic diseases and uveitis. An Sist Sanit Navar 2008;31:97–110.
5. El Maghraoui A. Extra-articular manifestations of ankylosing spondylitis: prevalence. Eur J Intern Med 2011; 22(6):554–60. Epub 2011 Jul 13.
6. Foster CS. Systemic lupus erythematosus, discoid lupus erythematosus, and progressive systemic sclerosis. Int Ophthalmol Clin 1997; 37:93–110.
7. Horai R, Caspi RR. Cytokines in autoimmune uveitis. J Interferon Cytokine Res 2011;10:733–44.
8. Levy RA, de Andrade FA, Foeldvari I. Cutting-edge issues in autoimmune uveitis. Clin Rev Allergy Immuno, 2011.
9. Papotto PH, Marengo EB, Sardinha LR, Goldberg AC, Rizzo LV. Immunotherapeutic strategies in autoimmune uveitis. Autoimmun Rev 2014;13:909–916.
10. Muñoz-Fernández S, Martín-Mola E. Uveitis. Best Pract Res Clin Rheumatol 2006;20:487–505.
11. Nguyen QD, Foster CS . Systemic lupus erythe-matosus and the eye. Int Ophthalmol Clin 1998; 38:33–60.
12. Selmi C. Diagnosis and classification of auto-immune uveitis. Autoimmun Rev 2014;13:591–4.
13. Tan EM, Cohen AS, Fries JF, et al: The 1982 revised criteria for the classification of systemic lupus erythematosus. Arthritis Rheum 1982; 25:1271–7.

7.2 OCULAR SARCOIDOSIS

Introduction and Epidemiology
- Introduction
- Epidemiology

Pathogenesis and Pathology
Pathogenesis
- Immunological process
- Causative antigens
Histopathology
- Sarcoid granuloma

Clinical Menifestations
Systemic features
- Pulmonary sarcoidosis
- Extrapulmonary sarcoidosis
- Childhood sarcoidosis
Ocular sarcoidosis
- Lacrimal gland and orbit lesions
- Eyelid, conjunctiva and corneal lesions
- Sarcoid uveitis

Diagnosis and Differential Diagnosis
Diagnosis
- Diagnostic criteria
- Investigations
Differential diagnosis
- D/D of granulomatous uveitis
- D/D of chorioretinal granulomas
- D/D of periphlebitis

Treatment
Treatment of ocular sarcoidosis
- Corticosteroids
- Immunospressive agents
Treatment of complication

INTRODUCTION AND EPIDEMIOLOGY

INTRODUCTION

Sarcoidosis is a chronic multisystemic granulomatous disorder caused by an exaggerated cellular immune response to a variety of self or non-self antigens in a genetically predisposed individual. It is characterised by non-caseating granulomas affecting many organs including the lung, lymph nodes, skin, liver, eye, heart and the muscles.[1,2]

Diagnosis is usually made on the basis of biopsy and a combination of typical clinical features and radiology findings in the absence of any condition that can cause similar clinicoradiological and pathological changes.

Ocular involvement was first observed by Schumacher in a patient with nodular iritis in 1909.[3] It is believed to occur in 25–60% of systemic sarcoidosis at some point of time. In 10–20% of patients, ocular involvement is the initial presentation before any other systemic manifestation.[4] Most patients with ophthalmic findings showed evidence of systemic involvement.

Sarcoidosis has been increasingly diagnosed in recent years, due to increased awareness of the disease and better availability of diagnostic modalities.
- *Ocular evaluations contribute in making a diagnosis* of systemic sarcoidosis.
- *Early diagnosis and appropriate, adequate treatment* reduces the visual morbidity in ocular sarcoidosis.

EPIDEMIOLOGY

Incidence. Sarcoidosis has an overall incidence of 6–10 per 100,000.[5]

Race and ethnic group. Although sarcoidosis occurs worldwide, it is more common in certain ethnic and racial groups like the Afrocaribbeans, Irish and Scandinavian populations.[5–7]

Age. Literature shows that the highest incidence of sarcoidosis is in the 20–40 years age group. Some studies show two peaks of incidence for ocular sarcoidosis at 20–30 years and at 50–60 years.[8]

Sex. There is also a higher incidence of ocular involvement in women.[5]

Incidence of ocular sarcoidosis. Reported incidence of ocular sarcoidosis varies according to the geography, patient population, diagnostic criteria employed and referral patterns of the reporting ophthalmologists.

- More than 25–60% of patients with sarcoidosis have ocular involvement with some reports being as high as 90%.[9]
- Earlier considered a disease of the developed world, ocular sarcoidosis is increasingly recognized from the developing world in recent years.[9,10] This may be due to the increasing awareness of this disease and availability of improved diagnostic modalities like computed tomography and trans-bronchial lymph node biopsies.
- Clustering of sarcoidosis in families has been reported in literature.[8]

PATHOGENESIS AND PATHOLOGY

PATHOGENESIS

Immunological process. Sarcoidosis is caused by antigenic stimulation. The process involves presentation of the antigen by antigen presenting cells in genetically susceptible individuals, activation of CD4+ T cells, production of cytokines, recruitment of immunocompetent cells, compartmentalisation at the site of inflammation sealing off the antigen and production of a granuloma.[8,11]

Causative antigen. Although bacterial, viral and environmental antigens have been studied, none have been proven to be the cause for sarcoidosis.
- Current literature evidence states that sarcoidosis may result from not a single agent, but multiple agents capable of generating a T_H1-mediated response in a genetically susceptible individual.
- *Mycobacterium tuberculosis (MTb) as antigen.* Although studies have demonstrated myco-bacterial DNA and RNA in sarcoid tissue, *Mycobacterium tuberculosis* (MTb) has not been isolated in culture from the sarcoid tissue. Recent detection of high frequency of *MTb* catalase peroxidase (mKatG) reactive, IFN-γ expressing T cells in patients with active sarcoidosis has renewed interest in myco-bacteria as a causative agent.[11,12]
- *Propionibacteria as antigen.* Recent studies reporting the occurrence of rRNA and DNA of propionibacteria in sarcoid tissue have supported the theory of propionibacteria as a causative agent.

- *Hepatitis C virus as antigen.* There are reports of the association of hepatitis C with sarcoidosis. Reports of sarcoidosis following the use of IFN-γ and antiviral therapies for hepatitis C are known. At the same time, reactivation of sarcoidosis in patients with pre-existing disease have been reported during treatment of hepatitis C with IFN- suggesting that the interferon is important in the patho-genesis of sarcoidosis.
- *Epstein-Barr virus, herpes virus and Helicobacter pylori* have also been reported as causative antigen as antibodies against these have also been found higher in sarcoid patients.[11]

Genetic implications. Although no gene has been demonstrated to be responsible for sarcoid.
- *HLADR17 and TNF polymorphisms* play a role in the disease severity and prognosis. High levels of TNF-α, associated with TNFA2 allele are found in Lofgren's syndrome, which is associated with good prognosis. Butyrophilin-like 2 gene, which is located near the HLA-DRB1 region has also been implicated as a susceptibility gene.[13]

HISTOPATHOLOGY

Sarcoid granuloma classically is made up of modified macrophages or epithelioid cells surrounded by a rim of lymphocytes and fibroblasts. This is similar to that of other granulomatous inflammations like tuberculosis, fungal infections like histoplasmosis and talc or beryllium granulomatosis.
- *Necrosis or caseation* is absent in sarcoid granulomas which is usually seen with tuber-culosis and fungal infections.
- Occasionally, as small foci.
- *Fibrinoid necrosis* may be present in sarcoidosis.
- *Immunohistochemical studies* demonstrate the presence of CD4+ T cells admixed with the epitheloid cells in the centre of the cellular infiltrate.
- This *localized accumulation of CD4+ T cells is* seen in the bronchoalveolar fluid and also in the eye.
- *Compartmentalisation of CD4+ T cells* at sites of the disease leads to markedly high CD4/CD8 ratio of more than 10.

- *An elevated BAL CD4/CD8 T cell ratio of greater than 3.5* predicts the diagnosis of sarcoidosis with 94% specificity and 53% sensitivity. This is also associated with a favourable prognosis.
- *Recent reports of increased CD4/CD8 ratio of vitreous infiltrating lymphocytes* greater than 3.5 provided a diagnosis of ocular sarcoidosis with a sensitivity of 100% and a specificity of 96.3%.[14]

CLINICAL MANIFESTATIONS[15-21]

- *Course of sarcoidosis* ranges from asymptomatic to severe disease.
- *Clinical manifestations* and the severity of the disease are strongly associated with racial and ethnic factors.
- *Acute and more severe disease* is seen in black patients. Prognosis of the disease is relatively benign. However, factors associated with poor outcome include black race, late onset, disease persisting longer than 6 months, involvement of more than 3 organs and stage 3 pulmonary disease.

SYSTEMIC FEATURES

The disease predominantly affects the lungs, thoracic lymph nodes, skin and eyes.[15-21] It might have either a self-limited or chronic course.

Pulmonary sarcoidosis

Symptoms include:
- *Asymptomatic disease* is more frequent and discovered by chest radiography.
- *Respiratory or constitutional symptoms,* like fever, malaise, fatigue and weight loss.

Staging of pulmonary sarcoidosis. Radiological findings are used to classify a pulmonary sarcoidosis.
- *Stage 1* includes bilateral hilar lymphadenopathy without parenchymal involvement.
- *Stage 2* is bilateral hilar lymphadenopathy with parenchymal involvement.
- *Stage 3* is pulmonary infiltrates, including cystic changes without hilar lymphadenopathy.

Acute Lofgren's syndrome comprises of a combination of erythema nodosum, arthritis and hilar lymphadenopathy.

Heerfordt's syndrome (uveoparotid fever) consists of fever, parotid swelling, uveitis and facial palsy.

Extrapulmonary sarcoidosis

Most common sites of extrapulmonary involvement include lymph nodes, skin and eye.

Skin lesions occur in about 25% of patients and include:
- *Erythema nodosum* is a common manifestation seen in sarcoidosis but is not diagnostic.
- *Lupus pernio* is an indurated, violaceous plaque usually seen on the face.
- *Other manifestations include* subcutaneous granulomas and nodules, maculopapular lesions, hyper- or hypopigmented plaques and even necrotising cutaneous vasculitis.

Lymph node enlargement could be generalised or localised to the thoracic region.

Hepatic involvement is usually subclinical with an occasional increase in liver enzymes. Occasional reports of liver failure requiring transplantation have been reported.

Renal involvement may be in the form of interstitial nephritis, calculus formation and renal failure.

Cardiac sarcoidosis is seen in less than 5%. It may be in the form of generalised myocardial involvement with heart failure, conduction abnormalities including paroxysmal ventricular arrhythmia or complete heart block and sometimes sudden cardiac death.

Arthropathy is seen in about of 20% of patients.

Neurological involvement is seen in 5–26% of patients. They include cranial nerve palsies, encephalopathy and disorders of hypothalamus and pituitary gland. Chiasmal syndromes, motility disorders, facial nerve palsy, optic nerve involvement either due to direct sarcoid tissue infiltration or compression by cerebral mass leading to optic nerve atrophy have been reported in sarcoidosis.[5,8]

Childhood sarcoidosis

In older children, it could be associated with generalized lymphadenopathy, eyes, skin, liver and lung involvement. Sarcoidosis usually manifests as a triad of rash, uveitis and arthritis in children less than 4 years of age.

Note. In the developing world where tuberculosis is endemic:

- Occurrence of generalised lymphadenopathy is usually mistaken for tuberculosis and many of the children are on antitubercular therapy.
- Childhood sarcoidosis may also be misdiagnosed as juvenile chronic arthritis.[8]

OCULAR SARCOIDOSIS

- About 15 to 50% of patients with systemic sarcoidosis develop ocular sarcoidosis.
- Patients may be asymptomatic or present with blurred vision, floaters, redness or discomfort.
- Ocular involvement may be acute or chronic. It is usually a chronic disease and has an insidious onset.
- *Ocular sarcoidosis* can involve the lacrimal glands, orbit, eyelids, conjunctiva, uveal tract and the optic nerve (Figs 7.2.1–7.2.8). Table 7.2.1 summarises the ocular findings in sarcoidosis.[4-10, 15-21]

Lacrimal gland and orbit lesions

- *Lacrimal gland involvement* is common and may present as a dry eye. Severe keratoconjunctivitis sicca is not uncommon.
- *Sarcoid-induced myositis* has also been reported.

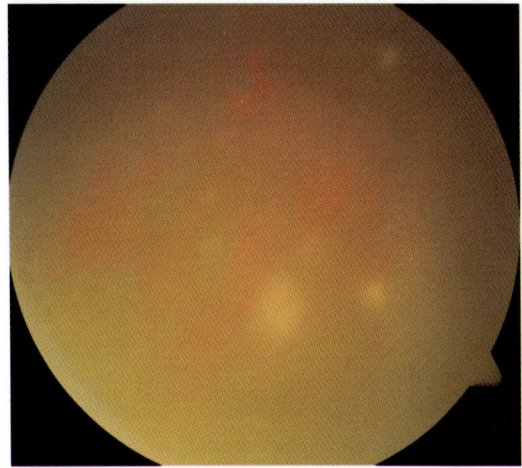

Fig. 7.2.2 *Fundus photograph showing vitritis with snowball opacities in the peripheral retina.*

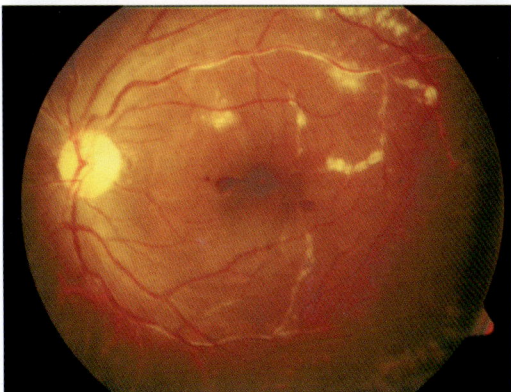

Fig. 7.2.3 *Fundus photograph showing the "candle wax drippings" perivasculitis.*

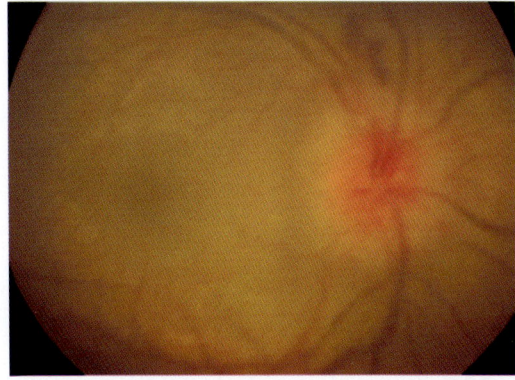

Fig. 7.2.4 *Fundus photograph showing disc oedema.*

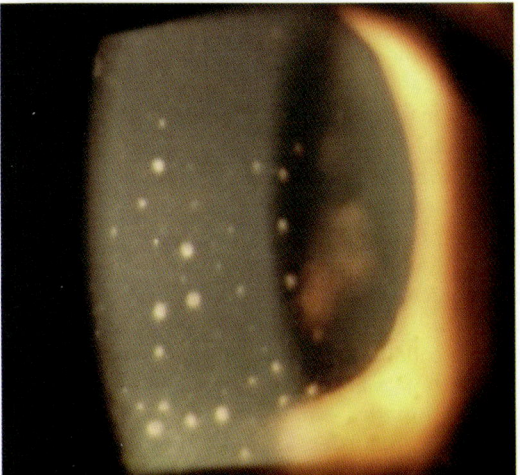

Fig. 7.2.1 *Slit-lamp photograph showing the granulomatous uveitis with medium-sized keratic precipitates.*

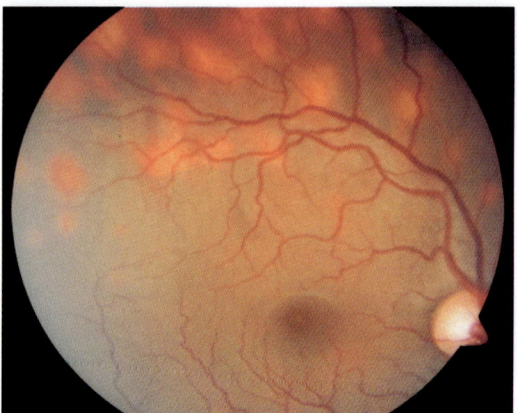

Fig. 7.2.5 *Fundus photograph showing multiple choroidal granulomas*

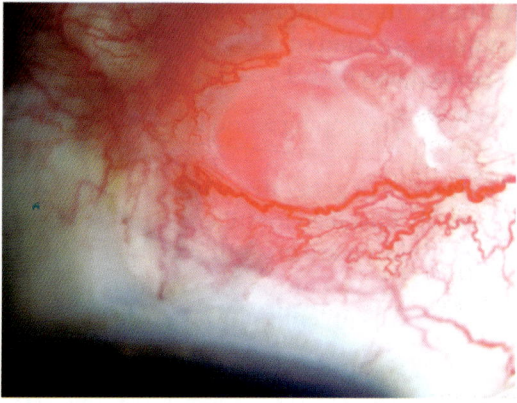

Fig. 7.2.8: *Slit-lamp photograph showing the scleral nodule.*

- *Sarcoidosis coexisting with Graves' disease* has also been reported.

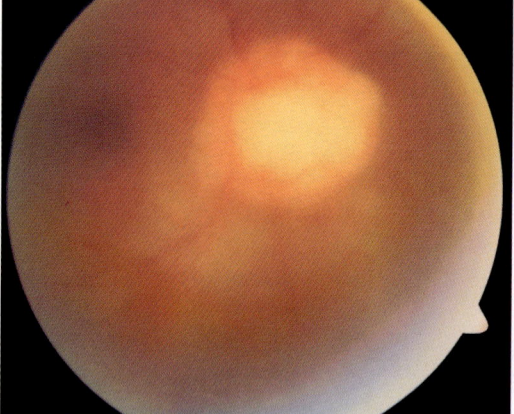

Fig. 7.2.6 *Fundus photograph showing the optic nerve granuloma.*

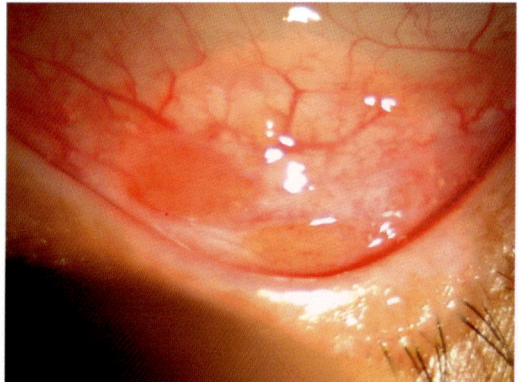

Fig. 7.2.7 *Slit-lamp photograph showing the conjunctival granulomas.*

Table 7.2.1 *Ocular findings in sarcoidosis*
Bilaterality
Eye lid and conjunctival granulomas
Lacrimal gland involvement
Keratoconjunctivitis sicca
Nongranulomatous anterior uveitis
Mutton-fat keratic precipitates
Iris and pupillary nodules/iris mass
Increase in IOP
Tent-shaped PAS
Nodules in trabecular meshwork
Intermediate uveitis
Snowballs/strings of pearls vitreous opacities
Multifocal peripheral chorioretinal lesions (active and atrophic)
Nodular and/or segmental periphlebitis (with or without candle wax exudate)
Retinal macroaneurysm
Choroidal granuloma
Haemorrhagic retinopathy with branch or central retinal venous occlusions
Acute posterior multifocal placoid pigment epitheliopathy and retinal pigment epithelial detachments
Optic disc nodules/granuloma/optociliary shunts/dilated collateral veins on the optic nerve head
Neurological manifestations: Cranial nerve palsies, encephalopathy, chiasmal syndromes, motility disorders, disorders of the hypothalamus and pituitary gland, optic atrophy either due to direct sarcoid tissue infiltration or compression by cerebral mass.

Eyelids, conjunctiva and corneal lesions

Conjunctival granulomas are millet-shaped to large cream nodular lesions, which can occur in sarcoidosis. They are usually asymptomatic. However, large conjunctival granulomas can cause diplopia. They respond generally to topical steroids. Eyelid granulomas are also seen in sarcoidosis.

• *Corneal band degeneration* especially in children may occur in patients with long-standing uveitis.

Sarcoid uveitis

Incidence. Sarcoid uveitis accounts for between 3 and 10% of all cases of uveitis.

Clinical types. Sarcoid uveitis can occur as anterior, intermediate, posterior or panuveitis.

Acute non-granulomatous anterior uveitis is a rare presentation but typically may affect patients with acute onset sarcoidosis.

Chronic anterior uveitis is more common and is known to affect older patients with chronic pulmonary sarcoidosis. It is typically a chronic bilateral uveitis and is characterized by granulomatous inflammatory reaction which includes mutton-fat keratic precipitates, iris nodules, trabecular meshwork nodules and tent-shaped peripheral anterior synechiae.

Intermediate uveitis characterized by snowball and/or string of pearls opacities in the vitreous may be associated with chronic anterior uveitis. Rarely it may occur perse even before the systemic manifestations.

Posterior uveitis may occur perse, or along with chronic anterior uveitis, or usually as a part of panuveitis. Posterior segment lesions occur in about 14 to 20% of patients with ocular sarcoidosis and include:

• *Nodular granulomas* measuring 1/4 to 1 disc diameter may occur in both retina as well as choroid. Usually the granulomas are multiple and characterised by small pale-yellow infiltration with punched-out appearance, seen more numerous in inferior quadrent. Rarely the large confluent amoeboid infiltration may be seen.

• *Perphlebitis* characterised by sheathing and irregular perivenous infiltrates known as candle wax dripping *taches de bougie* is typical of sarcoidosis.

• *Multifocal choroiditis* is characterised by multiple peripheral active or atrophic chorio-retinal lesions.

• *Occlusive retinal vascular disease*, especially branch retinal vein occlusions, and less commonly, central retinal vein occlusion together with peripheral retinal capillary non-perfusion, may lead to retinal neovascularisation and vitreous haemorrhage.

• *Cystoid macular oedema* is a frequent association.

• *Optic disc involvement* may occur as papillo-oedema (due to CNS involvement), persistent disc oedema (secondary to vitreoretinal lesions), and focal granuloma (which may not affect vision).

Complications. Most frequent complications include cystoid macular oedema (76%), cataract (49%), glaucoma (36%), retinal ischaemia (16%) and neovascularisations (11%). Corneal band shaped keratopathy occurs in long-standing cases of uveitis. Reports of inflammatory choroidal neovascular membranes have been described in sarcoidosis.

Scleral lesions

Scleral involvement has also been described in sarcoidosis.

DIAGNOSIS AND DIFFERENTIAL DIAGNOSIS

DIAGNOSIS

Diagnostic criteria

The First International workshop on ocular sarcoidosis in Tokyo in 2006 laid down diagnostic criteria for ocular sarcoidosis, consisting of 7 ocular signs (Table 7.2.2), 5 laboratory investigations (Table 7.2.3) and diagnostic criteria based on a combination of ophthalmic signs and laboratory investigations (Table 7.2.4).[18]

However, the above criteria need validation in different ethnic groups.

Investigations

Investigations supportive for diagnosis of ocular sarcoidosis[19-21, 23-27] are described below.

Table 7.2.2 *Clinical signs suggestive of ocular sarcoidosis*

1	Mutton-fat keratic precipitates and/or iris nodules at papillary margin or on stroma
2	Trabecular meshwork nodules and/or tent-shaped peripheral anterior synechiae
3	Snowballs/strings of pearls vitreous opacities
4	Multifocal peripheral chorioretinal lesions (active and atrophic)
5	Nodular and/or segmental periphlebitis (with or without candle wax exudate) and/or macroaneurysm
6	Optic disc nodules/granuloma and/or solitary choroidal nodule

Table 7.2.3 *Laboratory investigations in suspected ocular sarcoidosis*

1	Negative tuberculin test in a patient who either had BCG vaccination or previously had a positive tuberculin test
2	Elevated serum angiotensin-converting enzyme and/or elevated serum lysozyme*
3	Chest X-ray: Bilateral hilar lymphadenopathy
4	Abnormal liver enzyme tests (any 2: of alkaline phosphatase; aspartate transaminase; alanine transaminase
5	Chest CT scan in patients with normal chest X-ray

*Lysozyme is required in patients treated with ACE inhibitors

Table 7.2.4 *Diagnostic criteria for ocular sarcoidosis*

1	Biopsy supported diagnosis with compatible uveitis	Definite ocular sarcoidosis
2	Biopsy not done; bilateral hilar lymphadenopathy with compatible uveitis	Presumed ocular sarcoidosis
3	Biopsy not done; chest X-ray normal; 3 suggestive ocular signs and 2 positive investigational tests	Probable ocular sarcoidosis
4	Biopsy negative; 4 suggestive ocular signs and 2 positive investigations	Possible ocular sarcoidosis

Note. All other causes of uveitis—in particular, tuberculosis—are excluded. The term ocular sarcoidosis implies sarcoidosis within the eye, with or without associated systemic disease.

Fluorescein angiography. This technique allows detection of activity in lesions and complications like cystoid macular oedema and neovascularisation.

Indocyanine angiography. ICGA allows detection not only of bilaterality of disease but also of occult choroidal lesions.

Optical coherence tomography. OCT allows detection of choroidal granulomas and response to treatment by enhanced depth imaging and complications like cystoid macular oedema.

Tuberculin test. Depression of delayed type hypersensitivity manifesting, as a cutaneous anergy to tuberculin is a clinically important phenomenon occurring in sarcoidosis. Tuberculin sensitivity is depressed in sarcoidosis even in the background of high prevalence of TB. Thus negative tuberculin test in a BCG vaccinated patient or in a patient with a previously positive tuberculin skin test is a useful test in diagnosis of sarcoidosis.

Serum angiotensin-converting enzyme and lysozyme level. Elevated serum ACE is advocated by some as a good measure of granuloma activity but it is elevated in only half the patients with sarcoidosis. It is nonspecific and is also elevated in children and in other diseases like tuberculosis, leprosy, Gaucher's disease, chronic pulmonary disease, rheumatoid arthritis and histoplasmosis. Serum ACE in patients taking ACE inhibitors is known to be undetectable. In such cases, serum lysozyme is helpful.

Abnormal liver enzyme tests. The international criteria for the diagnosis of ocular sarcoidosis included abnormal liver enzymes: three times the upper limit of normal values for alkaline phosphatase or elevation twice over the upper limit of two of the following liver enzymes: aspartate aminotransferase (ASAT), alanine aminotransferase (ALAT) or alkaline phosphatase.

Radiology. Bilateral hilar lymphadenopathy on chest radiography is the most common finding in systemic sarcoidosis and is present in 50–89% of systemic sarcoidosis. Computed tomography of the thorax is more sensitive than a chest X-ray. CT scan detects presence of interstitial infiltrates and small lymph nodes. Contrast enhanced CT scan helps to distinguish the tubercular lymph node enlargement from that of sarcoidosis (Figs 7.2.9 to 7.2.11).

Gallium citrate scanning. Gallium-67 is a radioactive isotope, which is taken up by activated macrophages and marks areas where epitheloid cell granulomas are formed. Gallium uptake is assessed and graded in the lacrimal gland, salivary glands, thorax, spleen, liver and eyes 48 hrs after injection. However, this is non-specific and is also increased in tuberculosis and malignancies.

Bronchoalveolar lavage fluids. Examination of BAL fluid includes cytology. Lymphocytosis

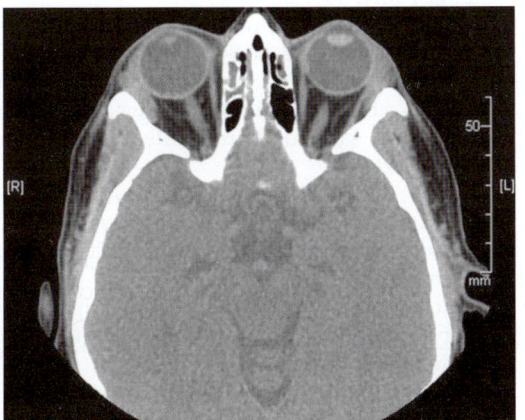

Fig. 7.2.9 *High resolution computed tomography of the orbits showing bilateral lacrimal gland enlargement.*

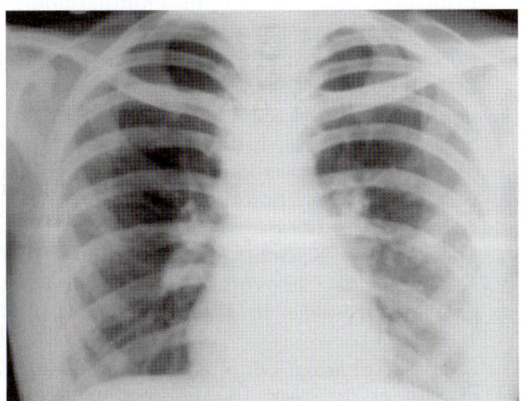

Fig. 7.2.10 *Chest X-ray showing bilateral hilar lymphadeno-pathy in a patient with sarcoidosis.*

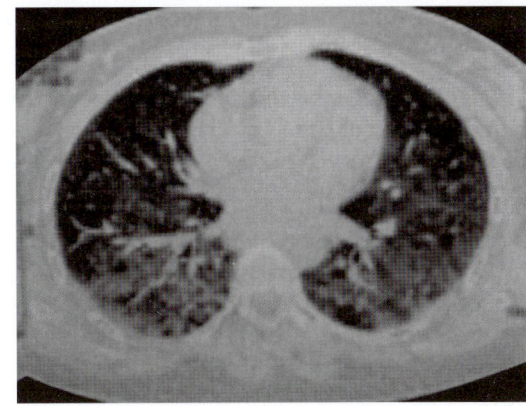

Fig. 7.2.11 *High resolution computed tomography of the thorax showing hilar lymphadenopathy with peribronchial thickening and interstitial opacities in sarcoidosis.*

and an increase of CD4/CD8 ratio in non-smoking individuals are considered to be characteristic in sarcoidosis. Smears and cultures may help to differentiate from tuberculosis.

Biopsy. Non-caseating granulomas are seen in sarcoidosis (Fig. 7.2.12). Endobronchial ultra-sound guided transbronchial lymph node biopsy is the most recently performed biopsy in sarcoidosis.

Hypercalcaemia. Hypercalcaemia occurs in fewer than 10% of patients with sarcoidosis and is of limited diagnostic value.

DIFFERENTIAL DIAGNOSIS

In addition to the clinical signs and laboratory tests indicative of sarcoidosis, exclusion of other

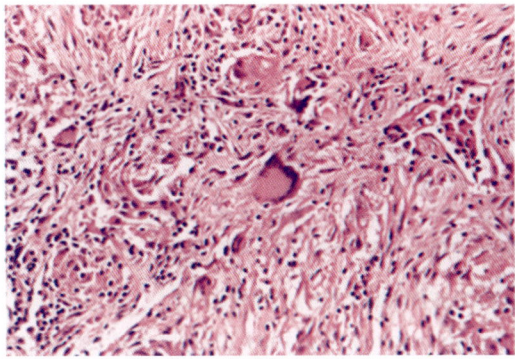

Fig. 7.2.12 *Photomicrograph of biopsy showing non-caseating granuloma with giant cells.*

entities is important for the diagnosis of sarcoidosis.

Differential diagnosis of granulomatous uveitis includes tuberculosis, syphilis, Vogt-Koyanagi-Harada syndrome, toxoplasmosis, herpetic uveitis and multiple sclerosis.[22]

Differential diagnosis of chorioretinal granulomas includes tuberculosis, syphilis, Vogt-Koyanagi-Harada syndrome, birdshot retinochoroidopathy, and primary intraocular lymphoma.

Differential diagnosis of periphlebitis includes tuberculosis, Behcet syndrome, cytomegalovirus retinitis.

TREATMENT[28-31]

TREATMENT OF OCULAR SARCOIDOSIS

Corticosteroids

There is no standardised therapy for ocular sarcoidosis associated uveitis. The mainstay of treatment is corticosteroids and is given in topical, periocular and systemic routes.

Periocular injections or intravitreal injections of steroids may be useful in unilateral disease in the absence of a systemic disease.

Systemic steroids are given in severe or resistant posterior uveitis.[28] Often higher doses of oral steroids with slow tapering are required to achieve remission.

Immunosuppressive agents

For corticosteroid-resistant or steroid-intolerant cases, steroid sparing immunosuppressive agents, like methotrexate, are effective.[29] Other immunosuppressives in the treatment of sarcoidosis include mycophenolate mofetil, azathioprine and cyclosporine.[30]

TNF-α blocking drugs have been used in resistant cases of sarcoidosis. Reports of treatment with rituximab in aggressive cases of sarcoid have been reported in literature.[31]

TREATMENT OF COMPLICATIONS

Neovascularisation may regress with systemic anti-inflammatory treatment and in some cases may require laser treatment.

Cystoid macular oedema. Intravitreal steroids or sustained steroid drug delivery devices, like dexamethasone implants, fluocinolone acetonide implants, are very useful in cystoid macular oedema.

Cataract and glaucoma occurring as complications need to be treated appropriately to prevent visual morbidity.

Inflammatory choroidal neovascular membranes (CNVM) and neovascularisation in sarcoidosis can be treated with intravitreal injections of anti-VEGF like bevacizumab and ranibizumab.

REFERENCES

1. Newman LS, Rose CS, Maier LA. Sarcoidosis. N Engl J Med 1997;336:1223–34.
2. Rothova A. Ocular involvement in sarcoidosis. Br J Ophthalmol 2000;84:110–6.
3. Schumacher G. Fall von beiderseitiger iridocyclitis chronica bei Boeckschem multiplem benignem sarkoid. Munch Med Wochenschr 1909:56:2664.
4. Usui Y, Kaiser ED, See RF, Rao NA, Sharma OP. Update of ocular manifestations in sarcoidosis. Sarcoidosis Vasc Diffuse Lung Dis 2002; 19(3): 167–75.
5. Jones N, Mochizuki M. Sarcoidosis: Epidemiology and clinical features. Ocular Immunology & Inflammation 2010;18(2):72–9.
6. Rothova A, Alberts C, Glasius E, et al. Risk factors for ocular sarcoidosis. Doc Ophthalmol 1989;72:287–96.
7. Hunter DG, Foster CS. Ocular manifestations of sarcoidosis. In: Albert DM, Jakobiec FA, eds. Principles and Practice of Ophthalmology. Philadelphia: WB Saunders, 1994:443–50.
8. Rothova A. Ocular involvement in sarcoidosis. Br J Ophthalmol 2000; 84:110–6.
9. Babu K, Kini R, Mehta R, Abraham MP, Subbakrishna DK, Murthy KR. Clinical profile of ocular sarcoidosis in a South Indian patient population. Ocul Immunol Inflamm 2010; 18(5): 362.
10. Pathanipitoon K, Goossens JHM, Tilborg TCV, Kunavisarut P, Choovuthayakorn J, Rothova A. Ocular sarcoidosis in Thailand. Eye 2010;24: 1669–1674.
11. Chan A, Sharma OP, Rao NA. Review for disease of the year: Immunopathogenesis of ocular sarcoidosis. Ocul Immunol Inflamm 2010;18(3):143–51.

12. Song Z, Marzilli L, Greenlee BM et al. Mycobacterial catalase peroxidase is a tissue antigen and target of the adaptive immune response in systemic sarcoidosis. J Exp Med 2005; 201(5): 755–67.

13. Grunewald J. Genetics of sarcoidosis. Curr Opin Pulm Med 2008;14(5):434–9.

14. Kojima K, Maruyama K, Inaba T, Nagata K, Yasuhara T, Yoneda K, Sugita S, Mochizuki M, Kinoshita S. The CD4/CD8 ratio in vitreous fluid is of highdiagnostic value in sarcoidosis. Ophthalmology 2012; 119(11): 2386–92.

15. Biswas J, Krishnakumar S, Raghavendran R, Mahesh L. Lid swelling and diplopia as presenting features of orbital sarcoid. Indian J Ophthalmol 2000;48(3):231–3.

16. Babu K, Kini R, Mehta R. Scleral nodule and bilateral disc edema as a presenting manifestation of systemic sarcoidosis. Ocul Immunol Inflamm 2010;18(3):158–61.

17. Verma A, Biswas J. Choroidal granuloma as an initial manifestation of systemic sarcoidosis. Int Ophthalmol. 2010;30(5):603–6.260.

18. Herbort CP, Mochizuki M, Rao NA. International criteria for the diagnosis of ocular sarcoidosis: results of the first international workshop on ocular sarcoidosis (IWOS). Ocul Immunol Inflamm 2009;17:160–169.

19. Kawaguchi T, Hanada A, Horie S, et al. Evaluation of characteristic ocular signs and systemic investigations in ocular sarcoidosis patients. Jpn J Ophthalmol 2007;51:121–6.

20. Papadia M, Herbort CP, Mochizuki M. Diagnosis of ocular sarcoidosis. Ocul Immunol Inflamm 2010;18(6):432–41.

21. Birnbaum AD, Chakrabarti A, Tessler H, Goldstein DA. Clinical features and diagnostic evaluation of biopsy proven ocular sarcoidosis. Arch Ophthalmol.2011; 129(4): 409–413.

22. Cowan CL. Differential diagnosis of ocular sarcoidosis. Ocul Immunol Inflamm 2010; 18(6): 442–51.

23. Mochizuki M, Takase H. The role of imaging in the diagnosis and management of ocular sarcoidosis. Int Ophthalmol Clinics 2012; 52(4): 113–20.

24. Jindal SK, Gupta D, Aggarwal AN. Sarcoidosis in developing countries. Curr Opin Pulm Med 2000;6:448–50.

25. Smith-Rohrberg D, Sharma SK. Tuberculin skin test among pulmonary sarcoidosis patients with and without tuberculosis: its utility for the screening of the two conditions in tuberculosis-endemic regions. Sarcoidosis Vasc Diffuse Lung Dis. 2006;23(2):130–4.

26. Ganesh SK, Roopleen, Biswas J, Veena N. Role of high-resolution computerized tomography (HRCT) of the chest in granulomatous uveitis: A tertiary uveitis clinic experience from India. Ocul Immunol Inflamm 2011Feb;19(1):51–7.

27. Agarwal R, Aggarwal AN, Gupta D. Efficacy and safety of conventional TBNA in sarcoidosis: A systematic review and meta-analysis. Respir Care 2012 Oct 8(epub ahead of print)

28. Shabbir Shafiq Jafferji, Biswas J. Optic nerve head sarcoid granuloma treated with intravenous methyl prednisolone. Oman Journal of Ophthalmology 2008;1(1):28–31.

29. Baughman RP, Lower EE, Ingledue R, Kaufman AH. Management of ocular sarcoidosis. Sarcoidosis Vasc Diffuse Lung Dis 2012; 29(1): 26–33.

30. Bhat P, Cervantes-Castañeda RA, Doctor PP, Anzaar F, Foster CS. Mycophenolate mofetil therapy for sarcoidosis-associated uveitis. Ocul Immunol Inflamm 2009; 17(3): 185–90.

31. Lower EE, Baughman RP, Kaufman AH. Rituximab for refractory granulomatous eye disease. Clin Ophthalmol 2012; 6:1613–8.

7.3 ADAMANTIADES-BEHÇET'S DISEASE

Introduction and etiopathogenesis
- Introduction
- Etiopathogenesis

Clinical features
- Systemic features
- Ocular features
- Complications

Diagnosis

Investigations
- Fundus fluorescein angiography
- Optical coherance tomography
- Pathergy test

Diagnostic criteria
- ISG criteria
- ICBD
- BRCJ

Treatment
- General considerations
- Therapeutics

INTRODUCTION AND ETIOPATHOGENESIS

INTRODUCTION

The first description of the syndrome was attributed to the Turkish dermatologist Hulusi Behçet in 1924. In 1930, the Greek ophthalmologist Benediktos Adamantiades reported a patient with inflammatory arthritis, oral and genital ulcers, phlebitis, and iritis,[1] so optly termed as Adamantiades-Behçet's disease.

Behçet's disease is observed to occur more commonly in countries along the old Silk Road, extending from Middle East to China. Countries most affected by Behçet's disease are Turkey, Iraq, Saudi Arabia, Iran, Afghanistan, Pakistan, northern China, Mongolia, the Koreas and Japan.

Males are more commonly involved and the mean age of onset in Behçet's disease is the third to fourth decades.

Turkey has the highest prevalence of Behçet's disease, with 420 cases per 100,000 population. The prevalence in Japan, Korea, China, Iran, and Saudi Arabia ranges from 13.5–22 cases per 100,000 population. The prevalence in North America and Europe is much less, with 1 case per 15,000–500,000 population.[2,3]

ETIOPATHOGENESIS

- *Autoimmune mechanism.* Current theories behind pathogenesis suggest an autoimmune mechanism. Many mechanisms play a role together including genetics, environmental conditions and infectious triggers.
- *Behçet's disease is a sporadic* disease, but carriers of HLA-B51/HLA-B5 have an increased risk of developing Behçet's disease compared with noncarriers.[4]
- *Cross-reactive immune response* after exposure to infectious agent especially herpes simplex virus (HSV), *Streptococcus* and other *Staphylococcus* species which inhabit the oral cavity have been postulated.
- *Systemic involvement* in Behcet's disease has pointed towards T lymphocytic response. Both CD4+ and CD8+ lymphocytes have been shown to be elevated.

CLINICAL FEATURES

SYSTEMIC FEATURES

1. Oral ulcer. Recurrent aphthous ulceration of the oral mucosa is characteristic. They occur in clusters and found not only on the gums but also on the lips, posterior pharynx, uvula, palate, and tongue. They are usually small but painful, and they heal in 7–10 days without scarring, but scarring occurs when a particularly large ulcer heals.

It has been suggested that in contrast to the regular flat borders of the aphthae seen in this disorder, the lesions in the Stevens–Johnson syndrome tend to be irregular, whereas in Reiter's syndrome they can have heaped-up edges.

2. *Skin lesions.* Many skin lesions have been described. These include:

- *Erythema nodosum* like lesions are frequently noted on the anterior surface of the legs, but can be seen on the face, neck, buttocks, and elsewhere. These lesions involute without ulceration after several weeks.

- *Psuedofollicultis* is common in Behcet's disease and often can be confused with acne- like eruptions associated with corticosteroid therapy.
- *Cutaneous hypersensitivity* is a characteristic feature of Behçet's disease. Dermatographs can be observed in one-third to one-half of patients. Scratching the skin with a needle or taking a blood sample often results in a pustule at that site. This phenomenon—pathergy—has become the basis for the 'prick'test.

3. *Genital ulcers.* Genital ulceration is seen in about 80% of the patients. These are typically painful punched out ulcers and are typically seen in the scrotum or vulva. These ulcaerations heal with scarring and scars are an indicator of old disease.

4. *Neurologic manifestations.* It gets involved usually late in the disease. Memory disturbances, behavioral changes, apathy or disinhibition occurs in about 54% of the patients.

5. *Vasculopathy.* Pulmonary arterial tree aneurysms are one of the most dreaded features seen in Behcet's disease. It mainly involves the veins and usually in the from of superficial thrombophlebitis. Vasculitis involving the arteries is mainly seen in males, but is rarely seen.

6. *Arthritis.* Around 50–60% patients show features of arthritis, mainly involving the lower extremity especially the knee. It is non-deforming and asymmetric in nature and can involve single or multiple joints.

7. *Gastrointestinal manifestations.* Seen in around 3–16% patients. Mainly involves the oesophagus and causes symptoms related to upper gastrointestinal tract.
- Genitourinary manifestations: It includes epididymitis, neurogenic bladder and urethritis.
- Renal manifestations: Associated with renal amyloidosis.
- Other manifestations include carditis, cardio-myopathy and pulmonary involvement.

OCULAR FEATURES

These have been described in 75% of the cases. It it the presenting feature of the disease in 10% of the patients. It can present as anterior, posterior or panuveitis. Posterior and panuveitis is usually seen in males.

1. *Acute anterior non-granulomatous uveitis with hypopyon.* The classic finding of Behçet's disease, iridocyclitis with hypopyon, is present in about one-third of cases (Fig. 7.3.1).

2. *Hypopyon.* Presenting finding in approximately 6% of ocular Behçet's disease cases.
- Generally visible to the naked eyes.
- Typically mobile in nature that shifts with gravity, head movement, or posture changes because the concentration of fibrinous exudates in the anterior segment is not profound in Behcet hypopyon.
- Need to r/o microhypopyon (visible only microscopically) and occult angle hypopyon (visible only gonioscopically)

Recurrent attacks may result in posterior synechiae, peripheral anterior synechiae, iris atrophy, and secondary glaucoma.

3. *Retinitis.* Retinal disease is the most serious complication of Behcet's disease. The classic fundus finding is retinal panvasculitis; that is it affects all vessels. Active periphlebitis is characterized by a fluffy white haziness surrounding the blood column with patchy involvement and irregular outside extensions, eventually resulting in vascular thrombotic occlusion with or without macular ischaemia. Severe vasculitis may lead to thrombosis and occlusive vasculopathy leading to secondary ischaemic retinal changes. Severe vitreous inflammation is seen in almost all the cases during acute phase. A funduscopic examination

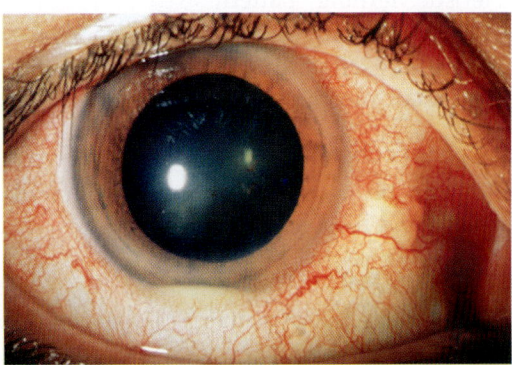

Fig. 7.3.1 *Behcet's disease presenting with non-granulomatous anterior uveitis with hypopyon.*

during the acute attack will, in addition, reveal areas of retinal haemorrhage and oedema, accompanied by an inflammatory response in the vitreous. The retinitis often has the appearance of a virally induced lesion, and the decision as to what has caused the lesion usually is based on the overall context in which it is being observed. Indeed, the disease can readily mimic acute retinal necrosis.

COMPLICATIONS

Most common complication of ocular BD is cystoid macular oedema, which is observed in about half of the patients. Secondary glaucoma is present in about 11% of BD patients.

Other complications include optic atrophy, macular ischaemia, recurrent inflammation and hypotony and pthisis bulbi.

DIAGNOSIS

INVESTIGATIONS

1. Fundus fluorescein angiography

Fundus fluorescein angiography shows diffuse retinal vascular leakage and occlusion of retinal vessels.

- Fluorescein leakage from retinal vessels may be seen.
- During acute inflammation, retinal vascular leakage is prominent, especially in the radial peripapillary area.
- Affected retinal and optic nerve vessels leak fluorescein profusely during early transit and their walls stain in late transit with a characteristic "ferning" pattern.
- Fluorescein angiography also may reveal macular ischaemia and cystoid macular oedema.

2. Optical coherence tomography

OCT can be used to quantify the macular oedema and response to treatment.

3. Pathergy test

The phenomenon of pathergy is the development of an aseptic non-specific hyper-reactivity, which varies from an indurated erythema to pustular formation on the skin following minor

trauma. If it is found to be positive, it can be of diagnostic value and is specific to Behçet's disease, which is very similar to erythematous papules or pustules that spontaneously appear in such patients. It is thought to denote increased neutrophil chemotaxis with an infiltration of PMNLs first followed by mononuclear and mast cells.

The pathergy test (Behçet line test) is performed by introducing a 20-gauge or smaller sterile needle 5 mm obliquely into the patient's flexor aspect of the avascular forearm skin without injection of saline under sterile conditions. At 24–48 hours after the pricking, the puncture site becomes inflamed and the test is considered positive, if there is an indurated erythematous small papule or pustule formation of more than 2 mm in diameter, which usually resolves within 3 or 4 days.

DIAGNOSTIC CRITERIA

In 1990, The International Study Group (ISG) for Behçet's Disease proposed a separate set of diagnostic criteria for Behçet's disease.

Behçet's syndrome international study group (ISG) criteria[5]

Diagnostic criteria include:
- Required criteria, and
- Minor criteria.

1. Required criteria. *Recurrent oral ulcerations:* Minor aphthous, major aphtous or herpetiform ulceration observed by physician or patient, which recurred at least 3 times in one 12-month period.

2. Minor criteria. *Recurrent genital ulceration:* Aphthous ulceration or scarring observed by physician or patient.

Eye lesion: Anterior uveitis, posterior uveitis, or cells in vitreous on slit-lamp examination or retinal vasculitis observed by ophthalmologist.

Skin lesions: Erythema nodosum observed by physician or patient, pseudofolliculitis or papulopustular lesions, or acneform nodules observed by physician in post-adolescent patients not on corticosteroid treatment.

Positive pathergy test (Behçet line test): Read by physician 24–48 hours.

Note. The ISG criteria for Behçet's disease have excellent specificity, but lack sensitivity. Thus, the International Criteria for Behçet's Disease (ICBD) was created in 2006, as a replacement to the ISG criteria.

International criteria for Behçet's disease (ICBD)[6]

Symptoms	Points
Ocular lesions (recurrent)	2
Oral aphthosis (recurrent)	2
Genital aphthosis (recurrent)	2
Skin lesions (recurrent)	1
Central nervous system	1
Vascular manifestations	1
Positive pathergy test	1

Scoring: Score ≥4 indicates Adamantiades-Behcet's disease.

Note. Though the main scoring system does not include the pathergy test, where pathergy test is conducted, a positive test may be included for 1 extrapoint.

Behçet's research committee of Japan (BRCJ) criteria

One diagnostic has been suggested by the Behçet's Research Committee of Japan.[7] In this criteria, there are 4 major and 5 minor criteria.

Major criteria
1. Recurrent oral aphthae
2. Skin lesions
3. Recurrent genital ulcers
4. Inflammation of the eye

Minor criteria
1. Arthritis
2. Ulceration of the bowel
3. Epididymitis
4. Vasculitis/vasculopathy
5. Neuropsychiatric symptoms

Types of ABD
- Complete (4 major)
- Incomplete (3 major or ocular involvement with one another major)
- Suspect (2 major with no eye involvement)
- Possible (1 major)

The committee also identified several special clinical types of ABD, depending on the predominant manifestation namely, neuro-Behçet, oculo-Behçet, intestinal-Behçet or vasculo-Behçet. Three laboratory tests have also been included in this system: a pathergy test (a skin prick), human leucocyte antigen (HLA) testing for HLA-B51 and a screening of non-specific factors indicative of immune system activation [elevated erythrocyte sedimentation rate (ESR), positive C-reactive protein (CRP) and an increase in peripheral blood leucocytes].

Undoubtedly, all the diagnostic systems have some degree of uncertainty, as any of the criteria may be manifested at different times during the clinical course of the disease.

TREATMENT

GENERAL COSIDERATIONS

Treatment approach depends on the individual patient, severity of disease, and major organ involvement. The European League Against Rheumatism (EULAR) recommendations for the management of Behçet's disease[8] were developed in 2008 and aid in the management of different aspects of Behçet's disease.

Goal of therapy is to treat acute episodes and to prevent recurrences of ocular inflammations; so as to prevent permanent damage.

Poor prognostic factors[9] include the following and should be aggressively treated.
- Complete ABD
- Involvement of the central nervous system
- Retinal involvement
- Vascular involvement
- Male sex
- Bilateral involvement
- Person hailing from Mediterranean Basin or Far East

THERAPEUTICS

I. Corticosteroids

Corticosteroids are being used in various forms for ABD like topical, local, systemic and even intra-articular. They are especially helpful in waning of the acute episodes of ocular inflammation in oral (1–1.5 mg/kg prednisone per day) or intravenous high dosage forms. But unfortunately, many patients of ABD show resistance towards corticosteroids and they need to be gradually tapered off before being shifted to immunosuppressive drugs. In some selected cases, low dose corticosteroids (≤10 mg/day) may be required along with immunosuppressive drugs. In anterior segment inflammations, topical steroids with or without periocular steroids may be required.

While giving corticosteroids especially for longer durations and higher dosages; their local and systemic side effects should be kept in mind and should be explained to the patient before starting them.

II. Immunomodulatory agents

Almost all patients of ABD will require immunomodulatory agents, as these patients show resistance towards corticosteroids. Various immunomodulatory agents used are given below:

Antimetabolites
- Azathioprine
- Mycophenolate mofetil

Cytotoxic agents
- Chlorambucil
- Cyclophosphamide

Calcineurin inhibitors
- Cyclosporine
- Tacrolimus
- Sirolimus

Biologic response modifiers
- Infliximab
- Adalimumab
- Daclizumab

Others
- Colchicine

1. Antimetabolites

Azathioprine. It is a purine analog that inhibits DNA synthesis, hence it affects the rapidly proliferating cells. Azathioprine alone is not effective in controlling ABD. Hence mostly used in combination therapy.

Mycophenolate mofetil. It is an agent which inhibits the enzyme inosine monophosphate dehydrogenase. Since it acts at the later stage of T cell cycle, it shows synergistic response when given with cyclosporin and hence used in combination theraphy.

2. Cytotoxic drugs

Chlorambucil. It is an alkylating agent. It was the first immunosuppressive drug used in ocular ABD. It is a slow-acting agent and takes around 2–3 months for its full action. But it is the single most efficacious agent capable of inducing long-term disease remission. However, because of its slow action, it should not be used in acute stages and is more useful in combination therapy in early course of the disease. Side effects, like azoospermia, low blood counts, should be kept in mind.

Cyclophosphamide. It is a faster-acting alkylating agent. It is thus useful in controlling acute uveitis, prevents relapse and maintains good visual acuity. It is useful in cases unresponsive to corticosteroids.

3. Calcineurin inhibitors

- *Cyclosporine.* It is an immunomodulatory agent which selectively inhibits CD4+ T cell-mediated immune response. The drug binds to cyclophilin and then binds and inhibits calcineurin. It is more effective and has less side effects when used in combination with corticosteroids. Renal toxicity is seen in almost all patients, if given in high doses.
- *Tacrolimus.* It is an immunosuppressive agent which has similar action to that of cyclosporine. It has a better safety profile than cyclosporin.

REFERENCES

1. Adamantiades B. A case of recurrent hypopyon iritis. Medical Society of Athens 1930;586–93.
2. Sakane T, Suzuki N, Takeno M. Innate and acquired immunity in Behcet's disease. 8th International Congress on Behcet's Disease. Reggio Emilia, Italy, 3-9 October 1998. Program and Abstracts: 56.

3. Krause I, Yankevich A, Fraser A, Rosner I, Mader R, Zisman D, et al. Prevalence and clinical aspects of Behcet's disease in the north of Israel. Clin Rheumatol 2007;26(4):555–60.

4. de Menthon M, Lavalley MP, Maldini C, Guillevin L, Mahr A. HLA-B51/B5 and the risk of Behcet's disease: a systematic review and meta-analysis of case-control genetic association studies. Arthritis Rheum 2009;61(10):1287–96.

5. International Study Group for Behcet's Disease. Criteria for diagnosis of Behcet's disease. Lancet 1990;335(8697):107–80.

6. The International Criteria for Behceti Disease (ICBD): **A** Collaborative study of 27 countries on the sensitivity and specificity of the new criteria. J Eur Acad Dermatol Venereol 2014; 28:338–47.

7. Behcet's Disease Research Committee of Japan. Behcet's disease: Guide to diagnosis of Behcet's disease. Jpn J Ophthalmol 1974;18:291–4.

8. Hatemi G, Silman A, Bang D, et al. EULAR recommendations for the management of Behcet disease. Ann Rheum Dis 2008;67(12): 1656–62.

9. Mishima S, Masuda K, Izawa Y, et al. Behcet's disease in Japan: ophthalmologic aspects. Trans Am Ophth 79;76:225–79.

7.4 VOGT-KOYANAGI-HARADA SYNDROME

INTRODUCTION AND PATHOGENESIS

INTRODUCTION

Vogt-Koyanagi-Harada syndrome is an idiopathic multisystem inflammatory disease of presumed autoimmune etiology that is characterised by bilateral granulomatous panuveitis that also involves the auditory system, meninges and skin.

Patients with bilateral anterior uveitis with vitiligo, poliosis, alopecia, and tinnitus were first described by Vogt (1906) and Koyanagi (1929) whereas Harada described a case of posterior uveitis with exudative retinal detachment and pleocytosis of cerebrospinal fluid in 1926. These spectra of diseases are now considered as a single systemic inflammatory condition and is known as Vogt-Koyanagi-Harada syndrome (VKH).[2-4]

PATHOGENESIS

• VKH is usually thought to be an autoimmune disease against melanocytes, and it is mainly mediated by cellular immune responses.[5]
• VKH is reported to occur more commonly in pigmented individuals and is rare in whites. But, interestingly, VKH is also rare in Africans.
• Genetic predisposition has been considered as major predisposing factor of this clinical condition.

• Genetic association to HLA-DR4 and HLA-Dw53 (most significant HLA-DRB1*0405) has been suggested.[6]
• VKH is hypothesised to be a T cell-mediated autoimmune disorder against melanocytes of various organs. Tyrosinase or tyrosinase-related proteins are implicated as target antigens on the melanocyte.[5]
• Histopathologically, there is diffuse non-necrotising granulomatous infiltration of the choroid sparing the choriocapillaris and thus VKH is often considered as primary stromal choroiditis.

CLINICAL FEATURES

Sex. Women are usually affected more often than men.

Age. VKH is most common in the third to fifth decades, but can affect individuals in all age groups.

PHASES OF VKH

Clinical manifestations of VKH can be divided into four phases, namely prodromal, uveitic, convalescent, and chronic or recurrent.

1. Prodromal phase is characterized by:
• Non-specific systemic symptoms like fever, headache, nausea, meningismus, vertigo, and dysacusis.
• Cerebrospinal fluid typically shows an increase in inflammatory cells with a pre-dominance of lymphocytes (pleocytosis).

2. Uveitic phase usually begins 3–5 days after the prodromal phase.

Symptoms. Uveitic phase is characterised by blurred vision, photophobia, and ocular pain.

Signs. Usually there occur bilateral, granulomatous uveitis characterised by following features:
• *Mutton-fat keratic* precipitates and inflammatory iris nodules can be seen.
• *Raised IOP.* Swelling of the ciliary body often displaces the lens-iris diaphragm forward and

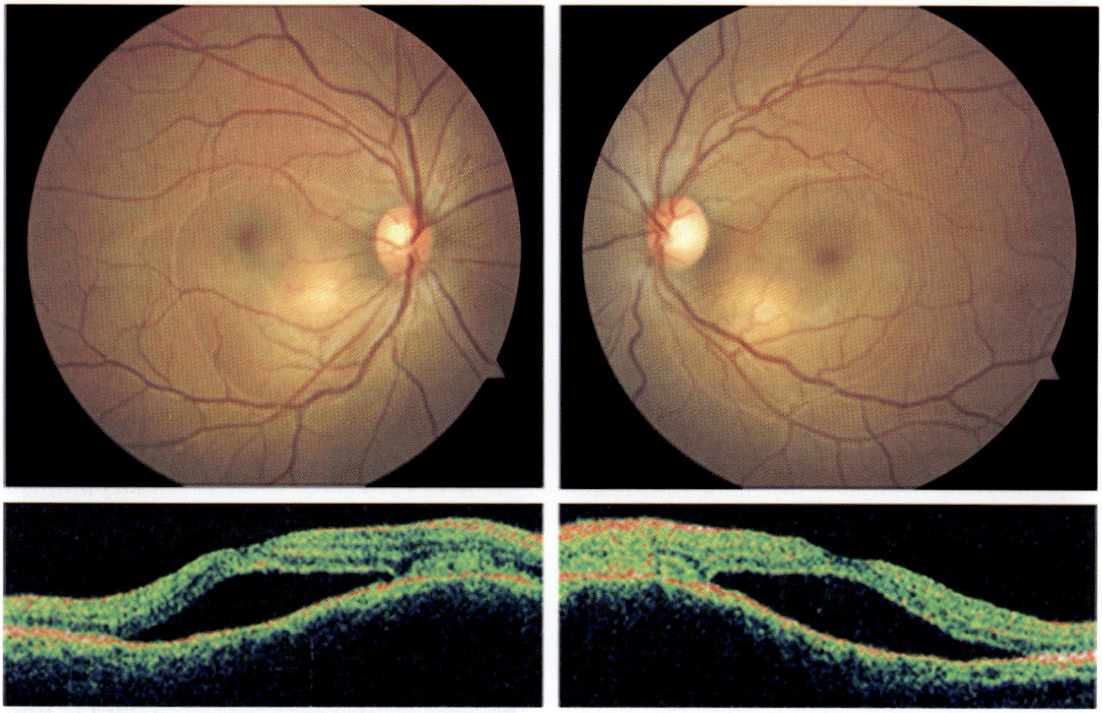

Fig. 7.4.1 *Fudus photograph and posterior segment OCT picture showing exudative retinal detachment in a patient with VKH syndrome.*

can lead to swallowing of the anterior chamber. This can result in episodes of angle closure and raised intraocular pressure.

- *Exudative retinal detachments* (Fig. 7.4.1) ranging from multiple pockets of subretinal fluid to bullous exudative retinal detachment can be seen.

- *Swelling and hyperaemia of optic nerve* can be seen.

- *Mild to moderate vitritis* with spillover of the inflammation into the anterior chamber is common.

Note. The ocular manifestations are clinically, histologically, and angiographically similar to those of sympathetic ophthalmia.

3. Convalescent stage usually starts with resolution of active inflammation and exudative retinal detachments with treatment. This stage is characterised by depigmentation that may be integumentary and/or uveal:

- *Depigmentation of the choroid* with loss of melanocytes produces the typical orange-red *"sunset glow"* appearance of the fundus.

- *Depigmentation of skin or vitiligo* can be observed in the face, eyelids, trunk and limbs (Fig. 7.4.2). Depigmentation can be seen in limbus also and is known as Suguira sign.

- *Multiple scattered, discrete, depigmented lesions* are seen in fundus and are called Dalen-Fuchs-like nodules, which represent localised absence of the retinal pigment epithelial cells.

4. Chronic recurrent stage is characterised by recurrent attacks of inflammation which can occur as part of the course of the disease or lack of adequate and prolonged immunomodulation. The chronic recurrent stage is usually charac-terised by mild to moderate panuveitis with

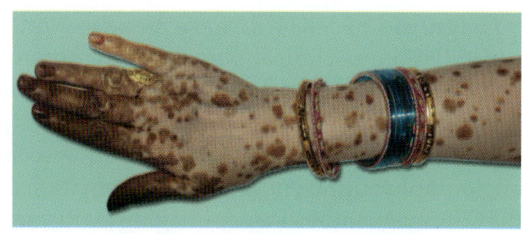

Fig. 7.4.2 *Depigmentation in VKH.*

anterior uveitis. It should be kept in mind that most vision-threatening complications occur in the chronic recurrent phase.

COMPLICATIONS

- *Choroidal neovascular membrane (CNVM)* is a major permanent vision-threatening complication of the disease.
- *Posterior synechiae, cataract* and *secondary angle closure* can develop because of the prolonged inflammation.
- *Subretinal fibrosis* may occur following posterior uveitis.
- *Neovascularization of the disc*
- *Pigmentary changes of the fundus* represent healed posterior uveitis.
- *Optic atrophy* may be secondary or consecutive.

SYSTEMIC MANIFESTATIONS

Neurological signs, such as meningismus, headache, malaise, fever, nausea, stiffness of neck and back, pleocytosis of the cerebrospinal fluid, cranial nerve palsies, hemiparesis and transverse myelitis.

Skin signs such as alopecia poliosis and vitiligo.

Internal ear disturbances such as tinnitus, and sensorineural deafness.

MANAGEMENT

DIAGNOSIS

Misdiagnosis of infectious uveitis can lead to inappropriate treatment and potential toxicity, while losing valuable ground without the needed steroid therapy. On the other hand, infectious uveitis misdiagnosed as VKH disease and treated with systemic immunosuppression can lead to disastrous results.

Diagnosis of VKH disease is based on a constellation of clinical signs and symptoms with no confirmatory tests. However, several diagnostic procedures may be useful in establishing the diagnosis, including fluorescein angiography, ultrasonography, examination of the CSF, magnetic resonance imaging (MRI), and electrophysiologic testing.

Investigations

1. *Fundus fluorescein angiography*[7,8] features are as below:

- *Acute VKH disease*: Fundus fluorescein angiography in arteriovenous phase of the disease shows multiple hyperfluorescent pin-head-like dots at the level of the RPE (Fig. 7.4.3.A), which gradually increases in size and shows placoid pooling of the dye in late phases (Fig. 7.4.3B).
- *Recovery phase of VKH disease* (after treatment with systemic corticosteroids): Most of the acute phase abnormalities, including exudative retinal detachment and disc oedema, resolve during this period. Fluorescein angiography may show persistent pinpoint areas of leakage and disc staining. Some patients may exhibit window defects and areas of mottled background hyperfluorescence.

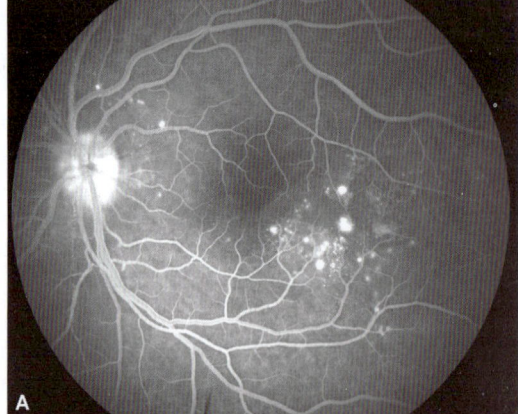

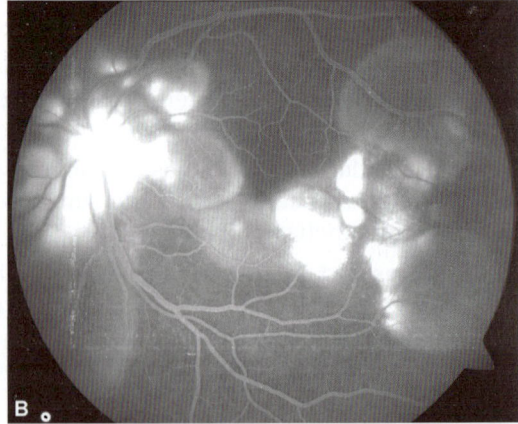

Fig. 7.4.3 *Fundus fluorescein angiography in acute VKH; A, Early frames of FFA showing pinhead leakage of the dye; B, Late frames of angiogram showing placoid pooling of the dye.*

- *Chronic VKH disease:* This is characterised clinically by depigmentation of the choroid. With angiography, signs of RPE atrophy are visible, such as a moth-eaten appearance, multiple window defects, and areas of alternating hyperfluorescence and hypo-fluorescence. Additional findings include choroidal neovascularisation, retinochoroidal and arteriovenous anastomoses, and neo-vascularisation of the disc. Macular oedema is rare in this disorder but may be seen in the chronic phase.

2. Indocyanine green angiography,[9,10] probably has limited diagnostic value but can be used for monitoring choroidal inflammation and response to therapy.

- *Acute VKH disease:* Indocyanine green angiography findings include delay of chorio-capillaris perfusion, as well as fuzzy and indistinct choroidal vessels, multiple hypo-fluorescent dark spots during the intermediate and late phases, and disc hyperfluorescence during the late phase.
- *Recovery phase of VKH disease (after treatment with systemic corticosteroids):* Most of the acute abnormalities resolve during this period. However, some of the hypofluorescent dark spots may persist for weeks.
- *Chronic VKH disease:* Findings include hypo-fluorescent areas during the intermediate and late phases.

3. Ultrasonography. The most characteristic feature seen on ultrasonography is low to medium reflective thickening of the posterior choroid. Other findings, like serous retinal detachment, mild thickening of sclera and mild vitreous opacities, can also be seen.

4. Optical coherence tomography (OCT) scanning. Early disease shows serous neuro-sensory retinal detachments with subretinal septa. Enhanced depth imaging (EDI) OCT and swept source OCT have revealed markedly increased choroidal thickness in patients with active VKH. OCT can be used for monitoring response to theraphy.[11]

Differential diagnosis

Sympathetic uveitis should be differentiated from VKH disease. The only difference between sympathetic uveitis and VKH disease is a history of penetrating ocular injury or intraocular surgery in patients with sympathetic uveitis and the absence of such a history in patients with VKH disease.

Central serous chorioretinopathy must be differentiated from the uveitic phase of VKH disease.

Posterior scleritis often shows exudative retinal detachment. Computed to mography scans and ultrasonography help to make the correct diagnosis, as they reveal thickening of the posterior sclera.

Other differential diagnoses to be kept in mind are:

- Intraocular lymphoma
- Bilateral diffuse uveal melanocytic proliferation
- Metastatic carcinoma
- Idiopathic uveal effusion syndrome
- Posterior scleritis

Diagnostic criteria

International Committee on Nomenclature established revised criteria for the diagnosis of VKH disease.[12]

Diagnostic criteria for Vogt-Koyanagi-Harada Disease

1. **No history of penetrating ocular trauma or surgery** preceding the initial onset of uveitis.
2. **No clinical or laboratory evidence suggestive** of other disease entities.
3. **Bilateral ocular involvement in which either part a or b must be met**, depending on the stage of disease when the patient was examined.

a. *Early manifestations of the disease:* There must be evidence of a diffuse choroiditis (with or without anterior uveitis, vitreous inflammatory reaction or optic disc hyperaemia) which may manifest as one of the following:

- Focal areas of subretinal fluid
- Bullous serous retinal detachment with equivocal fundus findings, both of the following must be present as well:
  i. Focal areas of delay in choroidal perfusion, multifocal areas of pinpoint leakage, large placoid areas of hyperfluorescence,

pooling within the subretinal fluid and optic nerve staining (listed in order of sequential appearance) by fluorescein angiography.

ii. Diffuse choroidal thickening, without evidence of posterior scleritis by ultrasonography.

b. *Late manifestations of the disease* history suggestive of prior presence of findings from 3a and either both 2 and 3 listed below or multiple signs from 3 ocular depigmentation (either of following manifestations is sufficient)

i. Sunset glow fundus

ii. Sugiura's sign

Other ocular signs (any of the following manifestations is sufficient)

i. Nummular chorioretinal depigmentation scars

ii. Retinal pigment epithelium clumping and/or migration

iii. Recurrent or chronic anterior uveitis

4. Neurological/auditory findings (which may have resolved by the time of examination). (Any of the following manifestations is sufficient)

i. *Meningismus* (malaise, fever, headache, nausea, abdominal pain, stiffness of the neck or back, or a combination of these factors. However, headache alone is not enough to meet a definition of meningismus).

ii. Tinnitus

iii. CSF pleocytosis

5. Integumentary findings (which do not precede the onset of central nervous system or ocular disease). (Any of the following manifestations is sufficient).

i. Alopecia

ii. Poliosis

iii. Vitiligo

Categories of VKH

The revised criteria defined the following three categories of disease:

1. *Complete VKH disease:* Criteria 1–5 must be present.

2. *Incomplete VKH disease:* Criteria 1–3 and either 4 or 5 must be present.

3. *Probable VKH disease:* Isolated ocular disease—criteria 1–3 must be present.

TREATMENT

Treatment consists of systemic steroids and immunosuppressants.

1. Systemic steroids

The key to successful therapy for VKH disease is early and aggressive treatment with systemic corticosteroids. Those patients who are treated later in the course of the disorder have a more guarded prognosis for recovery of visual acuity and probably have a greater risk for chronic inflammation.

The treatment of VKH disease should begin at the earliest stage to have better prognosis. Thus, it is critically important that the diagnosis of VKH be done accurately and as early as possible.

Intravenous methylprednisolone, 1 gm daily for 3 consecutive days may be required in patients with sight-threatening exudative retinal detachment.

Oral steroids are then required for long duration. Duration of treatment depends on the clinical response and should be individualised. Most patients will require at least 6 months of therapy before tapering of systemic corticosteroids. Early discontinuation has been associated with recurrences.

2. Immunosuppressants

In case of non-response to systemic steroids or intolerable adverse side effects, immunosuppressant drugs, like azathioprine, mycophenolate mofetil, cyclosporine, tacrolimus, or cyclophosphamide, can be started.[13–16]

Intravenous immunoglobulins and infliximab have also been used in patients of VKH.

REFERENCES

1. Jabs DA, Nussenblatt RB, Rosenbaum JT. Standardization of Uveitis Nomenclature (SUN) Working Group. Standardization of uveitis nomenclature for reporting clinical data. Results of the First International Workshop. Am J Ophthalmol 2005;140:509–16.

2. Vogt A. Fruhzeitiges Ergrauen der Zilien und Bemerkungen uber den sogenannten plotzlichen Eintritt dieser Veranderung. Klinische Monatsblatter fur Augenheilkunde, Stuttgart, 1906,44:228–42.

3. Koyanagi Y. Dysakusis, Alopecie und Poliosis bei schwerer Uveitis nicht traumatischen Ursprungs. Klinische Monatsblatter fur Augenheilkunde, Stuttgart, 1929,82:194–211.

4. Harada E. Clinical study of nonsuppurative choroiditis. A report of acute diffuse choroiditis. Acta Societatios phthalmologicae Japonicae, 1926.30: 356.

5. Andreoli CM, Foster CS. Vogt-Koyanagi-Harada disease. Int Ophthalmol Clin 2006;46(2):111–22.

6. Rajendram R, Evans MJ, Rao NA. Vogt-Koyanagi-Harada disease. Int Ophthalmol Clin 2005;45(2):115–34.

7. Arellanes-Garcia L, Hernhdez-Barrios M, Fromow-Guerra J, Cervantes-Fanning P. Fluorescein fundus angiographic findings in Vogt-Koyanagi-Harada syndrome. Int Ophthalmol 2007;27(2-3):155–61.

8. Wu W, Wen F, Huang S, Luo G, Wu D. Indocyanine green angiographic findings of Dalen-Fuchs nodules in Vogt-Koyanagi-Harada disease. Graefes Arch Clin Exp Ophthalmol 2007;245(7):937–40.

9. Bouchenaki N, Herbort CP. Indocyanine green angiography guided management of vogt-koyanagi-harada disease. J Ophthalmic Vis Res 2011;6(4):241–8.

10. da Silva FT, Hirata CE, Sakata VM, Olivalves E, Preti R, Pimentel S, et al. Indocyanine green angiography findings in patients with long standing Vogt-Koyanagi-Harada disease: a cross-sectional study. BMC Ophthalmol 2012;12(1):40.

11. Maruko I, Iida T, Sugano Y, Oyamada H, Sekiryu T, Fujiwara T, et al. Subfoveal choroidal thickness after treatment of Vogt-Koyanagi-Harada disease. Retina. 2011;31(3):510–7.

12. Read RW, Holland GNj Rao NA, Tabbara KFj Ohno S, Arellanes-Garcia L, et al. Revised diagnostic criteria for Vogt-Koyanagi-Harada disease: report of an international committee on nomenclature. Am J Ophthalmol 2001;131(5): 647–52.

13. Kim SJ, Yu HG. The use of low-dose azathioprine in patients with Vogt-Koyanagi-Harada disease. Ocul Immunol Ingamm 2007;15(5):381–7.

14. Agarwal M, Ganesh SK, Biswas J. Triple agent immunosuppressive therapy in Vogt-Koyanagi-Harada syndrome. Ocul Immunol Inflamm 2006;14(6):333–9.

15. Choudhary A, Harding SP, Bucknall RC, Pearce IA. Mycophenolate mofetil as an immuno-suppressive agent in refractory inflammatory eye disease. J Ocul Pharmacol Ther 2006;22(3): 168–75.

16. Nussenblatt RB, Palestine AG, Chan CC. Cyclosporin A therapy in the treatment of intraocular inflammatory disease resistant to systemic corticosteroids and cytotoxic agents; Am J Ophthalmol 1983;96(3): 275–82.

7.5 SYMPATHETIC OPHTHALMIA

General considerations
- Definition
- Changing trends in sympathetic ophthalmitis
- Incidence

Etiopathogenesis and pathology
Etiopathogenesis
- Predisposing factors
- Pathogenesis
Pathology

Clinical features
- Exciting eye
- Sympathizing eye

Treatment
- Prophylaxis

GENERAL CONSIDERATIONS

Definitions

Sympathetic ophthalmitis is a serious bilateral granulomatous panuveitis which follows a penetrating ocular trauma. Sympathetic ophthalmitis can also occur following an intraocular surgery. Fuchs' described it as a separate entity in 1905. The injured eye is called exciting eye and the fellow eye which also develops uveitis is called sympathizing eye.

Changing trends in sympathetic ophthalmitis

Over the years, lot of changes in sympathetic ophthalmitis have occurred. The changes worth taking into consideration[2] are summarised in Table 7.5.1.

Incidence

Incidence of sympathetic ophthalmitis has markedly decreased in the recent years due to meticulous repair of the injured eye utilizing microsurgical techniques and use of the potent steroids.

ETIOPATHOGENESIS AND PATHOLOGY

Etiopathogenesis

Etiology of sympathetic ophthalmitis is still not known exactly. However, the facts related with its occurrence are as follows:

A. Predisposing factors

1. It almost always follows a penetrating injury.
2. Wounds in the ciliary region (the so-called dangerous zone) are more prone to it.
3. Wounds with incarceration of the iris, ciliary body or lens capsule are more vulnerable.
4. It is more common in children than in adults.
5. It does not occur when actual suppuration develops in the injured eye.

Table 7.5.1 *Changing trends in sympathetic ophthalmitis worth taking into consideration*

Trend	Historical	Current
Cause	Post-trauma	Post-surgery (especially vitreoretinal)
Patients	Males and children (reflecting trauma peaks)	No sex preference (reflects positive impact of injury prevention programs) and increasingly elderly patients (reflects impact of ocular surgery)
Incidence	Considered disappearing 30 years ago	Probably increasing (underdiagnosed?)
Onset	For 65% within 2–8 weeks (for 90%, onset <1 year from trauma or most recent surgery)	Many delayed presentations (for significant percentage onset >1 year from trauma or most recent surgery)
Presentation	Granulomatous panuveitis	Any clinical uveitis
Outcome	Enucleation within 2 weeks for prevention of SO	Enucleation solely of SO prevention questionable
Visual prognosis	Poor	Reasonable due to modern immuno-suppression

B. *Pathogenesis*

The exact pathogenesis of sympathetic ophthalmia is still unknown. It is believed to be a result of autoimmune reaction generated by exposure of the choroidal melanocyte to immune system. It is characterised by a granulomatous inflammation predominantly by T lymphocytes, CD4+ helper T cells in early phase of the disease and CD8+ cytotoxic T cells in late phase of the disease. Choriocapillaris are typically spared in sympathetic ophthalmia and VKH.

Pathology

It is characteristic of granulomatous uveitis, i.e. there is:

- *Nodular aggregation* of lymphoctes, plasma cells, epitheloid cells and giant cells scattered throughout the uveal tract.
- *Dalen-Fuchs' nodules* are formed due to proliferation of the pigment epithelium (of the iris, ciliary body and choroid) associated with invasion by the lymphocytes and epitheloid cells.
- *Sympathetic perivasculitis*. Retina shows perivascular cellular infiltration.

Clinical features

Sympathetic ophthalmia presents as a bilateral diffuse uveitis. The clinical presentation of sympathetic ophthalmia covers a wide-spectrum depending on the severity of the disease.

I. Exciting (injured) eye. It shows clinical features of persistent low grade plastic uveitis, which include ciliary congestion, lacrimation and tenderness. Keratic precipitates may be present at the back of cornea (dangerous sign).

II. Sympathizing (sound) eye. It is usually involved after 4–8 weeks of injury in the other eye. Earliest reported case is after 9 days of injury. Most of the cases occur within the first year. However, delayed and very late cases are also reported. Sympathetic ophthalmitis, almost always, manifests as acute plastic iridocyclitis. Rarely it may manifest as neuroretinitis or choroiditis. Clinical feature of the iridocyclitis in sympathizing eye can be divided into two stages:

1. *Prodromal stage.*
- *Symptoms.* Sensitivity to light (photophobia) and transient indistinctness of near objects (due to weakening of accommodation) are the early symptoms.
- *Signs.* In this stage, the first sign may be presence of retrolental flare and cells or the presence of a few keratic precipitates (KPs) on back of cornea. Other signs includes mild ciliary congestion, slight tenderness of the globe, fine vitreous haze and disc oedema which is seen occasionally.

2. *Fully-developed stage.* It is clinically characterised by typical signs and symptoms consistent with acute plastic iridocyclitis.

- *Ciliary congestion and a granulomatous anterior chamber reaction* with mutton-fat keratic precipitates on the corneal endothelium is a characteristic feature of anterior uveitis seen in sympathetic ophthalmitis. However, it can present with non-granulomatous anterior uveitis also.
- *Posterior synechiae and raised* intraocular pressure are common.
- *Vitritis.* Fundus examination typically reveals a moderate to severe vitritis.
- *Optic disc involvement* in the form of papillitis or swelling and exudative detachment can occur.
- *Yellowish-white ocular lesions* may be seen in the posterior pole and mid-equatorial sub-RPE (Fig. 7.5.1A). They usually correspond to Dalen-Fuchs nodules seen on histopathological examination (Fig. 7.5.1B).

3. *Complications of sympathetic ophthalmia* include:

- Secondary glaucoma
- Cataract
- Chronic maculopathy
- Choroidal neovascularisation
- Optic atrophy
- Phthisis bulbi

Diagnosis

Diagnosis is mainly clinical and some ancillary testings, like FFA, ICG, USG B-scan and OCT, are very helpful in doubtful cases.

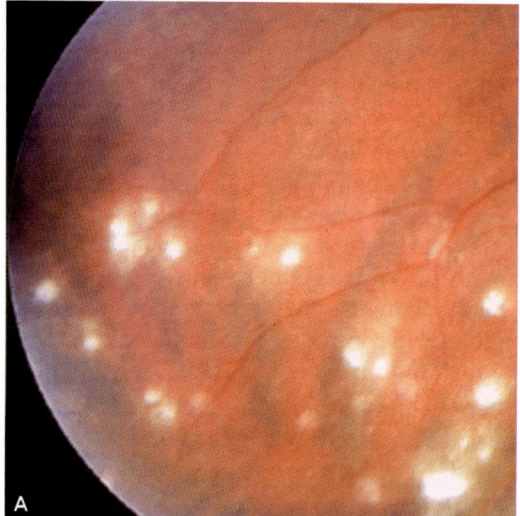

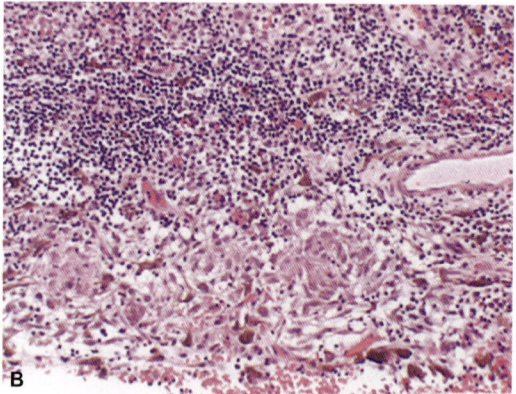

Fig. 7.5.1 *Dalen Fuchs' nodules in sympathetic ophthalmitis: A, Clinical appearance on fundus examination; B, Histological appearance.*

FFA. In acute phase, multiple subretinal hyper-fluorescent spots and pooling are seen. During healing phase, there is increased pigmentation and areas corresponding to Dalen- Fuchs nodules represent focal areas of atrophy and cause window defects.

ICG. Hypofluorescence is seen in the mid-phase followed by persisting hypofluorescence or gradual fading in later phases.

Treatment

A. Prophylaxis

I. *Early excision of the injured eye.* Prevention is the only known treatment whereby the injured eye may be enucleated within 2 weeks of trauma.

This is of course not the recommendation for the removal of an eye with useful vision.

II. *When there is hope of saving useful vision,* following steps should be taken:

1. *A meticulous repair of the wound* using micro-surgical technique should be carried out, taking great care that uveal tissue is not incarcerated in the wound.
2. *Immediate expectant treatment* with topical as well as systemic steroids and antibiotics along with topical atropine should be started.
3. *When the uveitis is not controlled after 2 weeks of expectant treatment,* i.e. lacrimation, photo-phobia and ciliary congestion persist and if KPs appear, this injured eye should be excised immediately.

B. Treatment of already supervened sympathetic ophthalmitis

I. Early excision (enucleation)

Once sympathetic ophthalmia develops, enucleation of the exciting eye is still a subject of controversy. However, enucleation may be done when the case is seen shortly after the onset of inflammation (i.e. during prodromal stage) in the sympathizing eye, and the injured eye has no useful vision, this useless eye should be excised at once.

II. Conservative treatment of sympathetic ophthalmitis

In all cases, once the diagnosis is established, aggressive treatment on the lines of acute iridocyclitis should be started immediately, as follows:

1. *Corticosteroids* should be administered by all routes, i.e. systemic, periocular injections and frequent instillation of topical drops. In severe cases, intravenous pulsed therapy of steroids should be considered. Intensive high dose oral steroids (1 mg/kg/day) are usually required. Aim is to reduce the steroids gradually over 2–3 months as per clinical response. Once below 10 mg, aim to maintain over 6–12 months.

2. *Immunosuppressant drugs.* In case of development of serious side effects or when refractory to steroids, other immunosuppressives should be considered, such as cyclosporine started at 5 mg/kg/day. Once the disease is under remission, a slow taper at 0.5 mg/kg/day

should be started and substituted with low dose corticosteroids. *Close monitoring* is necessary due to the side effect profile of hepatotoxicity, nephrotoxicity and neurotoxicity. Alkylating agents and antimetabolites can also be used, if the inflammation cannot be adequately controlled with corticosteroids and cyclosporine.
3. *Atropine* should be instilled three times a day in all cases.

Note. The treatment should be continued for a long time.

Prognosis

If sympathetic ophthalmitis is diagnosed early (during prodromal stage) and immediate treatment with steroids is started, a useful vision may be obtained. However, in advanced cases, prognosis is very poor, even after the best treatment.

BIBLIOGRAPHY

1. Fuchs E. Über sympathislerende Entzündung zuerst Bemerkungeen über seröse traumatische Iritis. Albrect Von Graefes Arch Ophthalmol 1905; 61:365–456.
2. Vote BJ, et al. Changing trends in sympathetic ophthalmia. Clin Exp Ophthalmol 2004; 32: 542–5.

7.6 FUCHS' UVEITIS SYNDROME

Etiology
• Idiopathic
• Associated condition
Clinical features
• Symptoms
• Signs
Diagnosis and treatment
Diagnosis
Treatment
• Treatment of uveitis
• Treatment of glaucoma
• Treatment of cataract
• Pars plana vitrectomy

ETIOLOGY

Idiopathic. Exact etiology of Fuchs' uveitis syndrome is not known.

Associations condition. Associations with ocular toxoplasmosis, herpes simplex virus, and rubella virus have been reported by some workers without any conclusive results.

CLINICAL FEATURES

Symptoms include:
• *Gradual blurring of vision* due to posterior sub-capsular cataract (PSC) is the most common presenting symptoms.
• *Floaters* and difference in the colour of the two eyes are other presenting symptoms.

Signs include:
1. *Keratic precipitates (KPs)* are typically fine stellate present all over the endothelium with filaments in between them, and possibly are pathognomonic of FUS (Fig. 7.6.1).
2. *Anterior chamber signs*
   • *Aqueous flare* is usually faint.
   • *Aqueous cells* are never more than +2
3. *Iris signs* include:
   • *Heterochromia iridis* is an important and common sign.
   • *Diffuse stromal atrophy* gives rise to washed-out appearance (moth-eaten appearance).

Radial iris vessel becomes more visible as stroma is atrophied.
• *Posterior pigment layer iris atrophy* is patchy and best detected by retroillumination as transillumination defects.
• *Iris nodules* may be present along the pupillary border.
• *Iris crystals.* Small, refractile iris crystals called Russell bodies can be seen on the surface of the iris. Russell bodies are aggregations of spherical immunoglobulin.
• *Rubeosis iridis* may be seen in the form of fine irregular fragile vessels on the iris surface. Recurrent hyphema may occur as a result of bleeding from the fragile vessels (Amsler's sign).
• *Posterior synechiae* are conspicuously absent.
4. *Cataract* (posterior subcapsular cataract) is a common complication of Fuchs' uveitis syndrome having a chronic long-lasting course. Most of the time, blurring of vision due to posterior subcapsular cataract is the presenting symptom.
5. *Glaucoma in FUS* occurs in about 30% of the cases, with following key features:
• *Mechanism.* Secondary open-angle glaucoma, occurring probably due to trabecular sclerosis. Prolonged steroid use may also contribute in causation of glaucoma as well as cataract.
• *Raised IOP*, initially intermittent, later becomes constant. Occasionally, the IOP rise may be precipitated by cataract surgery.
• *Gonioscopy* reveals open-angle with ± twig-like neovascularisation of the angle.

DIAGNOSIS AND TREATMENT

Diagnosis

Diagnosis is usually made from the typical signs in patients who mostly present with defective vision to complicated cataract.

Treatment

Treatment of uveitis. Uveitis in FUS is typically resistant to steroids, though steroids are still used to provide comfort.

- *Topical steroids* are all that is required. These can lessen the inflammation but does not resolve it, so aggressive treatment to eradicate the cellular reaction is not indicated.
- *Mydriatics* are not required since posterior synechiae are seldom formed.
- *Posterior subtenon injection of long-acting steroids* (triamcinolone) may be useful for the annoying floaters.

Treatment of glaucoma. Glaucoma is treated similar to POAG. However, pilocarpine and prostaglandin analogous are avoided.

- *Medical therapy.* Glaucoma is resistant to hypotensive agents in many cases (with 73% failing to respond to maximal medical therapy).
- *Surgery* (trabeculectomy with antimetabolites or a drainage device) is the main line of treatment.

Treatment of cataract. Cataract associated with Fuchs' uveitis can be well managed by cataract surgery with IOL implantation usually patients do well.

Pars plana vitrectomy may rarely be required in patients with associated vitreous opacification.

BIBLIOGRAPHY

1. Chee SP, Jap A. Presumed fuchshetero-chromiciridocyclitis and Posner-Schlossman syndrome: comparison of cytomegalovirus-positive and negative eyes. Am J Ophthalmol 2008; 146(6):883–9.e1.
2. Iesegang TJ. Clinical features and prognosis in Fuchs' uveitis syndrome. Arch Ophthalmol 1982; 100(10):1622–6.
3. Jones NP. Fuchs Heterochromic uveitis: A reappraisal of the clinical spectrum. Eye 1991; 5 (Pt 6):649–61.
4. Jones NP. Fuchs' heterochromic uveitis: an update. Surv Ophthalmol 1993;37(4):253–72
5. Loewenfeld IE, Thompson HS. Fuchs hetero-chromiccyclitis: A critical review of the literature. I. Clinical characteristics of the syndrome. Surv Ophthalmol 1973;17(6):394–457.
6. Melamed S, Lahav M, Sandbank U, et al. Fuchs' heterochromiciridocyclitis: an electron micro-scopic study of the iris. Invest Ophthalmol Vis Sci. 1978;17(12):1193–9.
7. Mohamed Q, Zamir E. Update on Fuchs' uveitis syndrome. Curr Opin Ophthalmol 2005;16(6): 356–63.
8. Schwab IR. The epidemiologic association of Fuchs' heterochromiciridocyclitis and ocular toxoplasmosis. Am J Ophthalmol 1991; 111(3):356–62.
9. Teyssot N, Cassoux N, Lehoang P, et al. Fuchs heterochromic cyclitis and ocular toxocariasis. Am J Ophthalmol 2005;139(5):915–6.
10. Toledo de Abreu M, Belfort R Jr, Hirata PS. Fuchs' heterochromiccyclitis and ocular toxo-plasmosis. Am J Ophthalmol 1982;93(6):739–44.
11. Van Gelder RN. Idiopathic no more: clues to the pathogenesis of Fuchs heterochromicirido-cyclitis and glaucomatocyclitic crisis. Am J Ophthalmol 2008;145(5):769–71.

7.7 POSNER-SCHLOSSMAN SYNDROME

Etiology
- Idiopathic
- Causes of acue rise in IOP
- Association with raised prostaglandins
- HLA-BW 54 association

Clinical features
- Presenting symptoms
- Signs
- Clinical course

Diagnosis
Clinical diagnosis

Treatment
- Treatment of uveitis
- Treatment of glaucoma

Posner-Schlossman syndrome (glaucomatico-cyclitic crisis) is characterised by recurrent attacks of unilateral acute rise of IOP. Both eyes may be involved at different times but very rarely contemporaneously.

ETIOLOGY

- *Idiopathic*, i.e. exact etiology of glucomato-cyclitic crisis is not known.
- *Cause of acute rise in IOP* is presumed to be acute trabeculitis, possibly secondary to HSV, CMV or *Helicobacter pylori*.
- *Association with raised prostaglandins.* A direct correlation between elevated levels of prostaglandins (prostaglandin E) in the aqueous humour and the level of IOP has been found during acute attacks of glaucomato-cyclitic crisis.
- *HLA-BW 54 association.* Condition typically affects young adult males much more than females, 40% of whom are positive for HLA-BW 54.

CLINICAL FEATURES

Presenting symptoms are vague and include mild discomfort, haloes around light and slight blurring of vision without any redness and pain.

Signs seen on examination:
- *No congestion*, i.e. the eye is typically white.

- *IOP is markedly raised* (40–50 mm Hg) during the attacks, but becomes normal in between the attacks. The rise of IOP is out of proportion to the severity of the uveitis, and this rise in IOP precedes the identifiable inflammatory reaction, often by several days.
- *Cornea* shows epithelial oedema due to a high IOP, and fine KPs on the back. Fine keratic precipitates appear after 2–3 days of elevated IOP and resolve rapidly. Fresh precipitates may appear with each episode of increased IOP.
- *Anterior chamber* shows few aqueous cells with minimal flare, no posterior synechiae.
- *Gonioscopy* reveals open-angle with no PAS (a differentiating point from other inflammatory glaucomas).

Course. The acute attack of the disease typically lasts from several hours to several days, and recurrences are common over many years.

The recurrent attacks are unilateral, however, about 50% patients do give history of bilateral attacks at times. The interval between the attacks becomes longer with time. Many patients develop chronic open-angle glaucoma as a result of damage to the trabecular meshwork caused by recurrent attacks.

DIAGNOSIS

Clinical diagnosis is made from typicall signs of mild uveitis associated with raised IOP. However, since the connectition is so rare, it should be diagnosed after excluding the common causes of hypertensive uveitis, such as herpetic uveitis.

TREATMENT

Treatment of uveitis. Uveitis is treated by:
- *Typical steroids* mainly.
- *Oral NSAIDs* may also be helpful.

Treatment of glaucoma. Glaucoma may be treated by:

- *Topical antiglaucoma drugs,* such as beta blockers, alpha-2 agonists, and carbonic anhydrase inhibitors.
- *Oral acetazolamide* may be added according to IOP level.
- *Hyperosmotic agents,* like intravenous mannitol, may be used during acute attack when IOP is very high.

Note. Pilocarpine should always be avoided, as it may exacerbate ciliary spasm.

BIBLIOGRAPHY

1. Dinakaran S, Kayarkar V. Trabeculectomy in the management of Posner-Schlossman syndrome. Ophthalmic Surg Lasers 2002; 33(4):321–2.

2. Kass MA, Becker B, Kolker AE. Glaucomatocyclitic crisis and primary open-angle glaucoma. Am J Ophthalmol 1973; 75(4):668–73.

3. Levatin P. Glaucomatocyclitic crisis occurring in both eyes. Am J Ophthalmol 1956; 41:1056.

4. Maeda H, Nakamura M, Negi A. Selective reduction of the S-cone component of the electroretinogram in Posner-Schlossman syndrome. Eye 2001; 15:163–7.

5. Posner A, Schlossman A. Further observations on the syndrome of glaucomatocyclitic crisis. Trans Am Acad Ophthalmol Otolaryngol 1953; 57:531.

6. Posner A, Schlossman A. Syndrome of unilateral recurrent attacks of glaucoma with cyclitic symptoms. Arch Ophthalmol 1948; 39:517.

7. Theodore FH. Observations on glaucomatocyclitic crisis. Br J Ophthalmol 1952; 36:207.

7.8 PHACOGENIC UVEITIS

Definition, epidemiology and etiopathogenesis
- Definition
- Epidemiology
- Etiopathogenesis

Pathology
- Histological features

Clinical profile
- Phacogenic uveitis
- Acute phacogenic uveitis
- Subacute phacogenic uveitis
- Phacolytic glaucoma
- Phacomorphic glaucoma

Diagnosis and differential diagnosis
- Clinical diagnosis
- Ultrasonography
- Anterior chamber tap

Treatment
- Medical treatment
- Surgical treatment
- Complications

DEFINITION, EPIDEMIOLOGY AND ETIOPATHOGENESIS

Definition

Phacogenic uveits or lens-induced uveitis is defined as anterior uveitis with or without vitreous inflammation caused by excessive release of lens proteins, occurring days to weeks after surgical or traumatic disruption of lens capsule, or spontaneously due to a hypermature cataract.[1,2] Over the years, many terms have been used interchangeably for lens-induced uveitis, like phacolytic, phacogenic, phacotoxic and phacoanaphylactic uveitis.

Epidemiology

Incidence. The occurrence of phacogenic uveitis is uncommon with an incidence rate as low as less than 1%.[4]

- *Sex.* Men are more affected than women.
- *Age.* The mean age of occurrence is between 60–70 years.
- *Geography.* Phacogenic uveitis is expected to be more prevalent in developing countries

where cataract is the leading cause of blindness.[5,6]
- It is generally coincidental with the time of cataract surgery.

Etiopathogenesis

Predisposing factors. Certain factors like mature/hypermature cataract, trauma (surgical and non-surgical) and abnormally developed eye precipitate phacogenic uveitis.

Pathogenes. The pathogenesis of lens-induced uveitis is not precisely understood. In fact, the terms phacoanaphylactic uveitis and phacotoxic uvetis, previously used seems misleading and misnomers. Since phacogenic uveitis lacks involovement of IgE, eosinophils, basophils and mast cells,[3] so it does not appear to be of type I hypersensitivity reaction or anaphylactoid reaction. Further, there is no evidence that lens proteins may be toxic to ocular uveitis.

PATHOLOGY

Histological features characteristic of phacogenic uveitis is zonal inflammation in and around the lens, more in the area of capsular rupture, if present.[7–9] The lymphocytes, neutrophils, epithelioid cells and giant cells are the inflammatory cells found.

CLINICAL PROFILE

As of today, most workers recomend descarding of the terms phacotoxic and phacoanaphylactic uveitis. The lens matter-induced uveitis (LIU) and phacogenic uveitis may be used as synonymous terms to denote the anterior uveitis occurring days to weeks after lens capsule disruption (either surgical or traumatic or spontaneously due to leakage of lens proteins in hypermature cataract). Further, since some uveal inflammation may be associated with lens induced glaucoma (LIG), so the clinical profile includes:
- Phacogenic uveitis,
- Phacolytic glaucoma, and
- Phacomorphic glaucoma.

Phacogenic uveitis

Phacogenic uveitis, as mentioned above, refers to anterior uveitis with or without vitreous inflammation caused by released or residual lens proteins. Phacogenic uveitis, though a rare condition, its incidence has increased following shift from intracapsular to extracapsular extraction techniques including phacoemulsi-fication. Phacogenic uveitis may manifest as:

• Acute phacogenic uveitis, and

• Subacute or chronic phacogenic uveitis.

Acute phacogenic uveitis

Acute phacogenic uveitis typically occurs within 24 hours of release of lens matter and manifests as severe acute granulomatous inflammation characterise by following features (Fig. 7.8.1):

Symptoms include unilateral:
• Ocular pain,
• Redness,
• Photophobia, and
• Visual loss.

Occurring typically following release of lens matter in the anterior chamber.

Signs include:
• *Keratic precipitates* (KPs), of mutton fat type, are generally present.
• *Anterior chamber cells and face* of moderate to severe degree.

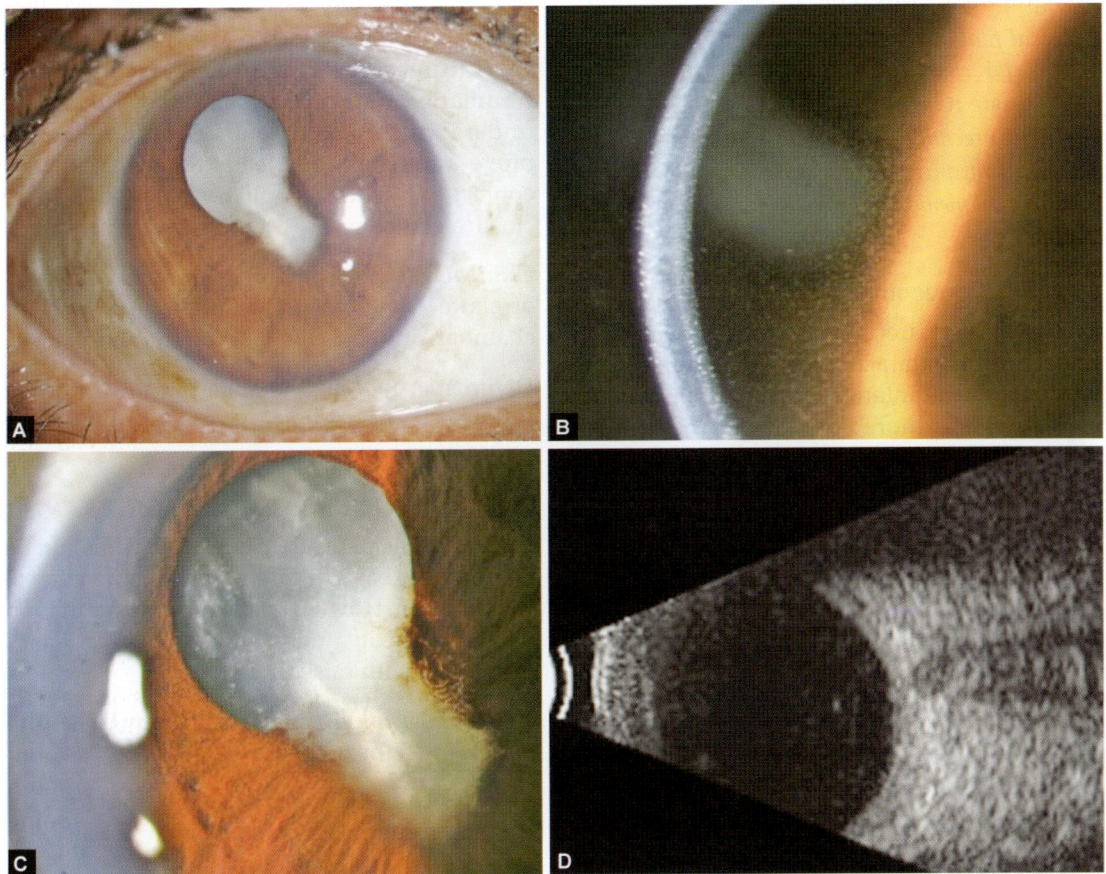

Fig. 7.8.1: *A case of 55-year-old man with complaints of diminution of vision in the right eye for a month, vision of projection of light positive showing: A, Irregular pupil and mature cataract; B, Fine keratic precipitates over the endothelium; C, Posterior synechiae and mature cataract with multiple white deposits within the cataractous lens, possibly macrophage laden lens matter; D, B-scan showing few vitreous echoes with normal optic nerve head and attached retina. The patient underwent cataract surgery under cover of topical and systemic steroids.*

- *Posterior synechia* formation is usually extensive.
- *Hypopyon* may be present.
- *Frangments of lens cortex* may be observed in the anterior chamber or in the vitreous cavity.
- *Vitritis* is usually severe, obscuring view of posterior segment.
- *Intraocular pressure* is often elevated due to blockage of trabecular mashwork by inflammatory cells and/or lens debris.

Subacute or chronic phacogenic uveitis

Subacute or chronic cases are usually less severe typically develop within 2–3 weeks after release or remnants of lens matter after cataract surgery or ocular trauma. Often the inflammation is of non-granulomatous type.

Clinical features include:
- *Anterior chamber cells* and flare of mild to moderate nature,
- *Keratic precipitates, posterior synechial,*
- *Intraocular pressure* can be raised,
- *Epiretinal membrane* and macular oedema may develop.

Phacolytic glaucoma

Phacolytic glaucoma is seen in cases of hypermature cataract where the lens proteins leak out into the anterior chamber from an intact capsule.[12] It is more common in the 6th–7th decade of life.

Clinical features (Fig. 7.8.2). Patients present with circumcorneal congestion, corneal oedema without any keratic precipitates, elevated intraocular pressure with an open angle, lens protein in the anterior chamber with a intact capsule around the hypermature cataract. Anterior segment inflammation consisting of lymphocytes, histiocytes, epithelioid cells, giant cells and polymorphonuclear leucocytes.[13] Inspite of lack of keratic precipitates, macrophages are found in the aqueous humour, although KPs are rare.[14] Treatment aims at reduction of IOP followed by cataract extraction.

Phacomorphic glaucoma

Pathogenesis. This type of glaucoma occurs due to the abnormality in the size of the lens due to

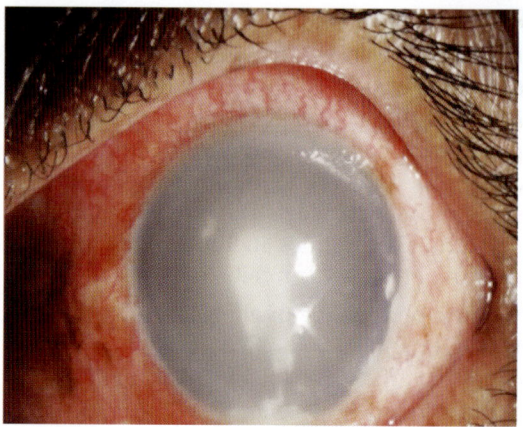

Fig. 7.8.2 *A case of 60-year-old male with phacolytic glaucoma showing circumcorneal congestion, corneal oedema, lens matter in the anterior chamber with elevated intraocular pressure.*

the intumescent lens in senile cataract or traumatic cataract. The suspensory ligament undergoes slackening and allows the lens to move anteriorly, this leads to iridolenticular contact and causes pupillary block and angle closure glaucoma.

Clinical features. The patient presents with signs of acute angle closure with shallow anterior chamber, anterior chamber inflammation.

Definitive treatment is aimed at lowering the IOP and inflammation and removal of cataractous lens.

DIAGNOSIS AND DIFFERENTIAL DIAGNOSIS

Clinical diagnosis of phacogenic uveitis can be made on the basis of careful history and clinical examination. However, additional examination like gonioscopy may be required in cases associated with raised IOP.

Ultrasonography, ocular B-scan, may be helpful in cases with hazy media.

Anterior chamber tap may be required in cases of doubt. Anterior chamber tap may reveal giant macrophages full of lens matter.

Differential diagnosis for the phacogenic uveitis includes:
- Toxic anterior segment syndrome
- Sympathetic ophthalmia

- Retained intraocular foreign body with traumatic endophthalmitis
- IOL-related uveitis
- Endophthalmitis
- Masquerades
- Primary uveitis (Fuchs' with mature cataract, other chronic uveitis with mature/hyper-mature cataracts)

TREATMENT

Medical treatment. Topical and systemic steroids and cycloplegics should be given. In cases of retained lens matter after surgery, only steroids are sufficient till the lens matter is fully resorbed.

Surgical treatment. In some cases, surgical removal through a limbal or a pars plana approach is needed when the lens matter do not resorb inspite of steroid therapy.[15]

Infact definitive treatment for phacogenic uveitis involves complete removal of lens matter.

Complications. If untreated, lens-induced uveitis result in chronic cystoid macular oedema, cyclitic membrane formation, tractional retinal detachment, and rarely phthisis bulbi.[4,16]

REFERENCES

1. Luntz MH, Wright R. Lens-induced uveitis. Exp Eye Res 1962;1:317–23.
2. Bloch-Michel E, Nussenblatt RB. International Uveitis Study Group recommendations for the evaluation of intraocular inflammatory disease. Am J Ophthalmol 1987;2:234–5.
3. Michel SS, Foster CS. Lens-induced uveitis. In: Foster CS, Vitale AT, eds. Diagnosis and treatment of Uveitis, Philadelphia: WB Saunders Co; 2002.
4. Forster David. Phacogenic uveitis. In: Myron Y, Jay SD, eds. Ophthalmology, 3rd edition. Mosby Elsevier; 2006.
5. Ronday MJ, Stilma JS, Barbe RF, et al. Blindness from uveitis in a hospital population in Sierra Leone. Br J Ophthalmol 1994;78(9):690–3.
6. Ronday M. Uveitis in Africa with emphasis on toxoplasmosis. Amsterdam: Netherlands Ophthalmic Research Institute of the Royal Netherlands, Academy of Arts and Sciences, Dept. of Ophthalmology; 1996.
7. Marak GE. Phacoanaphylactic endophthalmitis. Surv Ophthalmol 1992;36(5):325–39.
8. Thach AB, Marak GE, McLean IW, et al. Phaco-anaphylactic endophthalmitis: a clinicopatho-logic review. Int Ophthalmol 1991;15(4):271–9.
9. Muller-Hermelink HK. Recent topics in the pathology of uveitis. In: Kraus-Mackiwe E, O'Connor GR (Eds). Uveitis: Pathophysiology and Therapy. Stuttgart: Thieme; 1986, pp. 155–203.
10. American Academy of Ophthalmolog; 2011-2012; section 9; intraocular inflammation and uveitis; chapter 6: Noninfectious (Autoimmune) ocular inflammatory disease; 117–196.
11. Epstein DL. Diagnosis and management of lens-induced glaucoma. Ophthalmology 1982; 3:227–30.
12. Muller H. Phacolytic glaucoma and phacogenic ophthalmia (lens-induced uveitis). Trans Ophthal Soc UK 1963;83:689–704.
13. Jain P, Dokania P,Aggarwal R, Jain P, Manudhane A, Goyal J, Arora R. Phacogenic uveitis. Dos Times 2014;20(3):25–27.
14. Epstein DL, Jedziniak JA, Grant WM. Identification of heavy molecular weight protein in aqueous humor in human phacolytic glaucoma. Invest Ophthalmol 1978; 17:398–402
15. Shawkat Shafik Michel, Stephen Foster C. Lens induced uveitis. In: Foster S, Vitale AT, eds. Diagnosis and Treatment of Uveitis, 2nd ed. New Delhi: Jaypee Brothers Medical Publishers (P) Ltd; 2013.
16. Murthy S, Sangwan VS. Common pan uveitic entities. In: Dutta LC, Dutta NK, eds. Modern Ophthalmology, 3rd ed. New Delhi: Jaypee Publications; 2005, pp. 1276–98.

7.9 TRAUMATIC AND POSTSURGICAL UVEITIS

7.9.1 TRAUMATIC UVEITIS

Uveitis in mechanical ocular trauma
- Uveitis due to direct mechanical impact of trauma to the uveal tissue
- Phacogenic uveitis
- Haemophthalmitis
- Uveitis due to chemical effects of retained intra-ocular foreign body
- Uveitis due to microbial invasion in open globe trauma
- Traumatic chorioretinitis
- Sympathetic ophthalmitis

Uveitis in chemical injuries

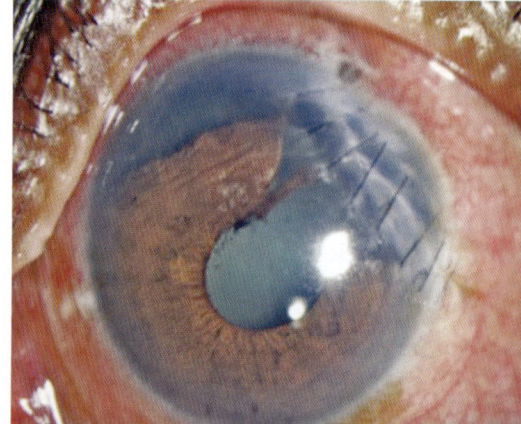
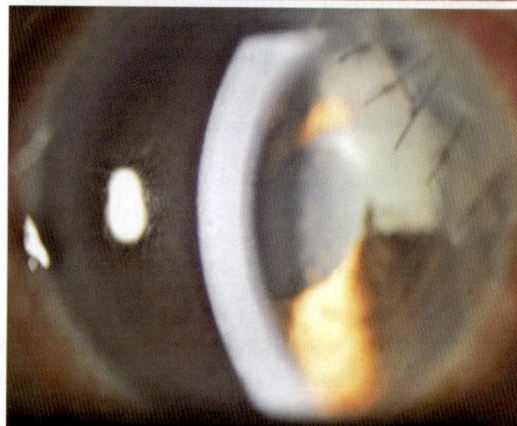

Fig. 7.9.1.1 *A case of ocular trauma showing: A, Corneal tear repair sutures, iridodialysis and sphincter tear; B, Fine keratic precipitates over the corneal endothelium.*

UVEITIS IN MECHANICAL OCULAR TRAUMA

Uveitis is a common manifestation of all types of mechanical ocular trauma including penetrating and non-penetrating injuries.

Penetrating trauma can cause catastrophic ocular consequences. The most frequent causes are assault, domestic and occupational accidents, and sports. It may results into corneal tear, hyphema, iridocyclitis, endophthalmitis, choroidal rupture (Figs 7.9.1.1 and 7.9.1.2). Late sequela includes narrow angle glaucoma, sympathetic ophthalmia, retinal and choroidal neovascularisation, and proliferative vitreoretino-pathy. Investigations, like fundus fluorescein angiography, may be helpful to examine the changes in the retina and vascular coating in traumatic and post-traumatic conditions. In all cases of penetrating trauma, intraocular foreign body should be ruled out.

Non-penetrating trauma. It is noticed that severe uveitis can even occur after minor non-penetrating ocular trauma. It is associated with hyphema, miosis, ocular hypotony, ciliary flush or hemorrhage with excessive fibrin in the anterior chamber. The impact of the blunt trauma causes an equatorial stretching of the globe and the iris–lens diaphragm absorbs this impact. It can cause tearing of structures near the angle and even anterior chamber bleed. It also causes an elevation in the IOP. It also causes sphincter tear and iridodialysis.

Mechanisms of trauma. Mechanical trauma to eyeball can induce uveal inflammation by one or more of the following mechanisms:

1. Uveitis due to direct mechanical impact of trauma to the uveal tissue
2. Phacogenic uveitis
3. Haemophthalmitis
4. Uveitis due to chemical effects of retained intraocular foreign body

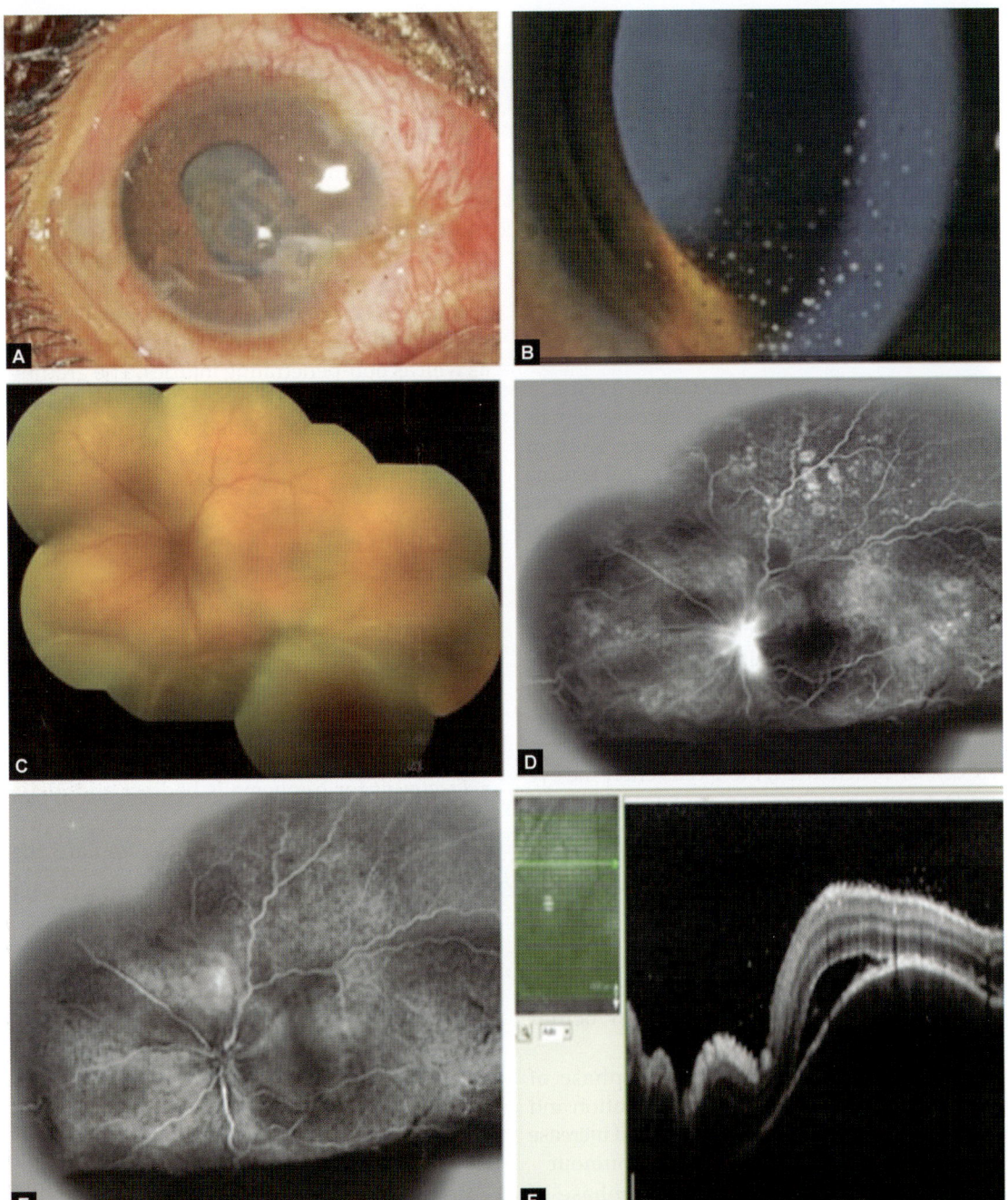

Fig. 7.9.1.2 *The case of a 13-year-old child with history of open-globe injury in the right eye showing: A, Circumcorneal congestion, corneal tear repair with sutures, posterior synechiae and pigment deposition on the anterior surface of lens in right eye; B, Six weeks later the left eye showed mutton-fat keratic precipitates, anterior chamber cells and flare grade 2; C, Fundus photograph of the left eye showing hazy media due to vitiritis, papillitis, and exudative retinal detachment; D, Fluorescein angiography of left eye showing disc leakage, multiple hyperfluorescence area with leakage and pooling in the late phase; E, Indocyanine green angiography of the left eye showing multiple hypofluorescence area with staining and leakage of choroidal vessels; F, Optical coherence tomography of left eye showing presence of posterior vitreous cells, internal limiting membrane (ILM) folds and exudative retinal detachment.*

5. Uveitis due to microbial invasion in open angle trauma
6. Traumatic chorioretinitis
7. Symapthetic ophthalmitis

1. UVEITIS DUE TO DIRECT MECHANICAL IMPACT OF TRAUMA TO THE UVEAL TISSUE

Mechanical injuries, both closed globe (blunt trauma) and open globe trauma, can induce uveal inflammation by direct mechanical impact of trauma and may involve tissues of iris, ciliary body and choroid.

Pathogenesis. Immune-mediated uveitis is triggered from autologus tissue damage signals which are known to occur following blunt or penetrating ocular trauma and surgical trauma from intraocular procedures such as cataract extraction, trabeculectomy and vitreoretinal procedures.

Following trauma or any other cause of tissue damage often there occurs accumulation of necrotic products at the site. As a result of tissue damage, and the ensuing enhanced release of sequestered self-antigen along with necrosis, there occurs activation of *antigen-presenting cells (APCs)*. Once activated, the T cells enter the eye tissue where they are exposed to the target antigen, and initiate the pathogenic process. Thus the necrotic cells promote immunopathogenecity by stimulating *'damage signals'* and pro-inflammatory process.

Role of leukotrienes, prostaglandins, cytokines and growth factors has been implicated in the pathogenesis of inflammation after ocular trauma.

- *Prostaglandins* are seen in early phase of inflammation. They cause vasodilatation and increase in capillary permeability and increase in protein content of the aqueous humour
- *Leukotrienes* are seen in the later phase of inflammation.

2. PHACOGENIC UVEITIS

Phacogenic uveitis, also known as lens induced uveitis, refers to anterior uveitis with or without vitreous inflammation caused by release of lens proteins occurring days to weeks after disruption of lens capsule. It can occur in both closed globe trauma as well as penetrating trauma. For details see Chapter 7.8, page 316.

3. HAEMOPHTHALMITIS

The term haemophthalmitis has been used in the literature to denote the uveal inflammation induced by blood products. In trauma, blood products are derived from the hyphema and/or vitreous haemorrhage. Anterior uveitis is a common accompaniment of hyphema. Blood in the anterior chamber is seen in both penetrating as well as non-penetrating injuries. The grading of hyphema is based on the extent and volume of anterior chamber filled with blood after layering of the red blood cells.

- Grade I: Less than one-third of the anterior chamber
- Grade II: One-third to one-half of the anterior chamber
- Grade III: One-half to nearly total
- Grade IV: Total ('eight ball')

Complications, like corneal blood-staining, ghost cell glaucoma and central retinal artery occlusion, result in permanent visual impairment.

- *Treatment* for hyphema is bedrest and globe protection.
- *Topical steroids* and *cycloplegics* remain the mainstay of treatment.
- *Anticoagulant and antiplatelet treatment* should be avoided.

4. UVEITIS DUE TO CHEMICAL EFFECTS OF RETAINED INTRAOCULAR FOREIGN BODY

The retained intraocular foreign bodies are associated with uveal inflammation due to autologus (tissue damage) signals as well as due to chemical effects of IOFB which include:

- *Local irritative reaction* produced by lead and aluminium particles
- *Specific reactions* produced by iron (siderosis bulbi) and copper alloys (chalcosis).

5. UVEITIS DUE TO MICROBIAL INVASION IN OPEN GLOBE TRAUMA

Microbes, especially bacteria and fungi, may invade the eyeball in open-globe trauma.

Depending upon the virulence of invading organism and the immune status of the host, uveal inflammation may occur by any of the following mechanisms:

Suppurative uveitis

Suppurative uveitis may soon develop as **exogenous endophthalmitis**. Post-traumatic infectious endophthalmitis accounts for 2–7% of all penetrating intraocular injuries. The most common organisms causing post-traumatic endophthalmitis are staphylococcal, streptococcal, and Bacillus species. A delay in the repair or medical therapy beyond 24 hours after injury or a purely corneal wound can lead to poor outcome. In cases of high risk or in established endophthalmitis cases, vitrectomy with anterior chamber and vitreous cultures and smears should be done.

Risk factors for poor prognostic outcome for a penetrating traumatic endophthalmitis are purely corneal wound, surgical primary repair more than 24 hours after injury and initiation of intravenous antibiotic therapy later than 24 hours after trauma. If risks are high or if endophthalmitis is present, vitrectomy with anterior chamber, vitreous cultures and smears is necessary.

For further details see page 388–391.

Non-suppurative uveitis

Non-suppurative uveitis may develop by uveitogenic immune processes which include:
- *Uveitis due to hypersensitivity reactions to microorganisms* or their products,
- *Microbial-induced autoimmune* uveitis,
- *Uveitis induced by exotoxins* and other secreting products of bacteria, and
- *Uveitis due to alternative pathway of inflammation induced* by material cell wall.

Note. For details of above mechanisms see Chapter 3.2 page 61–63.

6. TRAUMATIC CHORIORETINITIS

Traumatic chorioretinitis develops when the impact of blunt trauma is directed towards posterior pole of the eyeball. Traumatic chorioretinitis is associated with the following traumatic lesions involving choroid and retina:

Traumatic choroidal ruptures occur in closed-globe trauma. Choroidal rupture involves a tear in the inner choroid, Bruch's membrane and retinal pigment epithelium (RPE) due to the mechanical disruption by blunt trauma causing anterior posterior compression and subsequent horizontal expansion of the eye. The choroid is susceptible to rupture because of the inelastic characteristics of Bruch's membrane. The choroidal ruptures could be direct which are parallel to ora serrata and indirect, which are generally seen temporal to disc, and fovea (Fig 7.9.1.3). It is often associated with intrachoroidal, subretinal, and intraretinal hemorrhage.

Commotio retinae. The blunt non-tearing injury to retina is called as commotio retinae or Berlin's oedema. It is usually seen several hours after blunt ocular trauma. It is seen as a whitish grey appearance at the posterior pole and in retinal periphery. Retinal haemorrhages, pigment epithelial defect or choroidal rupture may also be seen. A cherry-red spot is seen in cases of macular involvement. Generally, it resolves spontaneously within 6 months or may lead to changes in pigment epithelium and even macular hole.

Other conditions in which traumatic chorioretinitis may occur include:
- Retinitis sclopetaria
- Purtscher's retinopathy
- Shaken baby syndrome

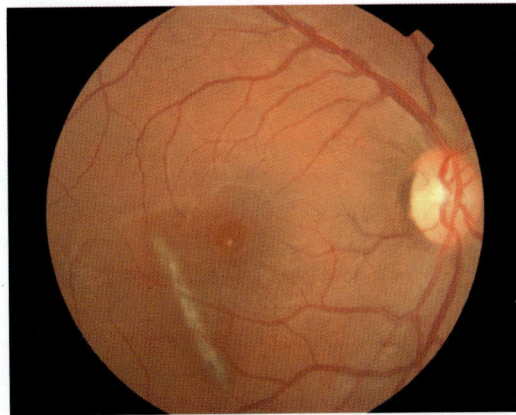

Fig. 7.9.1.3 *Choroidal rupture seen temporal to the disc and fovea.*

- Terson's syndrome
- Valsalva's retinopathy

7. SYMPATHETIC OPHTHALMITIS

Sympathetic ophthalmia is a rare, bilateral, granulomatous uveitis that follows penetrating ocular trauma or surgical insult to one eye and threatens sight in the fellow eye which develops inflammation. The injured eye is referred to as the exciting eye, while the fellow eye is called the sympathizing eye.

Risk factors. Ocular surgeries and penetrating trauma are considered as important risk factors for the development of sympathetic ophthalmia.

Incidence of sympathetic ophthalmia is 0.01% after intraocular surgery and 0.2–0.5% after trauma.

Pathogenesis of sympathetic ophthalmia includes:

Role of cell-mediated immune response to antigens from the retinal photoreceptor layer has been postulated in the etiopathogenesis of the disease.

Onset of sympathetic ophthalmia can be between 1 week to 66 years after the injury but most of the cases report within a year.

Patients present with bilateral anterior uveitis with mutton fat keratic precipitates, vitritis, choroiditis and papillitis. Sub-RPE nodular lesions that appear yellow-white, corresponding to histopathologic Dalen-Fuchs nodules are typical of sympathetic ophthalmia.

Complications of sympathetic ophthalmia include secondary cataract, glaucoma, and chronic maculopathy.

Treatment include:
- *High doses of oral corticosteroids* are recommended for 3 months and then tapered upon on improvement.
- *Other immunomodulatory* agents can be used in refractory cases or steroid intolerance.
- *Prevention of sympathetic ophthalmia* is enucleation of the injured eye before development of disease in the contralateral eye. However, it appears that preference for evisceration over enucleation is currently increasing with advancements in technique and greater perceived benefits. The debate for it still continues.
- *Nowadays, it is preferred to save* the eye instead of primay evisceration/enucleation due to the availability of good immunosuppressive therapy to control the inflammation in cases of sympathetic ophthalmia.

For further details, see Chapter 7.5 page 308.

UVEITIS IN CHEMICAL INJURIES

Chemicals causing injury especially alkalis penetrate deep inside the eyeball and can cause violent inflammation of the iris tissue. In severe cases, both iris and ciliary body are replaced by granulation tissue.

BIBLIOGRAPHY

1. Alfaro DV, Roth D, Liggett PE. Posttraumatic endophthalmitis. Causative organisms, treatment, and preventions. Retina 1994; 14:206.
2. Berlin R. Zur sogenannten commotio retinae. Klin Monatsbl Augenheilkd 1873;1:42.
3. Duch-Samper AM, Menezo JL, Hurtado- Sarrio M: Endophthalmitis following penetrating eye injuries. Acta Ophthalmol Scand 1997; 75:104–6.
4. Kilmartin DJ, Dick AD, Forrester JV. Prospective surveillance of sympathetic ophthalmia in the UK and Republic of Ireland. Br J Ophthalmol 2000;84(3):259–63.
5. Makley TA Jr, Azar. Sympathetic ophthalmia. A long-term follow-up. Arch Ophthalmol 1978;96(2):257–62.
6. Marak GE Jr. Recent advances in sympathetic ophthalmia. Surv Ophthalmol 1979;24(3):141–56.
7. Parrish CM, O'Day DM. Traumatic endophthalmitis. Int Ophthalmol Clin 1987;27:112.
8. Reich ME, Hanselmayer H. Intraocular infections in perforating eye injuries. Klin Monatsbl Augenheilkd 1981;179:411.
9. Rubsamen PE, Cousins SW, Martinez JA. Impact of cultures on management decisions following surgical repair of penetrating ocular trauma. Ophthalmic Surg Lasers 1997;28:43–9.
10. Yamana T. Retinochoroidal lesions in concussional injuries of the eyes. An experimental study. Acta Soc Ophthalmol Jpn 1986;90:1049.
11. Youssri AI, Young LH. Closed-globe contusion injuries of the posterior (segment. Int Ophthalmol Clin 2002;42:79–86.

7.9.2 POSTSURGICAL UVEITIS

Introduction
- Causes
- Complications

Clinico-etiological types of postsurgical uveitis
- Lens-induced uveitis
- Postoperative sympathetic ophthalmia
- IOL-related uveitis
- Execerbation of pre-existing uveitis
- Pseudophakic cystoid macular oedema
- Uveitis due to surgical trauma

Complications of postoperative uveitis
- Common complications
- Preventive measures

INTRODUCTION

Postsurgical intraocular inflammation is common and may vary depending on the type of surgical interventions. For the scope of this chapter, we will discuss uveitis post-cataract surgeries. Infectious postoperative uveitis (endophthalmitis) and uveitis due to non-infectious toxic substance (TASS) have been covered separately in chapter on endophthalmitis (page 395). Once exogenous endophthalmitis and TASS are ruled out other non-infectious causes of postoperative (PO) uveitis have to be considered (Fig. 7.9.2.1).

Causes. PO uveitis commonly occurs due to:
- Surgical trauma itself,
- Malposition of IOL,
- Retained lens fragments or lens matter, exacerbation of pre-existing uveitis or onset of uveitis in patients at risk (underlying systemic auto-immune disease), and rarely due to
- Sympathetic ophthalmia.

Note. Unless the cause of the inflammation is identified, management is difficult and time consuming.

Complications. Persistent chronic inflammation may lead to further complications, such as cystoid macular oedema, glaucoma, cyclitic membrane formation, tractional retinal detachment and eventually phthisis bulbi.

CLINICO-ETIOLOGICAL TYPES OF POSTSURGICAL UVEITIS

LENS-INDUCED UVEITIS

Lens-induced uveitis account for less than 1% of all cases of uveitis and is generally seen in elderly individuals.

Pathogenesis and pathology

Earlier it was thought that the lens protein is not recognised by the immune system and it mounts an inflammatory response when the lens protein is exposed to intraocular environment similar to the rejection of a foreign tissue graft.[1,2] But now it is known that lens-induced uveitis (LIU) is an *abrogation of tolerance of the immune system* towards the lens protein probably due to excessive lens proteins exposure or excessive antibody formation against lenticular antigen.[3] The failure of anterior chamber-associated immune deviation (ACAID) in the mechanism of LIU still remains unexplained.

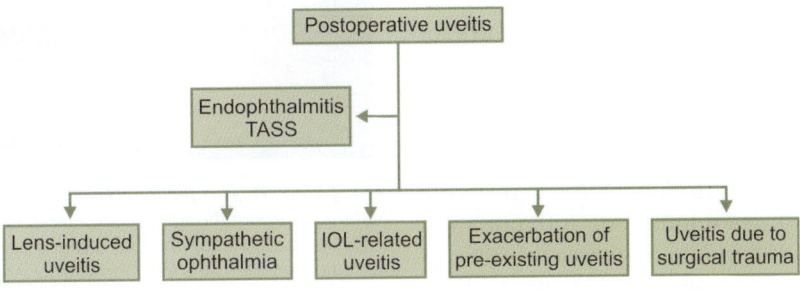

Fig. 7.9.2.1 *Classification of postoperative uveitis.*

Lens-induced inflammation can present as granulomatous or non-granulomatous uveitis.

Granulomatous uveitis. Previously the granulomatous variant was classified as phacoanaphylactic uveitis also known as phaco-anaphylactic endophthalmitis or phacoantigenic uveitis.

Non-granulomtous variant was earlier labelled as phacotoxic uveitis.

These terminologies are now considered as "misleading."

Phacoanaphylactic uveitis was first reported by Straub in 1919 when basic immunologic mechanisms were not completely understood and the term "anaphylaxis" was used to describe "sudden onset" of the inflammation. But now we know that lens proteins are present in low concentration in normal aqueous and phacoanaphylactic uveitis is an immune complex-mediated inflammation and not due to IgE cross-linking or histamine release as in type 1 hypersensitivity (anaphylactic) reaction.[1]

Phacotoxic uveitis was thought to be due to toxic substance released by lens on lens capsular rupture. Again no evidence was found for this hypothesis.[4]

Histopathologically, LIU is a zonal granulomatous inflammation characterized by polymorphonuclear leucocytes in the inner layer, surrounded by an intermediate mantle layer of epithelioid cells, macrophages, and giant cells. Seldom retained lenticular fragment can be seen in the centre of the granuloma.[5]

Clinical profile

Onset of inflammation may vary from 1 day to 59 years after disruption of the lens capsule.[1] In patients who have undergone cataract surgery in fellow eye, the onset may be acute and within 24 hours.[1,20]

Age. Patients are often in their 50s to 70s.

Inflammation varies from mild to severe. Acute cases manifest granulomatous inflammation frequently with hypopyon whereas chronic or subacute cases show non-granulomatous inflammation.

Lenticular debris or retained lens fragment is frequently seen in anterior chamber or in the vitreous or may be hidden behind iris or at the pars plana (Fig. 7.9.2.2).

Choroidal and retinal involvement has also been described by Tach, et al.[2]

Granulomatous LIU is generally unilateral but bilateral cases have been reported.[6]

Acute LIU is a differentiated clinically from acute endophthalmitis by its granulomatous and

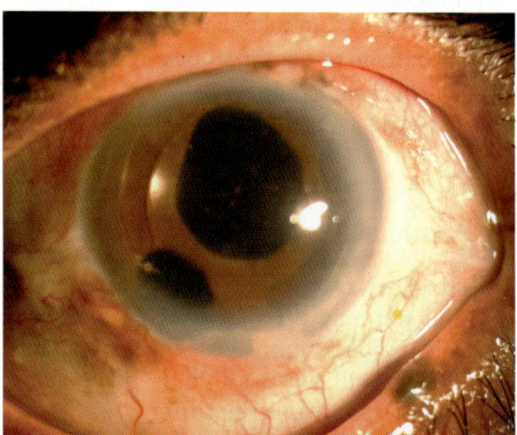

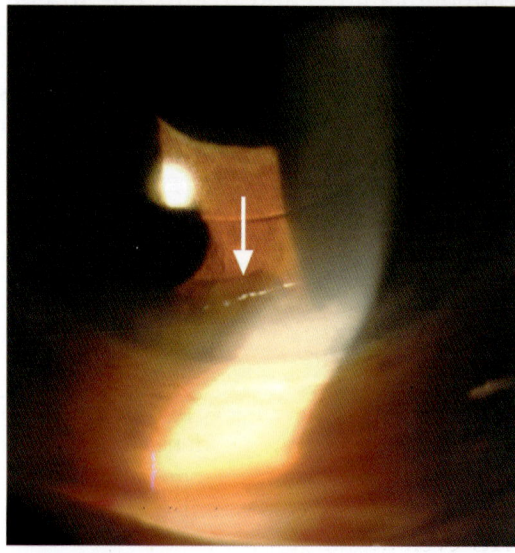

Fig. 7.9.2.2 *A, This patient had chronic inflammation after cataract surgery thought to be chronic endophthalmitis or AC-IOL-related inflammation; B, But a careful examination revealed retained lens fragment (arrow mark) in the anterior chamber, removal of which resulted in complete resolution of postoperative uveitis.*

less painful nature. Negative smear, culture and PCR analysis and predominance of macrophages on cytological analysis of aqueous fluid may support the diagnosis of LIU.

Subacute or chronic LIU cases are difficult to differentiate from cases of chronic endophthalmitis.

Discovery of retained lenticular fragment may aid to the diagnosis.

Differential diagnosis from sympathetic ophthalmia. LIU unlike sympathetic ophthalmia is generally unilateral and inflammation is predominantly anterior or around the lens matter whereas in sympathetic ophthalmia, choroid is primarily involved which can be well demonstrated on fundus fluorescein angiography and on EDI-OCT.

Treatment

LIU is potentially curable uveitis once diagnosed appropriately.

Steroids and cyloplagic drugs are quite effective in controlling lens-induced uveitis.

Removal of retained lens particles gives rewarding response to the steroids. Inflammation to minimal retained lens matter eventually resolves with steroids but larger lens fragments needs to be removed surgically.

Note. Failure to respond completely to surgical removal of lens matter should alert clinician to the possibility of endophthalmitis or sympathetic ophthalmia.[7]

POSTOPERATIVE SYMPATHETIC OPHTHALMIA

Sympathetic ophthalmia (SO) following surgery is a rare form of postoperative uveitis compared to non-surgical trauma. Incidence is estimated to be just 0.015%.[8] SO is known to occur not only after surgical interventions like evisceration, YAG cyclotherapy and retinal detachment surgery but also post-cataract surgery.[9-13]

Pathogenesis

Exact mechanism is unknown but exposure to melanin antigen as well as a genetic pre-disposition particularly HLA-A11 antigen expression has been proposed.[14] The onset of SO has been reported to vary from 5 days to 66 years after the trauma or surgery, but 90% of cases present within a year.[15]

It was formerly believed that purulent infection will destroy uveal tissue to such an extent that it will not incite SO and hence in past, purulent infection was induced in traumatized eyes of horses to prevent development of SO, but cases of SO post-endophthalmitis in exciting eyes have been reported by Rathinam et al.[16]

Clinical profile

Signs of inflammation. Bilateral granulomatous inflammation is characterised by keratic precipitates, generally without hypopyon (in contrast to LIU), with vitritis, disc oedema, retinal detachment, choroiditis, Dalen-Fuchs nodules and rarely vasculitis (Fig. 7.9.2.3).

Dalen-Fuchs nodules which represent collection of lymphocytes, histiocytes and pigment epithelium are generally seen at peripheral fundus but may also occur at posterior pole and are suggestive of more severe stage of the disease.[16,17]

Extraocular features, such as vitiligo, poliosis, hearing loss, alopecia, are not seen as frequently as in Vogt-Koyanagi-Harada syndrome.

Treatment

High dose of steroids (1–1.5 mg/kg) and early commencement of *immunomodulatory therapy* is recommended once the diagnosis of SO is made. Management of SO may sometimes be challenging when exciting eye harbours endophthalmitis.

Enucleation of exciting eye, the only preventive measure for development of SO, is controversial. Enucleation of exciting eye prior to development of immune response, classically within 14 days of penetrating trauma was recommended earlier by some authors. But now with advent of newer immunomodulatory drugs, advancement in technique of surgery, removal of exciting eye is less popular; moreover preference for evisceration over enucleation is increasing.[14]

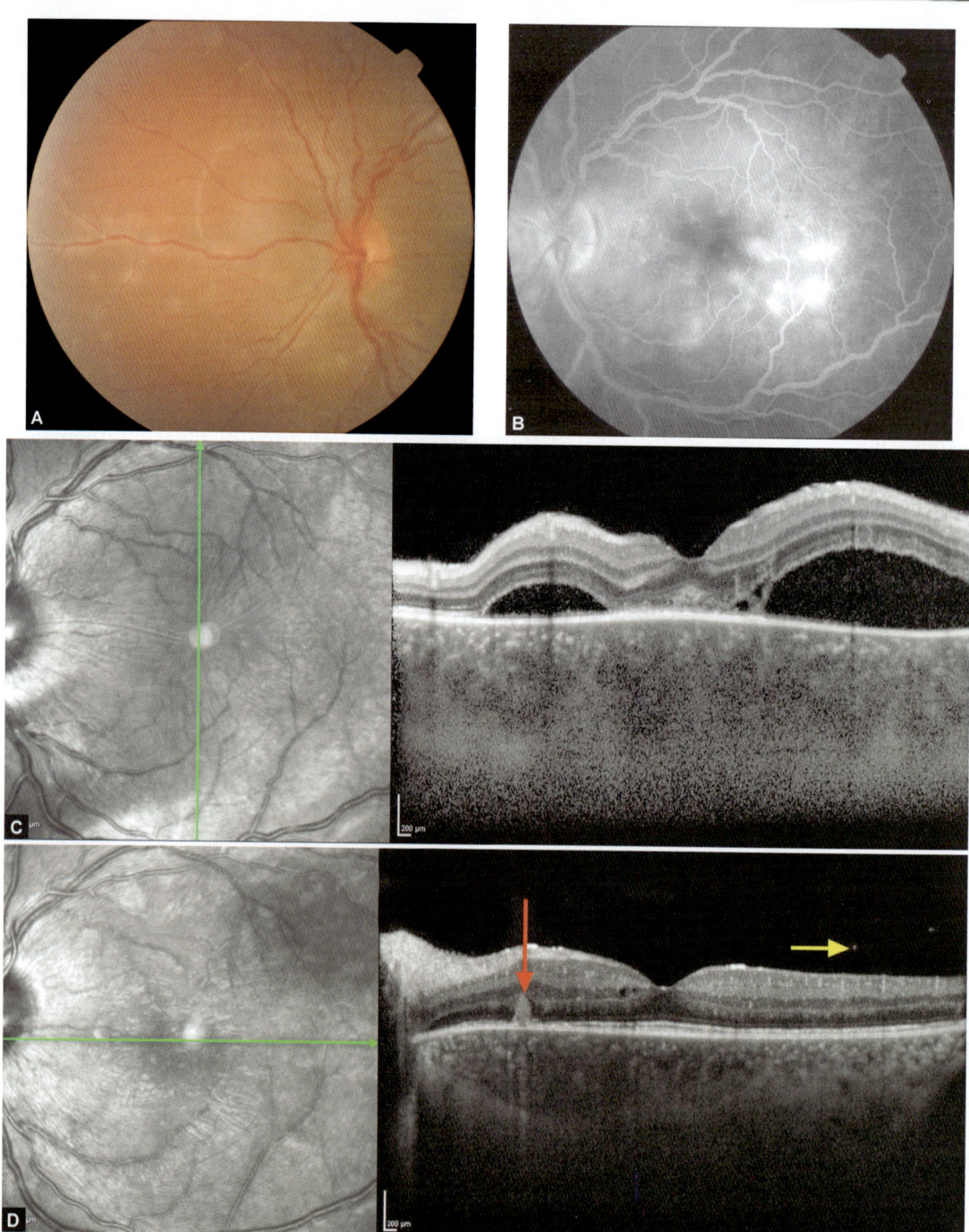

Fig. 7.9.2.3 *Postoperative sympathetic ophthalmitis: A, This patient had traumatic endophthalmitis in his right eye and underwent vitrectomy and lensectomy for same and subsequently developed sympathetic ophthalmia. Note multifocal serous detachments around the disc and subtle vascular sheathing; B, FFA shows multiple pinpoint leak at macula and vascular staining; C, EDI OCT shows vitreous cells, serous retinal detachment; posterior border of choroid is not well defined due to thickening; D, After starting steroids and immunomodulatory drugs, note the resolution of serous detachments, reduction in vitritis (horizontal arrow) and appearance of Dalen-Fuchs nodule (vertical arrow), few intraretinal cystic spaces suggestive of early cystoid macular oedema.*

IOL-RELATED UVEITIS

Occurrence of IOL-related uveitis has drastically decreased with the advancement in technology and better finishing of the implant.

Pathogenesis

Uveitis-glaucoma-hyphema (UGH) syndrome, earlier reported complications, has now become a rarity. UGH syndrome was first described by Ellingson who noted early generation IOL or anterior chamber IOL (AC IOL) causing mechanical irritation at the iris root resulting into uveitis, recurrent hyphema and glaucoma.[19] UGH syndrome may rarely occur with posterior chamber IOLs.

True inflammation due to mechanical rubbing with the iris tissue may also occur due to breakdown of blood aqueous barrier.
- *Constant rubbing of IOL* (AC IOL, scleral-fixated IOL, iris-fixated IOL) against iris tissue may cause release of pigments granules which may mimic uveitis and also may lead to iris transillumination defects or iris atrophy. These pigment dispersion should be differentiated from cells in the anterior chamber.
- *Malpositioned IOLs* may also be the cause of chronic inflammation due to constant rubbing. UBM and anterior chamber OCT can help to rule out IOL malposition. Chronic inflammation due to IOL malposition warrants its repositioning or explanation to achieve complete resolution of the inflammation.

Hypersensitivity reaction. Some authors have postulated that chronic inflammation post-IOL implantation could be because of hypersensitivity reaction or foreign body type response to the implant material. It has also been shown that IOL polymer may activate compliment system, specifically C5a.[19]

Treatment

Medical treatment with steroids and cylcoplegic may be effective.

IOL exchange. In case of chronic inflammation where infectious and other causes have been ruled out, one may consider exchange of IOL as a final solution to cure the inflammation.

EXACERBATION OF PRE-EXISTING UVEITIS

Uveitic eyes are known to mount increased inflammatory reaction to surgical intervention as compared to normal eyes with the only exception of Fuchs' uveitis.

Exacerbation of pre-existing uveitis can occur due to mishandling of iris tissue or due to release of extensive posterior synechiae. Hence it is utmost important that the uveitic eyes are quiet for at least 3 months prior to surgical intervention.

Severity of postoperative inflammation in uveitic eyes may vary depending upon type of uveitis, pre-existing uveitic complications, such as posterior synechiae, and type of surgical intervention.

Posterior uveitis, like serpiginous choroiditis or *multifocal choroiditis,* may not develop inflammation as severe as in case of anterior uveitis like *HLA-B27-related uveitis* or *juvenile idiopathic arthritis* (JIA)-associated uveitis in postoperative period. In these aggressive anterior uveitis, patient may develop severe anterior chamber inflammation very next day of the surgery and rapidly form posterior synechiae with IOL.

Differential diagnosis from endophthalmitis. Presence of hypopyon makes it difficult to differentiate from postoperative endophthalmitis. Inflammation generally remains confined to anterior segment in contrast to endophthalmitis where vitreous is frequently and severely involved. Negative ocular fluid investigations and better response to increased dose of steroids differentiate this uveitis from endophthalmitis.

Preoperative, intraoperative and postoperative preventive measures should be taken to avoid this type of uveitis. This aspect will be discussed in detailed in the Chapter on 'Cataract Surgery in Uveitis (*see* page 188).'

PSEUDOPHAKIC CYSTOID MACULAR OEDEMA (PCME)

This is in fact a complication of postoperative inflammation. Patients with uncomplicated cataract surgery and with usual postoperative inflammation can develop PCME but chances are higher when posterior capsule is ruptured. It was first described by Irvin in1953 and the cause of visual impairment was explained by Gass and Norton by demonstrating classical petalloid pattern at macula on fundus fluoroscein angiography (FFA).[22]

Incidence

Although incidence of PCME is decreased with the advent of small incision cataract surgery, on imaging it could be as high as 41% on OCT and 20–30% on FFA.[23,24] But incidence of clinical PCME, which is defined as best corrected visual acuity 6/12 or worse, is estimated to be 0.1–2.35% following phacoemulsification.[25, 26]

Pathogenesis

Pathogenesis is thought to be subclinical inflammation due to breakdown of blood–aqueous barrier (BAB) and blood–retinal barrier (BRB).

- *Can be associated with* diabetes, glaucoma and pre-existing uveitis, intraoperative complications, increased duration of surgery, photo-toxic effect of operating microscope.
- *Surgical manipulations* in the anterior chamber may lead to release of inflammatory mediators, like leukotrienes (IL2, IL10, TNF alpha) and prostaglandins. This in turn increases retinal vascular permeability and results into macular oedema.
- *Other factors* to be considered are mechanical traction of perifoveal capillaries due to contraction of posterior hyaloids as a result of inflammation and iridovitreal adhesions resulting into traction may develop CME. Muller cells plays important role by acting as metabolic pumps which keeps macula dehydrated but they in turn may accumulate fluid and impaired visual function.

Clinico-investigative profile

Onset. PCME often develops within 4–6 weeks post-surgery but can occur after several months to years. Acute CME occurs within 6 months and chronic after 6 months of cataract surgery.

One may not observe active inflammation clinically in the form of cells or flare in the anterior chamber or cells in the vitreous and fundus examination may remain unremarkable except for the presence of CME.

OCT and FFA are highly sensitive to pick up subclinical CME. FFA may additionally reveal mild disc leak and subtle capillary leaks at macula while OCT can demonstrate accumulation of fluid in the outer plexiform layer. OCT can also quantify the severity of CME by measuring macular thickness. OCT being a non- invasive diagnostic tool is useful for follow-up.

Treatment

Treatment of postoperative CME may include:

- *Topical non-steroidal anti-inflammatory drugs (NSAIDs)*, such as nepafenac, diclofenac and bromfenac, are frequently used for treatment of mild to moderate CME. Heier et al have noted better outcome with NSAID-steroid combination therapy.[27]
- *Carbonic anhydrase inhibitors* are also used for treatment of CME. But in large CME topical treatment alone may not help.
- *Periocular or intravitreal steroid injections* or intravitreal steroid injections or implants are needed in such cases.
- *Anti-VEGFs*, like bevacizumab, ranibizumab, have gain popularity recently in treatment of PCME.
- *PPV.* Refractory CME due to vitreomacular traction may require surgical intervention.[28]

UVEITIS DUE TO SURGICAL TRAUMA

Any form of trauma to any living tissue will induce inflammation. Uncomplicated ocular surgeries also cause mild to moderate inflammation in the eye depending upon the nature of the surgery. Larger the surgical incision and duration of the procedure, greater is the inflammation. With advent of small incision techniques, this type of uveitis is now-adays seen in milder form and resolves within few days to weeks with use of topical steroids.

COMPLICATIONS OF POSTOPERATIVE UVEITIS

Uncontrolled chronic inflammation can lead to various complications and transient or permanent damage to retina and optic nerve.

Common complications. In a large study of 1500 patients, incidence of posterior synechiae was 7.1%, pupillary block glaucoma was 1.5%, acute rise of intraocular pressure was 4.7% and among late postoperative complications posterior capsular opacity was found to be 34.5% and incidence of cystoid macular oedema was 3.2%.[20]

Rate of complications in patients with early onset postoperative inflammation is higher than overall cataract surgery results.[21]

Preventive measures, like preoperative medications, choice of IOL, intraoperative measures, will be discussed in detailed in the Chapter on 'Cataract Surgery in Uveitis.'

CONCLUSION

Postoperative uveitis is exasperating condition for both surgeon and for the patient. Mere ruling out infections is not enough but attempts to find other non-infectious causes should be made and managed appropriately. Adequately treated postoperative inflammation after cataract surgery does not result in significant visual loss.[20]

REFERENCES

1. Marak GE. Phacoanaphylactic endophthalmitis. Surv Ophthalmol 1992;36:325.
2. Thach AB, Marak GE, Jr, McLean IW, Green WR. Phacoanaphylactic endophthalmitis: A clinicopathologic review. Int Ophthalmol 1991;15: 271.
3. Khalil MK, Lorenzetti DW. Lens-induced inflammations. Can J Ophthalmol 1986;21:96.
4. Rao SM, Murthy SV, Geethamala K. An unsuspected case of lens-induced uveitis: A case report. J Clin Ophthalmol Res 205;3:100–2.
5. Spencer WH. Len. In; Spencer WH.ed, Ophthalmic Pathology: An Atlas and Textbook. Philadelphia: Sounders; 1985;473–5.
6. DeVeer JA. Bilateral endophthalmitis phaco-anaphylactica. Pathologic study of the lesion in the eye first involved and, in one instance, the secondarily implicated, or "sympathizing" eye. Arch Ophthalmol 1953;54:607.
7. Shawkat Shafik Michel C Stephen Foster. Lens indusced uveitis. In: Foster CS, Vitale AT (eds). Diagnosis and Treatment of Uveitis. Philadelphia: Sounders, 2002; pp 817–21.
8. Allen JC. Sympathetic ophthalmia, a disappearing disease. JAMA 1969;209:1090.
9. Green WR, Maumenee AE, Sanders TE, Smith ME. Sympathetic uveitis following evisceration. Trans Am Acad Ophthalmol Otolaryngol 1972; 76:625–44.
10. Lam S, Tessler HH, Lam BL, Wilensky JT. High incidence of sympathetic ophthalmia after contact 'and noncontact neodymium: YAG cyclotherapy. Ophthalmology 1992; 12:1818-22.
11. Wang WJ. Clinical and histopathological report of sympathetic ophthalmia after retinal detachment surgery. Br J Ophthalmol 1983; 67:150–2.
12. Das SP. Sympathetic ophthalmia. J All India Ophthalmol Soc 1968;16(3):134–8.
13. Lakhanpal V, Dogra MR, Jacobson MS. Sympathetic ophthalmia associated with anterior chamber intraocular lens implantation. Ann Ophthalmol 1991;23(4):139-43. 1972;76:625–44.
14. Xi K Chu, Chi-Chao Chan. Sympathetic ophthalmia: to the twenty first century and beyond. Journal of Ophthalmic Inflammation and Infection 2013;3:49.
15. Lubin JR, Albert DM, Weinstein M. Sixty-five years of sympathetic ophthalmia: A clinico-pathologic review of 105 cases (1913-1978). Ophthalmology 1980;87:109
16. Rathinam SR, Rao NA. Sympathetic ophthalmia following postoperative bacterial endophthalmitis: a clinicopathologic study. Am J Ophthalmol 2006;141(3):498–507.
17. Varghese M, Raghavendra R. Dalen-Fuchs nodules and serous retinal detachment on optical coherence tomography in sympathetic ophthalmitis. Indian J Ophthalmol 2013;61(5):245–6.
18. Jennings T, Tessler HH. Twenty cases of sympathetic ophthalmia. Br J Ophthalmol 1989; 73:140.
19. Apple DJ, Mamalis N, Loftfield K, Googe JM, Novak LC, Kavka-Van Norman D, Brady SE, Olson RJ. Complications of intraocular lenses. A historical and histopathological review. Surv Ophthalmol 1984; 29(1):1–54.

20. Mohammadpour M, Jafarinasab MR, Javadi MA. Outcomes of acute postoperative inflammation after cataract surgery. Eur J Ophthalmol 2007; 17(1):20–8.

21. Powe NR, Schein OD, Gieser SC, et al. Synthesis of the literature on visual acuity and complications following cataract extraction with intraocular lens implantation. Arch Ophthalmol 1994; 112: 1–15.

22. Gass JD, Norton EW. Cystoid macular edema and papilledema following cataract extraction. A fluorescein fundoscopic and angiographic study. Arch Ophthalmol 1966;76:646e61.

23. Lobo CL, Faria PM, Soares MA, et al. Macular alterations after small-incision cataract surgery. J Cataract Refract Surg 2004;30:752–60.

24. Gulkilik G, Kocabora S, Taskapili M, et al. Cystoid macular edema after phacoemulsification: risk factors and effect on visual acuity. Can J Ophthalmol 2006;41:699–703.

25. Henderson BA, Kim JY, Ament CS, et al. Clinical pseudophakic cystoid macular edema. Risk factors for development and duration after treatment. J Cataract Refract Surg 2007;33: 1550–8.

26. Loewenstein A, Zur D. Postsurgical cystoid macular edema. Dev Ophthalmol. 2010;47:148–59.

27. Heier JS, Topping TM, Baumann W, et al. Ketorolac versus prednisolone versus combination therapy in the treatment of acute pseudophakic cystoid macular edema. Ophthalmology 2000;107:2034–8.

28. Atul K, Anusha K, Bhavin Shah. Cystoid macular edema. In: Khurana AK (ed). Disorders of Retina and Vitreous. New Delhi: CBS, 2014, pp. 387–93.

7.10 WHITE DOT SYNDROME

7.10.1 WHITE DOT SYNDROME: AN OVERVIEW

- Definition and constituent conditions
- Salient features and differential diagnosis

DEFINITION AND CONSTITUENT CONDITIONS

White dot syndrome refers to a heterogenous group of idiopathic immunological disorders characterised by visual disturbances with descreate multiple, well-circumscribed whitish subretinal lesions in the fundus at the level of a outer retina, RPE and choroid. The term white dot syndrome, also known as *inflammatory chorioretinopathies of unknown etiology*, is a pot-pourri of following idiopathic disorders:

- Birdshot retinochoroidopathy
- Serpeginous choroidopathy
- Acute posterior multifocal placoid, pigment epitheliopathy (APMPPE)
- Acute zonal occult outer retinopathy (AZOOR)
- Multiple evanescent white dot syndrome (MEWDS)
- Punctate inner choroidopathy (PIC)
- Acute retinal pigment epitheliitis (ARPE)
- Acute idiopathic blind-spot-enlargement syndrome (AIBSES)
- Multifocal choroiditis and panuveitis (MCP) syndrome
- Subretinal fibrosis and uveitis (SFU) syndrome

SALIENT FEATURES AND DIFFERENTIAL DIAGNOSIS

Before describing the conditions included in the white dot syndrome, it will be worth while to have a brief view salient features and differential diagnosis of this group.

Salient features of white dot syndromes or inflammatory chorioretinopathies of unknown etiology are summarised in Table 7.10.1.1.

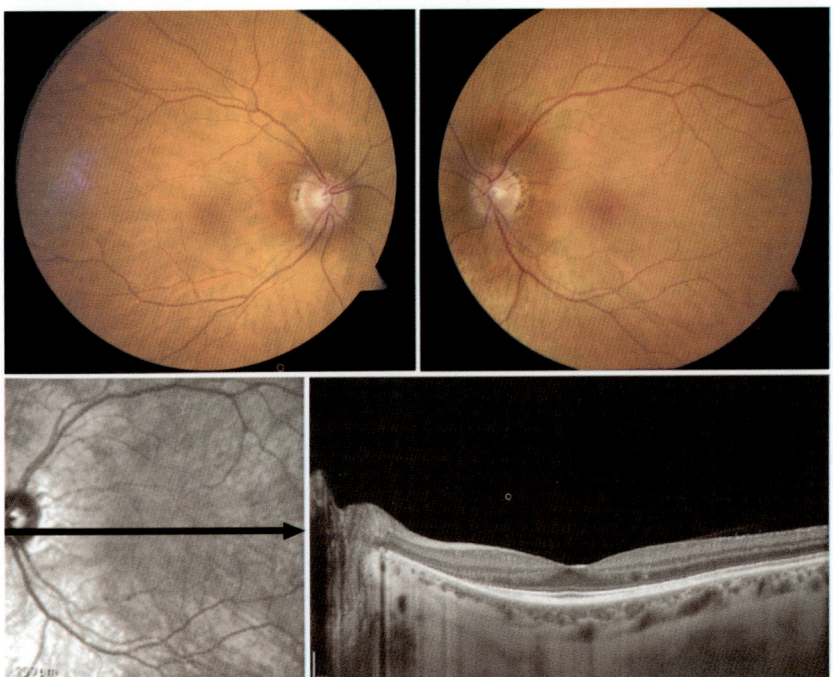

Fig. 7.10.1.1 *AIBSE: 36-year-old woman with temporal field defect and photopsias. VA 20/20 OU, normal fundus exam. Enlarged blind spot on left side with loss of peripapillary photoreceptors. (Courtesy: Dr Anita Aggarwal)*

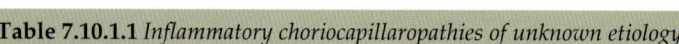

Table 7.10.1.1 *Inflammatory choriocapillaropathies of unknown etiology*

MEWDS and AIBSE (Fig. 7.10.1.1)	APMPPE (Fig. 7.10.1.2)	MFC and PIC (Fig. 7.10.1.3)
Young to middle-aged females, unilateral	Young adults, bilateral 20–50 yrs, unilateral or bilateral	Recurrent disease, bilateral (MFC) or unilateral (PIC)
Symptoms include visual loss, photopsias and field loss. Signs include normal fundus or discrete discolouration of midperipheral fundus	Symptoms include visual loss, field loss and photopsias. Signs include yellowish white lesions in the posterior pole and mild to moderate AC and vitreous inflammation in the acute stage and chorioretinal atrophic scars in the convalescent stage	Symptoms include moderate to advanced vision loss, photopsias and visual field loss. Signs include AC and vitreous inflammation and yellowish white retinal lesions of posterior pole and midperiphery. In convalescent stage chorioretinal scars
Preceded by viral flu-like illness in 50% cases	May be preceded by a flu-like illness.	Secondary CNVM in 30–40%
ICGA shows patchy and peripapillary hypofluorescence which persists in the late phase	ICGA shows geographic hypofluorescence which persists in late phase	ICGA shows early hypofluorescence persisting in late phase, which is more than in MEWDS or APMPPE
FFA shows early hypofluorescence and late hyperfluorescence or absence of findings. AIBSE are said to be subclinical or resolved counterparts of MEWDS	FFA shows early hypofluorescence and late hyperfluorescence	FA shows early hypo- and late hyperfluorescence in acute stage. Convalescent stage shows mixed hypo- and hyper-pattern
No treatment is needed as spontaneous recovery occurs in 6–10 weeks	Generally no treatment is needed, but some cases may result in scarring of the posterior pole and permanent visual loss in which case steroids may be considered	Systemic steroids for bilateral and sub-tenon steroids for unilateral disease along with immunosuppressant. CNVM requires anti-VEGFs and/or PDT

Serpiginous choroiditis	Serpiginous-like choroiditis (Fig. 7.10.1.4)	AZOOR
Recurrent, progressive bilateral autoimmune disease	Recurrent, progressive, may be unilateral or bilateral, secondary to tubercular hypersensitivity	Rare, middle-aged females.
Vision loss, visual field loss and photopsiae may occur	Vision loss and field loss	Sudden onset field loss with prominent photopsiae, which are worse in bright light and show movement
Peripapillary type is most common and begins as yellowish white lesions around the disc which spread in a amoeboid pattern. Macular type is rare but causes more severe visual loss. Ampiginous type starts a multifocal AMPPE-like lesions but gradually coalesce to classic serpiginous lesions	Multifocal type is most common and begins as discrete yellowish white subretinal lesions in the posterior pole and periphery which later coalesce to form SC-like lesions. Diffuse type is similar to SC right from the start. Mixed type has both types in two eyes	Fundus shows no abnormality in acute stage. In late stages, sectoral retinitis pigmentosa type picture may be seen
Lesions heal with extensive RPE pigmentation and cause diffuse chorioretinal atrophy and CNVM formation	Lesions heal with less RPE pigmentation and AC and vitreous inflammation is more marked	ICGA and FFA are normal if the fundus is normal. In late stages, FFA may show window defect in areas of RPE loss
ICGA shows early hypofluorescence persisting in the late phase	ICGA shows early hypofluorescence persisting in the late phase	Stabilization and partial recovery is seen at 4–6 months
FFA shows early hypo- and late hyperfluorescence in acute stage and window defect in chronic stage	FFA shows early hypo- and late hyperfluorescence in acute stage and window defect in chronic stage	
Pulse steroids in the acute stage along with immunosuppressant are strongly recommended to prevent severe vision loss. Anti-VEGFs and PDT are needed for CNVMs	Oral steroids are needed to control the inflammation and anti-tubercular treatment (ATT) are needed to prevent recurrences. 4 drug ATT is started and isoniazid and rifampicin are continued for 9–12 months. Pyrazinamide and ethambutol are stopped after 2–3 months.	No treatment is found to be particularly effective, however, anecdotal reports of improvement with steroids are there

Differential diagnosis of white dot syndrome includes following conditions:

i. *Infectious chorioretinopathies,,* such as:

- Syphili
- Diffuse unilateral subacute neuroretinitis (DUSN)
- Ocular histoplasmosis syndrome (OHS)
- Tuberculosis
- Toxoplasmosis
- Pneumocystic choroidopathy
- Candidiasis
- Acute retinal necrosis (ARN)
- Ophthalmomyosis

ii. *Non-infectious chorioretinopathies,* such as;

- Sarcoidosis
- Sympathetic ophthalmitis
- VKH syndrome

iii. *Intraocular malignancies,* e.g.

- Intraocular lymphoma

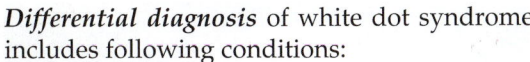

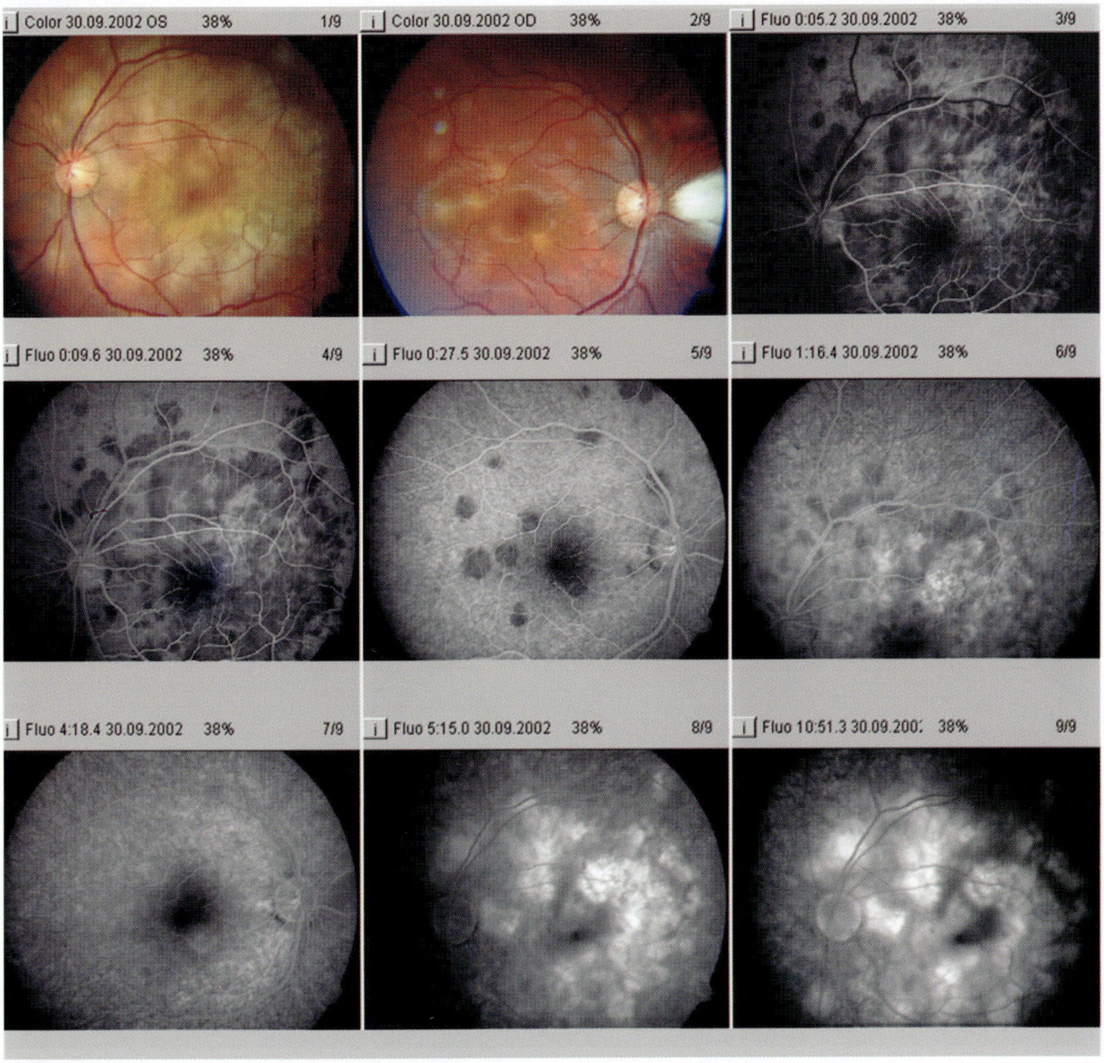

Fig. 7.10.1.2 *Young adult presenting with bilateral blurred vision showing bilateral multifocal yellowish lesions which showed early hypofluorescence and late hyperfluorescence on FFA consistent with APMPPE. The lesions healed without any pigmentation after a short course of steroids.*

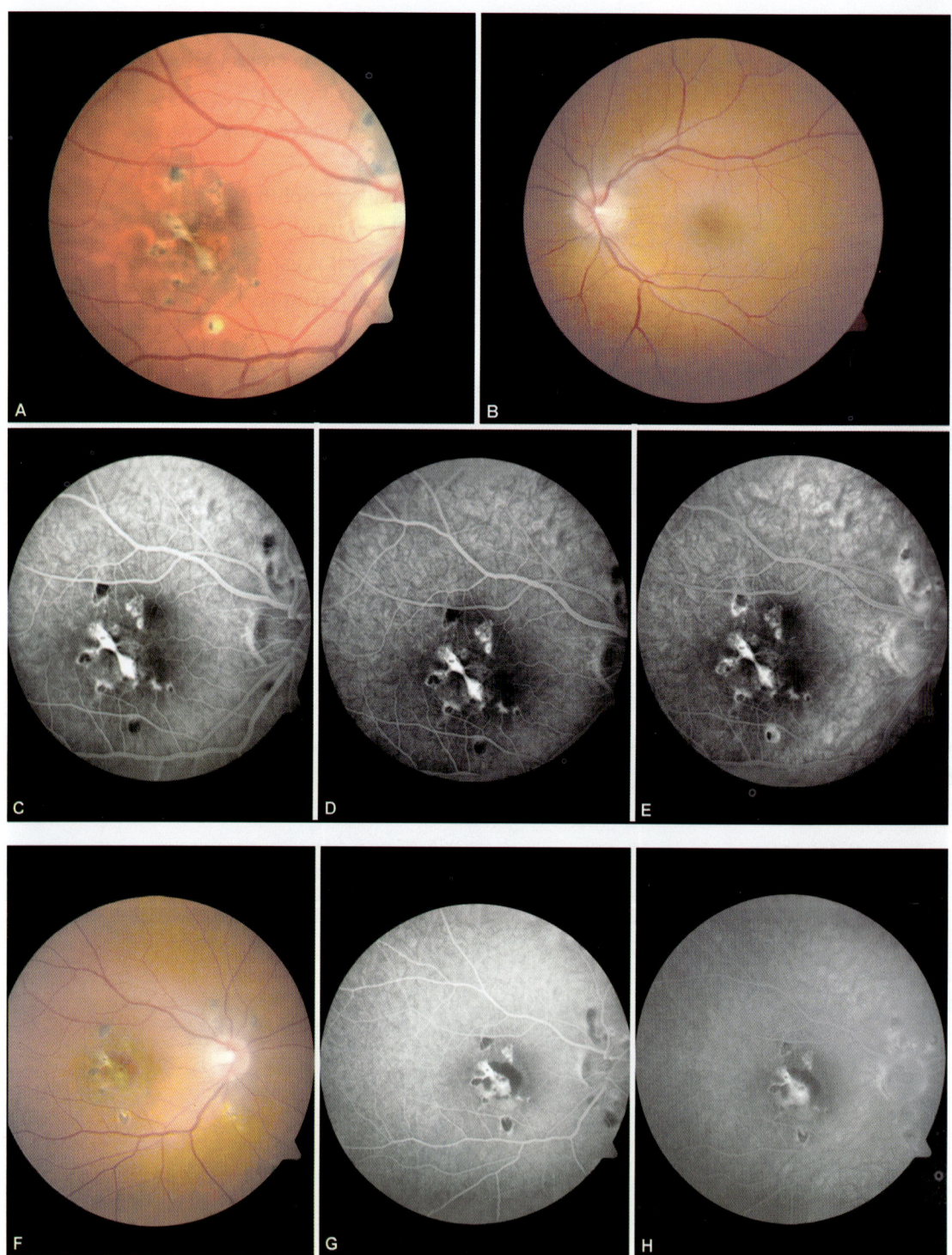

Fig. 7.10.1.3 A to E. *This patient is a 26-year-old woman with moderate myopia with PIC lesions in the right eye in 2003; F to H. She returned with central distortion, due to a type 2 CNVM with subretinal blood (Courtesy: Dr Anita Aggarwal).*

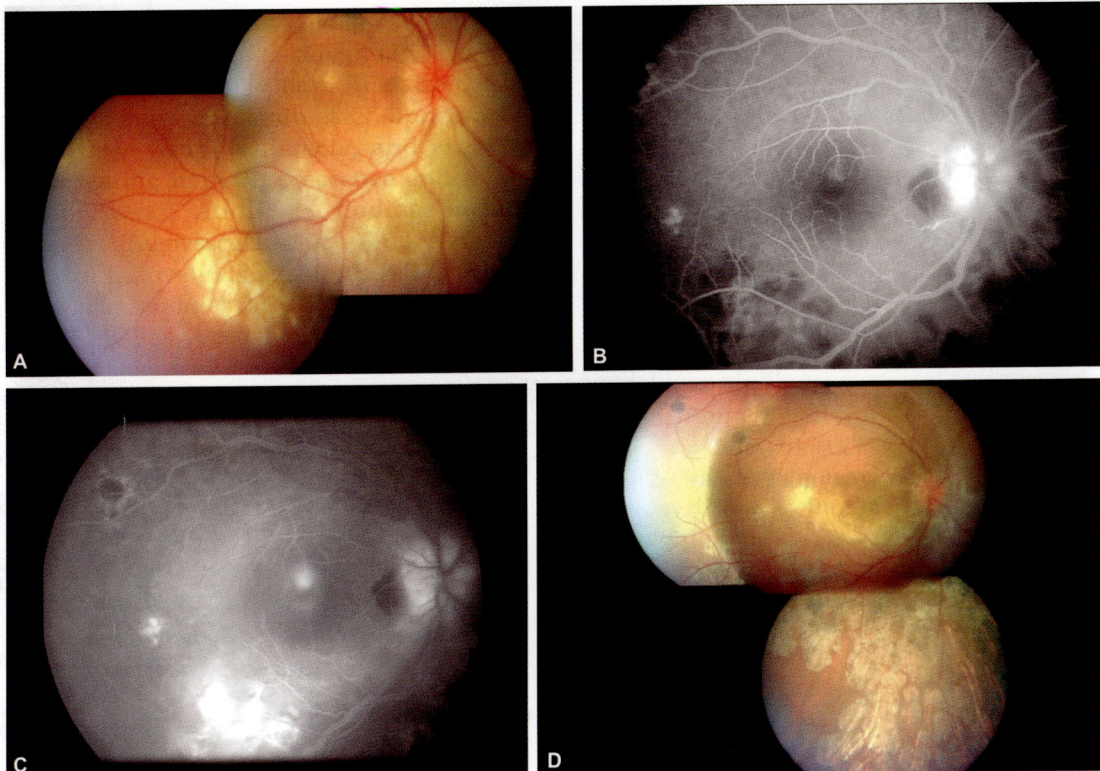

Fig. 7.10.1.4 *Biopsy proven case of abdominal tuberculosis: A, Fundus picture showing serpiginous like choroiditis; B and C, FFA showed classical hypofluorescence in early and hyperfluorescence in late phase; D, Fundus picture shows partial resolution after 3 weeks treatment of ATT and steroids.*

BIBLIOGRAPHY

1. Folk JC, Reddy CV. White dot chorioretinal inflammatory syndromes. In: Lewis H, Ryan SJ, (eds). Medical and Surgical Retina: Advances, Controversies, and Management. St Louis: Mosby-Year Book; 1994;385–400.

2. Gass JD. Acute posterior multifocal placoid pigment epitheliopathy. Arch Ophthalmol 1968; 80(2):177–85.

3. Jones NP. Acute posterior multifocal placoid pigment epitheliopathy. Br J Ophthalmol 1995; 79(4):384–9.

4. Mamalis N, Daily MJ. Multiple evanescent white-dot syndrome. A report of eight cases. Ophthalmology 1987; 94(10):1209–12.

5. Polk TD, Goldman EJ. White-dot chorioretinal inflammatory syndromes. Int Ophthalmol Clin 1999; 39(4):33–53.

6. Ryan SJ, Maumenee AE. Acute posterior multifocal placoid pigment epitheliopathy. Am J Ophthalmol 1972; 74(6):1066–74.

7. Savino PJ, Weinberg RJ, Yassin JG, Pilkerton AR. Diverse manifestations of acute posterior multifocal placoid pigment epitheliopathy. Am J Ophthalmol 1974; 77(5):659–62.

8. Slusher MM, Weaver RG. Multiple evanescent white dot syndrome. Retina 1988;8(2):132–5.

9. Spaide RF. White dot syndromes. In: Spaide RF, (ed). Diseases of the Retina and Vitreous. Philadelphia: WB Saunders Co; 1999;195–213.

10. Stangos A, Zaninetti M, Petropoulos I, Baglivo E, Pournaras C. Multiple evanescent white dot syndrome following simultaneous hepatitis-A and yellow fever vaccination. Ocul Immunol Inflamm 2006; 14(5):301–4.

7.10.2 BIRDSHOT CHORIORETINOPATHY

- Definition, etiopathogenesis and pathology
- Clinical features
- Diagnosis and differential diagnosis
- Treatment and monitoring

DEFINITION, ETIOPATHOGENESIS AND PATHOLOGY

Definition

It is an uncommon chronic posterior uveitis characterised by vitritis, multiple ovoid, hypopigmented spots concentrated in the posterior pole and midperiphery of the retina.

The term 'Birdshot chorioretinopathy' was given to this disease owing to the distinctive fundus lesions originally characterised as multiple, small white spots that frequently have the pattern similar to birdshot in the scatter from a shotgun.

Synonyms

- Birdshot retinochoroidopathy
- Birdshot chorioretinitis
- Birdshot retinochoroiditis
- Vitiliginous choroiditis
- Salmon patch choroidopathy

Etiology and pathogenesis

- The exact etiology of birdshot chorioretinopathy is not known.
- An autoimmune mechanism is suspected.
- Has a strong association with the human leucocyte antigen (HLA), the H29 allele.
- Autoimmunity is thought to play a mediating role in birdshot chorioretinopathy. Patients with birdshot chorioretinopathy may exhibit lymphocyte proliferation responses to several retinal autoantigens, including S antigen (S-Ag) and interstitial retinoid-binding protein (IRBP), which are antigenic proteins found in the photoreceptor layer of the retina.

Histology

Focal lymphocytic inflammation is observed in the choroid and adjacent to choroidal vessels. Accompanied by milder inflammation in the retina along the retinal blood vessels and around the optic disc.

CLINICAL FEATURES

Prevalence and demography

- *Prevalance.* Birdshot chorioretinopathy is an uncommon disease representing 0.6–1.5% of patients with uveitis seen at tertiary care centres and 6–8% of patients with posterior uveitis.
- *Age.* Unlike other forms of uveitis that typically occur in younger age groups, birdshot chorioretinopathy typically occurs during middle age.
- *Sex.* Have a slight female predominance.

Symptoms include:

- Blurred vision and floaters are common, followed by
- Nyctalopia, dyschromatopsia
- Abnormal contrast sensitivity
- Vibrating vision
- Metamorphopsia
- Decreased peripheral vision
- Difficulties with dark–light adaptation.

Clinical signs are as below:

- The eye appears 'quiet'
- A mild non-granulomatous anterior uveitis
- Intraocular pressures (IOP) are typically normal
- Mild cataract
- Diffuse, but low-grade, vitritis.

DIAGNOSIS AND DIFFERENTIAL DIAGNOSIS

Diagnosis

Diagnosis is made from following clinical findings and investigations:

Fundus examination shows following typical features (Fig. 7.10.2.1)

- Characteristic 'birdshot lesions', which are ovoid, orange to cream-coloured, hypopigmented spots concentrated in the posterior pole and mid-periphery of the retina.
- Typically symmetrically distributed and often assume a radial orientation.
- The borders of these hypopigmented lesions are ill-defined and are not 'punched out'.
- Optic disc oedema, diffuse oedema of the retina, retinal vasculitis, and cystoid macular oedema (CME) are common in this disease.

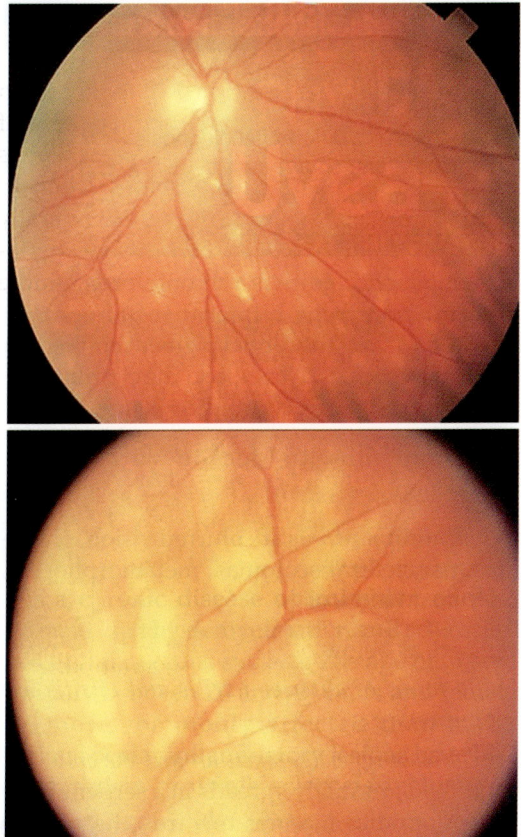

Fig 7.10.2.1 *Retinochoroidal lesions in birdshot chorioretinopathy (Courtesy: Jennifer E. Thorne Albert Jakobiec's Principles and Practice of Ophthalmology)*

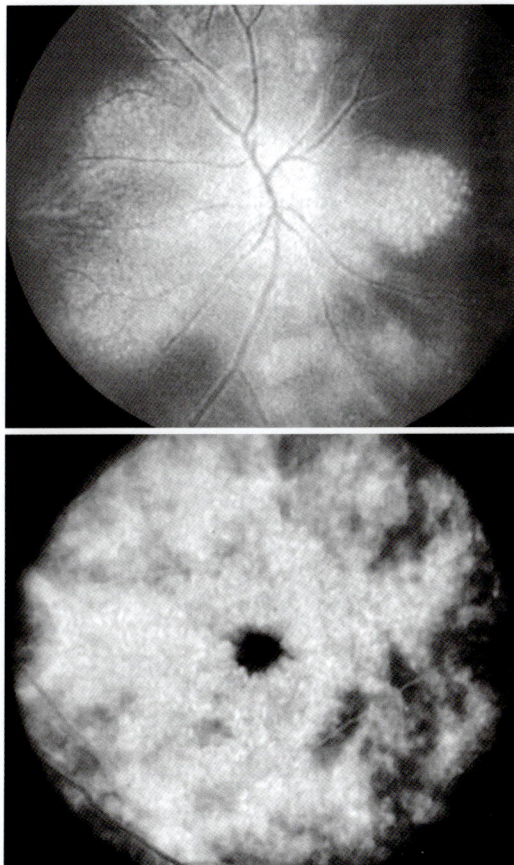

Fig. 7.10.2.2 *Peripapillary cystoid retinal oedema and the profound degree of CME often associated with active birdshot (Courtesy: Jennifer E. Thorne Albert Jakobiec's Principles and Practice of Ophthalmology)*

Fundus fluorescein angiography shows following features (Fig. 7.10.2.2):

• Leakage of fluorescein dye from the retinal vessels and capillaries.

• Birdshot lesions, which may be distinctive on fundoscopic examination, do not typically block the underlying choroidal phases of the fluorescein angiogram and show minimal hyperfluorescence and staining in the latter phases of the study.

Indocyanine green angiography (ICG). Birdshot lesions may be evident on ICG imaging as hypofluorescent dark dots even in the absence of birdshot lesions observed on the fundus.

Visual field. Abnormalities, such as generalised constriction of the field, may be seen in birdshot chorioretinopathy.

Electrophysiologic studies. May show a reduced electroretinogram (ERG) and normal electro-oculogram (EOG) responses.

Laboratory studies. Typically are used to rule out other uveitidies associated with chorioretinal lesions. Chest radiograph, purified protein derivative, skin testing for anergy, rapid plasma reagin (RPR) test, fluorescent treponemal antibody absorption (FTA-Abs) test, Lyme antibody, and complete blood count can help to rule out other diseases.

Differential diagnosis

Differential diagnosis includes:
• Infectious forms of uveitis, such as tuberculosis and syphilis
• Vogt–Koyanagi–Harada (VKH) syndrome

- Sympathetic ophthalmia
- Acute posterior multifocal placoid pigment epitheliopathy (APMPPE)
- Multiple evanescent white-dot syndrome (MEWDS)

TREATMENT AND MONITORING

Treatment

It remains unclear when treatment should be initiated. Treatment for birdshot chorioretinopathy includes:

- *Oral and periocular corticosteroids* have been used to treat CME, vitreous inflammation, and optic nerve oedema.
- *Cyclosporine* in doses ranging from 2 to 5 mg/kg/day often is associated with resolution of vitreous cells and marked restoration of the blood–ocular barrier.

Monitoring

The best method of monitoring patients with birdshot chorioretinopathy has not been established, although it appears that monitoring for central visual acuity loss and clinical signs of intraocular inflammation alone are observed.

BIBLIOGRAPHY

1. Gass JDM. Vitiliginous chorioretinitis. Arch Ophthalmol 1981;99:1778–87.
2. Gaudio PA, Kaye DB, Crawford J. Histopathology of birdshot chorioretinopathy. Br J Ophthalmol 2002;86:439–63.
3. Kaplan HJ, Aaberg TM. Birdshot retinochoroidopathy. Am J Ophthalmol 1980;90:773–82.
4. Nussenblatt RB, Mittal KK, Ryan S, et al. Birdshot retinochoroidopathy associated with HLA-A29 antigen and immune responsiveness to retinal S-antigen. Am J Ophthalmol 1982; 94:147–58.
5. Priem HA, Kijlstra A, Noens L, et al. HLA typing in birdshot chorioretinopathy. Am J Ophthalmol 1988;105:182–85.
6. Priem HA, Oosterhuis JA: Birdshot chorioretinopathy: clinical characteristics and evolution. Br J Ophthalmol 1988;72:646–59.
7. Ryan SJ, Maumenee AE. Birdshot retinochoroidopathy. Am J Ophthalmol 1980;89:31–45.
8. Shah KH, Levinson RD, Yu F, et al. Birdshot chorioretinopathy. Surv Ophthalmol 2005; 50:519–41.

7.10.3 SERPIGINOUS CHOROIDITIS

- Clinical features
- Diagnosis and differential diagnosis
- Treatment and course

CLINICAL FEATURES

Serpiginous choroiditis is a chronic, progressive, rare and recurrent bilateral inflammatory disease involving the retinal pigment epithelium (RPE), the choriocapillaris, and the choroid. The cause of serpiginous choroiditis is unknown.

Age group 5th–6th decade with no sex predilection.

Presenting symptoms are blurred vision, photopsias, paracentral scotomas, metamorphopsia, and visual field loss.

Signs are as below:

- *Mild forms of anterior uveitis and vitritis* are common.
- *The disease typically starts around the optic disc* and then gradually spreads in a serpentine or pseudopodial manner towards the macula and peripheral fundus (Figs 7.10.3.1 and 7.10.3.2).
- *Active lesions* are grey-white (Fig. 7.10.3.2) and may remain active for several months.
- *Inactive lesions* are characterised by scalloped, atrophic areas of choroidal and RPE atrophy.

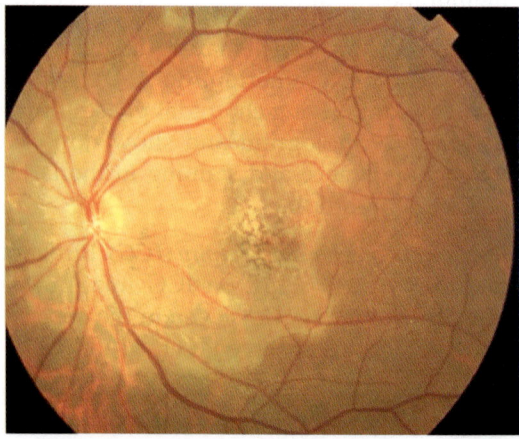

Fig. 7.10.3.1 *Left eye active serpiginous choroiditis.*

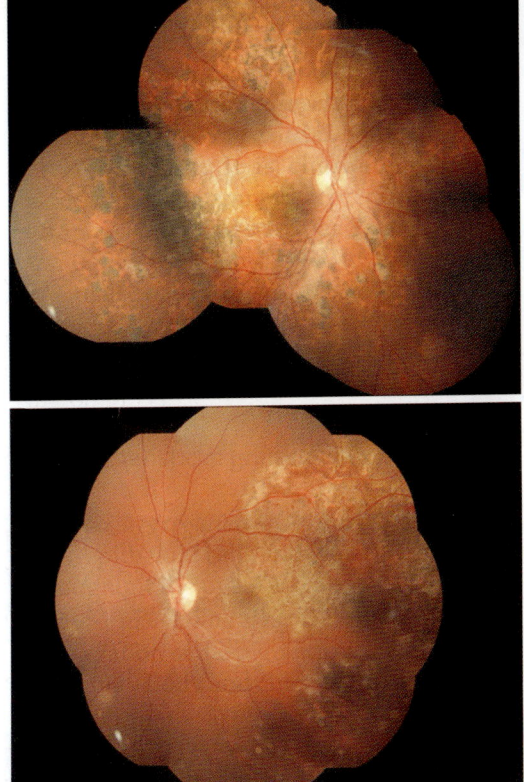

Fig. 7.10.3.2 *Colour fundus photograph in a case of bilateral serpiginous choroiditis.*

- *Recurrences* are characterised by yellow-grey extensions, contiguous or as satellites appearing in existing areas of chorioretinal scars.
- *Complications,* such as choroidal neovascular membrane and subretinal fibrosis can occur.

DIAGNOSIS AND DIFFERENTIAL DIAGNOSIS

Diagnosis

Typical clinical features and following investigations are helpful in making diagnosis:

Fundus fluorescein angiography (FFA) of active lesions shows early hypofluorescence and late hyperfluorescence, similar to APMPPE; inactive lesions show window defects (Fig. 7.10.3.3).

Fundus autofluorescence. Hyperautofluorescence corresponding to the areas of active edge in a case of active serpiginous choroiditis in the left eye (Fig. 7.10.3.4).

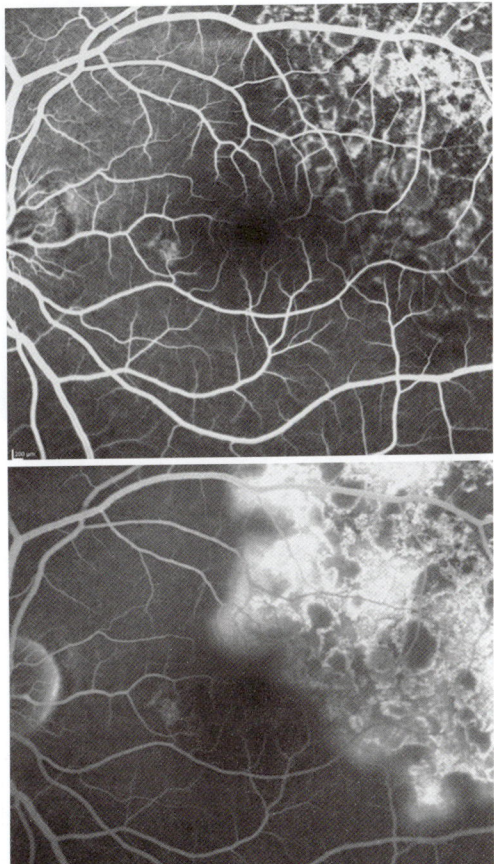

Fig. 7.10.3.3 *Fundus fluorescein angiography of a patient with serpiginous choroiditis.*

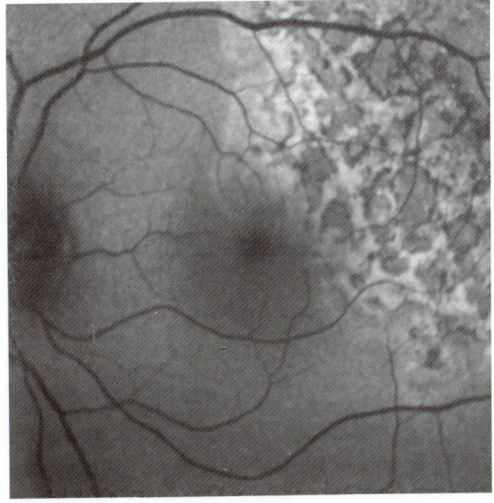

Fig. 7.10.3.4 *Fundus autofluorescence in a patient with active serpiginous choroiditis.*

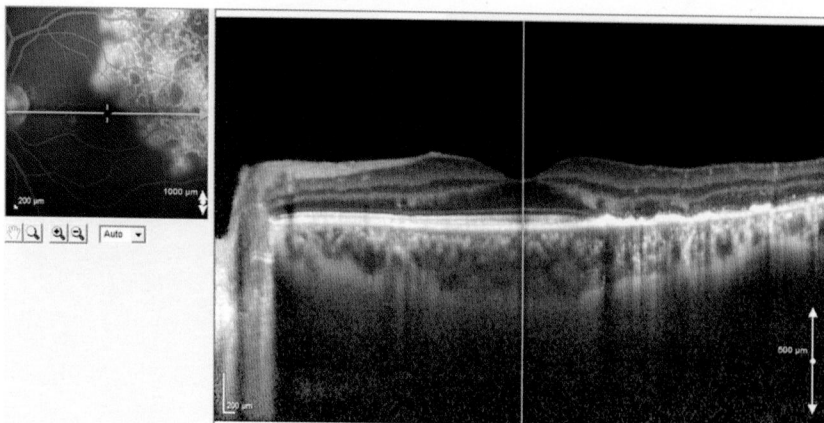

Fig. 7.10.3.5 *Optical coherance tomography of left eye of a patient with serpiginous choroiditis.*

Indocyanine green angiography (ICGA). Active lesions reveal marked hypofluorescence throughout all phases of the angiogram.

ERG may be abnormal in eyes with extensive retinal damage.

Optical coherence tomography. Optical coherence tomography of the left eye reveals hyperreflective echoes in the outer retina with disruption of IS/OS junction in the left eye with increased choroidal thickness (Fig. 7.10.3.5).

Differential diagnosis

- Serpiginous-like choroiditis
- Vogt-Koyanagi-Harada disease
- Central serous chorioretinopathy
- Multifocal choroiditis

TREATMENT AND COURSE

Treatment

- *Acute exacerbations* may respond to periocular or systemic steroids but this does not prevent recurrences.
- *Chronic cases* require long-term immuno-suppression with systemic steroids, azathio-prine and/or methotrexate.

Clinical course

The course lasts many years in an episodic and recurrent fashion and activity may recur after many months of remission, eventually resulting in extensive chorioretinal atrophy and development of CNVM.

BIBLIOGRAPHY

1. Chisholm H, Gass JDM, Hutton WL. The late stage of serpiginous (geographic) choroiditis. AmJ Ophthalmol 1876;82:343.
2. Hamilton AM, Bird AC. Geographical choroidopathy. Br J Ophthalmol 1974;58:784.
3. Hardy RA, Schatz H. Macular geographic helicoid choroidopath. Arch Ophthalmol 1987; 105:1237.
4. Laatikainen L, Erkkila H. A follow-up study on serpiginous choroiditis. Acta Ophthalmol 1981; 59:707.
5. Laatikainen L, Erkkila H. Serpiginous choroiditis. Br J Ophthalmol 1974;58:777.
6. Schatz H, Maumenee AE, Patz A. Geographic helicoid peripapillary choroidopathy: Clinical presentation and fluorescein angiographic findings. Trans Am Acad Ophthalmol Oto-laryngol 1974;78:747.
7. Weiss H, Annesley WH, Shields JA, et al. The clinical course of serpiginous choroiditis. Am J Ophthalmol 1979;87:133.

7.10.4 ACUTE POSTERIOR MULTIFOCAL PLACOID PIGMENT EPITHELIOPATHY

- Pathogenesis
- Clinical features
- Investigations, differential diagnosis and treatment

PATHOGENESIS

Acute posterior multifocal placoid pigment epitheliopathy (APMPPE) is a bilateral idiopathic condition, usually affects both sexes equally and it is associated with HLA-B7 and HLA-DR2.

It is a delayed type of hypersensitivity reaction due to sensitized T lymphocytes following vaccinations and various infections.

CLINICAL FEATURES

Presentation is in 20–30 years of age.

Symptoms. In about one-third of patients, it follows a flu-like illness with meningeal symptoms, decreased vision, central and paracentral scotomas.

Within several months, visual acuity usually recovers to normal or near-normal; occasionally paracentral scotomas persist.

Signs include:

- *Multiple, yellow-white, deep placoid lesions* which typically begin at the posterior pole and then extend to the post-equatorial fundus (Fig. 7.10.4.1A).
- *RPE disturbances.* After a few days, the lesions begin to fade centrally and are replaced by RPE disturbances (Fig. 7.10.4.1B).
- New lesions may appear, so that different stages of evolution may be seen.

INVESTIGATIONS

Differential diagnosis and treatment

Investigations include:

Fundus fluorescein angiography (FFA) of active lesions show early dense hypofluorescence associated with non-perfusion of the choriocapillaris (Fig. 10.4.2C) and late hyperfluorescence due to staining (Fig. 7.10.4.2B & C).

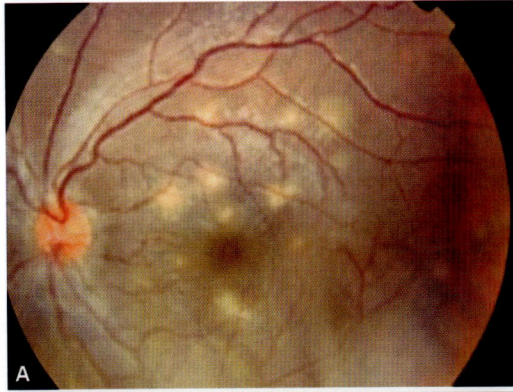
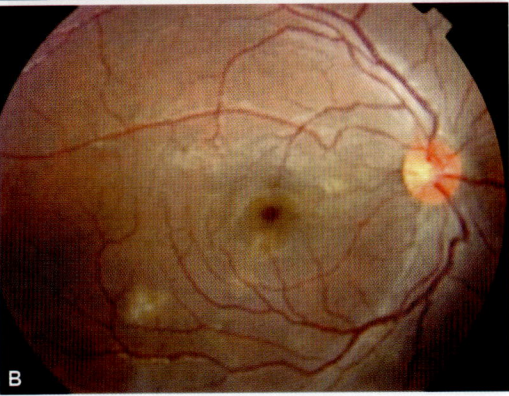

Fig. 7.10.4.1 *Acute posterior multifocal placoid pigment epitheliopathy showing multiple yellow-white lesions (A) and RPE disturbance (B).*

Indocyanine green angiography (ICG) shows more areas of hypofluorescence in the fundus corresponding to the areas of the yellowish lesions.

Optical coherence tomography (OCT) shows increased choroidal thickness with hyper-reflective echoes in the outer retina with or without localized serous detachment of the retina.

Differential diagnosis includes:

- Multifocal choroiditis.
- Serpiginous choroiditis.
- Birdshot chorioretinopathy.
- Vogt-Koyanagi-Harada syndrome.

Treatment is controversial. Spontaneous improvement in majority of the cases and systemic steroid therapy is indicated in severe cases.

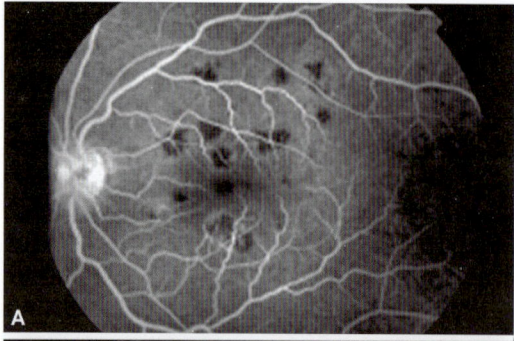
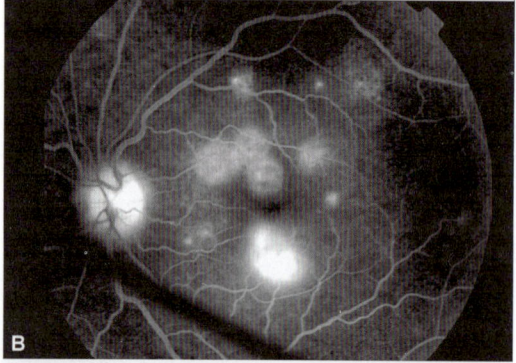
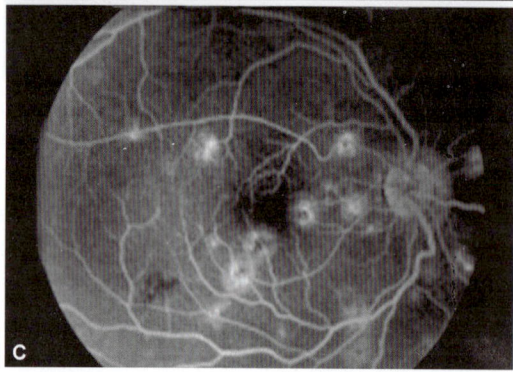

Fig. 7.10.4.2 *Fundus fluorescein angioraphy in a patient with APMPPE showing hypofluorescence associated with non-perfusion of choriocapillaris in activ lesion (A) and late hyperfluorescence due to staining (B & C).*

BIBLIOGRAPHY

1. Baxter KR, Opremcak EM. Panretinal acute multifocal placoid pigment epitheliopathy: a novel posterior uveitis syndrome with HLA-A3 and HLA-C7 association. J Ophthalmic Inflamm Infect 2013;3(1):29.
2. Borruat FX, Piguet B, Herbort CP. Acute posterior multifocal placoidpigment epitheliopathy following mumps. Ocul Immunol Inflamm 1998;6:189–93.
3. Gass JDM. Acute posterior multifocal placoid pigment epitheliopathy. Arch Ophthalmol 1968;80:177–85.
4. Williams DF, Mieler WF. Long-term follow-up of acute placoid multifocal pigment epitheliopathy. Br J Ophthalmol 1989;73:985–90.

7.10.5 ACUTE ZONAL OCCULT OUTER RETINOPATHY (AZOOR)

- Etiology
- Clinical features
- Investigations
- Treatment

ETIOLOGY

Acute zonal occult outer retinopathy (AZOOR) is a disease characterised by damage on the broad zones of outer retina.

- Exact etiology of AZOOR is unknown but possible pathogenesis includes a primary viral infection of photoreceptors or an autoimmune mechanism.
- A case of polycythemia vera and increased hemophilic factor VIII causing acute zonal occult outer retinopathy.
- Patients tend to be young women with unilateral or bilateral presentation with occasional recurrences.

CLINICAL FEATURES

Presenting symptoms are photopsias and acute visual field loss.

Signs. Ocular examination typically reveals vitreous cells with a normal-appearing fundus or attenuation of retinal vessels in the affected zone and occasionally periphlebitis.

- *Late fundus findings* are characterised by atrophy and migration of retinal pigment epithelium resulting in RPE clumps and arteriolar narrowing in the involved area (Fig. 7.10.5.1).

Clinical course. The majority of patients have one episode with good visual recovery while one-third of patients may develop recurrence with a poor visual outcome.

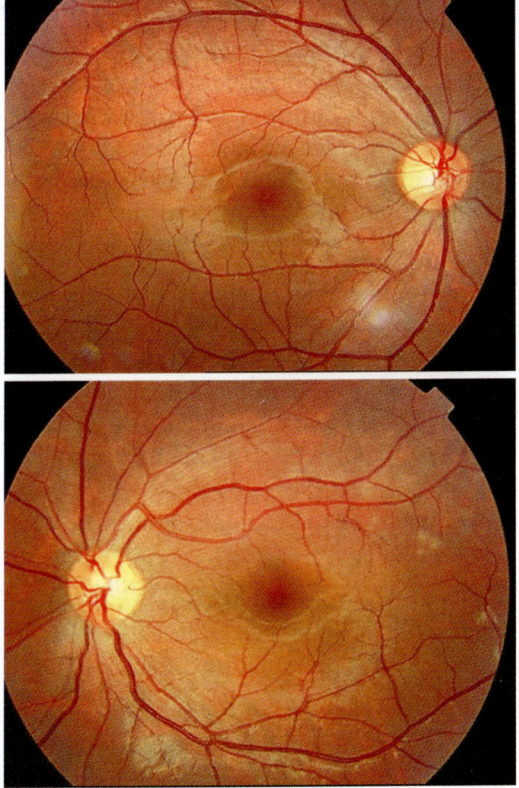

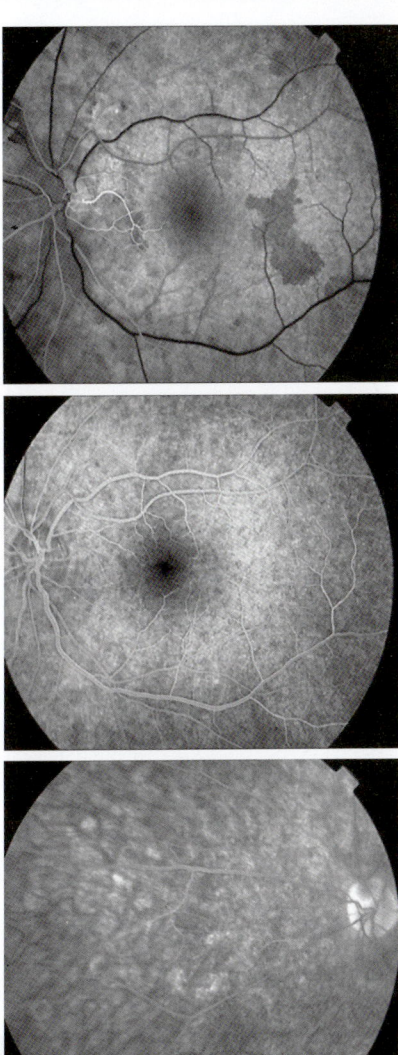

Fig. 7.10.5.1 *Fundus photograph of the right eye is normal and left eye reveales multiple ill-defined hypopigmented lesions in the midperiphery.*

INVESTIGATIONS

Investigations needed are:

Fundus fluorescein angiography (FFA). A revealed early choroidal blocked fluorescence, multiple hyperfluorescence spots in the fundus with late staining of the optic disc in the left eye (Fig. 7.10.5.2).

Perimetry should include both central and peripheral fields otherwise large peripheral zones of visual field loss may go undetected. Visual field loss does not correlate with retinal findings. *Temporal field defects* are common and usually central field is spared. The zones may enlarge, or remain the same or improve. In most of the cases, visual field loss stabilizes within 4–6 months (Fig. 7.10.5.3).

Electroretinography (ERG) is abnormal and can show either or both rod and cone dysfunction with a-wave and b-wave amplitude reduction and delayed 30 Hz flicker.

Fig. 7.10.5.2 *Fundus fluorescein angiography in patient with AZOOR.*

Electro-oculogram (EOG) shows absence or severe reduction of the light rise.

TREATMENT

Treatment is based on the patient's medical history, review of systems, and the presence or lack of inflammation. In general, patients with severe vitritis have been treated with systemic corticosteroids. The visual field defects have persisted in many patients despite therapy. No treatment has shown to effectively treat AZOOR.

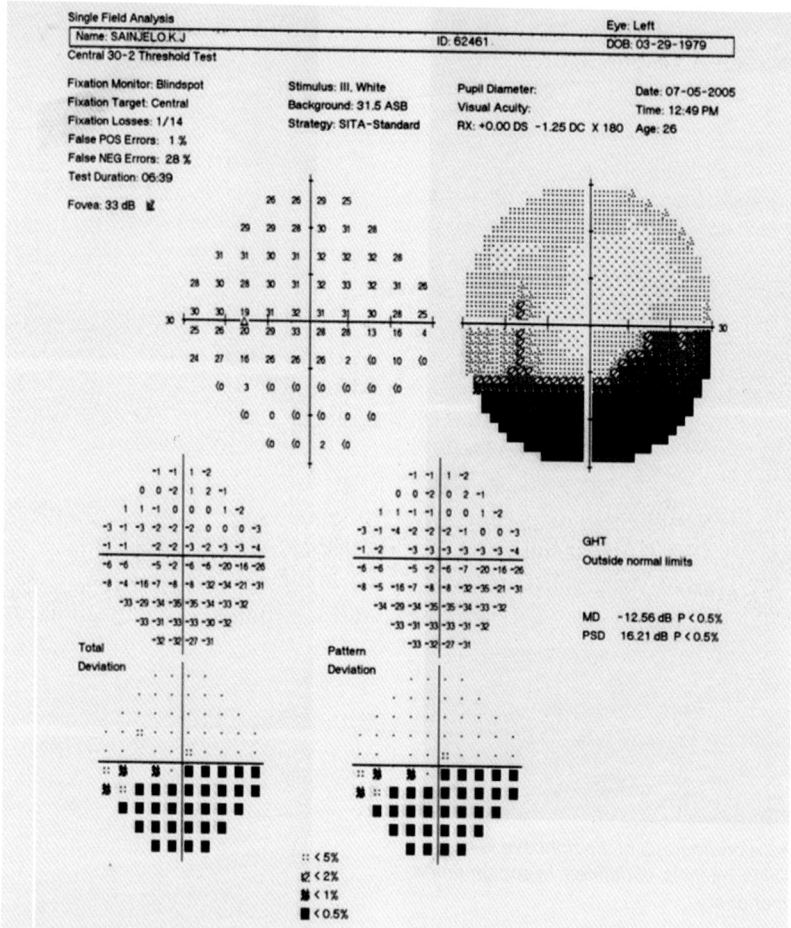

Fig. 7.10.5.3 *Inferior altitudinal hemianopia in the left eye in a patient with AZOOR.*

BIBLIOGRAPHY

1. Gass JDM, Acute zonal occult outer retinopathy, Journal of Clinical Neuro-Ophthalmology, vol. 13, no. 2, 79–97, 1993.
2. Gass JD, Agarwal A, Scott IU, Acute zonal occult outer retinopathy: a long-term follow-up study, American Journal of Ophthalmology, vol. 134, no. 3, pp. 329–39, 2002.
3. Gass JD, Are acute zonal occult outer retinopathy and the white spot syndromes (AZOOR complex) specific autoimmune diseases? American Journal of Ophthalmology, vol. 135, no. 3, pp. 380–81, 2003.
4. Mahendradas P, Shetty R, Avadhani K, Ross C, Gupta A, Shetty B. Polycythemia vera and increased hemophilic factor VIII causing acute zonal occult outer retinopathy: a case report. Ocul Immunol Inflamm 2010;18(4):319–21.

7.10.6 MULTIPLE EVANESCENT WHITE DOT SYNDROME

- Clinical features
- Investigations
- Treatment

CLINICAL FEATURES

Multiple evanescent white dot syndrome (MEWDS) is an uncommon, unilateral inflammatory choriocapillaropathy of idiopathic origin usually self-limiting disease, with a female preponderance. A flu-like viral illness may proceed the disease in one-third of patients.

Presentation: 3rd to 4th decade.

Symptoms: They present with the complaints of scotoma and decreased vision but most recover fully without any treatment in 1–2 months.

Signs include:
- *Vitritis is usually present*
- *Multiple yellowish white dots in the deep retina in the posterior pole and up to the mid-* periphery with foveal granularity (Fig. 7.10.6.1).

INVESTIGATIONS

- *Physiological blind spot is enlarged* (Fig. 7.10.6.2). Peripapillary nonperfusion is responsible for the enlarged blind spot.

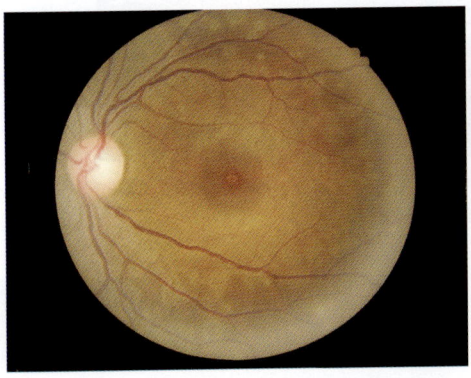
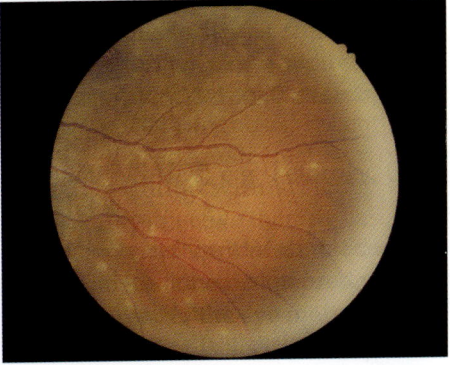

Fig. 7.10.6.1 *Fundus photograph showing multiple yellowish white dots in deep retina.*

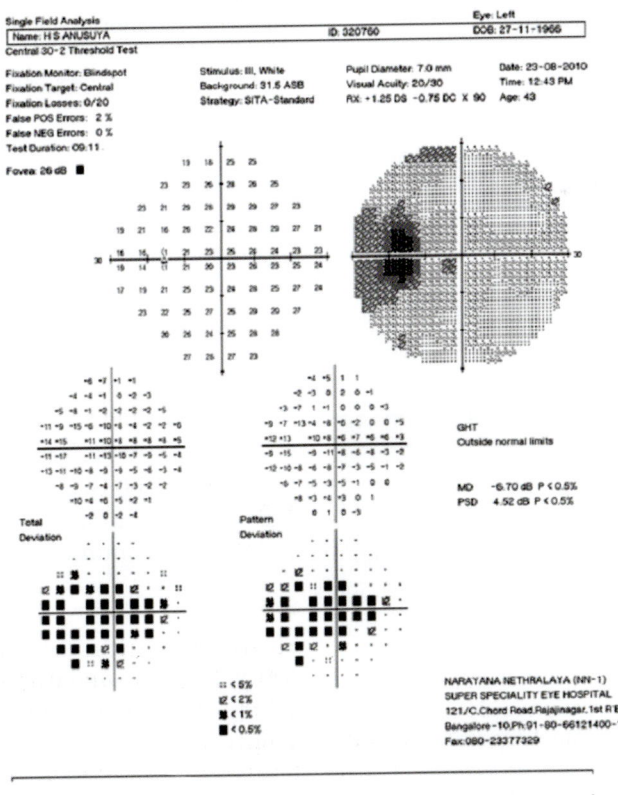

Fig. 7.10.6.2 *HFA visual field chart showing enlargement of blind spot.*

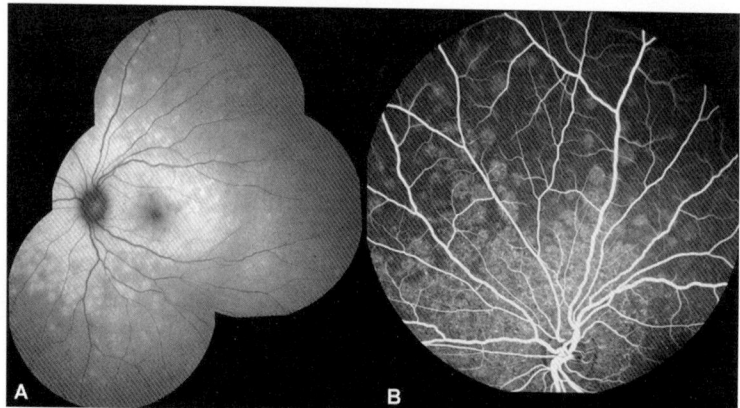

Fig. 7.10.6.3 *Multiple evanescent white dot syndrome: A, Fundus autofluorescence; B, Fundus fluorescein angiography showing stippled hyperfluorescence corresponding to the yellow white lesion.*

- *Fundus autofluorescence.* Many more lesions may be visible than seen clinically as hyperfluorescent areas (Fig. 7.10.6.3A).
- *Fluorescein angiography* shows stippled hyperfluorescence corresponding to the yellow white lesions (Fig. 7.10.6.3B).
- *ICGA* shows more numerous hypofluorescent spots than are apparent clinically or on fluorescein angiography.
- *ERG* shows a decrease in a-wave amplitude which returns to a normal pattern once the lesions disappear.

TREATMENT

Spontaneous improvement without any treatment.

BIBLIOGRAPHY

1. Crawford CM, Igboeli O. A review of the inflammatory chorioretinopathies: the white dot syndromes. ISRN Inflamm 2013;2013:783190.
2. Jampol LM, Sieving PA, Pugh D, et al. Multiple evanescent whitedot syndrome. 1. Clinical findings. Arch Ophthalmol 1984;102:671.
3. Ie D, Glaser BM, Murphy RP, et al. Indocyanine green angiography in multiple evanescent white-dot syndrome. Am J Ophthalmol 1994; 117:7.
4. Reddy CV, Brown J JI~ Folk JC, et al. Enlarged blind spots inchorioretinal inflammatory disorders. Ophthalmology 1996;103:606.

7.10.7 PUNCTATE INNER CHOROIDOPATHY

- Etiopathogenesis
- Clinical features
- Investigations
- Differential diagnosis and treatment

ETIOPATHOGENESIS

Punctate inner choroidopathy (PIC) is characterised by inflammation at the level of the RPE and outer retina. It does not appear to be a true choroiditis. Chorioretinal scars are left by the inflammation. The etiology and pathogenesis of this entity is unclear.

CLINICAL FEATURES

Punctate inner choroidopathy is a disease of young, relatively healthy, myopic women. Mean age at presentation is 30 years (range 15–55). Race—more common in Caucasians.

Symptoms

Scotomas are the most common presenting complaint, followed by:
- Blurred vision,
- Photopsias,
- Floaters,
- Metamorphopsia, and
- Decreased peripheral vision.

Signs

Fundus findings include (Fig. 7.10.7.1):

- Multiple grey or yellow, small round lesions are seen scattered throughout the posterior pole (Fig. 7.10.7.1)
- Occasionally, there is a linear pattern.
- The lesions are at the level of the outer retina, RPE, and inner choroid and a neurosensory detachment may be present.
- With time, these spots evolve into atrophic chorioretinal scars. After 2–3 years, they become more distinct and pigmented.

Other ocular findings. Generally, PIC is not associated with anterior or posterior segment inflammation.

Clinical course and prognosis

- Patients generally become asymptomatic after one month.
- The scars continue to become atrophic and pigmented over the next 2–3 years.
- These scars appear to involve the RPE and choriocapillaris.
- Recurrences are common.
- Some lesions disappear without sequelae.
- Choroidal neovascular membrane (CNVM) can occur.

INVESTIGATIONS

1. *Funuds fluorescein angiography* (Fig. 7.10.7.2) may show following features:

- PIC lesions can appear hyperfluorescent in the arterial phase or may appear as blocked fluorescence.
- In later phases, staining of the lesions can occur.
- More lesions are seen on FFA than clinically visible lesions. Tiny punctuate hyperfluorescent lesions may be seen scattered in the posterior pole (Fig. 7.10.7.2).
- Leakage of fluorescein into the subretinal space is also possible.

2. *Indocyanine green angiography (ICG)* may reveal (Fig. 7.10.7.3):

- As with other white spot diseases, the PIC lesions reveal hypofluorescence in the early, middle, and late phases of ICGA.

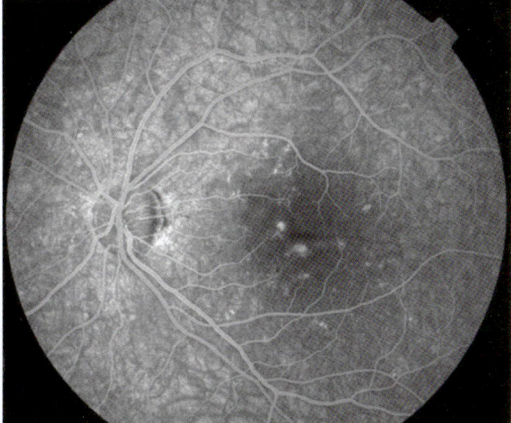

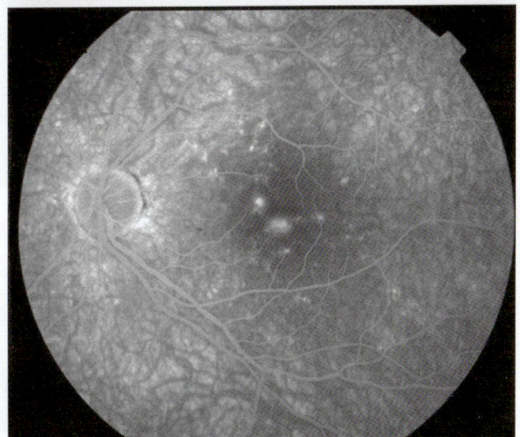

Fig. **7.10.7.2** *Punctate inner choroidopathy: Fluorescein angiography shows increasing fluorescence (staining) and some slight leakage of lesions is seen (Courtesy: Rukhsana G Mirza, Lee M Jampol, Stephen J Ryan. Textbook of Retina).*

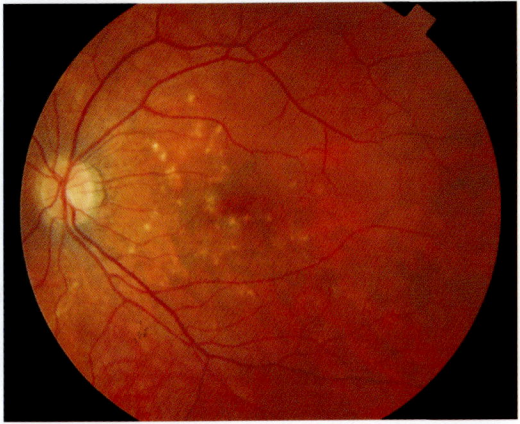

Fig. **7.10.7.1** *Punctate inner choroidopathy: Posterior pole showing small round lesions (Courtesy: Rukhsana G Mirza, Lee M Jampol, Stephen J Ryan. Textbook of Retina).*

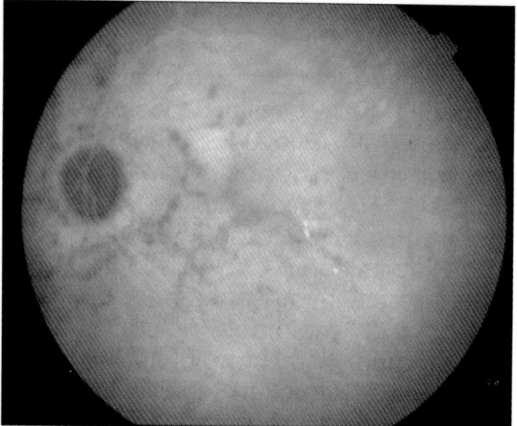

Fig 7.10.7.3 *Punctate inner choroidopathy: ICG shows numerous hypofluorescent spots (Courtesy: Rukhsana G Mirza, Lee M Jampol, Stephen J Ryan. Textbook of Retina).*

- Many more lesions are seen on ICGA than are clinically visible or seen in FFA.

3. *Optical coherence tomography* (Fig. 7.10.4):

- A homogenous thickening is seen overlying chorioretinal lesions.

- There is sub-RPE solid looking material that pushes up the RPE and may extend into the retina.

4. *Electrophysiology.* Asymmetry in b-wave amplitudes between the two eyes can be present on electroretinogram.

DIFFERENTIAL DIAGNOSIS AND TREATMENT

Differential diagnosis

- Sarcoidosis
- Vogt-Koyanagi-Harada syndrome
- Sympathetic ophthalmia
- Myopic degeneration of the macula
- Serpiginous choroiditis
- Birdshot chorioretinopathy.

Treatment

- Treatment is aimed at inflammation and its sequelae such as cystoids macular edema (CME) and choroidal neovascular membrane (CNVM).

- Significant anterior and posterior segments inflammation can be managed with topical, periocular, intraocular, and systemic corticosteroids.

- Steroid-sparing agents are used when steroids are not tolerated or recurrence is frequent.

- Although PIC is not associated with significant visible inflammation, the lesions do respond to immunosuppressives.

- CNVM can be managed with anti-VEGF therapy, steroids, photodynamic therapy and thermal laser if the lesions are extrafoveal.

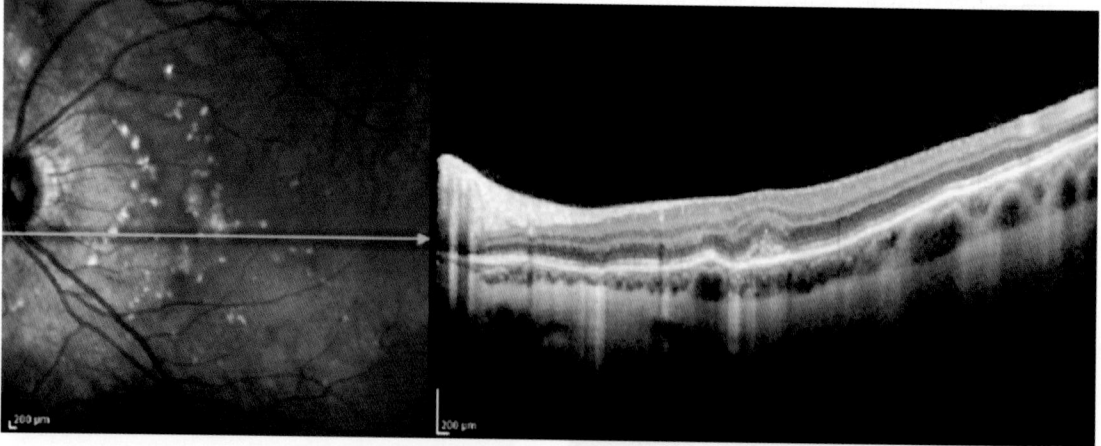

Fig. 7.10.7.4 *Punctate inner choroidopathy: OCT done through an active lesion in punctate inner choroidopathy (Courtesy: Rukhsana G Mirza, Lee M Jampol, Stephen J Ryan. Textbook of Retina).*

BIBLIOGRAPHY

1. Akman A, Kadayifçilar S, Aydin P. Indocyanine green angiographic findings in a case of punctate inner choroidopathy. Eur J Ophthalmol 1998; 8(3):191–4.
2. Amer R, Lois N. Punctate inner choroidopathy. Surv Ophthalmol 2011;56(1):36–53.
3. Atan D, Fraser-Bell S, Plskova J, et al. Punctate inner choroidopathy and multifocal choroiditis with panuveitis share haplotypic associations with IL10 and TNF loci. Invest Ophthalmol Vis Sci 2011;52(6):3573–81.
4. Brown J, Folk JC, Reddy CV, et al. Visual prognosis of multifocal choroiditis, punctate inner choroidopathy, and the diffuse subretinal fibrosis syndrome. Ophthalmology 1996;103(7): 1100-5.
5. Bryan RG, Freund KB, Yannuzzi LA, et al. Multiple evanescent white dot syndrome in patients with multifocal choroiditis. Retina 2002;22(3):317–22.
6. Essex RW, Wong J, Fraser-Bell S, et al. Punctate inner choroidopathy: clinical features and outcomes. Arch Ophthalmol 2010;128(8):982–7.
7. Gerstenblith AT, Thorne JE, Sobrin L, et al. Punctate inner choroidopathy: a survey analysis of 77 persons. Ophthalmology 2007;114(6):1201–4.
8. Levy J, Shneck M, Klemperer I, et al. Punctate inner choroidopathy: resolution after oral steroid treatment and review of the literature. Can J Ophthalmol 2005;40(5):605–8.
9. Olsen TW, Capone A, Sternberg P, et al. Subfoveal choroidal neovascularisation in punctate inner choroidopathy. Surgical management and pathologic findings. Ophthalmology 1996; 103(12):2061–9.
10. Patel KH, Birnbaum AD, Tessler HH, et al. Presentation and outcome of patients with punctate inner choroidopathy at a tertiary referral center. Retina 2011;31(7):1387–91.
11. Reddy CV, Brown J, Folk JC, et al. Enlarged blind spots in chorioretinal inflammatory disorders. Ophthalmology 1996;103(4):606–17.
12. Shimada H, Yuzawa M, Hirose T, et al. Pathological findings of multifocal choroiditis with panuveitis and punctate inner choroidopathy. Jpn J Ophthalmol 2008;52(4): 282–8.
13. Stepien KE, Carroll J. Using spectral-domain optical coherence tomography to follow outer retinal structure changes in a patient with recurrent punctuate inner choroidopathy. J Ophthalmol ePub 2011, 753741; doi: 10.1155/2011/753741.
14. Tiffin PA, Maini R, Roxburgh ST, et al. Indocyanine green angiography in a case of punctate inner choroidopathy. Br J Ophthalmol 1996; 80(1):90–1.
15. Watzke RC, Packer AJ, Folk JC, et al. Punctate inner choroidopathy. Am J Ophthalmol 1984; 98(5):572–84.

7.10.8 ACUTE RETINAL PIGMENT EPITHELIOPATHY (ARPE)

- Etiopathogenesis
- Clinical features
- Investigations
- Differential diagnosis and diagnosis
- Treatment

ETIOPATHOGENESIS

- The precise etiology is still unknown. A viral etiology has been postulated.
- ARPE presents as inflammation at the level of RPE. Some authors have concluded that it involves photoreceptor outer segments along with RPE.

CLINICAL FEATURES

Symptoms

- Acute visual disturbance
- Most commonly—unilateral blurred vision or metamorphopsia
- Central scotoma
- Rarely may be asymptomatic
- No preceding history of flu-like illness or viral prodrome

Signs

Visual acuity is typically 20/20–20/100

Anterior segment examination is normal.

Posterior segment examination shows:
- Round lesion at the macula, which is the hallmark of the disease (Fig. 7.10.8.1).
- There is a presence of cluster of discrete hyperpigmented dark grey spots at the level of RPE surrounded by a yellow-white halo. As the condition resolves, the dark grey spots may darken or fade away, displaying only the RPE changes.

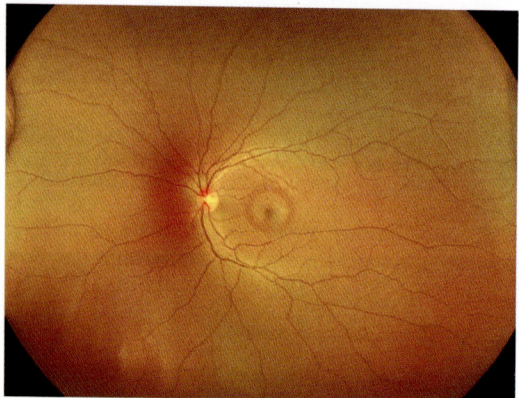

Fig. 7.10.8.1 *Wide field fundus photograph showing a halo like lesion at the fovea.*

- The optic nerve, retinal vessels and the rest of the retina are normal.
- A mild vitritis may be seen sometimes.

Natural history

ARPE is a benign condition with total or near-total resoultion observed over 6–12 weeks.

INVESTIGATIONS

1. *Amsler's grid* shows central scotoma or central metamorphopsia.
2. *Visual field examination* shows central scotoma.
3. *Colour vision abnormalities*
4. *Fundus fluorescein angiogram:* Hypofluorescence of the grey black spots with surrounding early hyperfluorescent halo that fades later (Fig. 7.10.8.2).
5. *Electrophysiology:* Abnormal electro-oculogram (EOG) with a normal electroretinogram (ERG) and visually evoked potential(VEP) in the acute stages which implies RPE dysfunction.

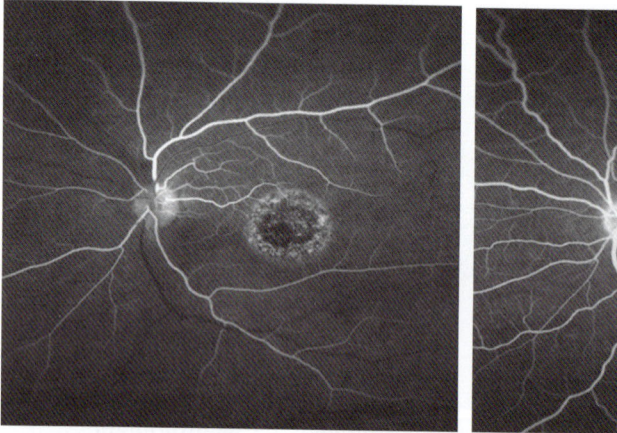
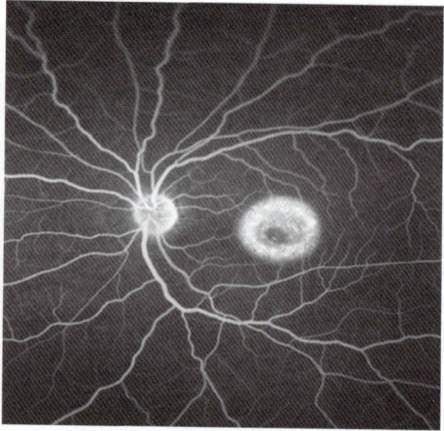

Fig. 7.10.8.2 *Fundus fluorescein angiogram showing hypofluorescent grey black spot with surrounding hyperfluorescent halo.*

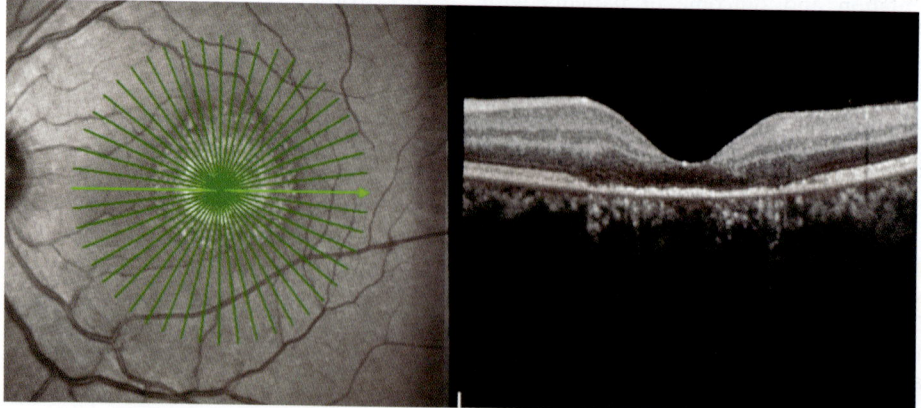

Fig. 7.10.8.3 *OCT shows disruption at the level of IS–OS junction and RPE.*

6. *ICG angiography* in the late phase, a hyper-fluorescent halo is seen with cockade-like appearance of the macula.

7. *OCT* shows disruption of photoreceptor outer segment–inner segment (IS–OS) junction associated with disruption of inner RPE (Fig. 7.10.8.3). As the disease resolves, there is restoration of the IS/OS and RPE integrity.

DIFFERENTIAL DIAGNOSIS AND DIAGNOSIS

Differential diagnosis

- Acute macular neuroretinopathy (AMN)
- Acute posterior multifocal placoid pigment epitheliopathy (APMPPE)
- Central serous chorioretinopathy (CSCR)
- Viral retinitis (especially rubella retinitis)

Diagnosis

The diagnosis of ARPE is purely clinical and based on a history of acute visual disturbance or metamorphopsia in an otherwise healthy adult in the 2nd or 3rd decade. Ancillary procedures (fundus fluorescein angiography, Amsler's grid and visual fields) and investigations (optical coherence tomography) aid in the diagnosis of the condition.

TREATMENT

ARPE is a self-limited disease with favourable visual outcomes. This is the reason why no treatment is advocated. However, corticosteroids can be used for treatment since the condition is inflammatory, but the effect of therapy is difficult to differentiate from the natural history.

Experimental treatment

Systemic treatment of Lewis rats with macrophage depleting agent has shown rapid disappearance of clinical signs of uveitis.

BIBLIOGRAPHY

1. Cho HJ, Lee DW, Kim CG, Kim JW. Spectral domain optical coherence tomography findings in acute retinal pigment epitheliitis. Can J Ophthalmol 2011:46(6);498–500.

2. Hsu J, Fineman MS, Kaiser RS. Optical coherence tomography findings in acute retinal pigment epitheliitis. Am J Ophthalmol 2007;143:163–5.

3. Krill AE, Deutman AF. Acute retinal pigment epitheliitis. Am J Ophthalmol 1972;74:193–205.

4. Pedro BA. Acute retinal pigment epitheliitis. Chapter 72. In diagnosis and treatment of uveitis. 2nd ed.

7.10.9 ACUTE IDIOPATHIC BLIND SPOT ENLARGEMENT SYNDROME (AIBSES)

- Clinical features
- Investigations and treatment

CLINICAL FEATURES

Acute idiopathic blind spot enlargement syndrome is a rare, self-limiting, condition which seems to exclusively affect women.

Symptoms

- Presentation is in the 3rd–6th decade with photopsia and decreased vision which can be misdiagnosed as migraine or optic neuritis.
- Occasionally, photopsia may precede visual loss by several weeks.

Signs

- *Relative afferent pupillary defect* (RAPD) may be present.
- *Blind spot enlargement* with steep margins but variable size is universal.
- *Mild disc swelling* or hyperaemia with peripapillary subretinal pigmentary changes in 50% of cases.

Clinical course

- Vision improves after a few weeks but the blind spot may remain permanently enlarged.
- *Recurrences* may occur in the same or fellow eye.

INVESTIGATIONS AND TREATMENT

FFA may show late staining of the optic nerve head.

Treatment is not required.

BIBLIOGRAPHY

1. Fletcher WA Imes RK, Goodman D, Hoyt WF. Acute idiopathic blind spot enlargement: a big blind spot syndrome without optic disc edema. Arch Ophthalmol 1988;10:644–49.
2. Hamed LA, Schatz NJ, Glaser JS, Gass JD. Acute idiopathic blind spot enlargement without optic disc edema. Arch Ophthalmol 1988; 106:1030–1.
3. Khorram KD, Jampol LM, Rosenberg MA. Blind spot enlargement as a manifestation of multifocal choroiditis. Arch Ophthalmol 1991; 109:1403–7.
4. Kimmel AS, Folk JC, Thompson HS, Strnad LS. The multiple evanescent white dot syndrome with acute blind spot enlargement. Am J Ophthalmol 1989;107:425–6.
5. Reddy CV, Brown J Jr, Folk JC, Kimura AE, Gupta S. Walker J. Enlarged blind spots in chorioretinal disorders. Ophthalmology 1996;103:606–617.
6. Rehman SU, Woon WH. An unusual case of acute idiopathic blind spot enlargement syndrome. Eye 1997;11:941–2.
7. Singh K, de Frank MP, Shults WT, Watzke RC. Acute idiopathic blind spot enlargement: a spectrum of disease. Ophthalmology 1991;98:497–502.

7.10.10 MULTIFOCAL CHOROIDITIS AND PANUVEITIS SYNDROME

- Etiology
- Clinical features
- Investigations and treatment

ETIOLOGY

The exact etiology of multifocal choroiditis and panuveitis sundrome (MCP) is unknown; however, some propose that antigens become sensitized in the retinal pigment epithelium and the retinal photoreceptors by an exogenous pathogen.

CLINICAL FEATURES

Multifocal choroiditis and panuveitis (MCP) syndrome is an uncommon, usually chronic/recurrent, bilateral, asymmetrical disease that predominantly affects myopic females.

- Affects women between the second and sixth decade of life.
- Most affected patients are in their 30s.

Symptoms

- Photopsias
- Floaters
- Metamorphopsia
- Paracentral or temporal scotomas
- Ocular discomfort
- Photophobia

Signs

Fundus findings include:

In the acute phase of MFC (Fig. 7.10.10.1)

- *Yellow round or oval lesions* are seen in the outer retina and RPE. They range in size from 50 to 1000 μm.
- They occur in the posterior pole, peripapillary region and midperiphery.
- The lesions can also be arranged in linear scars parallel to the ora in the periphery.
- Active lesions can be associated with subretinal fluid.
- As inflammation resolves, the lesions become atrophic with a variable amount of pigment ("punched out" appearance).

In recurrent episodes:

- *New chorioretinal lesions* may develop.
- *Optic disc oedema* can be seen and atrophy may occur.
- *Optic disc neovascularisation* can very rarely be seen.

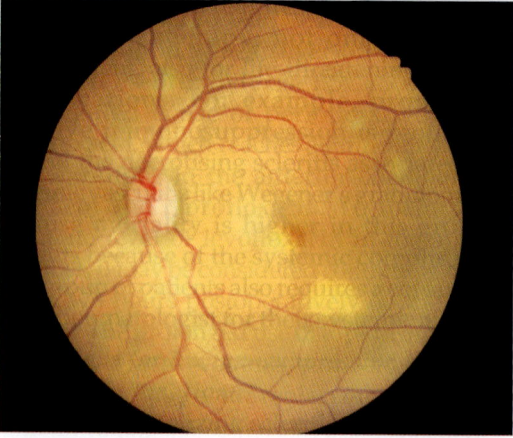

Fig. 7.10.10.1 *Fundus photograph of a patient with active multifocal choroiditis.*

- *Subretinal fibrosis.* The peripapillary region may have a characteristic subretinal fibrosis that has been described as a "napkin ring" configuration.
- *Periphlebitis* may develop.
- *Cystoid macular oedema* occurs in 10–20% of individuals.
- *CNV* develops in 25–30% of cases and can be the presenting sign.

Other ocular findings include:
- May have a mild to moderate *anterior uveitis.*
- Non-granulomatous keratic precipitates and *posterior synechiae* can be present.
- *Iris abnormalities,* such as neovascularisation.
- Vitritis, if present, is usually mild or moderate.

Systemic associations include:
- An association between MFC and Epstein–Barr virus (EBV) has been suggested.
- Some patients with MFC may also have or develop sarcoidosis. These individuals are often not distinguishable from those who have idiopathic MFC.

Clinical course and prognosis
- *MFC waxes and wanes,* but vision loss can occur.
- Most patients tend to have *recurrent episodes* that can involve the central or peripheral vision.
- These lesions *responds to immunosuppressive therapy.*
- Recurrent inflammation may cause *CME, vitreous haze,* and swelling around old scars.
- *CNV* is the most common cause of visual loss in MFC and can be seen with either inactive macular scars or recurrent inflammation.
- *Long-term visual prognosis* of MFC is variable.

INVESTIGATIONS AND TREATMENT

Investigations
Fundu fluorescein angiography (FFA) may show:
- In the acute phase, the clinical lesions appear hypofluorescent on (Fig. 7.10.10.2) FA.
- Late in the angiogram, the lesions stain (Fig. 7.10.10.3).

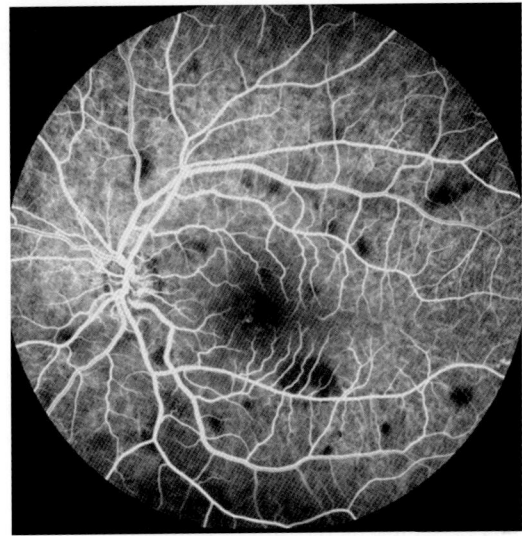

Fig. 7.10.10.2 *Multiple hypofluorescence lesions in the early phase of FFA in a patient with active multifocal choroiditis.*

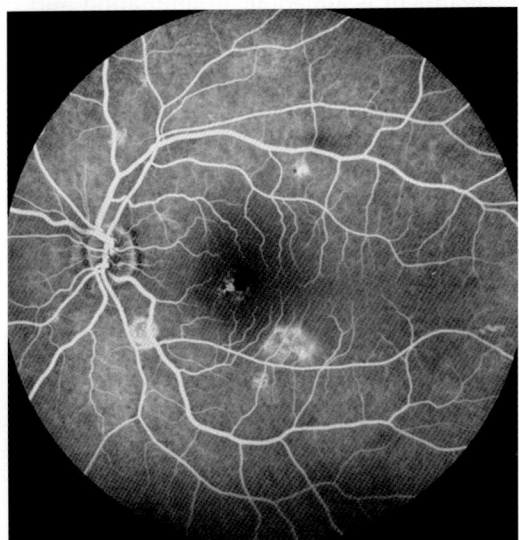

Fig. 7.10.10.3 *Multiple hyperfluorescence lesions in the late phase of FFA in a patient with active multifocal choroiditis.*

- CNV may be present in the peripapillary or macular areas. Most CNV is classic.
- In the healed phase, the lesions become atrophic and show a window defect on angiography.

2. *Indocyanine green angiography.* ICGA shows hypofluorescent round spots that may be far more numerous than seen on clinical examination and fluorescein angiography.

3. *Optical coherence tomography (OCT).* In the active phase, stratus OCT findings show an RPE irregularity corresponding to a clinical lesion. This RPE irregularity resolves with treatment.

The lesion disrupts the photoreceptor layer with potential normalization after treatment.

4. *Fundus autofluorescence* may reveal (Fig. 7.10.10.4):

- *Hyperautofluorescence* will be seen in the areas of fresh lesions which will resolve with immunosuppression.
- Punctate hypoautofluorescence spots will be seen on FAF corresponding to the areas of chorioretinal atrophy indicating inactive lesions.

5. *Visual field testing.* Blind spot enlargement may be seen which resolves with the treatment.

Treatment

- Treatment is aimed at inflammation and its sequelae such as cystoids macular edema (CME) and choroidal neovascular membrane (CNVM).
- Significant anterior and posterior segment inflammation can be managed with topical, periocular, intraocular, and systemic corticosteroids.
- Steroid-sparing agents are used when steroids are not tolerated or recurrence is frequent.

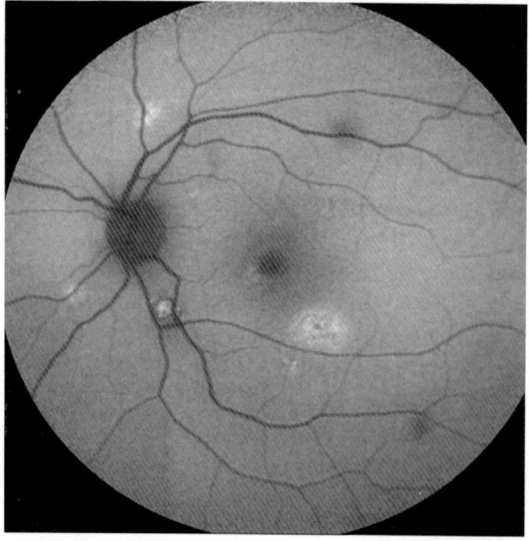

Fig. 7.10.10.4 *Multiple areas of hyperautofluorescence suggestive of active choroiditis.*

- Although punctate inner choroidopathy (PIC) is not associated with significant visible inflammation, the lesions do respond to immunosuppressives.
- CNVM can be managed with anti-VEGF therapy, steroids and photodynamic therapy.

BIBLIOGRAPHY

1. Borodoker N, Cunningham ET, Yannuzzi LA, et al. Peripheral curvilinear pigmentary streak in multifocal choroiditis. Arch Ophthalmol 2002; 120(4):520–1.
2. Brown J, Folk JC, Reddy CV, et al. Visual prognosis of multifocal choroiditis, punctate inner choroidopathy, and the diffuse subretinal fibrosis syndrome. Ophthalmology 1996;103(7): 1100–5.
3. Buerk BM, Rabb MF, Jampol LM. Peripapillary subretinal fibrosis: a characteristic finding of multifocal choroiditis and panuveitis. Retina 2005;25(2):228–9.
4. Cantrill HL, Folk JC. Multifocal choroiditis associated with progressive subretinal fibrosis. Am J Ophthalmol 1986;101(2):170–80.
5. Fonseca RA, Dantas MA, Kaga T, et al. Subretinal fibrosis and linear streaks in multifocal choroiditis. Arch Ophthalmol 2001;119(1):142.
6. Kedhar SR, Thorne JE, Wittenberg S, et al. Multifocal choroiditis with panuveitis and punctate inner choroidopathy: comparison of clinical characteristics at presentation. Retina 2007;27(9):1174–9.
7. Morgan CM, Schatz H. Recurrent multifocal choroiditis. Ophthalmology 1986;93(9):1138–47.
8. Parnell JR, Jampol LM, Yannuzzi LA, et al. Differentiation between presumed ocular histoplasmosis syndrome and multifocal choroiditis with panuveitis based on morphology of photographed fundus lesions and fluorescein angiography. Arch Ophthalmol 2001;119(2): 208–12.
9. Spaide RF, Yannuzzi LA, Freund KB. Linear streaks in multifocal choroiditis and panuveitis. Retina 1991;11(2):229–31.
10. Thorne JE, Wittenberg S, Jabs DA, et al. Multifocal choroiditis with panuveitis: Incidence of ocular complications and of loss of visual acuity. Ophthalmology 2006;113(12):2310–16.
11. Wiechens B, Nölle B. Iris angiographic changes in multifocal chorioretinitis with panuveitis. Graefes Arch Clin Exp Ophthalmol 1999; 237(11):902–7.

7.10.11 SUBRETINAL FIBROSIS AND UVEITIS SYNDROME

Etiopathogenesis
Clinical features
Diagnosis
Treatment

ETIOPATHOGENESIS

Progressive subretinal fibrosis and uveitis (SFU) syndrome is a chronic bilateral panuveitis which effects healthy young women in 3rd decade of life.

Idiopathic, i.e. exact etiology is unknown.

Immune mechanisms have been implicated in the etiopathogenesis of SFU because of following observations:

- *Antibodies* directed against the RPE are reported to be present locally.
- *Fas-fas legend* in the retina shows enhanced expression.
- *Granulomatous infiltration* in the choroid is noted.
- *Choroidal granulomas* are present.

CLINICAL FEATURES

Symptoms. Presenting symptoms include floaters and defective vision.

Signs. Disease is a chronic recurrent panuveitis characterised by:

- *Anterior uveitis which* is usually mild.
- *Vitritis* of mild to moderate degree is typically present bilaterally.
- *Subretinal lesions* include multiple white-yellow spots located in the posterior pole to mid-periphery at the level of RPE.
- *Serous retinal detachment,* CME and choroidal neovascularisation may also develop.
- *Subretinal fibrosis* eventually develops later when the active lesions fade, become atrophic and coalesce into lagre stellate zone of sub-retinal fibrosis.

DIAGNOSIS

Clinical diagnosis

Clinical diagnosis is made from the fundus findings; but the *differential diagnosis* has to be made from other causes of panuveitis and also from the conditions forming white-dot syndrome including sarcoidosis, OHS, APMPPE, syphilis, tuberculosis, sympathetic ophthalmitis, toxo-plasmosis, pathological myopia and birdshot retinochoroidopathy.

Investigations

Fundus fluorescein angiography (FFA) shows multiple areas of blocked choroidal fluorescence and hyperfluorescence in the early phase. In the late phase of FFA, staining of the lesions without leakage is seen.

ERG is usually decreased.

TREATMENT

Systemic steroids and *immunosuppressants* are used for treatment. Although steroids may benefit initially, the prognosis is poor as the progressive fibrotic subretinal lesions lead to severe and permanent visual loss.

BIBLIOGRAPHY

1. Adan A, Sanmarti R, Bures A, et al. Successful treatment with infliximab in a patient with diffuse subretinal fibrosis syndrome. Am J Ophthalmol 2007;143:53–534.
2. Gandorfer A, Ulbig MW, Kampik A. Diffuse sub-retinal fibrosis syndrome. Retina 2000; 20:561–3.
3. Gass JD, Margo CE, Levy MH. Progressive subretinal fibrosis and blindness in patients with multifocal granulomatous chorioretinitis. Am J Ophthalmol 1996;122:76–85.
4. Kaiser PK, Gragoudas ES. The subretinal fibrosis and uveitis syndrome. Int Ophthalmol Clin 1996;36(1):145–52.
5. Kaiser PK, Gragoudas ES. The subretinal fibrosis and uveitis syndrome. Int Ophthalmol Clin 1996;36:145–52.
6. Palestine AG, Nussenblatt RB, Parver LM, et al. Progressive subretinal fibrosis and uveitis. Br J Ophthalmol 1984;68:667–73.

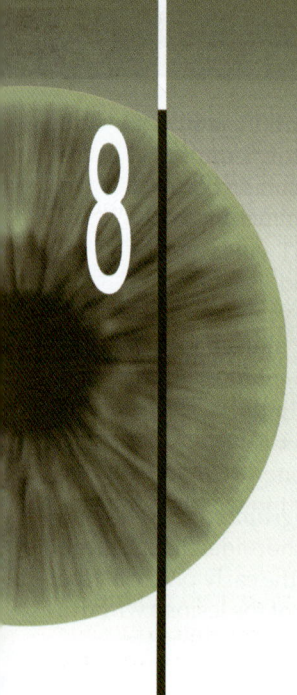

8

MASQUERADE SYNDROME

INTRODUCTION AND CLASSIFICATION

INTRODUCTION

Definition. Masquerade syndrome includes a group of malignant and non-malignant, primary or secondary ocular diseases, that clinically present or mimic as an intraocular inflammation or uveitis but are not due to any immune-mediated uveitic entities.[1]

The term masquerade syndrome of eye was first used to describe conjunctival malignancies mimicking chronic conjunctivitis.[2,3] Masquerade accounts for 5% of patients with uveitis in a tertiary care centre.

Masquerade syndromes should always be suspected in cases presenting as uveitis:
- At extremes of age.
- Ocular inflammations not responsive to corticosteroid treatment
- Undiagnosed uveitis with atypical presentation and course.

Making an early and correct diagnosis is vital as most cases are malignant. Primary intraocular lymphoma (PIOL), in particular, should be considered as a differential diagnosis in middle-aged patients as it is the commonest cause of masquerade syndrome.

Increased awareness together with the development of better diagnostic techniques has decreased the frequency of incorrect diagnoses. However, a correct diagnosis is not always established until a cytological, histopathological or newer, molecular-based laboratory examination is performed.

CLASSIFICATION AND CAUSES

Masquerade syndrome can be classified into of neoplastic and non-neoplastic etiologies.

A. *Neoplastic masquerade syndromes*

1. *Lymphomas*
- Primary intraocular lymphomas (PIOL)

- Non-Hodgkin's lymphoma of central nervous system or primary CNS lymphoma.
- Systemic metastasis from non-Hodgkin's lymphoma.
- Hodgkin's lymphoma

2. *Leukaemia*
- Acute myelomonocytic leukaemia
- Acute lymphocytic leukaemia

3. *Metastasis*
- Lung, breast and renal carcinomas.

4. *Childhood malignancies*
- Retinoblastoma
- Juvenile xanthogranuloma
- Medulloepithelioma

5. *Paraneoplastic syndromes*
- Carcinoma-associated retinopathy
- Melanoma-associated retrinopathy

6. *Uveal malignant melanoma*

B. *Non-neoplastic masquerade syndromes*
  1. Retained lens matter
  2. Infectious including chronic endoph-thalmitis
     - Fungal endophthalmitis
     - Propionibacterium acnes endophthalmitis
  3. Intraocular foreign body
  4. Retinitis pigmentosa
  5. Pigment dispersion syndrome
  6. Drugs
     - Rifabutin
     - Cidofovir
  7. Chronic peripheral rhegmatogenous retinal detachment
  8. Amyloidosis
  9. Central serous chorioretinopathy (CSCR)
  10. Vitreous hemorrhage
  11. Retinal vascular diseases
     - Ocular ischaemic syndrome
     - Hypertensive retinopathy
     - Coats disease
     - Vascular occlusive diseases
     - Diabetic retinopathy

NEOPLASTIC MASQUERADE SYNDROMES

Neoplastic masquerade syndromes account for 2–3% of all patients seen in tertiary uveitis referral clinics. The most common cause amongst the neoplastic conditions is the primary central nervous system lymphoma (PCNSL).

MASQUERADE SYNDROME AND INTRAOCULAR LYMPHOMAS

Primary central nervous system lymphoma (PCNSL)

Primary central nervous system lymphomas (PCNSLs), also known as non-Hodgkin's lymphoma of central nervous system (NHLCNS) or primary intraocular lymphoma (PIOL), are most commonly seen in people in their 5th-6th decades of life.
- In 30 to 50% of cases, ocular manifestations are the first presenting features in PCNSL.
- The 5-year survival rate is less than 5%.
- PIOL/PCNSL is frequently associated with immunosuppression especially HIV infection.[4]
- 95% of HIV-positive patients with PIOL/PCNSL have evidence of antibodies to Epstein-Barr virus (EBV) compared to only 20% of immunocompetent patients.[5]
- *Sites of ocular involvement* include vitreous, retina, and subretinal pigment epithelium.

Clinical features

Symptoms

Most common complaints are diminution of vision and floaters. Bilateral involvement may be seen.

Signs

Slit-lamp biomicroscopic examination shows
- Mild anterior chamber inflammation and rarely pseudohypopyon.
- Vitreous cells, occurring in sheets, are typical.
- Patients may have a variable degree of vitritis.

Fundus examination may reveal
- Multiple creamy yellowish subretinal infiltrates with overlying retinal pigment epithelial (RPE) detachments and no cystoid macular oedema (Fig. 8.1).
- Vasculitis with perivascular sheathing of overlying retinal vessels, disc oedema and exudative retinal detachments can be seen.
- Subretinal fibrosis and RPE atrophy are seen in resolved lesions.

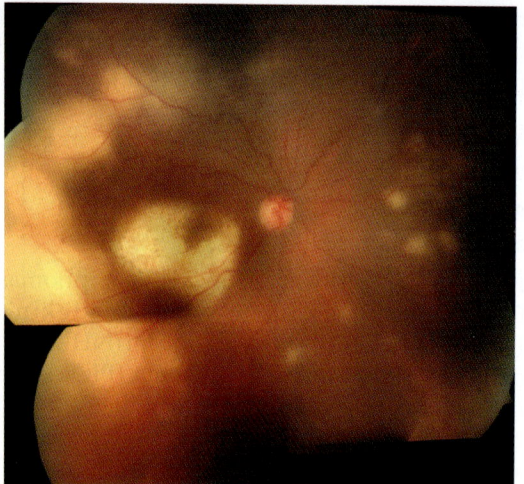

Fig. 8.1 *Right eye of a patient with intraocular lymphoma showing multiple creamy yellowish subretinal infiltrates.*

Diagnosis

Clinical suspicion. Patients, without any past ocular history, presenting with uveitis which is non-responsive to steroids, should arouse suspicion.

Ultrasonography will show choroidal thickening, vitreous debris, elevated chorioretinal lesions, disc oedema and serous retinal detachment.

FFA, hypofluorescence may be seen due to a sub-RPE tumour mass or from RPE clumping; or hyperfluorescence due to RPE atrophy and perivascular staining.[6]

Magnetic resonance imaging (MRI) brain is to be done in all suspected cases which may show isointense lesions on T1-weighted and isointense to hyperintense lesions on T2-weighted images. Multiple diffuse periventricular lesions which enhance with contrast can also be seen in MRI.

CSF tap may reveal lymphoma cells in about one-third of patients. Vitreous tap, vitreous biopsy or diagnostic vitrectomy is the standard investigation.[7,8]

Treatment

Intravenous plus intrathecal high dose (via Ommaya reservoir) methotrexate in combination with radiation therapy and intravenous cytarabine is a mode of therapy.

Combination of radiation therapy and chemotherapy is preferred for patients younger than 60 years.

Local ocular treatment with repeated intravitreal injections of methotrexate (400 μg) can also be used along with systemic treatment.[9] Intravitreal monoclonal antibody against the CD20 antigen on B cells (rituximab, 1 mg in 0.1 ml) is also being tried for this indication.

Chemotherapy alone is indicated for patients 60 years and older because of the potential toxicity and compromised quality of life from radiation (radiation retinopathy, optic neuropathy, dry eyes, cataracts, glaucoma, and dementia).

NEOPLASTIC MASQUERADE SYNDROMES SECONDARY TO LEUKAEMIA

Up to one-third of patients with acute leukaemia develop intraocular manifestations[10]

Presenting features. Masquerade syndrome secondary to leukaemia presents with intraretinal haemorrhage, cotton wool spots, white centred haemorrhages (Roth's spots), microaneurysms, and peripheral neovascularisation. If the choroid is involved, exudative retinal detachment may be present which is angiographically similar to Vogt-Koyanagi-Harada (VKH) syndrome.

Other presentations include hyphema, iris heterochromia, or a pseudohypopyon.

NEOPLASTIC MASQUERADE SYNDROMES SECONDARY TO SYSTEMIC LYMPHOMA

Ocular features include vitritis and creamy subretinal infiltrates of various size and extent, retinal vasculitis, necrotizing retinitis, and diffuse choroiditis or uveal mass. A positive history should arouse suspicion.

MASQUERADE SYNDROME WITH METASTASIS TO EYE

Metastatic cancer is the most common cause of intraocular malignancy.

Primary sites

Overall, breast (in female) and lung cancers (in male) are the most common primary cancers with metastases to eye.

Renal and lung carcinomas are the malignant conditions most likely to present with ocular metastases.

Breast carcinomas although frequently metastasize to the eye, in more than 90% of patients, the primary lesion is known at the time the ocular lesion is noted.

Sites of metastasis in eye

Anterior uveal metastasis may present with cells in the aqueous humour, iris nodules, rubeosis iridis, and elevated intraocular pressure (IOP). Anterior chamber paracentesis may confirm the diagnosis.

Choroidal metastases are typically bilateral, multifocal, creamy yellow lesions, usually posterior to equator, which may be associated with serous neurosensory detachment frequently not in proportion with the tumour size.

Globular vitreous opacities may be seen in cutaneous melanoma. Site is known in approximately two-thirds of cases at the time of diagnosis, with 17% of cases remaining unknown after thorough systemic evaluation.

Retinal metastases are extremely rare, most common primary cancers being cutaneous melanoma. Metastatic melanoma produces brown spherules in the retina, whereas other retinal metastatic cancers are white to yellow and result in perivascular sheathing, simulating a retinal vasculitis or necrotizing retinitis.

Period of survival

Period of survival ranges from 2 weeks to 5 years with an average of 9.5 months.

UVEAL MELANOMA

Incidence

Approximately 5% of patients with uveal melanoma present with unilateral ocular inflammation and may mimic uveitis.

Predisposing ocular disease

Predisposing ocular diseases are choroidal nevus, congenital ocular melanocytosis, dysplastic nevus syndrome, and xeroderma pigmentosa.

Clinical presentation

Melanomas involving the ciliary body can produce dilated episcleral vessels called sentinel vessels simulating episcleritis. Melanoma can cause anterior segment inflammation, complicated cataract and may be mistaken for an inflammatory granuloma or posterior scleritis.

Choroidal melanoma is the most common primary intraocular malignancy in adults.

- *Typical features that tilt the diagnosis in favour of choroidal melanoma* are old age, elevated, well circumscribed sub-RPE mass with variable pigmentation, i.e. from amelanotic (yellow-white) to darkly pigmented in colour, associated with overlying RPE changes like orange pigmentation (highly characteristic), drusen, or atrophy. It may be multi-lobed or can have a mushroom configuration with exudative retinal detachment.
- *It may also present as a dark diffuse mass without defined borders* (diffuse melanoma), vitreous cells, vitreous or subretinal hemorrhage, sentinel vessels (in anterior lesions), and conjunctival hyperpigmentation (trans-scleral extension).

Diagnostic signs on investigations

- *FFA* shows double circulation.
- *Ultrasonography.* Low internal reflectivity, acoustic hollowing, choroidal excavation and kappa sign on ultrasound usually confirms choroidal melanoma.

Treatment

Treatment of uveal melanomas comprises radiotherapy as brachytherapy (ruthenium or iodine is administered) or teletherapy (protons, gamma knife). More recently combinations of surgical and radiotherapeutic measures have been used.[11,12]

CHILDHOOD MALIGNANCIES

Retinoblastoma

- Retinoblastoma is the commonest primary intraocular malignancy in childhood. Approximately 1–3% of retinoblastomas may present with inflammation and most of which are diffuse infiltrating retinoblastoma.
- Older age group, poor visibility of fundus, andabsence of calcification on ultrasonography may result in diagnostic dilemmas.

• Patients may have conjunctival chemosis, endothelial dusting or deposits, vitritis and a pseudohypopyon (Fig. 8.2) which shifts with change in position.

Imaging techniques. Ultrasound of the eye, ultrasound biomicroscopy (UBM) of the eye (Fig. 8.3) and MRI of brain and orbit are required in suspected cases.[13]

Juvenile xanthogranulomas

Clinical profile

• Juvenile xanthogranulomas (JXGs) are small, benign, *elevated histiocytic tumours* that are usually multiple and can be found on the iris or skin and rarely in the viscera of the affected infants.

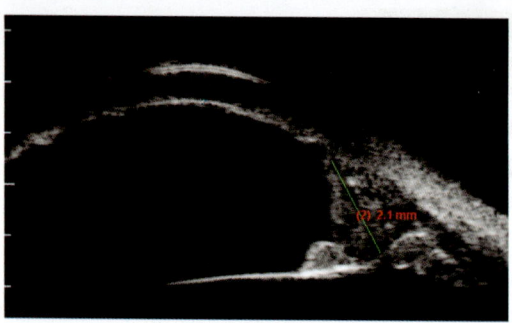

Fig. 8.3 *Ultrasound biomicroscopy (UBM) of the right eye of the patient in Fig. 8.2 revealed a medium reflective ciliary body mass measuring 3.6 mm from 3 to 6 clock hour in the inferonasal quadrant. Histopathological evaluation after enucleation revealed a poorly differentiated retinoblastoma involving the undersurface of cornea, anterior chamber, iris, ciliary body, trabecular meshwork and the vitreous adjacent to pars plana with no invasion of the choroids or the optic nerve and retina was also tumour free.*

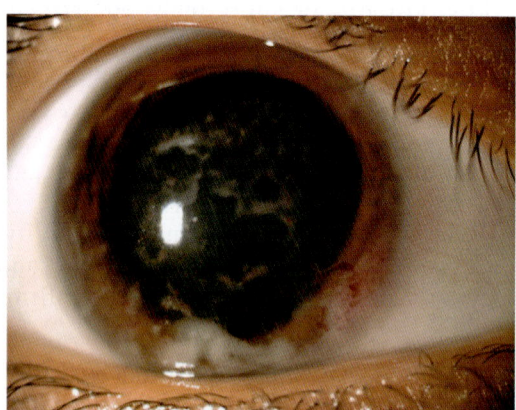

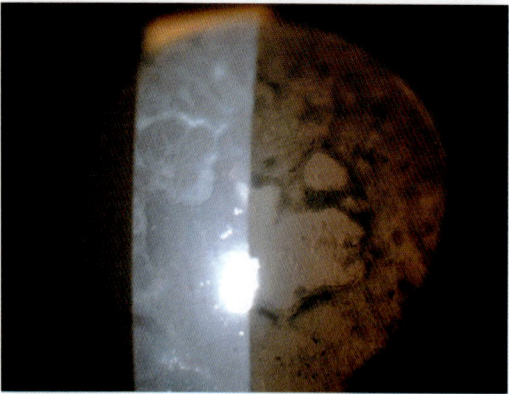

Fig. 8.2 *Anterior segment photograph of the right eye of an 11-year-old child presenting with fluffy exudates in the anterior chamber and with endothelial dusting. The child was initially treated as a case of endophthalmitis, but actually had diffuse infiltrating retinoblastoma.*

• *They are highly vascular*, which, along with the lipid content, contribute to their characteristic orange tint and have a propensity for spontaneous hyphema.

• *Iris nodules* can also be mistaken as secondary to granulomatous uveitis.

• *Histologic investigation* shows large histiocytes with foamy cytoplasm and Touton giant cells.

Treatment

Intraocular lesions may respond to topical, periocular, or systemic corticosteroid therapy. Resistant cases may require local resection, radiation, or immunomodulator therapy.

Medulloepithelioma

Medulloepithelioma (diktyomas) may also rarely masquerade as uveitis. It primarily affects the pediatric age group. It is typically cystic on its surface.

Common sites. It usually occurs from the ciliary body (non-pigmented ciliary epithelium) but has also been reported in the retina and optic nerve.

Cellular characteristics are strikingly similar to retinoblastoma with Homer Wright rosettes. Medulloepithelioma may show either benign or malignant histologic characteristics but is rarely metastatic.

NON-NEOPLASTIC MASQUERADE SYNDROMES

INTRAOCULAR INFECTIONS

Intraocular infections which may masquerade as uveitis include:

- *Bacterial uveitis* due to Nocardia species and Tropheryma whipplei (Whipple disease)
- *Fungal endophthalmitis* due to Candida species, Aspergillus species, or Coccidioides immitis, and late onset endophthalmitis due to Propionibacterium acnes sequestered in the capsular.

Diagnosis and treatment. Suspected cases should undergo AC or vitreous tap and, when diagnosed, should be treated accordingly with intravitreal antibiotic or antifungal or with vitrectomy.

DROPPED LENS MATTER IN VITREOUS CAVITY

Complicated cataract surgery with posterior capsular rupture and with retained lens matter in vitreous may present with anterior chamber cells, increased IOP and even sterile hypopyon with vitritis masquerading uveitis.

Diagnosis: History of recent and/or eventful cataract surgery, a posterior capsular defect on slit-lamp examination, and visualization of dropped lens matter by indirect ophthalmoscopy or ultrasonography helps in diagnosis.

ADVERSE DRUG REACTIONS

Uveitis can be caused or aggravated by a variety of medications, both systemic and local, like the prostaglandin analogues and hence, a patient with uveitis should be enquired about his/her drug history. In suspected cases, the drug should be stopped and the patient is to be kept under close watch.

PIGMENT DISPERSION SYNDROME

Pigment dispersion syndrome is characterized by:

Deposition of pigment released from the iris and/or ciliary body on the endothelium in a vertical spindle shape (Krukenberg's spindle); these granules may be confused with the cells of anterior uveitis.

Transillumination of mid-peripheral iris and a quiet vitreous is seen in such cases.

Raised IOP may be associated with such cases and needs treatment to prevent glaucomatous changes.

CHRONIC PERIPHERAL RHEGMATOGENOUS RETINAL DETACHMENT

Chronic peripheral rhegmatogenous retinal detachment can be associated with:

- *Anterior chamber cells* and flare and vitreous cells and pigments. Patient may have good vision that can sometimes deteriorate because of cystoid macular edema (CME).
- *IOP* may be low or even raised. The outer segments of photoreceptors may block the trabecular meshwork causing rise in intra-ocular pressure (IOP) (Schwartz syndrome) despite a rhegmatogenous retinal detachment.
- *Dilated fundus examination with scleral depression* is important in suspected cases and may reveal hypotony, retinal corrugations, peripheral pigment demarcation lines, sub-retinal bands, breaks, glial bands, proliferative vitreoretinopathy and peripheral retinal cysts may be present.
- *Ultrasound* is useful in suspected cases with media haze or in presence of shifting fluid and vitreous cells to rule out a mass lesion or exudative retinal detachment.
- *FFA* becomes important in some cases of retinal detachment to rule out exudative component.

RETINITIS PIGMENTOSA

- Patients with retinitis pigmentosa (RP) often have vitreous cells, complicated cataract and can develop cystoid macular edema (CME).
- *Clinical features* like history of nyctalopia, positive family history, waxy disc pallor, attenuation of arterioles, and bone-spicule and pigmentary changes clinch the diagnosis in favour of RP.
- *Cystoid macular oedema* does not leak on FFA and responds to oral acetazolamide therapy.
- *Intermediate uveitis* may rarely co-exist in retinitis pigmentosa with pars plana exudates,

snow balls, and leak at both disc and macula on FFA. Such cases require steroids or immunomodulator therapy.

INTRAOCULAR FOREIGN BODIES

- *Chronic intraocular inflammation* may be the presenting features in many patients with retained intraocular foreign body.
- *Ocular complications* such as proliferative vitreoretinopathy, endophthalmitis and siderosis or chalcosis may occur if the intraocular foreign body is not removed early.
- *Past history and signs of penetrating injury* should arouse suspicion.
- *Ultrasonography and CT scan* might be required in suspected cases.

AMYLOIDOSIS AND VITREOUS HAEMORRHAGE

- Amyloidosis and old vitreous haemorrhage may simulate vitritis or endophthalmitis rarely.
- *Uveitis is ruled out* by absence of signs of inflammation, though vitreous haemorrhage can be associated with vasculitis.
- *Uveitic etiologies should be strongly suspected* in young patients, especially males, presenting with sudden onset vitreous haemorrhage with no history of trauma.

CENTRAL SEROUS CHORIORETINOPATHY (CSCR)

- *CSCR may present with exudative retinal detachment that may mimic panuveitis* like VKH syndrome. Absence of inflammation and typical multifocal leaks on FFA in CSCR distinguishe it from the VICH. However, it should be kept in mind that a patient of uveitis under treatment with systemic steroids can develop concomitant CSCR.
- *Treatment.* Stopping any form of inciting factors or drug, i.e. steroids and treatment of the leaks by laser in non-resolving cases is the treatment of choice.

RETINAL VASCULAR DISEASES

Ocular ischaemic syndrome

Ocular ischemic syndrome results from hypoperfusion of the entire eye usually due to carotid artery obstruction.

Symptoms

Patients are typically males, 65 or older and present with decreased vision and mild ocular pain.

Signs

Anterior segment signs. Corneal oedema, flare out of proportion to anterior chamber cells, and neovascularisation of iris and of the angle and complicated cataract are the usual findings. IOP may be low from decreased aqueous production due to ischaemia or high due to neovascular glaucoma.

Posterior segment signs. Dilated fundus examination may show disc oedema associated with dilated (not tortuous) retinal venules, narrowed arterioles and medium to large intraretinal scattered blot haemorrhages in the midperiphery and far periphery of the retina. Neovascularisation of disc or elsewhere in the retina may be present.

Investigations

- *FFA* shows delayed arteriolar filling, diffuse leakage in the posterior pole as well as from the optic disc and areas capillary nonperfusion.
- *Diagnostic studies* include carotid Doppler ultrasonography. Ipsilateral carotid stenosis greater than 75% supports the diagnosis.

Treatment

- *Definitive treatment* includes carotid end-arterectomy.
- *Local treatment* consists of topical cortico-steroids and cycloplegics, as well as panretinal photocoagulation, if rubeosis or retinal neovascularisation is present.
- *Intraocular injection of vascular endothelial* growth factors (VEGF) inhibitors may also be considered.

Other vascular disorders

Hypertensive retinopathy with bilateral disc oedema, multiple cotton wool spots and a macular star may simulate neuroretinitis or viral retinitis in young patients.

- Absence of cells in anterior chamber and vitreous and elevated blood pressure helps in differentiating it from neuroretinitis.

• Renal function test, ultrasound of kidney, evaluation for pheochromocytoma and urgent control of blood pressure is to be done.

Diabetic retinopathy, vascular occlusions and *coats disease* may sometimes mimic posterior uveitis or retinitis. Absence of signs of inflammation along with typical clinical features help to make the diagnoses.

BIBLIOGRAPHY

1. Read RW, Zamir E, Rao NA. Neoplastic masquerade syndromes. Surv Ophthalmol 2002; 47:81–124.
2. Theodore FH. Conjunctival carcinoma masquerading as chronic conjunctivitis. Eye Ear Nose Throat Mon 1967l;46:1419.
3. Irvine AR. Diffuse epibulbar squamous cell epithelioma. Am J Ophthalmol 1968;64:550.
4. Fine HA, Mayer RJ. Primary central nervous system lymphoma. Ann Int Med 1993;119:1093–1104.
5. Paulus W, Jellinger K, Hallas C, Ott G, Muller-Hermelink HK. Human herpesvirus-6 and Ebstein-Barr virus genome in primary cerebral lymphomas. Neurology 1993;43:1591–3.
6. Chan CC, Wallace D. Intraocular lymphoma: Update on diagnosis and management. Cancer Control 2004;11:285–95.
7. Coupland SE, Bechrakis NE, Anastassiou G et al. Evaluation of vitrectomy specimens and chorioretinal biopsies in the diagnosis of primary intraocular lymphoma in patients with masquerade syndrome. Graefe's Arch Clin Exp Ophthalmol 2003;241:860–70.
8. Bechrakis NE, Foerster MH, Bornfeld N. Biopsy in indeterminate intraocular tumors. Ophthalmology 2002;109:235–42.
9. Smith JR, Rosenbaum JT, Wilson DJ et al. Role of intravitreal methotrexate in the management of primarycentral nervous system lymphoma with ocular involvement. Ophthalmology 2002; 109:1709–16.
10. Reddy SC, Jackson N, Menon BS. Ocular involvement in leukemia—a study of 288 cases. Ophthalmologica 2003;217:441–5.
11. Bornfeld N, Talies S, Anastassiou G, Schilling H, Schuler A, Horstmann GA. Endoresektion maligner Melanomeder Uvea nach präoperativer stereotaktischer Einzeldosis-Konvergenzbestrahlung mit dem Leksell-Gamma-knife. Der Ophthalmologe 2002;99:338–44.
12. Bechrakis NE, Foerster MH. Neoadjuvant proton beam radiotherapy combined with subsequent endoresectionof choroidal melanomas. Int Ophthalmol Clin 2006;46:95–107.
13. Bornfeld N, Schuler A et al.. Retinoblastom. Ophthalmologe 2006;103:59–76.

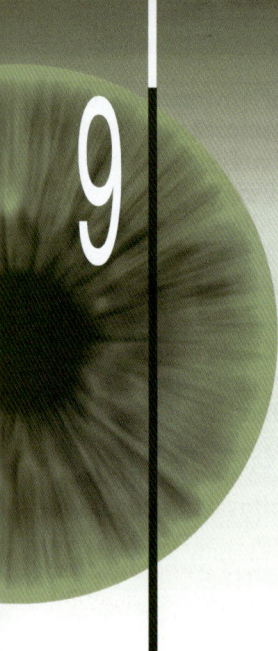

9 RETINAL VASCULITIS

DEFINITION, ETIOPATHOGENESIS AND TERMINOLOGY

DEFINITION

Inflammation of retinal vessel wall resulting in evident clinical manifestations, such as vascular sheathing, leakage and occlusion, is termed as retinal vasculitis.

ETIOPATHOGENESIS

Etiology

Retinal vasculitis can be either primary ocular disorder without any systemic disease or it can be a manifestation of a systemic disorder. It can be thus complication of infective, neurological or neoplastic disorder or in association with systemic inflammatory disease or else it can be idiopathic.

Retinal vasculitis without systemic disease (Idiopathic)

Eales disease, frosted branch angiitis, pars planitis, birdshot retinochoroidopathy, idiopathic retinal vasculitis aneurysms and neuroretinitis (IRVAN).

Retinal vasculitis with systemic diseases

1. *Infectious disorders* include:
• *Bacterial.* Tuberculosis, syphilis, brucellosis, lyme disease, cat-scratch disease, leptospirosis.
• *Viral disease.* Herpes simplex, herpes zoster, cytomegalovirus, hepatitis-B, C; HIV, acute retinal necrosis, progressive outer retinal necrosis, infectious mononucleosis, dengue fever virus.
• *Parasitic disease.* Toxoplasmosis, toxocariasis.

2. *Neurological disorder.* Multiple sclerosis.

3. *Neoplastic disorders.* Acute leukemia, ocular lymphoma, Susac syndrome (later is a micro-angiopathy of brain, retina and cochlea).

366

4. Systemic inflammatory disorders. Behcet's disease, sarcoidosis, systemic lupus erythematosis, Wegener's granulomatosis, polyarteritis nodosa, rheumatoid arthritis, relapsing polychondritis, HLAB-27 associated uveitis, Crohn's disease, dermatomyositis, polymyo-sitis, Takayasu's disease, Buerger's disease.

Pathogenesis

In spite of advances in the observation of microcirculation of retina, the pathophysiology of retinal vasculitis remains obscure. Although experimental animal models have been devised to assess that the clinical manifestations of sheathing and cuffing of vessels are probably due to type III hypersensitivity reaction, however, this hypothesis has not been fully proved. The evidence is more in favour of breakdown of blood–retinal barrier due to ocular or systemic inflammation causing the clinical features of the disease.

There have been number of reports in the available literature demonstrating the presence of focal or diffuse retinal perivascular proliferation of lymphoplasmocytic infiltrates and in diseases like sarcoidosis, there is collection of epitheloid cells. Characterisation of lymphocytic cells reveal the predominance of CD4+ T cells as compared to CD8+ T cells and B lymphocytes. There is an upregulation of various inflammatory cellular markers.

Despite large diversity among retinal vasculitis etiologies, the presentation of inflammatory changes resemble in number of ways. In infectious vasculitis, the organism such as *Mycobacterium tuberculosis* may be cultured from various systemic foci. The organism may involve the retinal vessels either by endothelium or there may be release of toxins, upregulating the molecules such as heat, shock, proteins (HPS) resulting in the activation of immunological pathways causing all the pathological manifestations. Thus the pathophysiology of retinal vasculitis continues to elude the research workers and it remains an open subject for the interested ophthalmologists to dwell further.

TERMINOLOGY

Although the term retinal vasculitis is popular worldwide, on the basis of available meager pathological data, it is more of retinal perivasculitis which can involve either veins predominantly or the arteries or the both. Accordingly on the basis of clinical examinations, following terms are used:

- *Periphlebitis*, where veins are predominantly involved as in tuberculosis, sarcoidosis, Behcet's disease, multiple sclerosis, Eales' disease and HIV.
- *Retinal arteritis* occurs predominantly in association with SLE, PAN, syphilis, HSV (acute retinal necrosis), VZV (progressive outer retinal necrosis), IRVAN (idiopathic retinal vasculitis, aneurysm and neuroretinitis).
- *Vasculitis*, when both retinal arteries and veins are involved in toxoplasmosis, frosted branch angiitis, relapsing polychondritis, Wegener's granulomatosis and Crohn's disease.

GENERAL CLINICAL FEATURES

SYMPTOM PROFILE

Retinal vasculitis can be asymptomatic, minimally symptomatic or sight-threatening. This is the one condition where timely diagnosis and proper treatment can prevent sightthreatening complications and provide gratifying results. Patient is asymptomatic initially, if the peripheral vessel is involved without vitreous involvement. Mostly patient present with painless rapid decrease in vision which may be at times preceded with floaters. Patient may have large area of scotoma relating to the area of ischaemia.

STAGES OF VASCULITIS

The retinal vasculitis mainly passes through four stages such as stage of active vasculitis, stage of occlusion, stage of neovascularisation and advanced stage of the disease.

1. Stage of active retinal vasculitis

Active vascular disease is characterised by sheathing or cuffing of blood vessels and vitreous cells. The veins are dilated, tortuous with perivascular exudates along with superficial flame-shaped and in more severe cases sheets of haemorrhages. Sheathing could vary from thin white lines to segmental heavy exudative sheathing. This could be associated with early signs of occlusion such as cotton wool spots, retinal oedema and intraretinal haemorrhages (Fig. 9.1).

2. Stage of occlusion

The lesion of active vasculitis may progress further and get occluded and may develop variable degree of capillary non-perfusion (CNP). Junction between perfused and non-perfused retina may show telengiectatic vessels, microaneurysms, venovenous shunts, hard exudates and cotton wool spots. Obliterated vessels may be seen as white lines.

3. Stage of neovascularisation

CNP areas release VEGF (vascular endothelial growth factors) because of hypoxia leading to neovascularisation. If less than 90° retina is hypoxic, then NVE (neovascularisation elsewhere) and if more than 90° retina is hypoxic

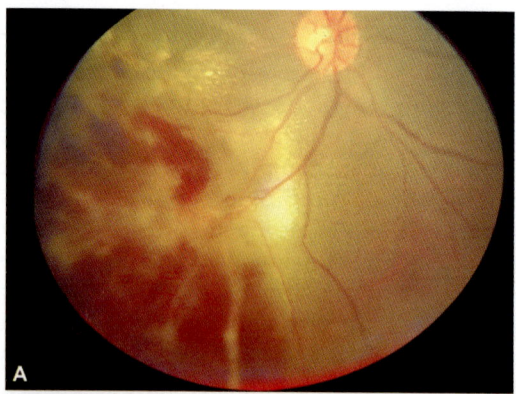

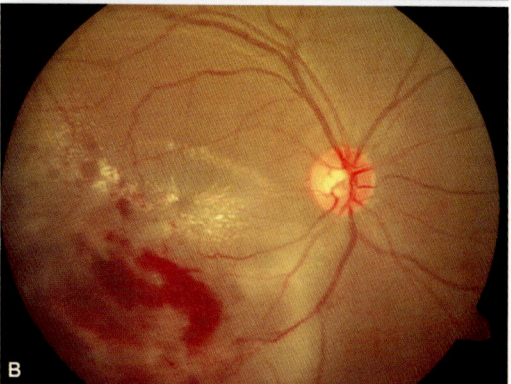

Fig. 9.1 A, Right fundus photographs showing sheathing of blood vessels, veins are dilated with perivascular exudates along with superficial haemorrhages suggestive of active periphlebitis; B, Macular oedema, however, the follow up picture shows some resolution.

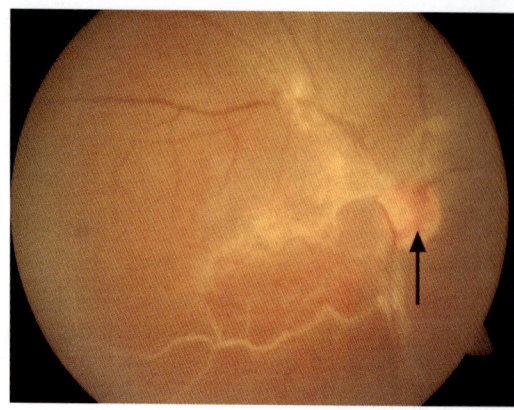

Fig. 9.2 Right fundus photograph showing stage of neovascularisation disc (NVD) in a case of vasculitis.

then NVD (neovascularisation disc) is likely to occur which is the Nature's way of healing by reperfusing the hypoxic area. NVE occurs at the junction of perfused and non-perfused areas (Fig. 9.2). However, new vessels are fragile and likely to break with trivial trauma like the movement of eye causing vitreous haemorrhage and rapid painless diminution of vision. In due course of time, the haemorrhage may settle down with propped up posture and process of resolution starts. This may lead to improvement in vision to be followed by another recurrent bleed (Fig. 9.3). Eventually, the fibrovascular gliosis may follow causing tractional retinal detachment (TRD).

4. Advanced stage of disease

Because of increasing hypoxia, the VEGF may permeate anteriorly causing rubeosis iridis

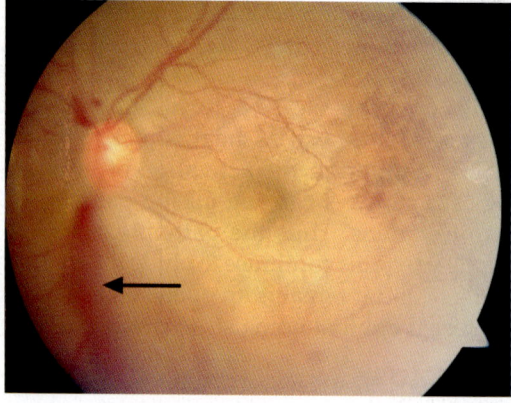

Fig. 9.3 Left fundus photograph showing vitreous haemorrhage from NVD in a case of vasculitis.

leading to neovascular glaucoma (NVG). Further traction may cause break in the retina causing combined retinal detachment. Vision is mainly affected by CME, vitreous haemorrhage and TRD.

SPECIFIC CLINICAL ENTITIES

DISORDERS ASSOCIATED WITH PERIPHLEBITIS PREDOMINANTLY

1. Tuberculosis

Ocular tuberculosis may be due to organismal invasion or due to hypersensitivity to myco-bacterial antigens mostly in the absence of active systemic disease. Although the most common ocular manifestation of tuberculosis is choroiditis, but retinal periphlebitis may be presenting sign of ocular tuberculosis. It

manifests as an obliterative periphlebitis with thick perivenous sheathing affecting the retina in multiple quadrants starting at or anterior to equator and progressing posteriorly. The inflammation-induced occlusion can lead to hypoxia and release of VEGF and consequent proliterative vascular retinopathy (Fig. 9.4).

The patient usually present with recurrent vitreal bleeding and in the advanced disease may develop TRD. It may be associated with active or healed focal choroiditis seen typically under the retinal vessel. Active periphlebitis may be associated with vitritis and mild to moderate AC reaction. The disease is mostly bilateral affecting healthy young adults in the 3rd and 4th decade of life involving men more often than women.

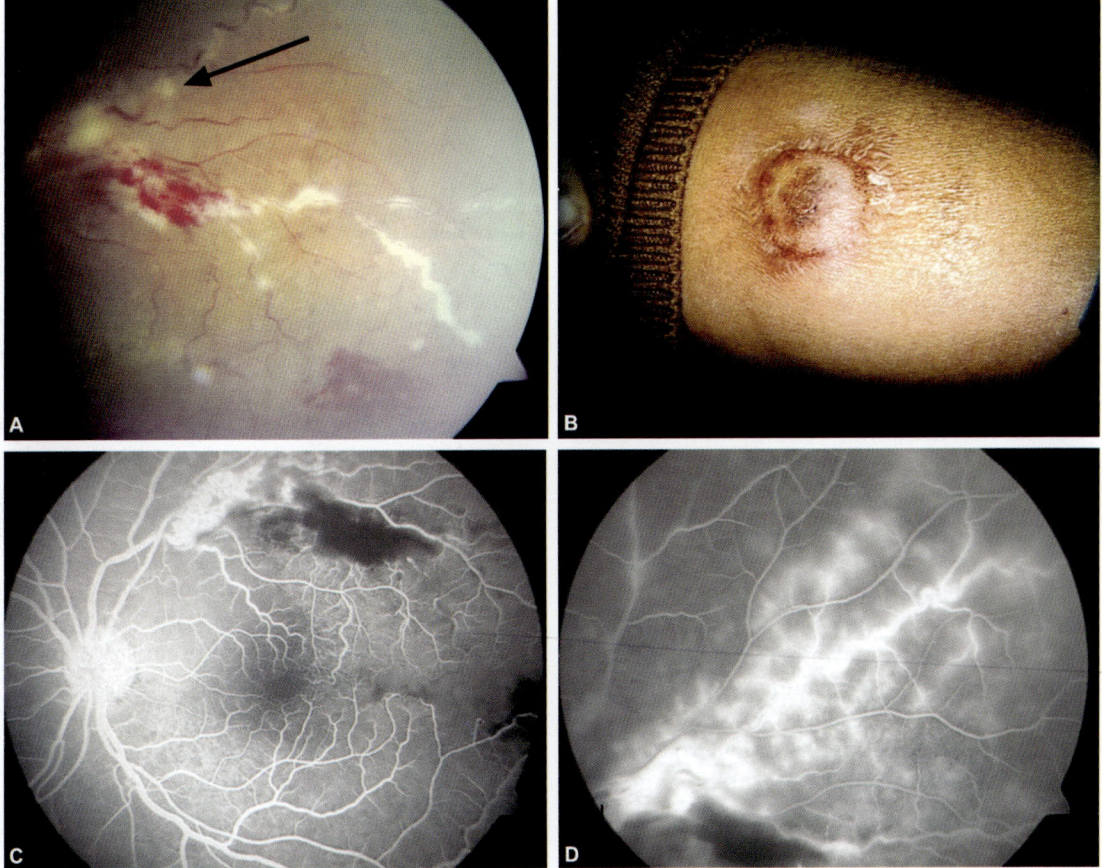

Fig. 9.4 *A, Left fundus photograph showing active tubercular periphlebitis with choroiditis (black arrow) with superficial haemorrhages; B, Mantoux test highly positive >15 mm; C, FFA shows hypofluorescence because of haemorrhage, hyperfluorescence suggestive of active periphlebitis; D, FFA showing areas of capillary non-perfusion (CNP) in the periphery.*

It is very uncommon to have associated active tubercular lesions but highly positive Mantoux test, positive PCR and quantiferon Tb gold test and characteristic vasculitis lesions with heavy exudation and patch of choroiditis (active or healed) underlying the retinal vessel usually clinch the diagnosis. The condition is treated with oral steroids and with appropriate anti-tubercular therapy. The proliferative stage of neovascularisation is treated by laser photo-coagulation. Patients with non-resolving vitreous haemorrhage and with TRD are treated with early pars plana vitrectomy and adequate endolaser photocoagulation. The prognosis of vision is usually good unlike PDR vitrectomy.

2. Sarcoidosis

It is seen mostly in young adults, females are more commonly affected than males and the patients usually present with bilateral hilar lymphadenopathy, ocular and skin lesions. Ocular involvement is seen in 60% of the systemic disease. In addition to anterior granulomatous uveitis and conjunctival nodule, the characteristic posterior segment findings include intermediate uveitis with vitritis and peripheral phlebitis. Retinal periphlebitis is of non-occlusive type with typical segmental cuffing. Sometimes there may be extensive sheathing and dense focal non-occlusive perivenous exudates which are termed as "Candle wax drippings". Multiple small round chorioretinal lesions are frequently seen in the peripheral fundus. The diagnosis is usually established with X-ray chest, negative Mantoux test, raised serum Ca and ACE levels. In doubtful cases, gallium 67 scan may be helpful in determining sites of inflammation for potential transbronchial biopsy. Combination of an abnormal gallium scan and raised ACE levels yield a specificity of 83–94% in patients with sarcoidosis. The treatment is oral steroids in the active stage, lasers in proliferative stage and PPV in patients of non-clearing VH and TRD (Fig. 9.5).

3. Behçet's disease

It is a multisystem inflammatory disorder involving oral and genital ulcerations and

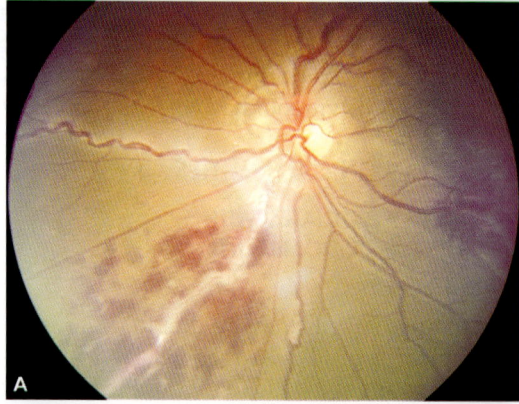

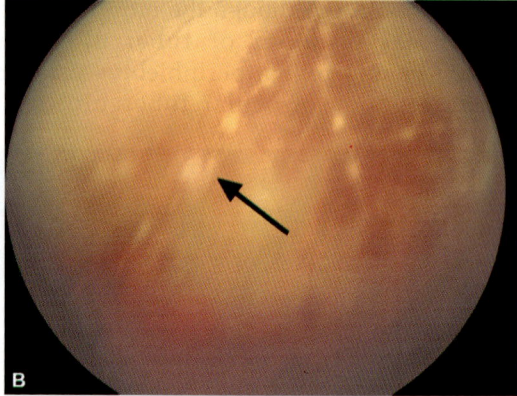

Fig. 9.5 *A, Left fundus photograph showing active periphlebitis in patient of sarcoidosis; B, Perivenous exudates which are termed as candle wax drippings (black arrow).*

inflammation of eye and skin. HLA-B51 is strongly associated with the susceptibility of the disease. Ocular involvement typically includes non-granulomatous panuveitis with or without hypopyon and retinal vasculitis. Veins are predominantly involved in the form of leaky periphlebitis and recurrent vaso-occlusive episodes which are the major cause of visual morbidity. Course of disease is characterised with recurrent explosive attacks and spontaneous remissions. The diagnosis is established by following the criteria proposed by the international study group for Behçet's disease in 1990. The criteria require recurrent aphthous ulcers of oral mucosa as an essential symptom plus two or more symptoms of genital ulceration, eye lesions, skin lesion and positive pathergy test.

Treatment. Corticosteroids are the mainstay of treatment. In severe cases, corticosteroids can be combined with immunosuppressive agents like cyclosporine since it leads to synergistic effect. Other immunosuppressives used are tacrolimus and azathioprine. Interferon-alpha has a role in treating in mild or moderate exacerbations of Behcet's disease. Here, it acts through immunomodualtory mechanism. Presently, the newer drug infliximab which acts by inhibition of tumour necrosis factor (TNF) is being tried. It is said to have a role in lowering the recurrence of the disease. However, its use is limited only to sight-threatening uveitis as the drug is costly and its side effects include pulmonary embolism and retinal evin thrombosis.

4. Multiple sclerosis

It is a chronic disease of unknown etiology characterised by demyelination and sclerosis in the central nervous system. The age of onset is typically between 20 and 40 years and females are more commonly affected than males. Various ocular inflammatory lesions have been described in multiple sclerosis inclusive of iridocyclitis, pars planitis, retinitis, periphlebitis and optic neuritis and some times these may be presenting sign of the disease. The disease is bilateral in 95%. Retinal periphlebitis may occur in 5–10% of cases of multiple sclerosis. In an active lesion, perivenular infiltrates are present which can progress to occlusive peripheral vasculitis leading to neovascularisation, vitreous haemorrhage and tractional retinal detachment (Fig. 9.6). These infiltrates are similar to what has been demonstrated in the brain where demyelination plaques encircle the venules in active stage. In addition, one can see the foci of granulomatous retinal inflammatory cells in the inner retina and overlying vitreous corresponding to the white plaques visible on the inner surface on gross examination. These round dot-like opacities of the diameter of medium-sized veins visible in the vitreous immediately overlying the retinal were described by Rucker and hence are known as Ruker's bodies. MRI scan that show periventricular foci of hyperintensity in conjunction with CSF oligocolonal bands are the

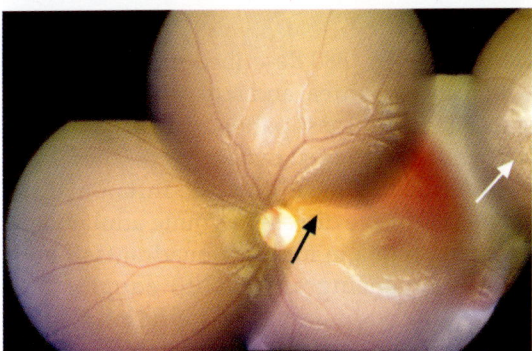

Fig. 9.6 *Left fundus photograph showing active periphlebitis (black arrow) and active pars planitis (white arrow) in a case of multiple sclerosis.*

most sensitive tests for detecting multiple sclerosis.

5. Human immunodeficiency virus (HIV)

Mostly perivasculitis in HIV patients is associated with cytomegalovirus (CMV) retinitis which is the most common opportunistic infection in these patients. The classical CMV retinitis is associated with scattered yellow-white areas of necrotising retinitis with haemorrhage described as "Pizza pie retinopathy". It is often associated with retinal phlebitis presenting as perivenous sheathing. However, in some cases of AIDS, perivasculitis of the peripheral vessels involving veins more often than arteries has been observed even without CMV retinitis (Fig. 9.7).

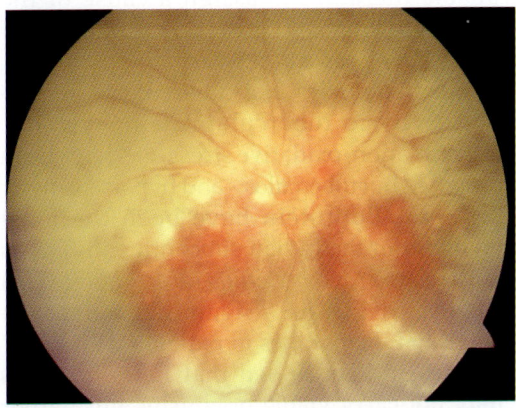

Fig. 9.7 *Right fundus photograph showing classical CMV retinitis in an HIV patient. It is associated with scattered yellow white areas of necrotising retinitis with haemorrhage termed as "Pizza pie retinopathy". Patches of periphlebitis are also seen.*

6. Eales' disease

Henry Eales in 1880 described five young men with recurring vitreal and retinal haemorrhages associated with constipation and epistaxis. The description has varied over the years, however, it is defined as an idiopathic inflammatory venous occlusive disease of young adult males, involving retina in multiple quadrants of both eyes commencing anterior to equator and progressing posteriorly. Non-perfusion leads to neovascularisation causing recurrent vitreous haemorrhage and tractional retinal detachment. The disease is mostly without vitritis, uveitis and obvious systemic disease. The condition is in essence diagnosis of exclusion.

Epidemiology

Eales' disease has been reported from various parts of the world including Canada, United States, United Kingdom, Germany, Greece, Korea, Turkey, etc. but is particularly prevalent in Indian subcontinent being reported in 1 in 200–250 ophthalmic patients. It predominantly affects males in the age range of 20–30 years. It is a bilateral disease (50–90%) though both the eyes may be involved asymmetrically with patient reporting symptoms in only one eye.

Etiopathogenesis

The condition is said to be idiopathic but there has been a continued effort as reported in the available literature to assign a cause of the disease and in this endeavour a number of theories have been put forward.

a. Various etiologies like tuberculosis, hypersensitivity to tuberculoprotein, systemic inflammation, oxidative stress, etc. have been proposed but tuberculosis and hypersensitivity to tuberculoprotein have been the most favoured in the Indian subcontinent. Biswas *et al* isolated *Mycobacterium tuberculosis* (MTb) genome by PCR in a significant number of epiretinal membranes in patients with Eales' disease and concluded that Eales' patients may not carry viable organisms but harbor non-viable antigens or DNA of Mtb in significant number of patients. In addition, certain phenotypes, like HLA DR1, DR4, HLA B5 (B51), show more predisposition to mount a cell-mediated reaction to sequestered tubercular antigen than others.

b. Increased levels of C-reactive protein, IL-6, CD 16+ monocytes and increased expression of cell surface toll like receptors TLR-2 have been implicated in the etiopathogenesis of the disease.

c. Oxidative stress as shown by increased levels of thiobarbituric acid reactive substances (TBRS) in vitreous and blood cells and weakening of antioxidant defense by superoxide dismutase, glutathione and glutathione peroxidase has also been proposed as one of the pathologies in the disease.

d. Increased levels of matrix metalloproteinase 9 (MMP9), increased VEGF/PEDF ratio, retinal S antigen and interphotoreceptor retinoic acid binding protein S also have been proven to play an important role in the disease manifestations.

Despite all these hypotheses, the hypersensitive reaction to tubercular proteins remains the most probable causative factor to date in the etiopathogenesis of the condition.

Clinical features

Patients may be asymptomatic or complain of floaters due to vitreous haemorrhage. Mild reduction of vision can be reported due to retinal vasculitis and marked and sudden visual loss is caused by vitreous haemorrhage.

Anterior uveitis is usually not found in Eales' disease, however, severe retinal periphlebitis can lead to some non-granulomatous reaction in anterior chamber. Similarly, vitritis is uncommon in Eales' disease. The hallmark features of the disease are—retinal periphlebitis, peripheral non-perfusion, and neovascularisation.

1. *Retinal phlebitis* is characterised by venous dilation and sheathing, perivascular exudates and superficial haemorrhages. Patches of active and healed perivasculitis can be seen in all quadrants. Other vascular anomalies include sclerosing and kinking of vessels, vessels pulled towards vitreous cavity, abnormal anastomosis, pigmentation around vessels, irregularities of vessel caliber, etc. Presence of granulomatous

inflammation and patches of active and healed choroiditis points towards other disease entities like tuberculosis, sarcoidosis or syphilis rather than Eales' disease.

Macular involvement is uncommon in Eales' disease, when it does occur (18%), it is known as central Eales' and is characterised by central periphlebitis causing cystoid macular oedema, macular exudates, epimacular membranes and rarely subhyaloid haemorrhage and hence early visual loss.

2. *Peripheral non-perfusion.* Vascular changes lead to peripheral non-perfusion which in turn leads to neovascularisation. The junction of perfused and non-perfused retina is marked by venovenous shunts, microaneurysms, venous beading, etc. The non-perfused area is much better delineated on fundus fluorescein angiography with the seemingly uninvolved eye showing areas of non-perfusion.

3. *Neovascularization.* Peripheral neovascularisation has been reported in 36–84% of cases with neovascularisation disc (NVD) occurring in 9% of eyes. This leads to recurrent vitreous haemorrhage which is a hallmark of the disease (Fig. 9.8a). Patient can have a single episode of vitreous haemorrhage which resolves over 6–8 weeks, but mostly patients have repeated episodes with fresh vitreous haemorrhage admixed with old bleed. There can be subsequent fibrovascular proliferation and tractional/combined retinal detachment. Other sequelae include complicated cataract, rubeosis iridis and neovascular glaucoma.

Staging of eales disease

A staging system has been proposed by Saxena and Kumar depending on the severity of the disease.

Stage 1a. Periphlebitis of small caliber veins

Stage 1b. Periphlebitis of large caliber vessels with superficial retinal haemorrhages

Stage 2a. Characterised by capillary non-perfusion

Stage 2b. Consists of neovascularisation disc/elsewhere.

Stage 3a. Includes fibrovascular proliferation

Stage 3b. Consists of vitreous haemorrhage

Stage 4a. Constitutes tractional/combined retinal detachment

Stage 4b. Consists of rubeosis iridis, neovascular glaucoma, complicated cataract and optic atrophy.

Investigations

1. *Fundus fluorescein angiography.* FFA shows staining of veins in early phases with leakage in late phases signifying active vasculitis. It not only helps in delineating areas of non-perfusion but also useful in monitoring response to treatment in subsequent angiograms. Neovascularisation disc and elsewhere show characteristic sea fan appearance with leakage of dye in late phases. FFA can also help detect doubtful macular oedema and delineate other vascular anomalies like venous obstruction and stasis, tortuous capillaries and venovenous shunts. Hence, FFA is useful in diagnosing, assessing the extent of disease and monitoring response to treatment.

2. *Ultrasonography.* Ultrasound is used in cases of opaque media like complicated cataract (to assess the status of posterior segment) and vitreous haemorrhage to look for any detachment of the retina, areas of traction and status of posterior vitreous detachment before taking up the patient for vitrectomy.

3. *Systemic work up.* Eales' disease is a diagnosis of exclusion hence systemic investigations to rule out other disease entities like tuberculosis, sarcoidosis, syphilis, etc. should be done.

Treatment

1. *Inflammatory stage*

- *Corticosteroids* have been found to be helpful in controlling the inflammation in the active perivasculitis stage of the disease. Since most of the patients show good response to steroids, this limits the use of immunosuppressive agents to the patients who cannot tolerate steroids or have associated complications.

- *Antitubercular therapy* (ATT) along with corticosteroids is indicated in patients with retinal periphlebitis and strongly positive Mantoux test in order to avoid reactivation of systemic TB. ATT in this condition has also been reported to reduce the frequency of recurrence of the disease. Macular oedema though rare can be treated with intravitreal or posterior subtenon depot steroid preparations.

2. Occlusive stage. In eyes with occlusion and capillary non-perfusion, FFA is done to delineate the non-perfused areas and monitor the response to treatment. Prophylactic laser photocoagulation to the ischemic areas helps to prevent/control subsequent neovascularisation and recurrent vitreous haemorrhage. In case of neovascularisation of the discs a panretinal photocoagulation is done (Fig. 9.8b).

3. Stage of neovascularisation. In eyes with fresh vitreous haemorrhage, a detailed indirect ophthalmoscopy or ultrasound in case of opaque media is done to look for attachment of retina. In case of attached retina, observation is recommended as vitreous haemorrhage resolves over 6–8 weeks and laser to capillary non-perfusion areas is done following resolution of vitreous haemorrhage. Anti-VEGF injections have also been seen to be useful in faster resolution of mild vitreous haemorrhage and prevention of rebleeds. In eyes with non-resolving vitreous haemorrhage or retinal detachment, vitrectomy is done. A standard 3-port pars plana vitrectomy followed by endolaser is effective in treating vitreous hemorrhage. Allied procedures, like lensectomy, membrane peeling, gas/silicon oil injection, are done as required for managing associated retinal detachment and other complications of the disease. Early surgey has been seen to improve outcomes in patients with Eales' disease.

Prognosis and natural course

The natural course in Eales' disease is variable with total remission in few patients and significant visual loss due to vitreous haemorrhage or retinal detachment in others. Blindness due to Eales' disease is rare. In a case series of 800 cases, only 4 eyes (0.5%) had visual acuity <6/60 and 8% had visual acuity between 6/36 and 6/60. Contrary to diabetic retinopathy, the prognosis of retaining vision is good in Eales' disease provided the patient is conscious of the threat to his vision and is under the care of a competent vitreoretinal surgeon. Visual loss in Eales' can be due to macular involvement (ischemia, oedema, subhyaloid haemorrhage) or vitreous haemorrhage with or without retinal detachment.

Conclusion

Eales' disease is a disease of young males characterised by perivasculitis, peripheral non-perfusion, neovascularisation and recurrent vitreous haemorrhage. Tuberculosis or hyper-sensitivity to tuberculoprotein has been implicated in the etiology of the disease. With timely diagnosis and appropriate management, the prognosis for these patients is good.

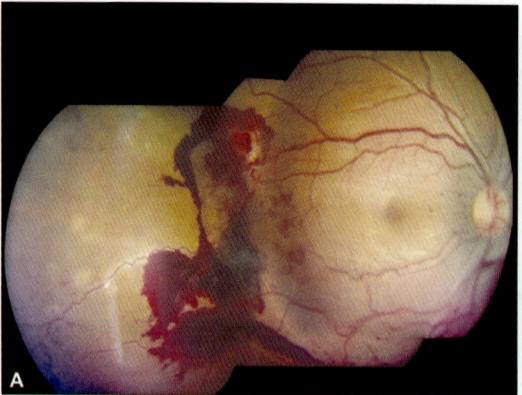
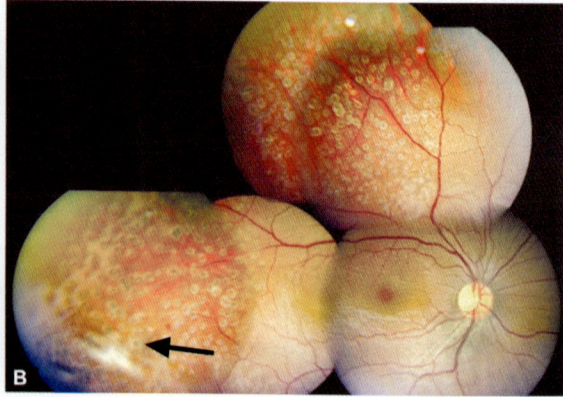

Fig. 9.8 *Right fundus photograph showing healed periphlebitis in a patient of Eales' disease: A, Stage of neovascularisation with preretinal bleeds; B, Regression (black arrow) after panretinal photocoagulation.*

DISORDERS ASSOCIATED WITH PERIARTERITIS PREDOMINANTLY

1. Syphilis

It is sexually transmitted disease (STD) caused by spirochete *Treponema pallidum*. Although leutic vasculitis is predominantly arterial but it needs to be excluded in any patient with retinal vasculitis as it is a great imitator and can mimic wide variety of ocular disorders. Since Treponema can thrive in all the layers of the eye thus it can cause variety of lesions such as focal or multifocal chorioretinitis, vitritis, retinal vasculitis, neuroretinitis, optic neuritis, intermediate and panuveitis and pseudoretinitis pigmentosa (Fig. 9.9A and B). Each and every patient of vasculitis is subjected to venereal disease research laboratory test (VDRL), fluorescent treponemal antibody absorption test (FTA-ABS) and microhaemagglutination *T. pallidium* test MHA – TP) to rule out syphilis. VDRL test is for screening syphilis and FTA-ABS and MHA-TP are for confirmation. Treatment includes IV Penicillin G 12–24 million units daily for 10–15 days or procaine Penicillin I/M 2.4 million units per day with oral probenecid.

2. Systemic lupus erythematosus (SLE)

It is an autoimmune disease characterised by multisystem involvement causing small vessel occlusion in different organs. The prevalence ranges from 3 to 29% and retinal vascular lesions are the most common ocular manifestation of SLE. It is due to periarteritis leading to arteriolar occlusion. The retinopathy consists of cotton wool spots with or without retinal haemorrhages not associated with hypertension. It can be focal or diffuse vascular disease. The former is more common where retinal artery or vein occlusion may occur. The later is less common but more severe characterised by diffuse arteriolar occlusion with extensive capillary non-perfusion.

The patients with SLE and with raised antiphospholipid antibodies (APLA) have a higher risk of retinal vascular occlusive disease. Exacerbations of disease activity might manifest in retina as a retinal vascular occlusion. The clinical manifestations and higher titres of anti-double stranded DNA antibody, raised anti-nuclear antibody, positive lupus erythematosus cell phenomenon, hypergammaglobulinemia, raised circulating immune complexes and reduced serum complement help in the diagnosis of SLE.

3. Polyarteritis nodosa (PAN)

It is a necrotising vasculitis of small and medium-sized arteries in various organs involving heart, kidney, liver, GIT and CNS. Ophthalmic involvement is observed in 10–20% of patients of PAN. Retinopathy which is primarily periarteritis consists of cotton wool spots, haemorrhages, oedema and central retinal artery occlusion. Other ocular manifestations

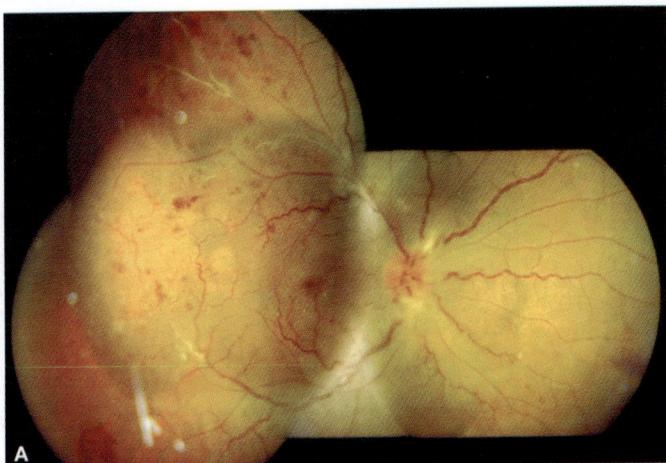 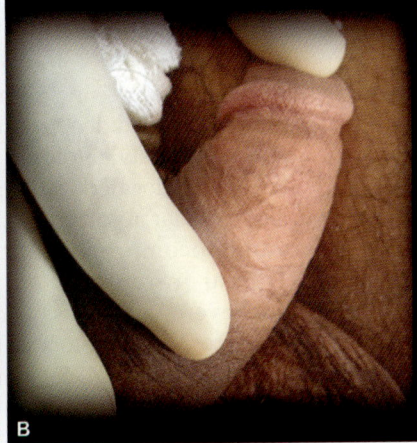

Fig. 9.9 *A, Right fundus photograph showing active vasculitis in a patient of syphilis; B, Chancre on the genitalia.*

include peripheral ulcerative keratitis, necrotising scleritis, non-granulomatous iritis, vitritis, papilitis and ischaemic optic neuropathy.

4. Acute retinal necrosis (ARN)

It is mainly caused by viruses such as varicella zoster, herpes simplex types 1 and 2. The clinical features included peripheral necrotising retinitis, retinal arteritis with severe vitritis and anterior chamber reaction. The typical fundus picture is that of vitritis with confluent areas of mid-peripheral retinal whitening with associated intraretinal haemorrhages. The earliest retinal lesions are subtle, isolated retinal opacities that may assume a patchy granular or a nummular configuration depending on their stage of evolution. Although macula is spared, but small nummular lesions may also be seen in posterior retina. As the disease progresses, the nummular lesions increase in size and coalesce to form confluent zones of full thickness retinal necrosis circumferentially. The diagnosis is mainly clinical, however, PCR may be done in doubtful cases. In addition, response to antiviral therapy is confirmatory. The vision loss usually occurs due to rhegmatogenous retinal detachment, macular involvement or optic neuropathy. Vasculitis is predominantly peripheral arteritis with closure probably at the beginning of the peripheral necrosis.

5. Progressive outer retinal necrosis (PORN)

It is a variant of necrotising herpetic retinopathy in immunocompromised patients. It is generally associated with reactivation of herpes zoster virus, although, herpes simplex (HSV-1) has also been reported to cause PORN. It presents as a rapidly progressive necrotising retinitis with early patchy choroidal and deep retinal lesions which progress relentlessly involving the whole retina. The lesions are located in the periphery with or without macular involvement. Since, the patient is immunocompromised, therefore, there is minimal intraocular or vascular inflammation. Severe visual loss occurs from diffuse retinal necrosis leading to hole formation and rhegmatogenous retinal detachment and optic atrophy in up to 70% cases. It has been observed that involvement of retinal vasculature occurs less commonly and in later stage of the

disease in PORN as compared to ARN. PORN should be differentiated from ARN.

DISORDERS ASSOCIATED WITH BOTH PERIARTERITIS AND PERIPHLEBITIS

1. Toxoplasmosis

It is caused by the obligate intracellular parasite *Toxoplasma gondii*. Infection may occur by either congenital or acquired route primarily affecting the retina. The characteristic retinal lesion is focal necrotising retinitis frequently involving the macula resulting into atrophic scar with pigmented borders. Reactivation is commonly seen adjacent to an old atrophic scar. Severe vitritis greatly impairs visualisation of the fundus, although, the inflammatory focus may be discernible which is labelled as *"headlight in the fog"* appearance. There may be an associated vasculitis near to or distant to the active retinochoroiditis. Recently frosted branch angiitis and occlusive vasculitis secondary to toxoplasma has also been reported. In addition, granulomatous anterior uveitis may be associated. Immunocompromised patients manifest more severe form of the disease (Fig. 9.10).

The diagnosis is based on characteristic fundus lesion and in a general population with evidence of *T. gondii* exposure and high prevalence of *T. gondii* antibodies (IgG), it is taken to be toxoplasmosis. However, in atypical cases, intraocular fluid samples may be subjected to PCR for toxoplasma DNA. Cytological evidence of *T. gondii* from vitreous specimens has also

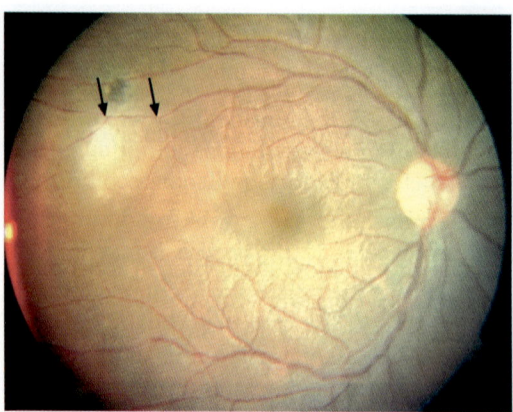

Fig. 9.10 *Right fundus photograph showing active lesion of retinochoroiditis adjacent to healed lesion of toxoplasmosis with adjoining perivasculitis.*

been reported. In addition, the authors have demonstrated the local synthesis of *T. gondii* antibodies in the eye by intraocular fluid analysis which may become a valuable diagnostic tool. Rarely, a chorioretinal biopsy is performed to show *T. gondii* organism.

2. Wegener's granulomatosis

It is a necrotising granulomatous vasculitis classically involving the kidneys and upper and lower respiratory tracts. Ocular involvement occurs in 28–58% patients which include retinal artery occlusion, choroidal arterial occlusion, retinal vein occlusion and optic nerve vasculitis. Other involvements are episcleritis, scleritis, corneal ulceration and paranasal granulomata. The diagnosis is established by antineutrophil cytoplasmic antibodies (ANCAs) and typical histopathological feature of inflammation of small vessels, necrosis and granuloma formation.

3. Frosted branch angiitis

It is an extreme form of diffuse perivasculitis involving both arteries and veins, however, predominantly veins, mostly bilateral, without any sex preference and occurs in young healthy individuals who typically have acute bilateral visual loss associated with anterior and posterior segment inflammation. Fundus appearance includes retinal oedema, severe sheathing of retinal vessels resembling the appearance of frosted tree branches. In addition, patient has retinal haemorrhages, hard exudates and serous retinal detachments of macula and periphery (Fig. 9.11A and B). Fundus fluorescein angiography demonstrates leakage of dye but no evidence of decreased blood flow or occlusion. Initially, the condition was considered to be idiopathic and patients respond to systemic corticosteroids with rapid resolution.

However, sufficient evidence exist that it can be associated with wide variety of conditions like lymphoma and leukaemia, viral infections and autoimmune diseases. It has also been reported to be associated with SLE, Crohn's disease, AIDS, HIV without CMV retinitis, HSV infection and with toxoplasma.

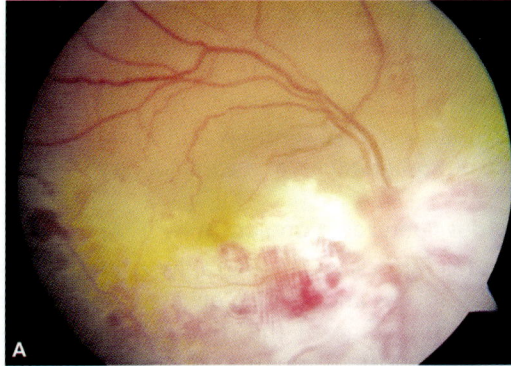
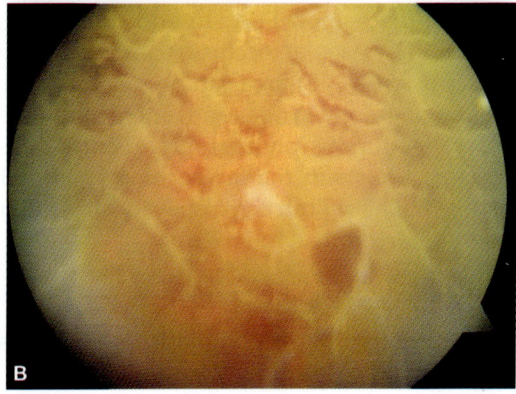

Fig. 9.11 *A, Retinal oedema, dilated tortuous vessels with severe sheathing and superficial haemorrhages in case of frosted branch angiitis; B, the sheathing of retinal vessels resemble the appearance of frosted tree branches, hence the name frosted branch angiitis.*

4. Crohn's disease

It is a chronic inflammatory bowel disease of unknown origin. The eye is involved in 4–10% of patients presenting with occlusive retinal arteritis and phlebitis.

MANAGEMENT

INVESTIGATIONS

The diagnosis of retinal vasculitis involves a multidisciplinary approach supported by laboratory investigations, detailed history, review of systems and physical examination which may help us to rule out infectious etiology. Once the infectious etiology is believed to be unlikely, then any associated systemic disease is considered and the diagnostic workout is tailored according to that disease. If, however, the patient has no signs and symptoms suggestive of systemic disease, then the diagnosis of idiopathic retinal vasculitis is most likely. In this situation, the basic work up of the patient includes FFA, total and differential leucocytic count, ESR, VDRL, FTA-ABS, Mantoux test, HIV serology and X-ray chest (to rule out tuberculosis and sarcoidosis).

Fundus fluorescein angiography (FFA)

Fundus fluorescein angiography demonstrates leakage of dye and staining of vessel wall during the active stage of the disease. Sometimes clinically normal looking vessels may show apparent disease on FFA. In addition, CME, NVE, NVD, vascular occlusion and capillary nonperfusion (CNP) area can be confirmed by using angiography. With the advent of ultrawide field (200°) fundus photography using Optos P200, the lesions in the far periphery can not only be diagnosed but can also be documented and monitored on all follow-up visits.

Other ancillary tests

Other ancillary tests as under are performed as and when indicated.
- Optical coherence tomography
- B scan ultrasonography
- Ultrasonic biomicroscopy

Tests for tuberculosis

Positive Mantoux test, findings on X-ray chest, raised ESR point towards tuberculosis. In suspected ocular TB cases, PCR from aqueous and quantiferon TB gold test from blood may clinch the diagnosis. If still there is ambiguity, vitreous biopsy can be performed.

Tests for sarcoidosis

Negative Mantoux test, raised serum calcium and serum ACE levels, CECT chest and transbronchial lung biopsy may help in obtaining the diagnosis of sarcoidosis.

Tests for other infectious diseases

Serology for toxoplasmosis, PCR from aqueous tap for VZV, HSV 1 and 2 and CMV retinitis in case of vasculitis associated with acute retinal necrosis and progressive outer retinal necrosis may be ordered.

Tests for systemic diseases

Patients with suspected systemic vasculitis can be diagnosed by ordering rheumatoid factor, antinuclear antibodies (ANA), antineutrophil cytoplasmic antibody (ANCA), antidouble stranded DNA antibodies C-reactive proteins, LE cell phenomenon test.

Other tests

HLA-B51 point towards Behçet's disease and *HLA-DRS* towards SLE.

Vitreous biopsy may help in suspected ocular lymphoma.

MRI and full neurological evaluation may establish multiple sclerosis.

Finally young adults with no known cause of vasculitis (Eales' disease) are labelled as idiopathic and managed as per the stage of presentation.

Liver and renal function tests

Certain tests, such as liver function tests (LFT), renal function tests (RFT), are performed before considering antimicrobial or immunosuppressive drugs.

COMPLICATIONS

These are cystoid macular edema (CME), vitreous haemorrhage, tractional retinal detachment (TRD), rubeosis iridis and neovascular glaucoma (NVG).

TREATMENT

Treatment of retinal vasculitis

In cases of active infectious vasculitis, oral steroids are started in the dose of 1 to 1.5 mg/kg b.w and are gradually tapered over 3-month period under the cover of specific antibacterial, antiviral or antiparasitic drugs.

Patients with tuberculosis or presumed ocular tuberculosis usually require ATT for 9 months with oral steroid. Similarly in cases of syphilis, appropriate antibiotics are instituted along with oral steroids.

In cases of active non-infectious vasculitis such as sarcoidosis, Behçet's disease and systemic arteritis, oral steroids are given and these entities may also require immunosuppressives for the control of disease.

- *Corticosteroids* help to control the inflammation and as the inflammation subsides these are tapered 5–10 mg/week within 2–4 weeks of starting the therapy. Once the eye is completely silent, these are further tapered down by 2.5–5 mg/week over few weeks and then are finally withdrawn. Posterior sub-tenon (PST) injections are considered for unilateral cases and for combating the complication of cystoid macular edema (CME). All the patients are monitored for ocular and systemic side effects of steroids at each follow-up visit.
- *Immunosuppressive drug.* In non-infectious vasculitis particularly in Behcet's disease (BD), sarcoidosis and systemic lypus erythematosus (SLE) when the condition is severe and sight-threatening, there may be requirement of immunosuppressive drugs like azathioprine (BD), methotrexate (sarcoid), and cyclo-phosphamide and mycophenolate (SLE).
- *Antitumour necrosis drugs* like infliximab and adalimumab have recently been successfully used in the management of sight-threatening vasculitis. These can be used when immuno-suppressive drugs are not giving desired results.
- In addition there have been reports of trial of drugs like interferon alpha in selected conditions to control the inflammation. However, the safety profile of these drugs is yet to be established and cost factor is another deterrent in the use of these drugs.

Treatment of complications of retinal vasculitis

1. *CME* may be managed by using posterior subtenon kenacort.

2. *Stage of neovascularisation* may require sector laser in cases of NVE and scatter laser (PRP) in cases of NVD.

3. *Advanced changes such as recurrent vitreous haemorrhage and tractional retinal detachment* can be managed by pars plana vitrectomy (PPV). Anti-VEGF drugs may have role prior to PPV in order to reduce the chances of intraoperative bleeding and for better visual prognosis after PPV.

4. *Rubeosis iridis and neovascular glaucoma* are managed by PRP and glaucoma filteration surgery.

PROGNOSIS

Prognosis of vision is relatively better than diabetic retinopathy since the patients are younger in age group and the macula remains healthy. However, macular oedema and macular ischaemia are significant causes for poor visual prognosis. In addition, inflammatory vascular occlusions are other factors detrimental to good visual prognosis. Recently it has been reported that adequate treatment of obliterative retinal vasculitis with systemic steroids and specific anti-infective therapy, laser application as and when required and early PPV when necessary, may result in improving the anatomic and visual outcome.

BIBLIOGRAPHY

1. Abu El-Asrar AM, AL Kharashi SA. Full PRP and early vitrectomy improves prognosis of retinal vasculitis associated with tuberculo-protein hypersensitivity (Eales' disease). Br J Ophthalmol 2002;86:1248–51.
2. Biswas et al. Eales' disease-current concepts in diagnosis and management. Journal of Ophthalmic Inflammation and Infection 2013; 3:11.
3. Biswas J, Mukesh BN, Narain S, Roy S, Madhavan HN. Profiling of HLA in Eales' disease. Int Ophthalmol 1998;21:277–81.
4. Biswas J, Sharma T, Gopal L, et al. Eales diseases-An update. Survey of Ophthalmology 47:197–214, 2002
5. Biswas J, Therese L, Madhavan HN. Use of PCR in detection of Mycobacterium tuberculosis complex DNA from vitreous samples of Eales' disease. Br J Ophthalmol 1999;83:994.
6. Biswas J. Eales disease-an update. Survey Ophthalmol 2002:47:197.
7. Chang TS, Aylward W, Davis JL, et al. Idiopathic retinal vasculitis, aneurysms and neuroretinitis. Ophthalmology 1995;102:1089–97.
8. Curi ALL, Freeman G, Pavesio C. Aggressive retinal vasculitis in PAN. Eye 2001;15:229–31.
9. Eales H. Primary retinal hemorrhages in young-men. Ophthalmol Rev 1882;1:41.

10. Eales H. Retinal haemorrhages associated with epistaxis and constipation. Brim Med Rev 1980; 9:262.

11. Elliot AJ. Thirty year observation of patients with Eales' disease. Am J Ophthalmol 1975;80: 404.

12. Geier SA, Nasemann J, Klauss V, Kronawitter U, Goebel FD. Frosted branch angiitis in a patient with AIDS. Am J Ophthalmol 1992;113:203–5.

13. Graham EM, Stanford MR, Sander MD, Kasp E, Dumonde DC. A point prevalence sudy of 150 patients with idiopathic retinal vasculitis: I. Diagnostic value of ophthalmological features. Br J Ophthalmol 1989;73:714–21.

14. Gupta A, Gupta V, Arora S, Dogra MR, Bambery R. PCR-positive tubercular retinal vasculitis. Clinical characteristics and management. Retina 2001;21:435–44.

15. Herbort CP, Limino L, Abu El-asrar AM. Ocular vasculitis: a multidisciplinary approach. Curr Opin Rheumatol 2005;17:25–33.

16. Kumar A, Tiwari HK, Singh RP, et al. Comparativeevalution of early vs deferred vitrectomy in Eales' disease. Acta Ophthalmol Scand 2000;78:77.

17. Nakao K, Ohba N. Human T cell lymphotropic virus type 1-associated retinal vasculitis in children. Retina 2003;23:197–201.

18. Perez VL, Chavala SH, Ahmed M, et al. Ocular manifestations and concepts of systemic vasculitides. Surv Ophthalmol 2004;49:399–418.

19. Puttamma ST. Varied fundus picture of central retinal vasculitis. Trans Asia Pacific Acad Ophthalmol 1970;3:520.

20. Quillen DA, Stathopoulos NA, Blankenship GW, Ferriss JA. Lupus associated frosted branch periphlebitis and exudative maculopathy. Retina 1997;17:449–51.

21. Rothova A. Ocular involvement in sarcoidosis. Br J Ophthalmol 2000;84:10–6.

22. Samuel MA, Equi RA, Chang TS, et al. Idiopathic retinitis, vasculitis aneurysms and neuroretinitis (IRVAN): new obervations and a proposed staging system. Ophthalmology 2007;114:1526–9.

23. Saxena S, Kumar D. A new staging system of idiopathic retinal periphlebitis. Eur J Ophthalmol 2004;14:236–9.

24. Spaide RF, Vitale AT, Toth IR, Oliver JM. Frosted branch angiitis associated with CMV retinitis. Am J Ophthalmol 1992;113:522–8.

25. Vine AK. Severe periphlebitis, peripheral retinal ischaemic, preretinal neovascularization in patients with MS. Am J Ophthalmol 1992;113: 28–32.

26. Ysasaga JE, Davis J. Frosted branch angiitis with ocular toxoplasmosis. Arch Ophthalmol 1999; 117:1260–1.

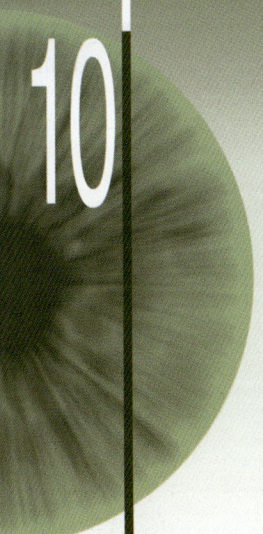

10

ENDOPHTHALMITIS AND PANOPHTHALMITIS

10.1 ENDOPHTHALMITIS

DEFINITION AND CLASSIFICATION

DEFINITION

Endophthalmitis is defined as inflammation of the anterior or posterior segment or both, with involvement of the adjacent ocular wall or as, an inflammatory reaction occurring as a result of intraocular colonisation by bacteria, fungi, or rarely parasites.

CLASSIFICATION

Endophthalmitis is classified as infectious and non-infectious (sterile) endophthalmitis. The infectious endophthalmitis is further classified as endogenous and exogenous, whereas non-infectious endophthalmitis has been termed as toxic anterior segment syndrome (TASS).

Endogenous endophthalmitis. Endogenous is also known as metastatic endophthalmitis. It is due to haematogenous spread of microorganisms to eye.

Exogenous endophthalmitis is due to inoculation of organism from extraneous source after surgery or trauma.

- *Postoperative endophthalmitis* incidence is 0.05–0.28%.
- *Post-traumatic endophthalmitis* accounts for 2.4–18.4% of open globe injuries.
- *Bleb-relatd endophthalmitis* incidence is reported to be 0.2 to 1.3%.

ENDOGENOUS ENDOPHTHALMITIS

INCIDENCE

Endogenous or metastatic endophthalmitis is a potentially blinding complication of haemato-genous spread of microorganisms to eye. It accounts for 2–17% of all cases of endoph-thalmitis and is misdiagnosed in more than 50% cases. It can be classified as anterior (focal or diffuse), posterior (focal or diffuse) and pan-ophthalmitis.

MICROBIAL SPECTRUM AND RISK FACTORS

More than 40% cases may not have any evident systemic source of infection and ocular disease may be due to transient bacteraemia and fungaemia. There is predisposition for diabetics, immune compromised patients, patients with malignancy, organ transplant, neutropenia, or those on intravenous hyperalimentation, intravenous or indwelling catheter, haemo-dialysis, and contaminated intravenous infusion (Fig. 10.1.1). The common sites of extraocular infection are liver abscess, pneumonia, endo-carditis, meningitis, soft tissue infection, gastrointestinal or urinary tract infection, renal abscess, pyonephrosis, brain abscess, etc. The bacteria responsible for endogenous endo-phthalmitis include *Streptococcus sp, Staphylococcus aureus, Bacillus* and *Serratia*. The common fungal isolates include *Candida* and *Aspergillus*. The studies from Asia show that *Klebsiella* liver

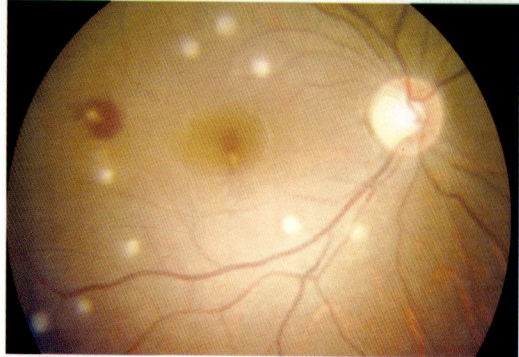
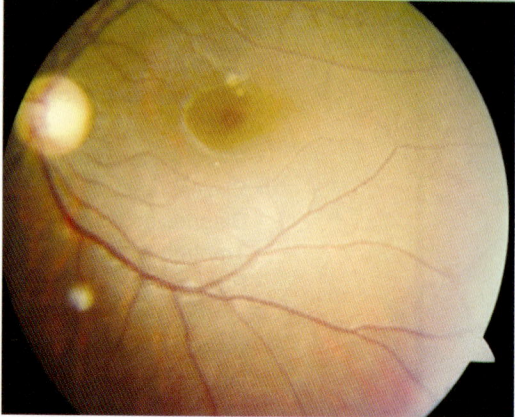

Fig. 10.1.1 *Fundus picture showing multiple retinal abscesses in IV drug abuser with Candida septicaemia.*

abscess in a diabetic is the commonest cause of endogenous endophthalmitis. In India, aspergillus endophthalmitis 4–6 weeks after single intravenous fluid injection has also been reported frequently (Fig. 10.1.2). Schiedler et al demonstrated, in his series from the USA, fungal etiology as a common cause of endogenous endophthalmitis (62% of cases positive for *Candida albicans*).

CLINICAL FEATURES

The disease is binocular in 15% cases. The male preponderance is seen and the peak age is in 3rd decade in bacterial and less than 1 year and middle age in fungal. The right eye is twice as often prone for a focus of infection than the left, because of comparatively direct blood flow to the right carotid artery.

The patient typically presents with ocular pain, blurred vision, lid swelling, discharge, injected and chemosed conjunctiva, elevated

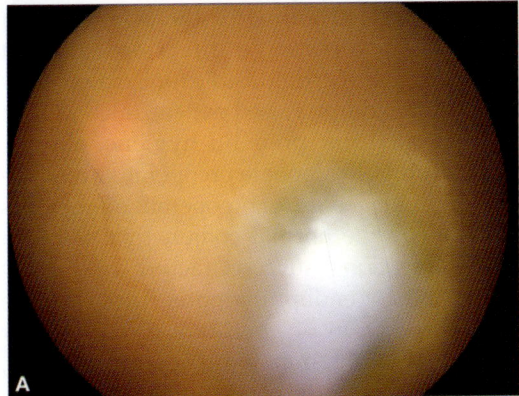

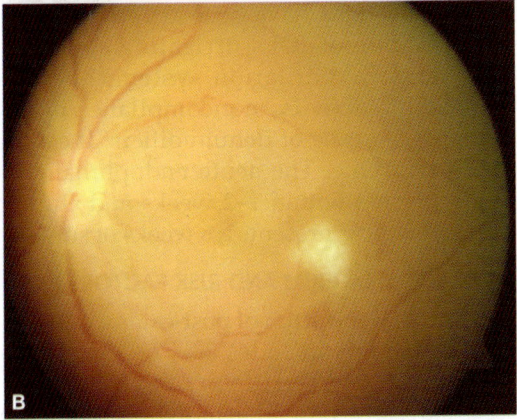

Fig. 10.1.2 *A, Fundus picture of a patient with history of intravenous dextrose 3 weeks prior to decreased vision showing fluff ball exudates and subretinal abscess; B, The same eye after PPV and intravitreal amphotericin B showing resolution with macular scar formation.*

IOP, corneal oedema, anterior chamber and vitreous reaction including hypopyon, reduced red reflex, retinal cotton wool spots, Roth's spots, haemorrhages, choroidal abscess or vitreous abscess. *B. cereus* is the common cause of metastatic endophthalmitis in drug abusers. The patients may exhibit a ring-shaped corneal ulcer with brownish anterior chamber exudates. If brownish hypopyon occurs without corneal involvement then *Listeria monocytogenes* should be considered as diagnosis. Endophthalmitis could be grouped as anterior focal, anterior diffuse, posterior focal, posterior diffuse, panophthalmitis. It is commonly misdiagnosed as granulomatous uveitis, fungal endophthalmitis, angle closure glaucoma, mucor mycosis, cavernous sinus thrombosis or orbital cellulitis.

DIAGNOSIS

B-scan ultrasonography is a useful adjunct to the clinical evaluation of infectious endophthalmitis especially in an eye with opaque media as it tells about for vitritis and retinal detachment.

- *Vitreous exudates* are seen as low to moderate intensity point like echoes in vitreous cavity.
- *Membranous structure* seen on USG is thick posterior vitreous detachment (PVD) or retinal detachment (RD).

Blood cultures which give higher positivity rate up to 94% compared to intraocular samples. (Vitreous culture positivity rate is 44–70%.)

Cultures from intraocular samples. It is necessary to take cultures from multiple sites and also repeated samples if suspicion of endogenous endophthalmitis is strong. Intraocular specimen for cultures can be taken as aqueous tap and vitreous sample by needle aspiration or cutter. The centrifuged deposit of vitreous sample should be used for Gram stain and cultures should be set up for aerobic and anaerobic bacteria and fungi. The samples should be incubated for at least a week before giving a negative report.

Polymerase chain reaction is being increasingly used nowadays for quick differentiation of bacterial from fungal endophthalmitis. PCR helps in quicker assay in small quantity samples.

TREATMENT

Thorough history taking and examination is recommended to look for the primary focus of infection once diagnosis of metastatic endophthalmitis is suspected. The primary focus of infection is the source of the ocular infection and is presumed to be **bacterial.**

Empiric broad-spectrum antibiotic therapy is given with vancomycin and an aminoglycoside or a third generation cephalosporin. The antibiotic therapy can later be tailored depending on the culture reports, if the patient does not respond. The patients with culture-positive endogenous endophthalmitis are more likely to have fungal isolates with a predominance of Candida.

In case of fungal endophthalmitis, antifungal of choice is intravitreal amphotericin 5–10 µg along with systemic triazoles. Systemic voriconazole and caspofungin are newer options.

Prompt treatment with intravitreal antibiotics and vitrectomy can result in improvement in ocular signs and visual acuity in majority of the patients. It has been seen that eyes that undergo pars plana vitrectomy are three times likely to retain useful vision and more than three times less likely to require enucleation or evisceration. It has also been seen that intravitreal antibiotics lowers chances of evisceration and enucleation. *Definite indications for vitrectomy* are:

- Worsening of signs and symptoms
- Rapid progression
- Retinal necrosis
- Extensive, subretinal abscess
- Retinal detachment.

PROGNOSIS

The poor prognosticators for endogenous endophthalmitis include delayed diagnosis and treatment (>4 days), poor initial visual acuity <20/200, presence of hypopyon and more virulent microorganisms. The visual outcomes are poor especially when it is *Klebsiella* species. *Aspergillus* has worse prognosis than *Candida*. Evisceration/enucleation is required in 25% cases. Only 5% of eyes with bacterial endogenous endophthalmitis can achieve visual acuity of 20/20 and 69% have vision worse than counting fingers.

EXOGENOUS ENDOPHTHALMITIS

POSTOPERATIVE ENDOPHTHALMITIS

INCIDENCE

The incidence of postoperative endophthalmitis decreased from 5–10% in early 20th century to 0.13–0.7% in 21st century. As over 2 million cataract surgeries are performed each year, endophthalmitis is encountered most commonly after cataract extraction. Penetrating keratoplasty has been associated with the highest incidence of postoperative endophthalmitis (0.38%).

Endophthalmitis could present as cluster infection or isolated cases. A cluster infection is described as the occurrence of two or more than two infections at a time or the occurrence of repeated postoperative infections. Patient factors are mainly responsible for isolated cases like immune compromised patient, uncontrolled diabetes mellitus, poor lid hygiene, chronic dacryocystitis, inadequate preoperative medications or prolonged use of preoperative antibiotics which alters the normal conjunctival flora. In cluster infections, surgeon factors are mainly responsible for endophthalmitis. These include poor sterilization of operation room (OR) or instruments, contaminated irrigating solution, viscoelastic agents or other consumables. Cluster infections have been reported due to contamination of IOLs, irrigating solutions, viscoelastics, ventilation system, hospital construction activity, noncompliance of OR standards as reuse of dehumidifiers. It can be acute or chronic. The acute endophthalmitis mostly present within 1–2 weeks and chronic endophthalmitis presents ≥ 6 weeks of surgery.

MICROBIAL SPECTRUM AND RISK FACTORS

The microbial spectrum of post-cataract surgery endophthalmitis includes 33–77% coagulase-negative staphylococci (CNS), 0.9–21% *Staphylococcus aureus*, 9–19% β-haemolytic streptococci (BHS), *S. pneumoniae*, a haemolytic, streptococci including *S. mitis* and *S. salivarius*, 6–22% gram-negative bacteria including *P. aeruginosa* (occurs rarely), up to 8–18.6% fungi (*Candida* sp., *Aspergillus* sp., *Fusarium* sp.). A study from South India, however, shows higher percentage of gram-negative and fungi accounting for 29.2% and 18.6% respectively and lesser per-centage (37.2%) of CNS compared to Western data (Table 10.1.1).

Delayed postoperative capsule bag endophthalmitis is primarily due to *Propionibacterium acnes*, corynebacteria including *C. macginleyi*. The most common organism of postoperative (glaucoma surgery) endophthalmitis is CNS (67%).

Factors that increase the risk of POE from cataract surgery include patient-related factors (male sex, concomitant diabetic retinopathy, same day cataract surgery combined with another intraocular surgery) and surgeon-related factors (low surgical volume, limited experience, prolonged operating time, operating on patients who are most prone to adverse events).

Table 10.1.1 *Microbial spectrum of postoperative endophthalmitis*

	S. India %ge	Endophthalmitis vitrectomy study (EVS)%
S. epidermidis	37.2	70
S. aureus	0.9	9.9
Staphylococcus sp.	2.7	0
Streptococcus sp.	11.5	9
Bacillus sp.	4.4	0.3
Propionibacterium sp.	2.7	0.6
Gram-negative	29.2	5.9
Filamentous fungi	18.6	0

The multi-centre randomized control trial by European Society for Cataract and Refractive Surgery Study (ESCRS) of antibiotic prophylaxis of endophthalmitis found that patients receiving the clear corneal incision were 5.88 times more likely to experience endophthalmitis than patients receiving scleral tunnel. The ESCRS study also demonstrated that patients experiencing complications at the time of surgery and the patients receiving a silicone intraocular lens had a 4.95 times and 3.13 times higher risk of infection, respectively.

CLINICAL FEATURES

In microbial endophthalmitis, three phases of infection can be observed: an incubation phase, an acceleration phase and a destructive phase. A clinically inapparent incubation phase is of at least 16 to 18 hours duration. The incubation phase is determined mainly by the generation time of the pathogen (e.g. *Pseudomonas aeruginosa* it is up to 10 min and *Propionibacterium* sp. > 5 hours) and toxin production.

Intraocular bacterial inoculation above a critical level then leads to breakdown of the aqueous barrier with fibrin exudation and cellular infiltration. With *Staphylococcus epidermidis* (CNS) and *Staphylococcus aureus*, the greatest infiltration is observed only three days after infection. Thus acute early endophthalmitis after cataract operations commences between the first postoperative day and approximately two weeks after the operation.

Acute Postoperative Endophthalmitis

The initial symptoms of **acute postoperative endophthalmitis** are usually pain and decreased vision. The presence of unexpectedly high intraocular inflammation is pointer towards endophthalmitis. Lid oedema is seen in 35% cases. Congestion is almost universal in more than 80% cases and hypopyon is seen in 75–86% cases. Media clarity decreases and there is loss of red reflex due to vitreous clouding. The poor prognosticators are poor initial visual acuity, relative afferent pupillary defect, corneal involvement and rubeosis iridis. The endophthalmitis is sometimes preceded for days or weeks by eyebrow pain, headache, blepharitis and conjunctivitis. In fungal endophthalmitis, usually long incubation period is reported, but the largest series from India on fungal endophthalmitis reports fungi even in acute cases. The typical fluff ball exudates and string of pearls appearance may be seen (Fig. 10.1.3A and B).

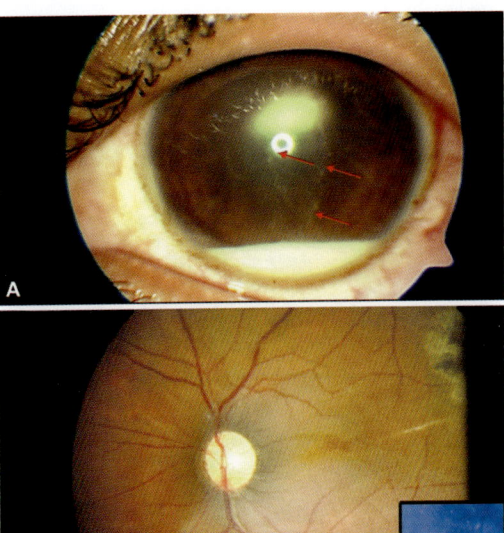

Fig. 10.1.3 *A, Anterior segment picture of a case of Aspergillus fungal endophthalmitis showing convex hypopyon fluff balls and string of pearls appearance (arrow); B, Fundus picture after pars plana lensectomy and vitrectomy with antifungal agents; inset showing acutely branching hyphae from vitreous biopsy.*

Chronic Late Endophthalmitis

Chronic late endophthalmitis after cataract operations commences only after two weeks, but may also take many months to appear. It is usually caused by *Propionibacterium acnes, S. epidermidis* (CNS), diphtheroids and fungi. The whitish plaques are seen in capsular bag in 40–89% cases of chronic endophthalmitis especially in propionibacterium endophthalmitis. Corneal oedema is present in 48% cases and keratitis in 26% cases of chronic postoperative endophthalmitis (Fig. 10.1.4).

POE needs to be differentiated from **toxic anterior segment syndrome** (TASS) is an acute inflammation of the anterior chamber of the eye. TASS may be related to any of the irrigating solutions, medications, or materials that gain access to the eye during anterior segment surgery. In addition, factors related to the cleaning and sterilisation of instruments. Some cases have been related to heat stable endotoxins from overgrowth of gram-negative bacilli in water baths of ultrasonic cleaners. TASS rarely occurs in one patient only, but usually in three or more, because most or all the patients have been exposed to the incriminating toxin during one or two operating sessions. Patients present within 12 to 48 hours of cataract surgery. The common signs include blurred vision, marked increase in anterior segment inflammation, including hypopyon formation as well as fibrin in the anterior chamber of the eye. There may be diffuse corneal oedema, classically from limbus to limbus, with endothelial cell damage. It is always Gram stain and culture negative. TASS responds well to intense topical corticosteroid treatment.

MANAGEMENT

Diagnosis

Apart from clinical features, microbiological results, ultrasonography guides us in treatment. In hazy media, it is required to rule out retinal detachment, choroidal detachment. The presence of vitreous membranes on ultrasonography is poor prognosticator.

Prophylaxis of postoperative endophthalmitis

It has been shown in the past that 85% of endophthalmitis cases could be traced to the patient by comparing DNA profiles of vitreous isolates of bacteria with those collected from the lid and skin flora of the patient. Thus proper perioperative antisepsis significantly decreases incidence of endophthalmitis. The use of **5% povidone-iodine** 3 minutes prior to surgery decreases the incidence of postoperative endophthalmitis to 0.06% from 0.24% in the control group in which silver-protein solution was used as prophylaxis. ESCRS study has investigated if use of perioperative **topical levofloxacin,** which reaches significantly higher concentrations in the anterior chamber than ofloxacin and ciprofloxacin. To maintain an adequate level of levofloxacin in the anterior chamber, it may be considered continuing to dose every two hours postoperatively on the day of surgery. The prolonged use of topical antibiotics, however, is not recommended before surgery. This is associated with replacement of normal ocular flora with resistant strains in conjunctival sac. **Intravenous antibiotic** prophylaxis is not used for conventional intra- and extraocular

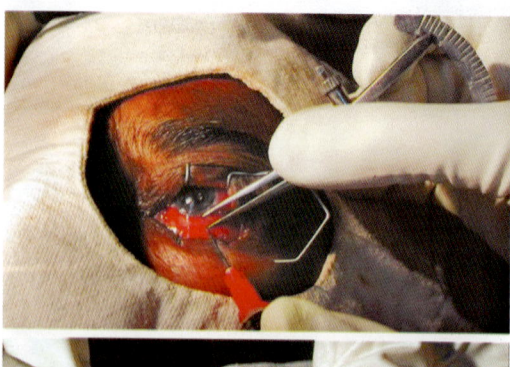
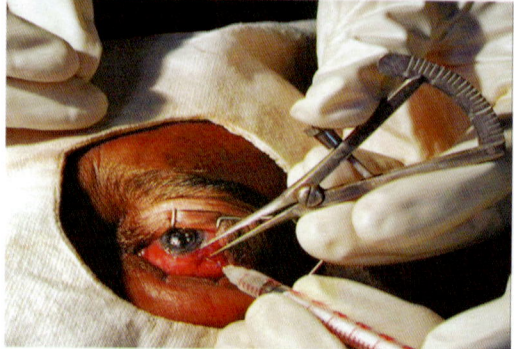

Fig. 10.1.4 *Vitreous tap and injection with 30 G needle 3 mm from limbus in pseudophakic patient.*

procedures and is not proven to be of benefit against postoperative endophthalmitis. The routine cataract surgery does not require oral prophylaxis unless the patient has severe atopic disease when the lid margins are more frequently colonised with *S. aureus*. ESCRS has shown periocular use **of intracameral injection of cefuroxime** at the end of surgery has lowered the incidence of endophthalmitis by fivefolds.

The use of topical quinolone is recommended 24 or 48 hours prior to surgery and one drop one hour prior to surgery and one drop one half-hour prior to surgery into conjunctival sac. It is recommended that after scrubbing the doctor should wear sterile gloves and patient's eyelashes should not be trimmed but covered with plastic sterile adhesive drapes.

Treatment

Endophthalmitis vitrectomy study (1990–1995) based initial management for acute post-operative endophthalmitis on the basis of presenting visual acuity. It was 3-port pars plana vitrectomy if patients present with vision worse than hand motions, but that an initial vitreous tap/biopsy with intravitreal antibiotics should generally be sufficient if presenting vision is hand motions or better (Fig. 10.1.5). Systemic antibiotics were not found of benefit in this study. The major limitations of this study were given as follows.

- It only included cases of acute postoperative endophthalmitis, 70% of which were due to *Staph. epidermidis*. The results cannot be extrapolated to other forms of endophthalmitis and to postoperative endophthalmitis in countries where gram-negative organisms and fungal infection form a big chunk.

- Amikacin and ceftazidime were the only systemic antibiotics evaluated in the EVS. Although patients in the EVS derived no demonstrable benefit from these systemic antibiotics, the study made no recommendations regarding treatment with additional anti-microbial agents (e.g. systemic fluoroquino-lones) or systemic antimicrobial agents for other types of endophthalmitis (e.g. chronic, bleb related)

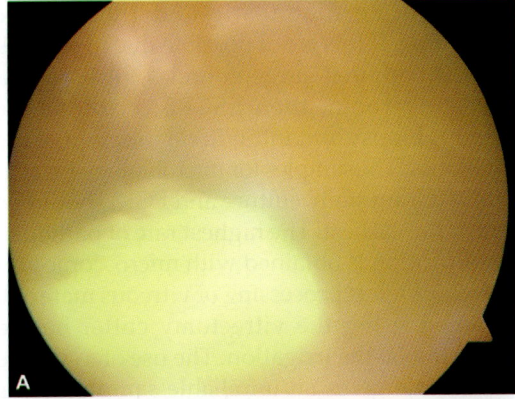

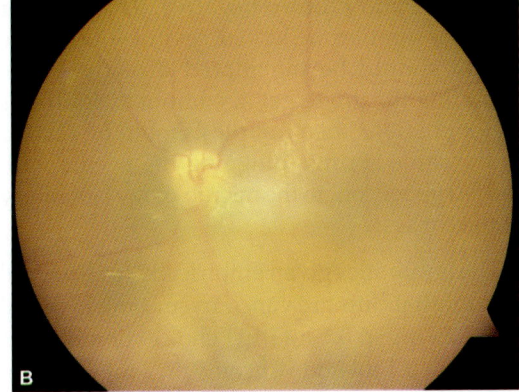

Fig. 10.1.5 *A, Fundus picture of a case of chronic post-operative fungal endophthalmitis showing retinal abscess; B, Fundus picture of the same patient 6 weeks after PPV with voriconazole.*

- Follow-up EVS analyses showed differences between diabetics and non-diabetics. Diabetics with a visual acuity of hand movements or better obtained vision of 20/40 more often (57%) by vitrectomy than after vitreous tap (40%) but the results ultimately were not statistically significant because of the low number of diabetic participants in the study.

There has been change in EVS guidelines for endophthalmitis management after report of ESCRS. In acute virulent POE, there is an achievement of only one metre vision in 44–53% cases with bacterial infection and 41–70% for fungal infection. To improve the anatomical and functional outcome in endophthalmitis, ESCRS gives guidelines for management of endophthalmitis. They recommend prompt action in such cases. The gold standard treatment is immediate diagnostic and therapeutic vitrectomy. If this is not possible due to the lack of a vitreoretinal surgeon and a vitreoretinal operating room, then ESCRS recommends vitreous biopsy and intravitreal injection of the antibiotics. The samples for microbiology investigation (Gram stain, culture and PCR) should be sent at the earliest. The highest rate of pathogen identification is obtained with microscopic and microbiological processing of vitreous material, obtained using the vitrectomy cutter before switching on the irrigation. The use of a syringe and needle gives an unreliable sample that is often dry and culture-negative. The anterior chamber samples are less successful. The culture media should be inoculated directly in the operating theatre to get maximum yield. If this is not possible, then samples should be carried in the same syringe plugging the needle with sterile rubber cork to the microbiology laboratory at the earliest.

The antibiotics given empirically for bacterial endophthalmitis are vancomycin 1 mg in 0.1 ml and 2.25 mg in 0.1 ml (first choice) or amikacin 400 µg in 0.1 ml and vancomycin 2 mg in 0.1 ml (second choice) in separate syringes with 30 G needle. The needle has to be directed away from macula into the mid-vitreous. This could be given in combination with intravitreal dexamethasone (400 µg in 0.1 ml) as it is the inflammation which is the basic culprit in endophthalmitis. For acute virulent endophthalmitis, ESCRS recommends systemic therapy with the same antibiotics as those used intravitreally for 48 hours to maintain higher levels within the posterior segment of the eye. The corticosteroids should also be given orally to control inflammation (prednisolone 1 or even 2 mg/kg/day).

Vitrectomy should also be the treatment of choice in chronic endophthalmitis, fungal endophthalmitis, deterioration of signs after initial management. The intravitreal antibiotics may be repeated at 48 hours, if required.

In cases of **chronic endophthalmitis,** early vitrectomy is advisable. A trial of therapy should be given with clarithromycin 250 mg twice daily which can be effective without surgery because the drug is well absorbed and concentrated 200 times into macrophages and other cells.

Special considerations in PPV

While doing pars plana vitrectomy in endophthalmitis

1. Use of 6 mm infusion cannula due to thickened retinochoroid in inflamed eye.
2. AC maintainer is needed to clear AC exudates and exudative membrane to visualize posterior segment cannula before starting pars plana infusion.
3. Before starting the infusion we must collect undiluted vitreous sample from mid-vitreous cavity.
4. The aim is to clear only core vitreous.
5. A small posterior capsulotomy helps as it makes anterior and posterior segments one unit and proper circulation of antibiotics is there.
6. The IOL explantation is done only in cases of gross infection, plaques in the capsule, recurrent endophthalmitis.

For **P. acnes endophthalmitis,** intravitreal vancomycin 1 mg/0.1 ml may be given into the capsular bag during first PPV and if it fails to respond then vitrectomy may be combined with total capsulectomy and IOL explantation.

In case of **fungal endophthalmitis**, amphotericin B (5–7.5 µg) is the only fungicidal antibiotic available for intravitreal injection, but its spectrum does not cover all fungi; in particular *Pseudallescheria boydii* is resistant to it but sensitive to miconazole which can be used instead. Miconazole is fungistatic but can be given intravitreally. Systemic antifungal therapy is also required and the source of the infection needs to be identified.

POST-TRAUMATIC ENDOPHTHALMITIS

INCIDENCE

Post-traumatic endophthalmitis (PTE) along with postoperative endophthalmitis is the second commonest form of endophthalmitis. The incidence of endophthalmitis after trauma is 100 times more than after surgery. The reported incidence ranges from 3.1–11.9% of open globe injuries in the absence of an IOFB.

The incidence in cases with an IOFB ranges from 3.8–48.1%, with higher infection rates reported in eyes with retained IOFBs contaminated with organic matter from a rural setting. In a study, the occurrence of post-traumatic endophthalmitis was reported in 30% in rural districts in contrast to 11% in non-rural districts. Post-traumatic endophthalmitis comprises approximately 25–30% of all cases of infectious endophthalmitis.

The prognosis is poorer in PTE because of various reasons. The diagnosis is delayed as signs of endophthalmitis are often masked due to disrupted anatomy, polymicrobial infection is seen in 20–42% cases and more virulent organisms including *Bacillus* are cultured from 20–40% cases (Fig. 10.1.6).

MICROBIAL SPECTRUM AND RISK FACTORS

PTE can be categorized as culture-independent or culture positive. The former includes all clinically diagnosed cases of endophthalmitis and the latter includes only culture-positive cases. The overall incidence of culture-independent post-traumatic endophthalmitis is higher than culture-positive endophthalmitis cases. It must be understood that the presence of positive cultures following open-globe trauma is not synonymous with the development of post-traumatic endophthalmitis. Ariyasu et al cultured 30 ruptured globes. Although one-third of these patients had positive anterior chamber fluid cultures, no patient developed endophthalmitis. In our experience, contamination after OGI was seen in 26% cases but only 18% developed endophthalmitis. Similar to post-operative endophthalmitis, two-thirds of the bacteria in PTE are gram-positive and 10–15% are gram-negative and 15% are fungi. Culture positivity is seen in 38–60% cases of post-traumatic endophthalmitis. In contrast to postoperative endophthalmitis, virulent *Bacillus* species are the common pathogens in post-traumatic endophthalmitis. Polymicrobial infection is seen in 20–30% cases.

Microbial spectrum of PTE is depicted in Table 10.1.2.

The major risk factors for PTE include rural setting trauma, vegetative matter associated injury, delayed repair after 24 hours, dirty wound, age greater than 50 years, female gender, large wound size, location of wound, ocular tissue prolapse, placement of primary intraocular lens (IOL), extent of injury, lens disruption. Thompson and coworkers reported endophthalmitis in 13.6% of 88 ruptured globe cases with lens disruption and in only 0.9% (1 case) of 117 cases with an intact crystalline lens. In their series, when both an IOFB and lens rupture were present, 15.6% of cases developed endophthalmitis. Delayed repair beyond 24 hours is another risk factor for PTE. The risk of PTE was 2.3% versus 15.7% if the repair was delayed by >24 hours. The sports-related injuries like due to fish hook or homemade bow and arrow are at high risk of endophthalmitis. Seventy-five per cent of bow and arrow injuries in India develop endophthalmitis. The presence of IOFB leads to 2-fold increase in relative risk

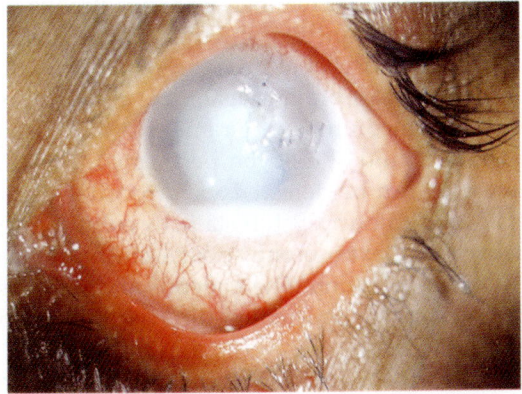

Fig. 10.1.6 Anterior segment picture of a case of zone 1 injury showing corneal sutures and hypopyon.

Table 10.1.2 *Microbial spectrum of post-traumatic endophthalmitis (Kunimoto et al 2007)*

	S. India	West
S. epidermidis	21.2	8–21
S. aureus	4.4	6
Staphylococcus sp.	0.9	0
Streptococcus sp.	26.5	8–21
Bacillus sp.	17.7	17–32
Gram-negative	22.1	11–18
Filamentous fungi	17.7	4–14

of PTE Wood IOFBs (18%) may be associated with a statistically higher risk of infectious endophthalmitis compared to metallic IOFBs (9%).

CLINICAL FEATURES

The start, course and symptoms of endophthalmitis after trauma are very varied, corresponding to the causative organisms. Symptoms of extreme pain with hypopyon and vitritis indicate an infection until proven otherwise. It is present at initial presentation in 50% cases of post-traumatic endophthalmitis. The peak interval between trauma and endophthalmitis is 3–6 days. The signs and symptoms of endophthalmitis may occur days, weeks, months, and even years after the injury (Fig. 10.1.6). Fungi are the causative organisms in 10–15% of cases of endophthalmitis after trauma. Fungal endophthalmitis usually commences only weeks to months after the injury. The initial symptoms are usually pain, purulent discharge, photophobia out of proportion to the injury and visual loss increasing intraocular inflammation, hypopyon, corneal oedema, loss of a red reflex, lid oedema, proptosis, and vitreous clouding, periphlebitis or gas bubbles (Fig. 10.1.6). Inflammation that progresses slowly following primary repair may be indicative of fungal endophthalmitis. In fungal endophthalmitis, string of pearls appearance or fluff ball opacities may be seen.

Metallic non-magnetic IOFBs (e.g. copper) can cause non-infectious inflammation, termed **reactive endophthalmitis**, if left in the eye. A 100% **copper IOFB** can cause a rapid sterile endophthalmitis-like reaction with hypopyon. Lower per cent copper IOFBs can cause chalcosis that includes chronic uveitis-related complications such as hypotony and phthisis. Green discolouration of iris, greenish-brown discolouration of the peripheral cornea (Kayser-Fleisher ring, due to copper deposition in Descemet's membrane), sunflower cataract, and copper. Plain radiography and computed tomography scans are then used to detect IOFBs. In order to detect small objects by computed tomography, the cut width should be less than 2 mm. B scan ultrasound may be used to help locate radiolucent foreign bodies such as glass

or plastic. Extreme caution should be used, if there is any suspicion of an open globe. Minimal pressure should be applied during echography, and the probe should be placed on the eyelid and not directly on the ocular surface. IOFBs containing greater than 85% copper can cause severe vision loss.

IOFBs with **free iron** content can cause siderosis; the iron ions interact with the epithelial cells causing cytotoxicity with cell degeneration and visual loss. Glass, plastic, and porcelain are inert materials that generally are well tolerated in the eye. However, all IOFBs (inert or non-inert) increase the risk of endophthalmitis because they may be contaminated with infectious material.

MANAGEMENT

Diagnosis

Any inflammation in a case of trauma more than anticipated should be tabken as endophthalmitis. All PTE cases where the view of posterior segment is not possible must be subjected to a gentle ultrasound to rule out the presence of intraocular foreign body (high echnogenicity with after shadow). It also gives information regarding retina and other membranes. If not possible, CT scan may also need to be done for proper localization of foreign body.

Prophylaxis

At the time of repair, the wound should be properly irrigated to clean any debris on it. Any dead or dirty looking tissue should be sent for cultures. Cultures may be obtained from the wound, anterior chamber, and/or vitreous as well as the conjunctiva, and they may be plated on blood and chocolate agar. Thioglycolate broth and heart-brain infusion are also used as a culture medium, and Gram stain of excised tissue or fluid should be performed. Fungal infection can be detected via Grocott's silver stain, periodic acid-Schiff stain, by culturing on Sabaroud's dextrose, or by potassium hydroxide (KOH) preparation. The aqueous and vitreous samples can be inoculated directly into blood culture bottles.

After repair, systemic antibiotics in addition to topical with wider organism coverage should be used routinely for prophylaxis against PTE.

Quinolone may be administered orally if access to the operating room is delayed and if intravenous antibiotics are not immediately available. The use of **prophylactic intravitreal injections** is debatable. The decision to use at the time of initial repair depends on whether the patient is a high-risk case for endophthalmitis—provided that the injections can be given safely and reliably into the vitreous cavity. In our experience, prophylactic intravitreal antibiotics in absence of foreign body decreases the incidence of post-traumatic endophthalmitis to negligible. The use of subconjunctival steroids should be considered along with antibiotics at the time of surgical repair of a ruptured globe.

In our practice, prophylactic **intravenous quinolones** are given in trauma cases for at least 3 days. These antibiotics cross the blood–ocular barrier reasonably well and may reach therapeutic levels in the eye. Their entry into the eye is also aided by the weakening of the blood–ocular barrier that results from infection and trauma-induced inflammation. After 5 days of intravenous antibiotics, the patient (after discharge) is placed on 1 week of oral quinolones.

Treatment

The principles of management are the same for post-traumatic and acute postoperative endophthalmitis, but the visual outcome is poorer. After the diagnosis of PTE is considered, early pars plana vitrectomy is recommended as soon as possible provided the corneal clarity permits. If the same is not possible, at least vitreous biopsy/tap must be done and vitreous samples sent for microbiological evaluation and PCR. The antibiotics given include combination of intravitreal vancomycin (1 mg/0.1 ml and intravitreal ceftazidime (2.25 mg/0.1 ml through pars plana. The type and nature of the injury may guide the choice of antibiotics. For example, *Clostridium* should be considered if soil contamination of the wound is present, and fungal infection should be considered if there is contamination with vegetable matter. Results of the culture, if obtained at the initial open-globe repair, may also direct the choice of antibiotics. For injuries that run a high risk of contamination with *Bacillus* species (homemade bow and arrow injuries), intravitreal clindamycin (0.5 mg/0.1 ml)

may also be given. Subconjunctival cefazolin (100 mg) or vancomycin (25 mg) with subconjunctival ceftazidime (100 mg) may be given after the procedure. Topical fortified cefazolin (50 mg/ml) or fortified vancomycin (50 mg/ml) every 1–2 h, alternating with fluoroquinolones (0.3%) may be used after surgery.

A related disorder is **sympathetic ophthalmia** in which injury to the eye, especially the uveal tract, can result in a harmful autoimmune T cell-mediated response. The inciting event is trauma to one eye, which is then followed by involvement of the sympathising eye.

The causes of poor visual outcome include recurrent/chronic endophthalmitis, macular infarction, optic atrophy, epiretinal membrane, macular oedema.

BLEB-RELATED ENDOPHTHALMITIS

INCIDENCE

Bleb-related endophthalmitis (BRE) is the second most frequent (16.7%) cause of postoperative endophthalmitis after acute and chronic post-cataract surgery endophthalmitis. The incidence of isolated blebitis is 2% with average follow-up of 2.7 years (range, 0.3 to 7.3). Early postoperative endophthalmitis following glaucoma surgery has an incidence of about 0.1%. However, the majority of cases of endophthalmitis after glaucoma surgery occur after months or years; the incidence is reported to be between 0.2 and 1.3%, and is more common with the use of antiproliferative agent (up to 3%) and even higher when the bleb is placed inferiorly (up to 9.4%). With antiproliferative use, one of every 100 patients developed endophthalmitis each year and 4% of patients developed a bleb-related complication consisting of a bleb leak, blebitis or endophthalmitis.

MICROBIAL SPECTRUM AND RISK FACTORS

Bleb leakage has been shown to increase 26-fold the risk of bleb infection. Most believe that bleb-related infections begin secondary to bleb leakage, which allows bacteria from the tear film and the periocular structures access into the eye. Early leakage is defined as leakage within the first 3 months following surgery, while late-onset leakage is defined as that occurring more than 3 months following surgery. Early leakage is most commonly caused by wound dehiscence or incomplete conjunctival closure. Late-onset leakage has been associated with the use of adjunctive antimetabolites, which are used to prevent fibrosis and scarring of the scleral flap and bleb in order to promote long-term patency. The use of Mitomycn-C (MMC) has been associated with a 15% risk of leak at 5 years. The use of antimetabolites, such as 5-fluorouracil (5-FU) and MMC, reduces the population of goblet cells, which produce mucin that serves as a protective barrier against leakage and bacteria. Their use also promotes general conjunctival thinning, reduced cellularity, and avascular blebs.

Blebitis describes an isolated bleb infection with signs of anterior segment inflammation, without vitreous involvement. It may represent a limited form or early stage of endophthalmitis. If untreated, blebitis progresses into endophthalmitis.

If inflammatory or infectious material in a blebitis extend beyond the anterior chamber, the diagnosis is bleb-associated endophthalmitis. BRE can be grouped into early onset (within 6 weeks) or late onset (after 6 weeks). BRE can have a clinical presentation similar to blebitis, except that the vitreous is involved. A positive vitreous culture is pathognomonic for BRE.

Coagulase-negative staphylococci (CNS) are responsible for endophthalmitis in 67% cases of early BRE. Delayed BRE is caused by streptococci species and gram-negative organisms especially *Haemophilus influenzae* (23%).

CLINICAL FEATURES

Prodromal signs and symptoms have been identified days or weeks before the diagnosis of blebitis or endophthalmitis is made. These include browache, headache, external eye inflammation or infection such as blepharitis or conjunctivitis. One must always maintain a high index of suspicion and pay careful attention to any of the above complaint in a patient who has undergone trabeculectomy. Blebitis must be differentiated from bleb-related endophthalmitis (BRE) depending on the vitreous involvement. The patients with endophthalmitis have more

rapidly progressive presentations, often with worsening pain, redness and decreasing visual acuity over a period of hours. Endophthalmitis can occur years after the initial filtering surgery. The defining feature of endophthalmitis is the presence of vitritis.

Like other forms of endophthalmitis, BRE usually presents with decreased visual acuity, redness, pain, lid swelling, diffuse conjunctival congestion, opalescent blebs (typical white on red appearance) with intense fibrin and/or hypopyon in the anterior chamber, and florid vitritis. These signs may be influenced by different variables and factors such as time to initial treatment, causative organism, wound leak (seidel's positive) and the presence of a vitreous wick.

MANAGEMENT

No clear management algorithm has been established for bleb-associated endophthalmitis.

The use of fluoroquinolones alone in the initial management of isolated blebitis. These could also be used in combination with one or two other fortified antibiotics for gram-negative and gram-positive organisms such as an aminoglycoside, vancomycin or cephalosporin.

The use topical corticosteroids is con-troversial till such time improvement of the blebitis is noted or once topical antibiotic therapy is well-established. There is no consensus regarding obtaining conjunctival cultures at initial diagnosis of blebitis.

Agressive treatment of endophthalmitis. Cases in which the vitreous is not well-visualized or in which the diagnosis of isolated blebitis is in doubt, should be treated for potential endophthalmitis. Aggressive treatment is important to prevent poor outcomes. Early PPV with intravitreal vancomycin (1 mg/0.1 ml) and either ceftazadime (2.25 mg/0.1 ml) or amikacin (0.4 mg/0.1 ml) with subconjunctival antibiotics is the preferred approach.

OUTCOME

Blebitis typically responds to therapy within 24 to 48 hours, both clinically and symptomatically. Most patients in one study noted a marked improvement in pain with rapidly improving anterior chamber reaction and conjunctival injection within 24 to 48 hours of the initiation of therapy.

In contrast, BRE has a poor visual prognosis even with aggressive medical and surgical treatment. Retrospective studies have shown that 94% of cases of endophthalmitis resulted in visual acuity of 20/200 or less. Busbee et al showed that 35% of patients had no light perception, and only 10% achieved 20/40 or better. They also demonstrated that those with a positive vitreal culture had poorer outcomes, likely due to a higher bacterial load at time of diagnosis. Additionally, poorer outcomes are thought to be the result of more virulent organisms, such as gram-negative bacteria that produce exotoxins and *Streptococcus* species. A significant number of eyes with BRE can end up being eviscerated or enucleated due to pain.

FUNGAL ENDOPHTHALMITIS

INCIDENCE

Fungal endophthalmitis results more commonly from exogenous infection and less commonly from endogenous infection. Exogenous fungal infections secondary to trauma or surgery are reported in much higher number of cases from India than West. Fungi comprise of 18.6– 21.8% of culture positive postoperative cases and 17.7% of post-traumatic culture positive cases in India. Endogenous fungal endophthalmitis results from intraocular dissemination of a systemic fungal infection.

MICROBIAL SPECTRUM AND RISK FACTORS

Normally, the blood–ocular barrier prevents invasion from infective organisms but if this is breached (directly through trauma or indirectly due to a change in its permeability secondary to inflammation), infection can occur.

Candida albicans is by far the most common cause of fungal endogenous endophthalmitis. They are commensal organisms that reside in the human body and are found normally in the female genital tract, the gastrointestinal tract, and the respiratory tract. When a breakdown in the host's immune system occurs, fungi may spread throughout the body. However, immunosuppression alone does not increase significantly the risk of fungi entering the bloodstream. Patients who are at risk include patients with long-standing indwelling catheters; persons who use intravenous drugs; postpartum women; premature infants; patients undergoing hyperalimentation; patients with a history of recent abdominal surgery; and patients with debilitating diseases, such as diabetes mellitus, postorgan transplantation, or malignancies.

Exogenous fungal endophthalmitis are mostly caused by filamentous fungi. *Aspergillus flavus* and *Aspergillus fumigatus* are the most common pathogenic organisms in humans. Its conidia, the asexual spores of aspergilli organisms are airborne and trauma and surgery are important routes of entry into the human body. In patients who are at risk, such as those patients with uncontrolled diabetes mellitus, chronic pulmonary diseases or those patients with orthotopic liver transplants, renal transplants, leukaemia and other haematologic disorders, Goodpasture syndrome, alcoholism, prematurity, and bone marrow transplants, disseminated aspergillosis may result. Other less common causes include cryptococcal endophthalmitis which is caused by inhalation of spores in pigeon droppings.

CLINICAL FEATURES

Endogenous endophthalmitis Diminished visual acuity, severe vitreous inflammation with persistent iritis, whitish puff balls and strands seen in *Candida* and *Aspergillus* infections. Choroidal neovascularisation in *C. albicans* endophthalmitis is a potential cause of late visual loss in patients who have had sepsis and endogenous chorioretinitis. It also shows macular chorioretinal abscess, subretinal hypopyon and final outcome is very poor due to frequent macular involvement.

Postoperative endophthalmitis is more locallised and exhibits focal choroiditis, "string of pearls" infiltrates and puff balls in AC and vitreous. It is usually delayed presentation after surgery, however, acute cases as early as 24 hours after surgery are also reported from India. It probably depends on the load of innoculum in the eye.

Post-traumatic fungal endophthalmitis is usually after trauma with vegetative matter. Classical signs of fungal endophthalmitis may not be there as anatomy of the globe is disrupted after trauma.

MANAGEMENT

Diagnosis

A presumptive diagnosis of endogenous fungal endophthalmitis can be made if the fungus is isolated from anywhere in the body and the typical intraocular findings are present. Vitreous biopsy is taken and direct examination of fungi with Giemsa, Gomori-methenamine-silver (GMS), and periodic-acid-Schiff (PAS) stains should be obtained. Vitrectomy samples are more sensitive for fungal cultures than vitreous needle biopsies. Vitreous biopsy by pars plana vitrectomy is important in obtaining undiluted specimens for culture and sensitivity. Vitreous samples should be concentrated either by centrifugation or by millipore filtration.

If *C. neoformans* is suspected, the sample should be stained with mucicarmine and undergo membrane filtration cytology.

A useful, recently introduced diagnostic tool for fungal endophthalmitis is the polymerase chain reaction (PCR). The main advantages of PCR over conventional fungal cultures are the higher sensitivity and the rapid results obtained with PCR. Where available, DNA microarray analysis may be useful for obtaining a rapid diagnosis.

Treatment

The following drugs are used in treating of fungal endophthalmitis:

- Amphotericin B
- Fluconazole
- Ketoconazole
- Miconazole
- Flucytosine
- Itraconazole
- Caspofungin

Systemic amphotericin has been the treatment of choice because of its broad-spectrum coverage; however, the penetration of the vitreous cavity is poor. Doses of 5 to 10 mg intravitreal amphotericin have been used. Retinal toxicity has been reported in animal models at these doses thus it must be combined with intravitreal dexamethasone 400 mg to combat macular toxic effects. Fluconazole and flucytosine have good intraocular penetration, but Candida species show high resistance to flucytosine.

A new systemic treatment is voriconazole; when administered orally or intravenously, it has good intravitreal concentrations. Intravitreal administration of voriconazole also seems safe without evidence of retinal toxicity with concentrations up to 25 mg/ml. The echinocandins (caspofungin, micafungin, and anidulafungin) are newer agents that exert their antifungal activity by inhibiting D-glucan synthase, an enzyme involved in fungal cell wall synthesis. Because mammalian cells lack a cell wall, it also represents an ideal and specific target for antifungal therapy. Echinocandins exert antifungal activity against *Candida* and *Aspergillus* species.

In *endogenous fungal endophthalmitis*, it is important to initiate systemic broad-spectrum antibiotics to treat the primary source of infection, but if the response to medical therapy is poor, pars plana vitrectomy along with amphotericin 5–10 µg along with systemic triazoles is instituted. Systemic voriconazole and caspofungin are newer options. It has been seen that eyes that undergo pars plana vitrectomy are three times likely to retain useful vision and more than three times less likely to require enucleation or evisceration. It has also been seen that intravitreal antibiotics lower chances of evisceration and enucleation. For Candida endophthalmitis treatment has been recommended by Sato et al. They recommend PPV only if vitreous is involved in the form of vitreous exudates and no antibiotic response. The use of steroids is controversial and should be used with extreme caution.

In *exogenous fungal endophthalmitis*, as a general rule, moderate-to-severe vitreous involvement requires vitrectomy because most systemic antifungals have poor vitreous penetration. The advent of pars plana vitrectomy has improved the treatment results of fungal endophthalmitis. The advantages of pars plana vitrectomy are that it provides material for culture, removes viable organisms and inflammatory end products from the infected vitreous, and provides intravitreal access to antifungal agents (e.g. amphotericin B).

Given the narrow therapeutic range of amphotericin B, it should not be given in a gas-filled eye.

The prognosis following fungal endophthalmitis depends on the virulence of the organism, the extent of intraocular involvement, and the timing and mode of intervention.

TOXIC ANTERIOR SEGMENT SYNDROME

The toxic anterior segment syndrome (TASS) is an acute inflammation of the anterior chamber of the eye. TASS is an acute sterile anterior chamber inflammatory reaction that develops 12–48 hours after anterior segment surgery. TASS is a form of sterile, non-infectious endophthalmitis with or without pain.

PATHOPHYSIOLOGY

The etiology of TASS is multifactorial. TASS may be related to any of the irrigating solutions, medications, or materials that gain access to the eye during anterior segment surgery. The causes could be inflammatory reaction to intraocular irrigating solutions with abnormal pH, osmolarity or ionic composition, denatured ophthalmic viscosurgical devices (OVD), intraocular medications (antibiotics in the irrigation solutions or intracameral antibiotics), topical ointments, inadequate sterilisation of surgical instruments and tubing, inadequate flushing of instruments between cases resulting in build-up of ophthalmic viscosurgical devices (OVD), preservatives, metallic precipitate, and rarely bacterial endotoxins or particulate contamination of balanced salt solutions.

It is always Gram stain and culture-negative.

CLINICAL FEATURES

It is associated with early marked decrease in vision 12–24 hours after surgery. There is diffuse corneal oedema that extends limbus to limbus associated with endothelial cell damage, severe anterior chamber reaction, occasionally with hypopyon.

TASS rarely occurs in one patient only, but usually in three or more, because most or all the patients have been exposed to the incriminating toxin during one or two operating sessions. If an outbreak occurs, then the surgeon must stop operating and investigate for the source of the problem.

TREATMENT

The focus should be primary prevention. This can be done by following proper protocol during surgery. Proper balance salt solution (BSS) with the correct pH, osmolarity, and ionic composition should be used. We should avoid use of intraocular solutions, intracameral medications or irrigating solutions with preservatives. Adequate sterilisation of instruments and tubing according to the manufacturer's protocol should be done.

Most patients do well with medical management using topical steroids (1% prednisolone acetate) given hourly. In rare cases, depending on the severity, there may be a need for systemic steroid treatment. The clearing may take up to 3–6 weeks which is a longer response than in mild cases. In the severe case, there may be permanent damage, persistent corneal oedema, chronic persistent inflammation, fixed dilated pupil, refractory glaucoma secondary to trabecular meshwork damage and cystoid macular oedema. In severe cases, there may be a need for systemic steroid treatments.

The severe cases may have compromised recovery and may need cornea transplant, glaucoma surgery or both.

TREATMENT OUTCOME IN ENDOPHTHALMITIS

The treatment outcome as improved treamendously in present ear. In EVS study, visual acuity of 20/40 or better was achieved in 33% cases of acute endophthalmitis after vitrectomy, and 20/100 or better acuity was achieved in 56% patients. In a recent review article, the visual outcome of 20/40 or better could be achieved in up to 56% of postoperative endophthalmitis patients. Significant factors associated with poor visual outcome are corneal involvement, hypopyon larger than 1.5 mm, detection of bacterial species other than a CNSP, the absence of fundus visibility, neovascularisation of iris and relative afferent papillary defect and above all the virulence of the causative organisms. Endophthalmitis due to gram-negative organisms, fungi and polymicrobial infections are associated with poor visual outcomes. Fungal infection is associated with a more unfavourable prognosis where more than 20% patients have severe visual impairment (worse than 5/200).

Visual prognosis is poorer in post-traumatic endophthalmitis than postoperative endo-phthalmitis. It is further poorer in geriatric and paediatric age group.

The late sequelae of endophthalmitis include macular oedema, disc oedema, optic atrophy, epiretinal membrane, macular infarction and scarring (Fig. 10.1.7).

PREPARATION OF ANTIBIOTICS AND CLINICAL TRIALS

PREPARATION OF ANTIBIOTICS (Adopted from ESCRS)

The antibiotics should be supplied freshly diluted by the hospital pharmacy department.

However, for emergency cases, a method for diluting the drugs in the operating theatre is given below. The procedure must use sterile equipment and be undertaken on a sterile surface; ideally, the hospital makes up sterile packs with drugs, bottles for dilution and instructions in advance for this purpose. All drugs should be mixed by inverting or rolling the bottle 25 times, avoiding frothing.

Some important "Dos" and "Don'ts"

- Never return diluted drugs to the same or original vial for further dilution
- Never dilute at greater than 1 in 10
- Do not use syringes more than once
- Do not reuse bottles
- Avoid use of drugs with preservatives, if possible
- Do inject the drugs slowly over 1 to 2 minutes prior to preparing the dilutions. It is mandatory to check the amount of the antibiotic in the vial as the same antibiotic may be sold in different strengths in each europlan country.

Important antibiotics

1. *Vancomycin.* Dose for use = 1000 mg. Reconstitute one vial of 250 mg and make up to 10 ml with sterile normal (0.9%) saline (SNS) in a sterile bottle with lid. Mix well. Withdraw 2 ml

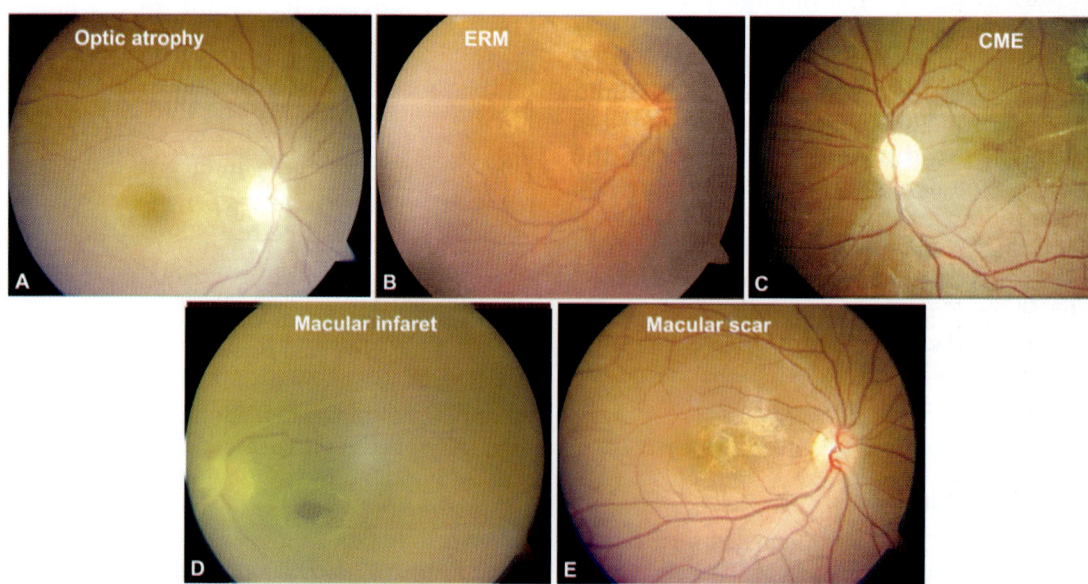

Fig. 10.1.7 *Fundus pictures showing sequelae of exogenous endophthalmitis: A, Optic atrophy; B, Epiretinal membrane; C, Cystoid macular oedema; D, Macular infarct induced by gentamicin; E, Macular scar.*

Table 10.1.3 *Clinical trials in endophthalmitis*

Enrollment	Criteria	Number	Endpoint	Aim Follow-up	Intervention	Results
Endo-phthalmitis vitrectomy study (EVS)	1990–1995	Acute post-cataract or sec IOL endophthal-mitis within 6 weeks of presentation Pt with clear cornea, Visual acuity (VA) <ETDRS 36 letters at 4 m, >PL and media clarity to obscure view of second order vessels	420 patients	Visual acuity and clarity of ocular media, final outcome assessment was at 9 months. Bacterial endoph-thalmitis.	• To determine the role of initial pars plana vitrectomy in the management of postoperative bacterial endophthalmitis. • To determine the role of intravenous antibiotics in the management of vitreous tap/biopsy • To determine which factors, other than treatment, predict outcome in postoperative bacterial endophthalmitis	Eyes received either (1) initial pars plana vitrectomy with intra-vitreal antibiotics, followed by retap and reinjection at 36–60 hours for eyes that did poorly as defined in the study or (2) initial anterior chamber and chance of va> 20/ with injection of intravitreal antibiotics, followed by vitrectomy and reinjection at 36–60 hours in eyes doing poorly. In addition, all eyes were randomized to either treatment or no treatment with intra-venous antibiotics.	Only 11% had visual acuity (VA) LP only, 33% chance of 20/40 vision with ppv than without ppv (11%) and double chance of receiving 20/100 final VA 20/40 eyes with better than LP 40 in 66% vs 62% with or without ppv; 20/100 in 86% vs 84% No diff in media clarity or VA outcome with systemic a/b
ECRS	2003–2006		16,603 patients treated at 24 clinical centres in nine European countries		• To evaluate the prophylactic effect of intracameral cefuro-xime with or without perioperative topical levofloxacin on post-operative endophthal-mitis after cataract surgery	Four treatment groups. One group received vehicle drops peri-operatively and no intracameral injection. The second group received placebo drops and an intra-cameral injection of	Injection of the antibiotic cefuroxime at the end of surgery reduced the incidence of endophthalmitis by nearly five-fold.

(Contd.)

Table 10.1.3 *Clinical trials in endophthalmitis (Contd.)*

Enrollment	Criteria	Number	Endpoint	Aim Follow up	Intervention	Results
				• Secondary questions included finding a more reliable estimate of the true rate of endophthalmitis and identifying risk factors for the complication.	1.0 mg of cefuroxime in 0.1 ml saline at the end of surgery. The third group received levofloxacin eyedrops perioperatively but no intracameral injection and the fourth group received both peri-operative levofloxacin eyedrops and intra-cameral cefuroxime. All groups received povidone iodine pre-operatively and topical levofloxacin post-operatively for six days.	The use of clear corneal incisions increased the risk for the complica-tion by nearly eight-fold and the implantation of silicone IOLs increased the risk by over three-fold. Other risk factors identified included the sex of the patient, with men being nearly three times more likely than women to develop the complication, and the occurrence of complications during surgery which increased the risk nearly fivefold.
Traumatic endoph-thalmitis Trial research group	Prophylaxis of traumatic endo-phthalmitis.	346 eyes	Occurrence of endophthalmitis within 2 weeks.	• Evaluate the efficacy of intraocular gentamicin sulphate and clindamycin in the prevention of acute post-traumatic bacterial endo-phthalmitis following penetrating eye injuries.	Randomized to intra-cameral or intravitreal injection of 40 µg of gentamicin sulphate and 45 µg of clindamycin (cases) vs balanced salt solution (controls).	

accurately and add to 3 ml of SNS in a sterile bottle with lid. Mix well (= 10 mg/ml). Use 0.1 ml = 1000 mg.

2. *Ceftazidime* (or other cephalosporin)   Dose for use = 2000 mg. Reconstitute one vial of 500 mg and make up to 10 ml with SNS in a sterile bottle with lid. Mix well. Withdraw 2 ml accurately and add to 3 ml of SNS in a sterile bottle with lid. Mix well (= 20 mg/ml). Use 0.1 ml = 2000 mg.

Note: The percentage of drug precipitation is less when using SNS instead of BSS.

3. *Amikacin.* Dose for use = 400 mg. Reconstitute one vial of 500 mg and make up to 10 ml with SNS or balanced salt solution (BSS) in a sterile bottle with lid. Mix well. Withdraw 0.8 ml, using a 1 ml syringe, and add to 9.2 ml of SNS or BSS in a sterile bottle with lid. Mix well (= 4.0 mg/ml). Use 0.1 ml = 400 mg.

4. *Clindamycin.* Dose for use = 1000 mg. Transfer the contents of a 2 ml ampule containing 300 mg to a sterile bottle and add 1 ml SNS or BSS, replace lid, and mix well. Withdraw 1 ml, using a 1 ml syringe, and add to 9 ml of SNS or BSS in a sterile bottle with lid. Mix well (=10 mg/ml). Use 0.1 ml = 1000 mg.

5. *Amphotericin.* Dose for use = 5 mg. Reconstitute a 50 mg vial with 10 ml water for injection. Withdraw 1 ml, using a 1 ml syringe, and add to 9 ml of water in a sterile bottle with lid for injection. Mix well. Withdraw 1 ml of this dilution, using a 1 ml syringe, and add to 9 ml of dextrose in a sterile bottle with lid, to complete a dilution of 1/100. Mix well (= 50 mg/ml). Use 0.1 ml = 5 mg. (A dose of 10 mg has been used by some clinicians.)

CLINICAL TRIALS

Important trials include:

European Society for Cataract and Refractive Surgery Study (ESCRS), Endophthalmitis Vitrectomy Study (EVS). These are summarised in Table 10.1.3.

BIBLIOGRAPHY

1. Aboltins CA, Allen P, Daffy JR. Fungal endophthalmitis in intravenous drug users injecting buprenorphine contaminated with oral Candida species. Med J Aust 2005;182:427.

2. Ayyala RS, Bellows AR, Thomas JV, et al. Bleb infections: clinically different courses of "blebitis" and endophthalmitis. Ophthalmic Surg and Lasers 1997; 28:452–60.

3. Bucci FA. An in vivo study comparing the ocular absorption of levofloxacin and ciprofloxacin prior to phacoemulsification. Am J Ophthalmol 2004:137,308–12.

4. Carolee M, Cutler Peck, Jacob Brubaker, Sue Clouser, Chris Danford, Henry E. Edelhauser, Nick Mamalis Toxic anterior segment syndrome: Common causes Journal of Cataract and Refractive Surgery July 2010; Vol. 36(Issue 7): 1073–108

5. Colin J, Simonpoli S, Geldsetze K, Ropo A. Corneal penetration of levofloxacin into the human aqueous humour: a comparison with ciprofloxacin. Acta Ophthalmol Scand 2003;81: 611–613.

6. Connell PP, et al. Endogenous endophthalmitis-10 years experience at a tertiary referral center. Eye 2011;25(1):66–72.

7. Endophthalmitis Vitrectomy Study Group: Results of the Endophthalmitis Vitrectomy Study. A randomized trial of immediate vitrectomy and of intravenous antibiotics for the treatment of post-operative bacterial endophthalmitis. Arch Ophthalmol 1995; 113: 1479–96.

8. Engstrom RE Jr, Mondino BJ, Glasgow BJ, Pitchekian-Halabi H, Adamu SA. Immune response to Staphylococcus aureus endophthalmitis in a rabbit model. Invest Ophthalmol Vis Sci 1991;32;1523–33.

9. ESCRS Endophthalmitis Study Group: Prophylaxis of postoperative endophthalmitis following cataract surgery: results of the ESCRS multi-center study and identification of risk factors. J Cataract Refract Surg 2007;33:978–88.

10. ESCRS guidelines on prevention investigation and management of postoperative endophthalmitis-Peter Barry, Wolgang Behrens-Baumann, Uwe Pleyer and David Seal. August 2007.

11. Holladay JT. Proper method for calculating average visual acuity. J Refract Surg 1997; 13: 388–91.

12. Keswani T, Ahuja V, Changulani M. Evaluation of outcome of various treatment methods for endogenous endophthalmitis. Indian J Med Sci 2006;60:454–60.

13. Kobayakawa S, Tochikubo T, Tsuji A. Penetration of levofloxacin into human aqueous humor. Ophthalmic Res 2003:35.

14. Koch HR, Kulus SC, Roessler M, Ropo A, Geldsetzer K. Corneal penetration of fluoro-quinolones: aqueous humour concentrations after topical application of levofloxacin 0.5% and ofloxacin 0.3% eye drops. J Cataract Refract Surg 2005:31:1377–85.

15. Kunimoto DY, Das T, Sharma S et al. Micro-biologic spectrum and susceptibility of isolates: part I. Postoperative endophthalmitis. Endophthal-mitis Research Group. Am J Ophthalmol 1999; 128(2):240–2.

16. Kunimoto DY, Das T, Sharma S, et al. Micro-biologic spectrum and susceptibility of isolates: part II. Post-traumatic endophthalmitis. Endophthalmitis Research Group. Am J Ophthalmol 1999;128(2):242–4.

17. Michael S, Kresloff MD, Castellarin AA, Zarbin MA. Endophthalmitis-Major review. Surv Ophthalmol 1998;43:193-224.

18. Mochizuki K, Jikihara S, Ando Y, et al. Incidence of delayed onset infection after trabeculectomy with adjunctive mitomycin C or 5-fluorouracil treatment. Br J Ophthalmol 1997;81:877–83.

19. Narang S, Gupta A, Gupta V, Dogra M R, Ram J, Pandav SS, Chakrabarti A. Fungal endo-phthalmitis following cataract surgery: Clinical presentation, microbiological spectrum, and outcome. Am J Ophthalmol 2001;132:609–17.

20. Narang S, Gupta A, Gupta V, et al. Fungal endophthalmitis following cataract surgery: clinical presentation, microbiological spectrum, and outcome. Am J Ophthalmol 2001;132:609–17.

21. Narang S, Gupta V, Gupta A, Dogra MR, Pandav SS, Das S. Role of prophylactic intravitreal antibiotics in open globe injuries. Indian J Ophthalmol 2003;51:39–44.

22. Narang S, Gupta V, Simalandhi P, Gupta A, Raj S, Dogra MR. Pediatric open globe injuries. Visual outcome and risk factors for endophthal-mitis. Indian J Ophthalmol 2004;52:29–34.

23. Peyman G, Lee P, Seal DV. Endophthalmitis-diagnosis and management. Taylor and Francis, London: 2004;1–270.

24. Pflugfelder SC, Flynn HW Jr, Zwickey TA, Forster RK, Tsiligianni A, Culbertson WW, Mandelbaum S. Exogenous fungal endophthal-mitis. Ophthalmology 1988;95:19–30.

25. Schiedler V, Scott IU, Flynn Jr HW, Davis JL, Benz MS, Miller D. Culture-proven endogenous endophthalmitis: clinical features and visual acuity outcomes. Am J Ophthalmol 2004; 137:725–31.

26. Seal DV, Barry P, Gettinby G, Lees F, Peterson M, Revie CW, Wilhelmus KR. ESCRS study of prophylaxis of postoperative endophthalmitis after cataract surgery: Case for a European multi-center study. J Cataract Refract Surg 2006; 32:396–406.

27. Seal DV, Barry P, Gettinby G, Lees F, Peterson M, Revie CW, Wilhelmus KR. ESCRS study of prophylaxis of postoperative endophthalmitis after cataract surgery: Case for a European multi-center study. J Cataract Refract Surg 2006; 32:396–406.

28. Seal DV, Reischl U, Behr A, Ferrer C, Alio J, Koerner R, Barry P. ESCRS Endophthalmitis Study Group: Laboratory management of endophthalmitis: comparison of microbiology and molecular biology methods in the European multi-center study and appropriate chemo-therapy. Manuscript in preparation.

29. Smith RS, Kroll AJ, Lou PL, et al. Endogenous bacterial and fungal endophthalmitis. Int Ophthalmol Clin 2007;47:173-83.

30. Soheilian M, Rafati N, Mohebbi MR, Yazdani S, Habibabadi HF, Feghhi M, Shahriary HA, Eslamipour J, Piri N, Peyman GA. Traumatic Endophthalmitis Trial Research Group: Pro-phylaxis of acute posttraumatic bacterial endo-phthalmitis: a multi-center, randomized clinical trial of intraocular antibiotic injection, report 2. Arch Ophthalmol 2007;125:460–5.

31. Speaker MG, Menikoff JA. Prophylaxis of endophthalmitis with topical povidone-iodine. Ophthalmology 1991;98:1769–75.

32. Yan H, Chen S, Zhang JK, Yu JG, Han JD. Treatment of postoperative endophthalmitis following cataract surgery without intraocular lens removal. Zhonghua Yan Ke Za Zhi 2009;45:684–7.

33. Yoon YH, Lee SU, Sohn JH, Lee SE. Result of early vitrectomy for endogenous Klebsiella pneumoniae endophthalmitis. Retina 2003;23: 366–70.

34. Zhang YQ, Wang WJ. Treatment outcomes after pars plana vitrectomy for endogenous endo-phthalmitis. Retina 2005;25:746–50.

10.2 PANOPHTHALMITIS

DEFINITION

Panophthalitis is an intense purulent inflammation of the whole eyeball including the Tenon's capsule. The disease usually begins either as purulent anterior or purulent posterior uveitis; and soon a full-fledged picture of panophthalmitis develops, following through a very short stage of endophthalmitis.

ETIOLOGY

Panophthalmitis is an acute bacterial infection.

Modes of infection

1. *Exogenous infections.* Purulent inflammations are generally caused by exogenous infections following perforating injuries, perforation of infected corneal ulcers or as postoperative infections following intraocular operations.

2. *Endogenous or metastatic infections.* It may occur rarely through bloodstream from some infected focus in the body such as caries teeth, generalised septicaemia and puerperal sepsis.

3. *Secondary infections from surrounding structures.* It is very rare. However, cases of purulent intraocular inflammation have been reported following extension of infection from the orbital cellulitis, thrombophlebitis and infected corneal ulcers.

Causative organisms

The most frequent pathogens causing acute bacterial suppurative infections are gram-positive cocci, i.e. *staphylococcus epidermidis* and *Staphylococcus aureus*. Other causative bacteria include *Streptococci, Pseudomonas, pneumococci* and *Corynebacterium*.

CLINICAL FEATURES

Symptoms include:
- *Pain* in the eye and surrounding area is severe and often associated with headache
- *Loss of vision* is complete
- *Watering* from the eyes is present is profuse
- *Purulent discharge*

- *Marked redness* and swelling of the eyes, and
- *Associated constitutional symptoms* malaise fever, nausea and vomiting are after present

Signs are as follows (Fig. 10.2.1):
1. *Lids* show a marked oedema and hyperaemia.
2. *Eyeball* is slightly proptosed, ocular movements are limited and painful.
3. *Conjunctiva* shows marked chemosis and ciliary as well as conjunctival congestion.
4. *Cornea* is cloudy and oedematous.
5. *Anterior chamber* is full of pus.
6. *Vision* is completely lost and perception of light is absent.
7. *Intraocular pressure* is markedly raised.
8. *Globe perforation* may occur at limbus, pus comes out and intraocular pressure falls.

Complications include:
- Orbital cellulitis
- Cavernous sinus thrombosis, and
- Meningitis or encephalitis.

TREATMENT

There is little hope of saving such an eye and the pain and toxaemia lend an urgency to its removal.

Medical treatment

1. *Anti-inflammatory and analgesics* should be started immediately to relieve pain.

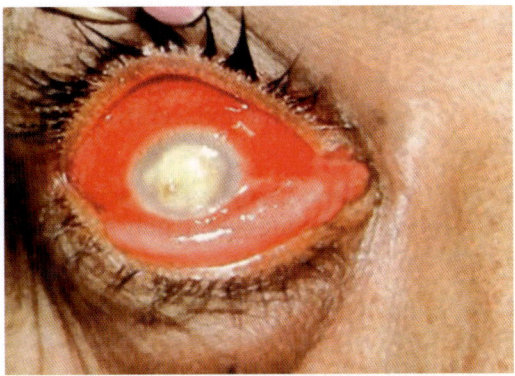

Fig. 10.2.1 *Panophthalmitis.*

2. *Broad-spectrum antibiotics* should be administered intravenously to prevent further spread of infection in the surrounding structures.

3. Topical antibiotic should also be given.

Evisceration

Evisceration operation should be performed to avoid the risk of intracranial dissemination of infection. In evisceration removal of the contents of the eyeball leaving behind the sclera is done. Frill evisceration is preferred over simple evisceration. In it, only about 3 mm frill of the sclera is left around the optic nerve, and rest of the sclera is removed.

Surgical steps of frill evisceration

Separation of conjunctiva and Tenon's capsule. Conjunctiva is incised all around the limbus with the help of spring scissors. Undermining of the conjunctiva and Tenon's capsule is done combinedly all around up to the equator, using blunt-tipped curved scissors. This manoeuvre exposes the extraocular muscles.

Separation of extraocular muscles. The rectus muscles are pulled out one by one with the help of a muscle hook and a 3–0 silk suture is passed near the insertion of each muscle. Each muscle is then cut with the help of tenotomy scissors leaving behind a small stump carrying the suture. The inferior and superior oblique muscles are hooked out and cut near the globe.

Removal of cornea. A cut at the limbus is made with a razor blade fragment or with a no. 11 scalpel blade and then the cornea is excised with corneoscleral scissors.

Removal of intraocular contents. The uveal tissue is separated from the sclera with the help of an evisceration spatula and the contents are scooped out using the evisceration curette (Fig. 10.2.2).

Removal of sclera. Using curved scissors, the sclera is excised leaving behind only a 3 mm frill around the optic nerve.

Closure of conjunctiva and Tenon's capsule is done separately. Tenon's capsule is sutured horizontally with 6-0 vicryl or chromic catgut. Conjunctiva is sutured vertically so that

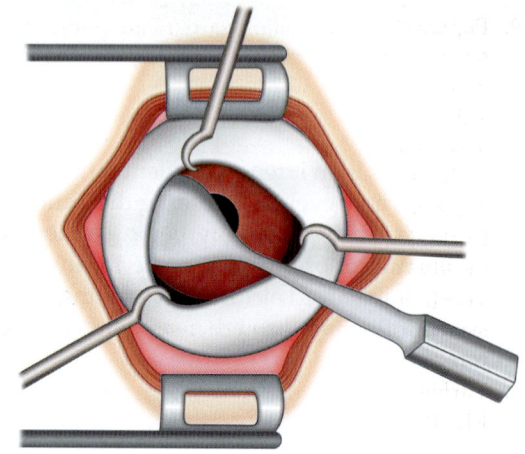

Fig. 10.2.2 *Surgical technique of evisceration.*

conjunctival fornices are retained deep with 6–0 silk sutures which are removed after 8–10 days. After completion of surgery, antibiotic ointment is applied, lids are closed and dressing is done with firm pressure using sterile eye pads and a bandage.

BIBLIOGRAPHY

1. Bouza E, Grant S, Jordan MC. Bacillus cereus endogenous panophthalmitis. Arch Ophthalmol 1979; 97:498–9.

2. Davenport R, Smith C. Panophthalmitis due to an organism of the Bacillus subtilis group. Br J Ophthalmol 1952; 36:389–92.

3. Farrar WE. Serious infection due to 'non-pathogenic' organisms of the genus Bacillus. AmJ Med 1963; 34:134–41.

4. Francois JM. Le bacille subtilique en pathologie oculaire. Bull Soc Ophtalmol Fr 1934; 47:423–6.

5. Gordon R. Endospore-forming rods and cocci. In: Buchanan RE, Gibbons NE, eds. Bergey's Manual of Determinative Bacteriology. 8th ed. Baltimore: Williams and Wilkins, 1974: 529-49.

6. Hatem G, Merritt JC, Cowan CL. Bacillus cereus panophthalmitisafterintravenous heroin. Ann Ophthalmol 1979; 11:431–40.

7. Ihde DC, Armstrong D. Clinical spectrum of infection due to Bacillus species. Am J Med 1973; 55:839–45.

8. Kerkenezov N. Panophthalmitis after a blood transfusion. Br J Ophthalmol 1953; 37:632–6.

9. Poplawska S. Zur Aetiologie der Panophthalmie nach Verletzung durch Fremdkorper. Fortschr Med 1890; 8:489–92.

10. Tabbara KF, O'Connor GF. Ocular tissue absorption of clindamycin phosphate. Arch Ophthalmol 1975; 93:1180–5.

11. Tuazon CU, Murray HW, Levy C, Solny MN, Curtin JA, Sheagren JN. Serious infections from Bacillus species. JAMA 1979; 241:1137–40.

12. Turnbull PCB, French TA, Dowsett EG. Severe systemic and pyogenic infections with Bacillus cereus. Br Med J 1977; i: 1628–33.

13. Turnbull PCB, Jorgensen K, Kramer JM, Gilbert RJ, Parry JM. Severe clinical conditions associated with Bacillus cereus and the apparent involvement of exotoxins. J Clin Pathol 1979; 32:289–93.

14. Turnbull PCB, Kramer JM, Jorgensen K, Gilbert RJ, Melling J. Properties and production characteristics of vomiting diarrheal and necrotizing toxins of B. cereus. Am J Clin Nutr 1979; 32: 219–28.

15. Van Bijsterveld OP, Richards RD. Bacillus infections of the cornea. Arch Ophthalmol 1965; 74:91–5.

16. Young EJ, Wallace RJ, Ericsson CD, Harris RA, Claridge J. Panophthalmitis due to Bacillus cereus. Arch Int Med 1980; 140:555–60.

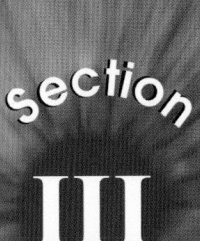

Degenerations and Dystrophies of Uvea

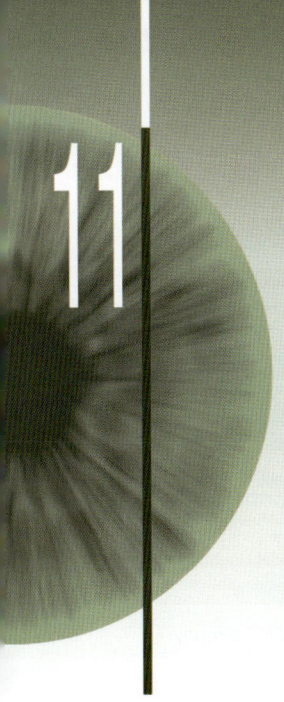

DEGENERATIONS AND DYSTROPHIES OF IRIS

11

DEGENERATIONS OF IRIS
Simple iris atrophy
• Primary
• Secondary
Essential iris atrophy
• Characteristic features

Iridoschisis
• Etiology
• Characteristic features
Pigment dispersion syndrome
• Pathogenesis
• Clinical features
• Treatment

DEGENERATIONS OF IRIS

Degenerations of iris include:
• Simple iris atrophy
• Essential iris atrophy
• Iridoschisis
• Pigment dispersion syndrome

SIMPLE IRIS ATROPHY

Simple iris atrophy is of two types: primary and secondary.

Primary simple iris atrophy

Primary simple iris atrophy is an idiopathic age-related degenerative condition of the iris seen in old people.

Characteristric features include depigmentation and thinning of iris stroma (Fig.11.1), usually in both eyes.
• *Small patches of depigmentation* are usually seen near the papillary margin. These may occur as small triangular patches or radial fissures.
• *Irregular lacunae in the pigmentary epithelium* may often be seen on retroillumination with a slit-lamp or transillumination by contact illumination.

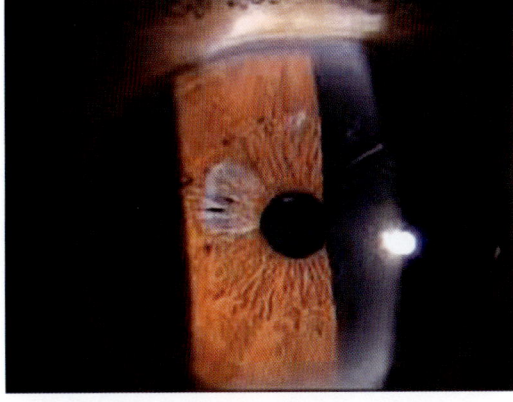

Fig. 11.1 *Primary simple iris atrophy.*

Differential diagnosis is to be made from secondary simple iris atrophy which is usually unilateral.

Secondary simple iris atrophy

Causes. Secondary simple iris atrophy occurs due to some ocular disease such as:
• Healed iridocyclitis
• Glaucoma
• Post-traumatic (surgical or otherwise)
• Neurogenic due to lesions of ciliary ganglion

Characteristic features
- *Small patches of depigmentation* (Fig. 11.2), one or more usually in one eye, but may be bilateral when the underlying disease involves both eyes.
- *Associated signs* of primary ocular disease are usually present.

ESSENTIAL IRIS ATROPHY

Essential atrophy of the iris, also known as progressive iris atrophy, is one of the three conditions included in iridocorneal endothelial (ICE) syndromes.

Characteristic features (Fig. 11.3) are as below:
- *Idiopathic* slowly progressive iris atrophy of rare occurrence involving usually one eye.
- *Age and sex*. The condition typically affects young adult females 5 times more than the males.
- *Iris atrophy changes* start insidiously and progress slowly.
- *Corectopia*, i.e. initially there occurs displacement of pupil away from the atrophic zone.
- *Lacunae in iris tissue*, which may be seen on retroillumination on slit-lamp examination or on transillumination, are formed by coalescence of areas of atrophy.
- *Ectropion uveae, dyscoria* (abnormal shape of pupil), and *pseudopolycoria* (more than one

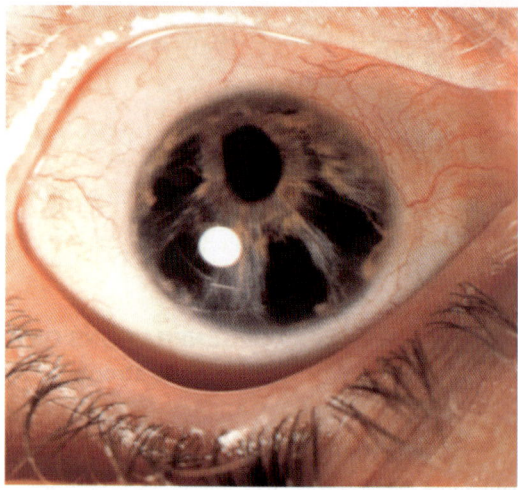

Fig. 11.3 *Essential iris atrophy.*

pupil due to secondary holes in the iris) may develop over the time due to progressive melting away of the iris tissue.
- *Intractable glaucoma* may supervene in advanced cases due to downgrowth of an endothelial membrane over the tissue at the angle of anterior chamber (typical of ICE syndrome).
- *Vision* is eventually lost due to progressive and intractable glaucoma.
- *Prognosis* is thus very poor, but fortunately as mentioned in the beginning the condition is unilateral.

IRIDOSCHISIS

Iridoschisis literally mean splitting of iris tissue.

Etiology. It is rare bilateral atrophy occurring as a senile degeneration of iris tissue in patients over 65 years of age. It may also occur as a later effect of iris trauma during intraocular surgery or otherwise.

Characteristic features (Fig. 11.4):
- *Formation of cleft* between the anterior and posterior stroma of the iris.
- *Strands of anterior stroma,* as a consequence, float into the anterior chamber, as if teased out by a needle. Occasionally, detachment of anterior layer of cleft may become extensively due to progressive atrophy of the iris tissue.
- *Glaucoma*, usually of angle-closure type, may develop over the period is about 50% of cases.

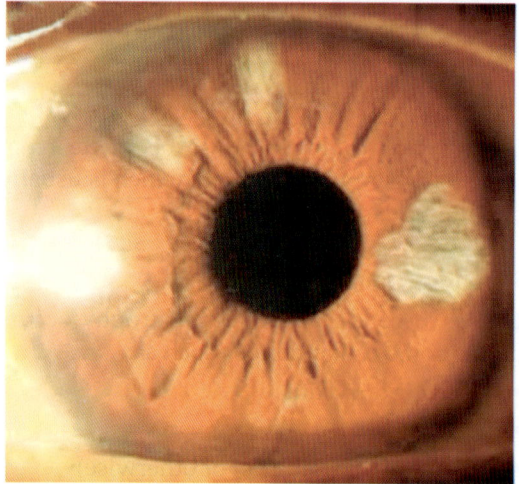

Fig. 11.2 *Secondary simple iris atrophy following attacks of acute glaucoma.*

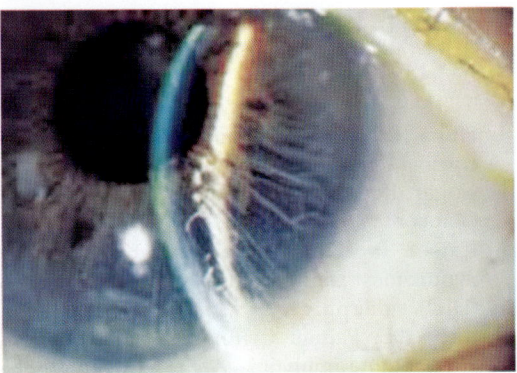

Fig. 11.4 *Iridoschisis.*

PIGMENT DISPERSION SYNDROME

Pigment dispersion syndrome (PDS), probably a degenerative condition of iris, is associated with pigmentary glaucoma in about 50% of cases.

Pathogenesis. Exact mechanism of pigment shedding is not known. It is believed that, perhaps, pigment release is caused by mechanical rubbing of the posterior pigment layer of iris with the zonular fibrils.

Clinical features (Fig. 11.5) include:
- *Young myopic males* typically develop this glaucoma.
- *Characteristic glaucomatous features* are similar to primary open-angle glaucoma (POAG), associated with.
- *Deposition of pigment granules* in the anterior segment structures such as iris, posterior surface of the cornea (Krukenberg's spindle), trabecular meshwork, ciliary zonules and the crystalline lens.
- *Gonioscopy* shows pigment accumulation along the Schwalbe's line especially inferiorly (Sampaolesi's line)
- *Iris transillumination* shows radial slit-like transillumination defects in the mid-periphery (pathognomonic feature).

Treatment of pigmentary glaucoma when associated with PDS is exactly on the lines of primary open-angle glaucoma.

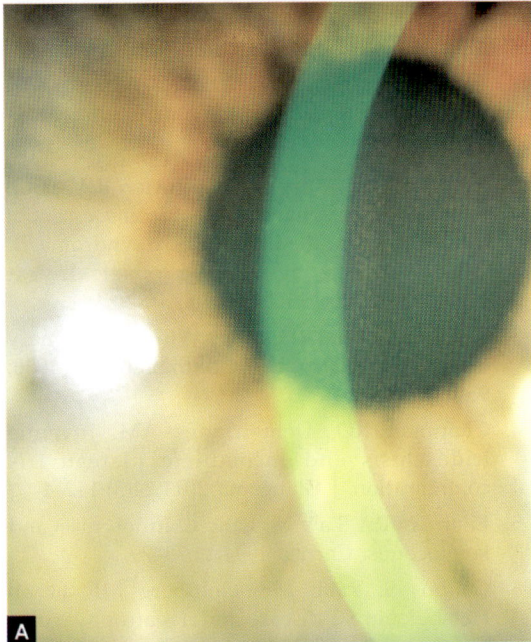

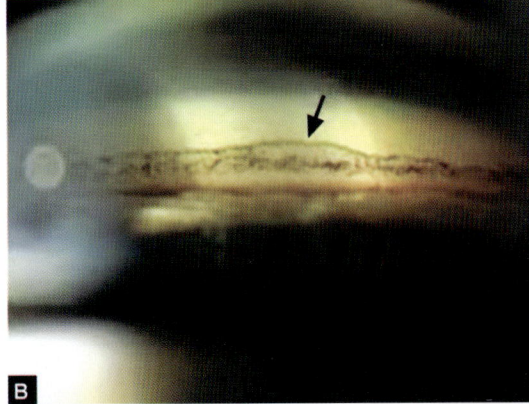

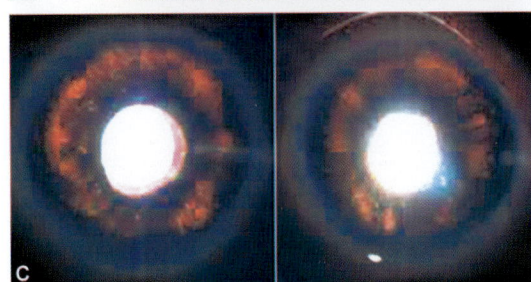

Fig. 11.5 *Pigment dispersion syndrome showing: A, Krukenberg spindle at back of cornea; B, Sampaolesi's line seen on gonioscopy; C, Slit-like transillumination defects in iris.*

BIBLIOGRAPHY

1. Acheson RW, Ford SM, Maude GH, et al. Iris atrophy in sickle cell disease. Br J Ophthalmol 1986;70:516.

2. Alvarado JA, Murphy CG, Juster RP, et al. Pathogenesis of Chandler's syndrome, essential iris atrophy and the Cogan-Reese syndrome. II. Estimated age at disease onset. Invest Ophthalmol Vis Sci 1986;27:873–82.

3. Brooks AM, West RH, Gillies WE. Acute primary ischemic iris atrophy. Ophthalmology 1988; 95:1234.

4. Chapman KO, Demetriades AM. Juvenile iridoschisis and incomplete plateau iris configuration. J Glaucoma 2011;24(5):142–4.

5. Eiferman RA, Law M, Lane L. Iridoschisis and keratoconus. Cornea 1994;13:78–79.

6. Galinos S, Rabb MF, Goldberg MF, et al. Hemoglobin SC disease and iris atrophy. Am J Ophthalmol 1973;75:421.

7. Gogaki E, Tsolaki F, Tigania S, Skatharoudi C, Balatsoukas, D. Iridoschisis: case report and review of the literature. Clin Ophthalmol 2011; 5:381–4.

8. Huna R, Barak A, Melamed S. Bilateral iridocorneal endothelial syndrome presented as Cogan-Reese and Chandler's syndrome. J Glaucoma 1996;5:60–2.

9. Kaiser P. Iridocorneal Endothelial (ICE) Syndromes. Digital Journal of Ophthalmology (DJO). nd. 2pp.

10. Knox DL, Palmer C, English F. Iris atrophy after quinine amblyopia. Arch Ophthalmol 1966; 76:359.

11. Lakosha HM, Pavlin CJ, Simpson ER. Essential Iris atrophy mimicking iris neoplasm: an ultrasound biomicroscopic study. Can J Ophthalmol 2000;35:390–3.

12. Loewenstein A, Foster J. Iridoschisis with multiple rupture of stromal threads. Br J Ophthalmol 1945;29:277–82.

13. Schmitt A. Ablosung des vorderen irisblattes. Augenh Klin Mbl 1922;68:214–5.

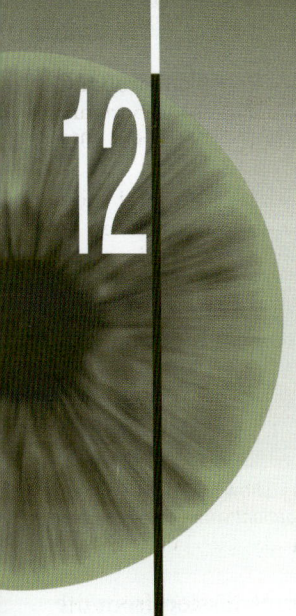

12

CHOROIDAL DYSTROPHIES AND DEGENERATIONS

CHOROIDAL DYSTROPHIES

GENERAL CONSIDERATIONS

DEFINITION

The term 'dystrophy' literally means faulty or inadequate nutrition or development. The term 'choroidal dystrophy' implies a primary degenerative process involving the choroidal circulation. While primary choroidal diseases like choroideremia do occur, various retinal degenerations also affect the choroid in the late phases of the diseases. The recent evidence suggests that defect in retinal pigment epithelium (RPE) plays an important role in the disorders that are categorized as choroidal dystrophy.

CLASSIFICATION

The hereditary choroidal dystrophies can be classified into three subtypes, namely:
- Choroidal atrophy phenotypes
- Gyrate atrophy of the choroid and retina
- Choroideremia (CHM).

Choroidal atrophy phenotypes can further be subclassified into the following three subtypes:
- Central areolar choroidal dystrophy (CACD),
- Peripapillary choroidal dystrophy, and
- Diffuse choroidal dystrophy

GENERAL FEATURES

These include retinal pigment epithelium (RPE) degenerative changes in the early stages that progresses to involve the choriocapillaris, the photoreceptor cell layer and in later stages, the larger choroidal vessels.

These changes may be generalised or localised, stationary or progressively expanding.

CHOROIDAL ATROPHY PHENOTYPES

Sorsby further subdivided this group on the basis of predominant geographical distribution into three clinical phenotypes. These include:

- Central areolar
- Choroidal peripapillary, and
- Diffuse/generalised choroidal atrophy.

Inheritance can either be as autosomal dominant or recessive traits.

CENTRAL AREOLAR CHOROIDAL DYSTROPHY (CACD)

Central areolar choroidal dystorphy (also termed as macular regional choroidal dystorphy; or circulate, annular choroidal atrophy; or central choroidal sclerosis; or central progressive areolar choroidal dystrophy), is a slowly progressive autosomal dominant disease,[1,2] involving the macula that manifests in the second to fourth decade of life. CACD was first described by Nettleship in 1884. Few reports of autosomal recessive traits have been reported.[3,4]

Clinical features

Clinical features are as below:

- *Initial symptoms* include diminished central vision presenting latter part of second decade.
- *Early changes* include mild granularity of the RPE in the foveal region.
- *With disease progression* a characteristic bilateral well demarcated circular or ovoid atrophic lesion is seen due to atrophy of the photoreceptors, RPE and choriocapillaris (Fig. 12.1). The lesion characteristically does not involve the peripapillary region or extend beyond the vascular arcades. The rest of the retina and underlying choroidal vessels are normal.

Investigations

Fluorescein angiography at the early stages of the disease show hyperfluorescence (window

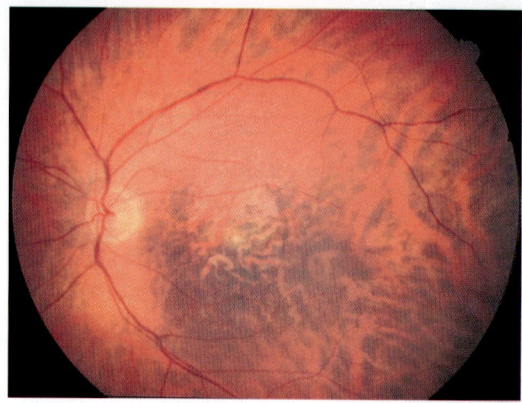

Fig. 12.1 *Central atrophic retina shows ribbon-like large vessels coursing through it in a patient with central areolar choroidal dystrophy.*

defect) due to increased transmission from the underlying normal choriocapillaris (Fig. 12.2).

Electroretinography. The disease depicts a normal full-field electroretinography (ERG). Multifocal ERG can show reduced amplitude in the affected areas before obvious clinical atrophic changes are visible.[6]

Genetic linkage analysis of the disease had mapped the locus to choromosome 17p25. A novel mutation in the peripherin/ RDS (retinal degeneration slow) gene has been identified in a Japanese family with an autosomal dominant form of CACD.[5]

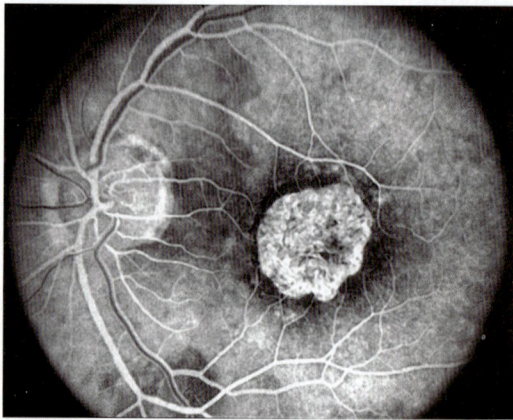

Fig. 12.2 *Central areolar choroidal dystrophy: Fluorescein angiography shows hyperfluorescence (window defect) due to increased transmission from the underlying normal choriocapillaris.*

Differential diagnosis

Similar pathologic characteristics may occur in *age-related maculopathy*, characterized by degenration and thinning of the RPE, associated with changes in Bruch's membrane and subsequent atrophy of the underlying choriocapillaris.

CACD-like macular lesion/phenotype can be seen in other conditions like Stargardt disease, advanced cone dystorphy, North Caroline mauclar dystrophy, pattern dystrophy and age-related macular degeneration.

PERIPAPILLARY CHOROIDAL DYSTROPHY

Inheritance is usually as an autosomal recessive trait,[7] although some reports of autosomal dominant transmission have been described.

Clinical features. The peripapillary from of choroidal dystrophy phenotypically resembles CACD but differs from it primarily in its location. It begins in the region surrounding the optic disc and slowly enlarges eventually occupying the posterior pole (Fig. 12.3).

Investigations include:

- *Electrophysiological testing* shows that the full-field ERG is either normal or in extensive cases, sligtly reduced amplitudes.
- *Fluorescein angiography* shows an intact choriocapillaris that differentiates it from those with choriocapillaris loss.[7]

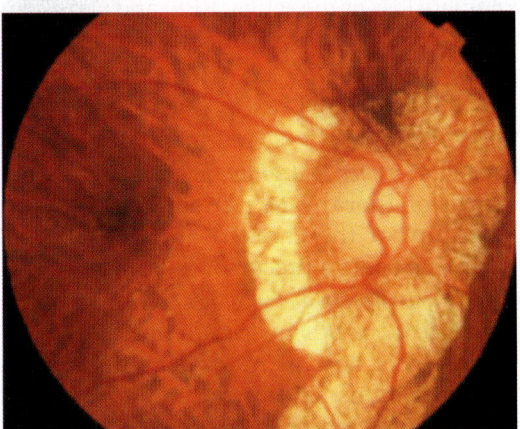

Fig. 12.3 *Peripapillary choroidal dystrophy.*

Differential diagnosis of peripapillary choroidal dystrophy includes serpiginous choroiditis, which usually begins in the peripapillary region and extends peripherally in a finger-like extensions, including in some cases, the macula.

DIFFUSE CHOROIDAL DYSTROPHY

Inheritence. It is inherited as autosomal dominant trait,[8] however, autosomal recessive transmission may occur.

Clinical features

It is a diffuse disorder involving the RPE and choriocapillaris with onset of symptoms in the fourth to fifth decade of life.

- *Patient* may present with dimness of vision or night vision impairment or both.
- *Fundus examination* in early stages shows a predilection for the posterior pole with retinal pigment mottling and hypopigmentation which progresses to a more diffuse phenotype. In late phases, there is atrophy of RPE, the choriocapillaris and later the large choroidal vessels sparing the retinal vessels.[9]

Investigations include:

- *Electrophysiological test* reveals a subnormal to undetectable full-field ERG recordings.
- *Visual fields.* There is a concentric peripheral constriction of visual fields.
- *Fluorescein angiography* shows a loss of the choriocapillaris with patchy choroidal flush due to some remnant choriocapillaris.

Differential diagnoses of the late stages of the disease include thioridazine retinal toxicity and advanced stages of Stargardt disease.

GYRATE ATROPHY OF CHOROID AND RETINA

It is a rare choroidal disease with low prevalence characterised by progressive chorioretinal atorphy especially in peripheral retina. The first case of this disease was described in 1888 by Jacobsohn[10] as an example of "atypical retinitis pigmentosa". The disease was first recognised as a distinct entity by Cutler[11] and Fuchs.[12]

INHERITANCE AND BIOCHEMICAL ABNORMALITIES

The disease is inherited as autosomal recessive trait,[9] due to a gene defect for a mitochondrial-encoded enzyme ornithine aminotransferase (OAT)[13]. A number of different mutations have been identified within the OAT gene on chromosome 10q26.[17-19] Ornithine aminotransferase—an enzyme with pyridoxal phosphate (vitamin B$_6$) as a cofactor, catalyzes inter-conversion of ornithine, glutamate and proline. This leads to hyperornithinaemia, and reduced levels of plasma lysine, glutamine, glutamate and creatinine.[14–16]

CLINICOINVESTIGATIVE PROFILE

Symptoms usually begin in the second to third decades of life and include poor night vision and constriction of peripheral field of vision with high myopia. Since the disease is progressive and spreads from periphery to centre, macula may be involved in later phases and hence, dimness of vision is a late presentation.

Associations frequently seen include myopia, posterior subcapsular cataracts and vitreous opacities.[20]

Fundus changes involve characteristic well circumscribed patches of chorioretinal atrophy with hyperpigmented margins that begin in the midperipheral and peripheral retina with thinning and atorphy of RPE with either normal or sclerotic underlying choroidal vessels.
• *Lesions typically* have scalloped margin between the affected and unaffected retina and are distinct to begin with, but later become confluent as they progress both centrally and peripherally (Fig. 12.4).
• *In later stages*, the retinal vessels may be attenuated when the optic nerve may appear pale.
• *Cystoid macular oedema* has been reported in patients with gyrate atrophy.[21–23] Intravitreal injection of 4 mg triamcinolone acetonide for macular oedema in gyrate atrophy has shown short-term therapeutic effects, with recurrence of oedema after drug clearance.[23]

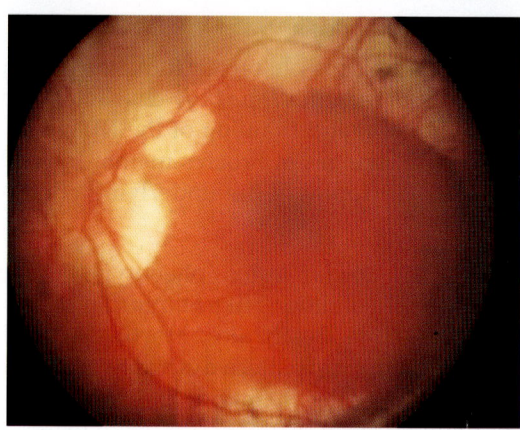

Fig. 12.4 *Gyrate atrophy lesions typically have scalloped margin between the affected and unaffected retina.*

Visual field testing most commonly shows a concentric peripheral constriction of the visual field. Annular ring or paracentral scotomas may be seen in later stages. Central scotoma is seen, if the fovea is involved.

Electrophysiological test findings are as below:
• *Full-field ERG* in early stages shows only a mild abnormality in rod and cone amplitude which deteriorates and may become undetectable as the disease progresses. In early stages, rods are more affected, but later both cone and rods are severely imapired.[24,25]
• *Electro-oculography* (EOG) light peak to dark trough ratio may become markedly reduced at later stages.

Histopathology is remarkable in that there is complete loss of the retina, RPE, and choroid in the affected areas, with an abrupt transition to unaffected retina.[26]

MANAGEMENT

• *A diet restricted in arginine has been advised* as a form of therapy in patients with gyrate atrophy of the choroid and retina since arginine being a precursor of ornithine.[27–29]
• *Rigid low-protein diet with near total elimination of arginine with supplementation of essential amino acid* has been advocated by some investigations since ornithine is produced from other amino acids as well. Dietary approach to reducing plasma ornithine levels

in patients with gyrate atrophy showed varied effectivity in various studies.[27-30]

- *Oral pyridoxal phosphate* (vitamin B_6) may be affective in some cases of gyrate atrophy with resultant decrease in plasma ornithine levels. Others may be non-responsive to B_6 and are called as non-responders.[30] Overall, ERG responses are better maintained by B_6-responders compared to non-responders.[27,31]

CHOROIDEREMIA (CHM/PROGRESSIVE TAPETOCHOROIDAL DYSTROPHY)

Choroideremia is a slowly progressive, X-linked condition that leads to generalised degeneration of the RPE, retina and choroid.

INHERITANCE

It is inherited as X-linked recessive condition,[37] the clinical features of which were first described by Mauthner in 1872.[36] It is caused by the mutations to the CHM gene located on Xq13-22 that codes for Rab escort protein (REP-1) that is required for the function of Rab geranylgeranyl-transferase in intracellular vesicular transport.[38,39]

CLINICOINVESTIGATIVE PROFILE

- The disease manifests in first or second decade and progresses slowly over several years.
- Patients complains of constriction of visual-field and nightblindness. Central vision is spared for a long time.
- Severe visual impairment with loss of central vision occurs in their fifth to sixth decades.[47]

Fundus changes begin in the midperipheral, equatorial or paramacular regions and include:

- *Granular pigment changes in the periphery and focal atrophy of the RPE* (clinically resembling gyrate atrophy in early stages). These early changes are also evident in female carriers that exhibit mosaicism.
- *Atrophy of RPE and choriocapillaris progresses* resulting in diffuse atrophy with exposure of large choroidal vessels. Towards the late stages, only islands of intact choroid remain in the macular area (Fig. 12.5). The rate of progression is variable in different individuals and family.

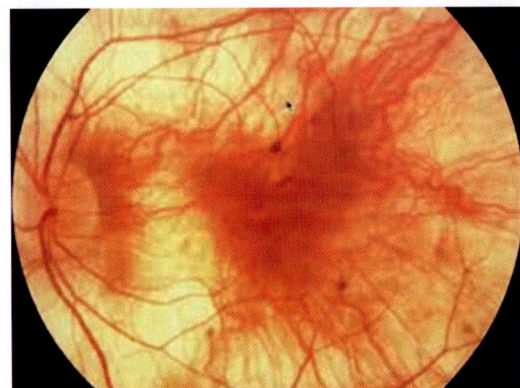

Fig. 12.5 *Choroideremia shows marked RPE atrophy and that of inner choroid.*

- *Cystoid macular oedema* has also been described recently to be present in some patients.[40]

Fluorescein angiography shows early window defects and hyperfluorescence, with later hypofluorescence (due to atrophy of choriocapillaris).[41,42]

Histopathological examination shows areas of RPE loss with overlying absence of photo-receptors and underlying choriocapillaris distrubance.[42-44] Capillary basement membrane fragmentation of choroidal vessels is seen in uninvolved pigmented fundus. Fragmentation and loss of Bruch's membrane is seen with outer retinal atophy and degeneration in areas of marked choriocapillaris atrophy. The phagocytic activity of the RPE cells results in overlying chorioretinal adhesions in the gliotic retina and resultant epiretinal membranes. Mild T lymphocyte infiltration within the choroid has been reported.[46]

Electrophysiology shows abnormal to undetect-able photopic and scotopic ERG response. ERG may be normal in early course of the disease.[45] EOG shows an abnormally low light peak to dark trough ratio (Arden's ratio) .

DIFFERENTIAL DIAGNOSIS OF CHOROIDAL DYSTROPHIES

Clinical phenotypes resembling hereditary choroidal diseases include:

1. X-linked retinitis pigmentosa (XLRP)

Retinitis pigmentosa—a group of inherited disorders of RPE and photoreceptors leading to night blindness, restriction of peripheral field and progressive vision loss may be inherited as AD, AR or X-linked manner. The fundus in later stages of CHM may resemble end-stage XLRP, however, the evidence of pigment migration into the retina in XLRP differentiates it from CHM.

2. Bietti's crystalline dystrophy

Both diffuse and localized form of retinal degenerative changes involving both RPE and choriocapillaris atrophy may be seen in this condition. The clinical picture may thus resemble choroidal dystrophy.

Bietti's crystalline dystrophy most commonly presents with glistening crystalline-like changes in the posterior pole associated with cholesterol or cholesterol ester crystals in superficial corneal stroma. The disease may be transmitted as autosomal recessive trait.

3. Thioridazine retinal toxicity

Thioridazine is a piperidine typical antipsychotic drug belonging to the phenothiazine drug *group*. Patients receiving high doses may complain of night blindness and dimness of vision. In earlier stages, a pigment granularity or mottling occurs in macular or paramacular region. Later may lead to extensive degenerative changes of RPE, choriocapillaris and photoreceptors, thus phenotypically resembling CHM, gyrate atrophy or diffuse choroidal dystrophy depending upon extent of degenerative process.

4. Stargardt disease

Stargardt disease typically leads to loss of central vision with a characteristic "beaten bronze" appearance of the macula, with yellowish-white flecks scattered at the posterior pole. Fluorescein angiography shows masking of the fluorescein from choroidal circulation (dark choroid) (Fig. 12.6).[31–34]

The most common mode of inheritance being autosomal recessive.[35] The advanced stages of Stargardt disease may show extensive atrophy of the RPE and choroid at the posterior pole.

5. Pattern macular dystrophy

Pattern macular dystrophy involves accumulation of lipofuscin within RPE cells with subsequent degeneration accompanied by choriocapillaris loss. It is an autosomal dominant disorder with variable fundus picture. In late stages, diffuse disorder may resemble CHM and a localised RPE and choroidal atrophy may resemble CACD.

REMARKS ON MANAGEMENT STATUS OF CHOROIDAL DYSTROPHIES

General considerations

Remarks: No defined treatment for hereditary choroidal dystrophies is there in current scenario.

- *Patients need to be explained* regarding the prognosis and need periodic follow-up to look for progression and amount of visual function loss.
- *A holistic approach by* a team of ophthalmologist, dietician, low-vision services, physician and genetic counsellor is essential.
- *Low-vision services* may be useful to help optimize the use of remaining visual function in patients with severe visual impairment.
- *Cataract surgery* may help clear the media and improve visual function, in some cases.

Genetic counselling and gene therapy

- *Genetic counselling* may help patients to understand the genetic implications and to make informed personal decisions.
- *Gene therapy.* With advent of biotechnological aids and mapping of genes for most of the dystrophies, individualised gene therapy for hereditary choroidal dystrophy is likely to be a viable treatment option in near future.

CHOROIDAL DEGENERATIONS

Only a few choroidal degenerations are mentioned here.

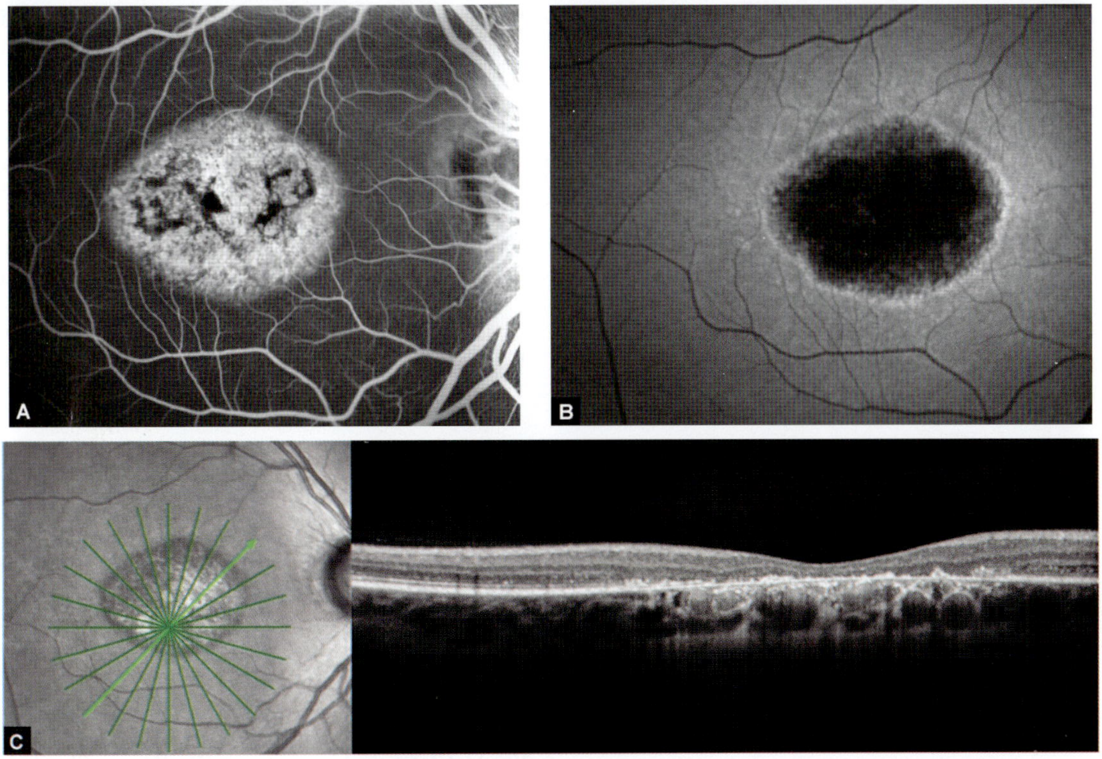

Fig. 12.6 *Stargardt's dystrophy: A, Fluorescein angiography reveals hyperfluorescent well-circumscribed lesion; B, Autofluorescence reveals dark central area signifying total loss of RPE; C, SD-OCT shows retinochoroidal atrophy in the same eye.*

I. PRIMARY CHOROIDAL DEGENERATIONS

1. Senile central choroidal atrophy

It is characterised by formation of multiple drusens (colloid bodies) which look as yellowish spots. These are scattered throughout the fundus, but more marked in the macular area.

2. Myopic chorioretinal degeneration

Degenerative changes in retina and choroid are common in progressive myopia (Fig. 12.7). These are characterized by:

- *Chorioretinal atrophic patches* at the macula with a little heaping up of pigment around them.
- *Foster-Fuchs' spot* (dark red circular patch due to subretinal neovascularisation and choroidal haemorrhage) may be present at the macula.
- *Cystoid degeneration* may be seen at the periphery.
- *Lattice degeneration* and or snail track lesions with or without retinal holes/tears may be present; which later may be complicated by retinal detachment.

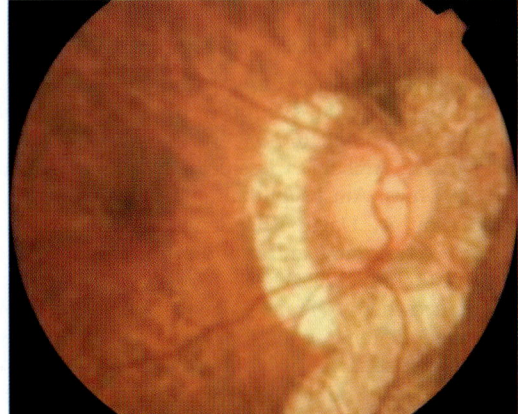

Fig. 12.7 *Myopic chorioretinal degeneration.*

- *Total retinal atrophy*, particularly in the central area may occur in an advanced case.

Posterior staphyloma due to ectasia of sclera at posterior pole may be apparent as an excavation with the vessels bending backward over its margins.

Degenerative changes in vitreous include: Liquefaction, vitreous opacities, and posterior vitreous detachment (PVD) appearing as Weiss' reflex.

II. SECONDARY CHOROIDAL DEGENERATION

Sencondary choroidal degeneration occurs following inflammatory lesions of the fundus. It is characterised by scattered area of chorioretinal atrophy and pigment clumping. *Ophthalmoscopic picture* resembles retinitis pigmentosa and hence also labelled sometimes as *'pseudoretinitis pigmentosa.'*

REFERENCES

1. Carr RE. Central areolar choroidal dystrophy. Arch Ophthalmol 1965;73:32–5.
2. Sandvig K. Familial, central, areolar, choroidal atrophy of autosomal dominant inheritance. Acta Ophthalmol (Copenh) 1955;33:71–8.
3. Waardenburg PJ. Familial angiosclerosis of the choroid. J Genet Hum 1952;1:83–90.
4. Sorsby A, Crick RP. Central areolar choroidal sclerosis. Br J Ophthalmol 1953;37:129–39.
5. Yanagihashi S, Nakazawa M, Kurotaki J, et al. Autosomal dominant central areolar choroidal dystrophy and a novel Arg195Leu mutation in the peripherin/RDS gene. Arch Ophthalmol 2003;121:1458–61.
6. Nagasaka K, Horiguchi M, Simada Y, et al. Multifocal electroretinograms in cases of central areolar choroidal dystrophy. Invest Ophthalmol Vis Sci 2003;44:1673-9.
7. Krill AE, Archer D. Classification of the choroidal atrophies. Am J Ophthalmol 1971;72:562–85.
8. Sorsby A, Davey JB. Generalized choroidal sclerosis; course and mode of inheritance. Br J Ophthalmol 1955;39:257–76.
9. Franceschetti A, Francois J, Babel J. Chorioretinal heredodegenerations. Springfield, Ill: Charles C Thomas; 1974.
10. Jacobsohn E. Ein fall von Retinitis pigmentosa atypica. Klin Monatsbl Augenheilkd 1888;26:202–6.
11. Cutler C. Dri ungewohnliche Falle von retinochoroideak Degeneration. Arch Augenheilkd 1895;30:117.
12. Fuchs E. Ueber awei der Retinitis pigmentosa verwandte Krankheiten (retinitis punctate albescens und atrophia gyrate chorioideae et retinae). Arch Augenheilkd 1896;32:111.
13. Simell O, Takki K. Raised plasma-ornithine and gyrate atrophy of the choroid and retina. Lancet 1973;1:1031–3.
14. Valle D, Walser M, Brusilow SW, et al. Gyrate atrophy of the choroid and retina: amino acid metabolism and correction of hyperornithinemia with an arginine-deficient diet. J Clin Invest 1980;65:371–8.
15. Valle D, Walser M, Brusilow S, et al. Gyrate atrophy of the choroid and retina. Biochemical considerations and experience with an arginine-restricted diet. Ophthalmology 1981;88:325–30.
16. Kaiser-Kupfer MI, de Monasterio FM, Valle D, et al. Gyrate atrophy of the choroid and retina: improved visual function following reduction of plasma ornithine by diet. Science 1980;210:1128–31.
17. Inana G, Hotta Y, Zintz C, et al. Expression defect of ornithine aminotransferase gene in gyrate atrophy. Invest Ophthalmol Vis Sci 1988;7:1001–5.
18. Mitchell GA, Brody LC, Siplia I, et al. At least two mutant alleles of ornithine delta-aminotransferase cause gyrate atrophy of the choroid and retina in Finns. Proc Natl Acad Sci USA 1989;86:197–201.
19. McClatchey AI, Kaufman DL, Berson EL, et al. Splicing defect at the ornithine amino-transferase (OAT) locus in gyrate atrophy. Am J Hum Genet 1990;47:790–4
20. Takki KK, Milton RC. The natural history of gyrate atrophy of the choroid and retina. Ophthalmology 1981;88:292–301.
21. Feldman RB, Mayo SS, Robertson DM, et al. Epiretinal membranes and cystoid macular edema in gyrate atrophy of the choroid and retina. Retina 1989;9:139–42.
22. Oliveira TL, Andrade RE, Muccioli C, et al. Cystoid macular edema in gyrate atrophy of the choroid and retina: a fluorescein angiography and optical coherence tomography evaluation. Am J Ophthalmol 2005;140:147–9.
23. Vasconcelos-Santos DV, Magalhães EP, Nehemy MB. Macular edema associated with gyrate atrophy managed with intravitreal triamcinolone: a case report. Arq Bras Oftalmol 2007;70:858–61.
24. Weleber RG, Kennaway NG. Clinical trial of vitamin B6 for gyrate atrophy of the choroid and retina. Ophthalmology 1981;88:316–24.
25. Raitta C, Carlson S, Vannas-Sulonen K. Gyrate atrophy of the choroid and retina: ERG of the neural retina and the pigment epithelium. Br J Ophthalmol 1990;74:363–7.

26. Wilson DJ, Weleber RG, Green WR: Ocular clinicopathologic study of gyrate atrophy. Am J Ophthalmol 1991: 111:24-33.

27. Berson EL, Hanson 3rd AH, Rosner B, et al. A two year trial of low protein, low arginine diets or vitamin B$_6$ for patients with gyrate atrophy. Birth Defects Orig Artic Ser 1982;18:209–18.

28. Kaiser-Kupfer MI, Caruso RC, Valle D. Gyrate atrophy of the choroid and retina. Long-term reduction of ornithine slows retinal degeneration. Arch Ophthalmol 1991;109:1539–48.

29. Vannas-Sulonen K, Simell O, Sipilä I. Gyrate atrophy of the choroid and retina. The ocular disease progresses in juvenile patients despite normal or near normal plasma ornithine concentration. Ophthalmology 1987;94:1428–33.

30. Weleber RG, Kennaway NG. Clinical trial of vitamin B6 for gyrate atrophy of the choroid and retina. Ophthalmology 1981;88:316–24.

31. Fishman GA, Farber M, Patel BS, et al. Visual acuity loss in patients with Stargardt's macular dystrophy. Ophthalmology 1987;94:809–14.

32. Rotenstreich Y, Fishman GA, Anderson RJ. Visual acuity loss and clinical observations in a large series of patients with Stargardt disease. Ophthalmology 2003;110:1151–8.

33. Armstrong JD, Meyer D, Xu S, et al. Long-term follow-up of Stargardt's disease and fundus flavimaculatus. Ophthalmology 1998;105:448–57.

34. Aaberg TM. Stargardt's disease and fundus flavimaculatus: evaluation of morphologic progression and intrafamilial co-existence. Trans Am Ophthalmol Soc 1986;84:453–87.

35. Allikmets R, Singh N, Sun H, et al. A photoreceptor cell-specific ATP-binding transporter gene (ABCR) is mutated in recessive Stargardt macular dystrophy. Nat Genet 1997;15:236–46

36. Mauthner L. Ein Fall von Chorioideremie. Berl Natur-med. Ver Innsbruck 1872;2:191.

37. McCulloch C, McCulloch RJP. A hereditary and clinical study of chorioideremia. Trans Am Acad Ophthal Otolaryngol 1948;52:160.

38. Nussbaum RL, Lewis RA, Lesko JG. Choroideremia is linked to the fragment length polymorphism DXYS1 at Xq13-21. Am J Hum Genet 1985;37:473.

39. Seabra MC, Brown MS, Slaughter CA, et al. Purification of component A of Rab geranylgeranyltransferase: possible identity with the choroideremia gene product. Cell 1992; 70:1049–57.

40. Genead MA, Fishman GA. Cystic macular oedema on spectral-domain optical coherence tomography in choroideremia patients without cystic changes on fundus examination. Eye (Lond) 2011;25:84–90.

41. McCulloch CL. Chorideremia and other choroidal atorphies. In: Newsome DA, ed. Retinal Dystrophies and Degenerations. New York: Raven; 1988:285–95.

42. Rodrigues MM, Ballintine EJ, Wiggert BN, et al. Choroideremia: a clinical, electron microscopic, and biochemical report. Ophthalmology 1984; 91:873.

43. Cameron JD, Fine BS, Shapiro I. Histopathologic observations in choroideremia with emphasis on vascular changes of the uveal tract. Ophthalmology 1987;94:187.

44. Flannery JG, Bird AC, Farber DB, et al. A histopatholgic study of a choroideremia carrier. Invest Ophthalmolo Vis Sci 1990; 31:229.

45. Francis PJ, Fishman GA, Trzupek KM, et al. Stop mutations in exon 6 of the choroideremia gene, CHM, associated with preservation of the electroretinogram. Arch Ophthalmol 2005;123:1146–9.

46. MacDonald IM, Russell L, Chan CC. Choroideremia: new findings from ocular pathology and review of recent literature. Surv Ophthalmol 2009;54:401–7.

47. Roberts MF, Fishman GA, Roberts DK, et al. Retrospective, longitudinal, and cross sectional study of visual acuity impairment in choroideraemia. Br J Ophthalmol 2002;86:658–62.

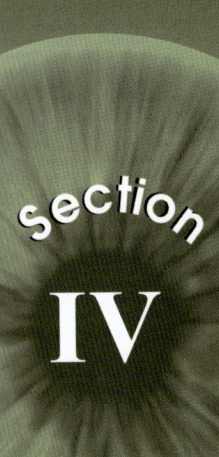

Tumours of Uvea

13. Tumours of Uveal Tract

TUMOURS OF UVEAL TRACT

13

INTRODUCTION AND CLASSIFICATION

INTRODUCTION

Uveal melanoma (UM) is the most common primary, malignant intraocular tumour in adults and account for 75% of malignant intraocular tumours. The incidence of UM is 5 per 1,00,000; approximately 0.003% of all cancers.[1] There is a slight male preponderence with average age of diagnosis in the 6th and 7th decades of life.[2] The mean reported age of diagnosed uveal melanoma is 44 years in Chinese, 52 years in American blacks, 55 years in Japanese, and 52 years in the Hispanic population.[2,3] In the Collaborative Ocular Melanoma Study (COMS),

1302 patients eligible for the study had a mean age of 60 years. Only 14% of patients were below 50 years of age. Hispanic, Blacks, Japanese, and Chinese patients have been noted to be younger at the time of diagnosis.[1] In a study conducted in Sankara Nethralaya by Biswas et al, the mean age at presentation was 45.7±14.2 years (range: 14 to 82 years) and 50% of patients were less than 45 years of age.[4]

The most common neoplasm is observed in the choroid accounting for 80% of all uveal melanomas followed by ciliary body (10%) and iris (10%).[1] Uveal melanoma has a high tendency to metastasize, the common sites being liver (89%), lung (29%) and bone (17%).[5] The median survival ranges between 6 and 12 months.[1]

Conditions predisposing to early onset of uveal melanomas are:[6-7]

- Ocular melanocytosis,
- Nevus of Ota,
- Dysplastic cutaneous nevi,
- Familial melanoma, and
- Neurofibromatosis-I.[6-7]

Melanocytosis

'Oculodermic melanocytosis' or nevus of Ota is a dermal melanocytic hamartoma (Fig. 13.1).[6]

Age. The age of onset of nevus of Ota is either at or soon after birth and family history is uncommon.

Race. It is fairly common in the Asian population with a rare occurrence in Caucasians, Chinese and African-American population.

Sex. There is a higher preponderance amongst the females with a male:female ratio of 1:4.8.

Triggering stimuli include puberty, trauma, sex hormones, infection and UV exposure.[6, 7]

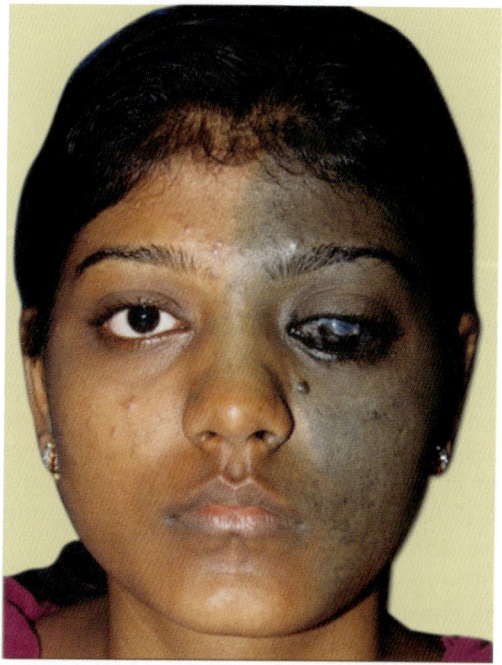

Fig. 13.1 *Nevus of Ota:* *An 18-year-old girl presented with grey-black skin pigmentation over left half of face since infancy. Left eye has ocular melanocytosis, anterior staphyloma, and buphthalmos due to secondary glaucoma.*

Pathogenesis. The occurrence of nevus of Ota is due to abnormal migration of the neural crest cells which results in formation of nevoids cells from Schwann cells.

Extent of involvement depends upon the embryological stage at which the abnormality occurs.

Histopathologically, it consists of elongated dendritic melanocytes which are scattered in the papillary to mid-reticular dermis.

Clinical features. Clinical appearance of nevus of Ota is usually unilateral, blue-black or slate grey macules along the 1st and 2nd branch distribution of the trigeminal nerve. Nevus of Ota was classified by Tanino according to cutaneous involvement:

- *IA:* Upper/lower eyelid; periorbital and temporal
- *IB:* Infrapalpebral, nasolabial fold and zygomatic region
- *IC:* Forehead
- *ID:* Nasal
- *II:* Over upper and lower eyelids, periocular, zygomatic, cheek and temple
- *III:* Scalp, forehead, eyebrow and nose
- *IV:* Bilateral

Associations. It is associated with pigmentation of sclera, iris and conjunctiva, increased intraocular pressure with or without glaucoma, asymmetric cupping of the optic nerve, uveitis, cataracts and rarely orbital melanoma.[6]

Differential diagnosis includes:

- Café-au-lait spot,
- Nevus spilus, and
- Nevus of Ito.

Treatment includes:

- *Camouflage therapy.* Colour correctors are available to correct and counterbalance the pigmented area.
- *Cryotherapy.* It causes cryonecrosis of the dermal melanocytes. It is done using liquid nitrogen with freezing temperature up to minus 218°C.
- *Derma-abrasion.* Removes the epidermal and superficial dermal melanin.

• *Laser surgery.* Photothermolysis using 1064 Nd:YAG Q-switched laser with short pulse durations causes profound beneficial lightening of the skin pigmentation. The initial side effects include slight transient hyper-pigmentation. The recurrence rate is 0.2 to 1.2%.[6-8]

CLASSIFICATION OF UVEAL TUMOURS

Tumours of uveal tract can be classified as below:

Tumour of iris

I. *Benign tumours of iris*
• Benign iris cyst
• Iris nevus
• Iris granuloma
• Naevoxanthoendothelioma

II. *Malignant tumours of iris*
• Iris melanoma
• Iris metastasis

Tumours of ciliary body

Tumour of non-pigmented ciliary epithelium
Benign tumours
• Adenoma
• Medulloepithelioma

Malignant tumours
• Adenocarcinoma

Myogenic tumour
• Leiomyoma

Melanocytic tumour
Benign
• Naevus

Malignant
• Ciliary body melanoma

Tumours of choroid

Primary tumours of choroid
Benign tumours of choroid
• Choroidal nevus
• Melanocytoma of choroid
• Choroidal haemangioma
• Choroidal osteoma

Melignant primary tumours of choroid
• Malignant melanoma
• Reticulum cell sarcoma
• Choroidal lymphoma

Secondary tumours of choroid
• Metastatic carcinomas of choroid
• Systemic lymphoma
• Leukaemic infiltration
• Local extension of retinoblastoma

TUMOURS OF IRIS

Primary iris tumours arise from the pigmented layer of neuroepithelium or from the melanoblasts of neural crest cells. The most common iris tumours arise from melanocytic stromal proliferations. The lesions may vary from simple nevi to melanoma to xantho-granuloma to metastasis. Tumours of iris can be divided into benign and malignant.

BENIGN TUMOURS OF IRIS

The common benign lesions of iris can be sub-divided as:
• Iris cyst,
• Iris freckle, and
• Iris nevus.

IRIS CYSTS
Clinical profile

Iris cysts are either primary or secondary in origin.

A. *Primary iris cysts*

The primary iris cysts arise from the pigment epithelium or the stroma of the iris. They have a benign natural course and usually cause no visual disturbance.[2]

Primary cysts of iris pigment epithelium (IPE) have a higher incidence in adults. Depending upon location, the iris cysts can be divided as below:

1. *Peripheral (iridociliary) cysts* are most common in women in the age group of 15–60 years. These are more commonly observed

temporally in the iris and allow transmission of light.

2. *Mid-zonal cysts* are visualised better after pupillary dilation and appear as rounded dark brown mass just posterior to the pupillary border which assume a fusiform, elongated shape after complete dilatation. They have characteristic thin walls and do not allow complete transmission of light. The mid-zonal cysts were observed in 9% of the subjects with a higher male preponderance.

3. *Central (pupillary) cysts*. These account for only 5% cases.

4. *Dislodged iris cysts* can be fixed or free floating. Most of these cysts are asymptomatic but can cause increased intraocular pressure, corneal oedema, cataract, lenticular astigmatism and iritis.[10]

Primary cysts of iris stoma. Primary cysts of the iris stroma characteristically occur in children but are not so common. Histopathologically, stromal cysts consist of pigmented layers with no evidence of connective or vascular component. These can be:

• Congenital, or
• Acquired.

B. Secondary iris cysts

Secondary iris cysts are more aggressive in clinical course and cause decrease in visual acuity, glaucoma, cataract and uveitis. These include:

I. *Epithelial cysts*

• Epithelial downgrowth which can be post-surgical or post-traumatic
• Pearl cysts
• Drug induced

II. *Cysts secondary to intraocular tumours*, e.g. secondary

• Medulloepithelioma
• Uveal melanoma

III. *Parasitic iris cysts*

Management

Diagnosis and confirmation can be made using ultrasound biomicroscopy (UBM) and anterior segment optical coherence tomography (AS-OCT). It also helps in differentiating between the solid and cystic anterior segment tumours.[2, 9]

Differential diagnosis includes primary iris cyst, epithelial inclusion cyst, iris melanoma, iris nevi, ciliary body melanoma and metastasis.

Treatment depends upon the site, size, local extent and growth pattern of the iris cysts.

Primary iris cysts resolve spontaneously.

Secondary cysts are treated if they obscure the visual axis or cause pupillary distortion, iridocyclitis or corneal decompensation.

Modalities of treatment available are:

• Excision
• Mitomycin injection into cyst with needle aspiration with endodiathermy
• Nd:YAG laser cystotomy
• Intracystic ethanol irrigation

IRIS NEVUS

The iris nevi present as flat or slightly elevated focal areas of iris pigmentation[5] (Fig. 13.2). Iris nevi are most common primary tumours of iris accounting for 49–72% of all iris tumours.[2]

Diagnostic features on ultrasonography of iris nevi are:

• Fusiform thickening of iris,
• Diffuse elongated thickening of the iris, and

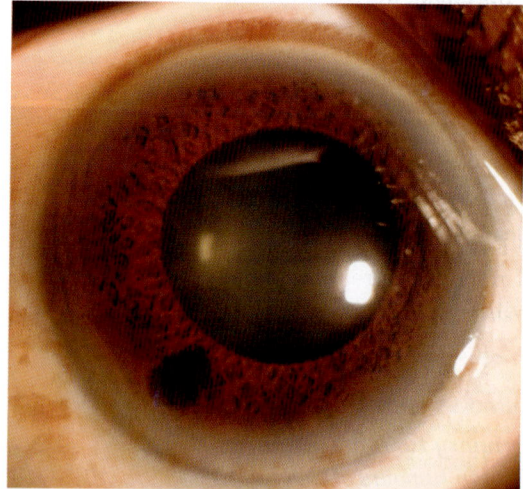

Fig. 13.2 *Iris nevus:* *A 45-year-old lady presented for a routine examination when an iris nevus was noted as a coincidental finding in right eye. Iris nevi appear as flat pigmented lesion. Ths lesion appeared to have been stable in size since several years.*

- Focal thickening of the iris surface with a sharp border between lesion and iris giving a "stuck on appearance".

Differential diagnosis from melanoma. Nevus showing ectropion uvea, neovascularization, sectoral cataract and iris distortion should be clinically differentiated from melanoma.[5]

Treatment. Iris freckles and nevi do not need to be treated but require close observation and monitoring. Suspicious lesions that show growth or increase in size require transcorneal fine needle aspiration biopsy or excisional biopsy.

IRIS GRANULOMA

Causes

- *Neurofibromatosis-I,* the iris granuloma can be observed as 'Lisch nodules' which appear as diffuse nodular nevi.
- *Cogan-Reese dystrophy,* nodules are small, dark-pigmented, pedunculated nodules—diffuse or focal in distribution.[5]
- *Non-infectious uveitis.* Iris nodules are observed in sarcoidosis, Vogt-Koyanagi-Harada syndrome, multiple sclerosis, Fuchs' hetero-chromic iridocyclitis, and infectious uveitis (Fig. 13.3).
- *Infectious uveitis.* Some bacterial species are associated with uveitis and iris nodules such as *Mycobacterium, Treponema,* and *Rickettsia.* Also, many fungal agents, such as *Crypto-coccus,* coccidioidomycosis, and *Candida,* have reported associations with iris nodules.[13]

Naevoxanthoendothelioma

It is a rare flashy vascular lesion seen in babies. It may cause recurrent hyphema. It is treated with X-ray or steroids.

MALIGNANT TUMOURS OF IRIS

IRIS MELANOMA

Epidemiology

Iris malignancy accounts for 5–10% of uveal tumours. It is three times more common in light irides (blue/grey).[2] The typical age of presentation is in the 4th–5th decade of life. The gender predilection is equal.

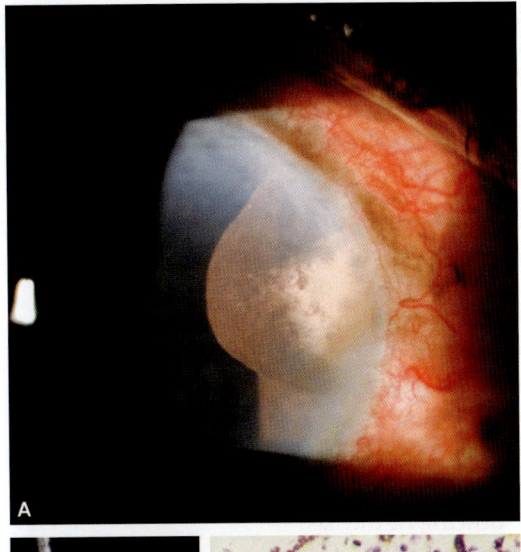

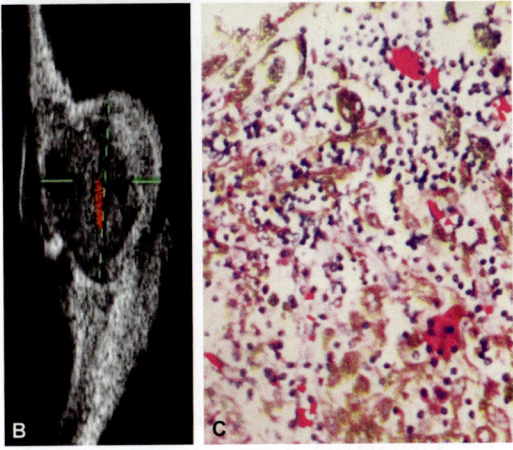

Fig. 13.3 *Iris granuloma: A partially melanotic, iris mass 3.3 × 4 × 4 mm in size extending between 2'30 and 3'30 meridian (A) was observed in a 65-year-old male. Transillumination was negative. Gonioscopy revealed no evidence of angle seeds of feeder vessel. Ultrasound biomicroscopy (UBM) confirmed the solid nature of the lesion (B). Excision biopsy was done and histopathology revealed inflammatory cells (C).*

Clinical features

Majority of the iris tumours arise from the pre-existing iris nevi or from the iris stroma. It is usually unilateral in presentation with a greater occurrence in the inferior quadrant.

Characteristic features of iris melanoma are inferior quadrant location (45%), and partially or completely pigmented (90%) tumour. Other less common features include corectopia (45%), glaucoma (35%), angle seeding (28%), ectropion uveae (24%), hyphema (3%), and extraocular extension (3%). Ring melanoma is a variant of iris tumour which tends to grow around the iris in a circular shape and shows a diffuse pattern of growth.

Clinical presentation of these patients can be asymptomatic and detected on routine evaluation from following signs:

- Pupillary distortion
- Pigment dispersion
- Sectoral cataract
- Ectropion uvea
- Tumour vascularisation
- Secondary glaucoma
- Bowing of the iris

Risk factors predictive for iris nevi growth to melanoma was created with ABCDEF guide which aids in the early identification and treatment:

A: Age
B: Blood
C: Clock hour inferior
D: Diffuse configuration
E: Ectropion
F: Feathery margin

American Joint Committee on Cancer (AJCC) classification of iris melanoma is as below:

- T-1: Limited to the iris
- T-2: Tumour extension to ciliary body and choroid
- T-3: Extension to sclera
- T-4: Extrascleral extension

Histological features

Modified callender classification is as below:

- *Spindel cell melanoma.* Spindle cells have a plump elongated nucleus with mild coarse chromatin with eosinophilic nucleus.
- *Epithelial cell melanoma.* The epitheloid cells are larger and pleomorphic with abundant eosinophilic cytoplasm and distinct cell borders with a high cytoplasm to nuclear ratio and absent nucleoli and no mitotic activity.
- *Mixed cell melanoma* has features of both spindle and epithelial cell melanoma.

Management

Clinical evaluation and investigations

Clinical evaluation. When evaluating a case of iris mass, a complete careful and detailed history about the lesion, slit-lamp evaluation, gonioscopy to rule out ciliary body involvement, anterior segment photography, and indirect ophthalmoscopy with a scleral depression is essential.[5]

Ultrasonic biomicroscopy (UBM). The diagnosis is made using UBM which shows typical low to medium reflective and nodular spikes arising from the iris surface.[12] The iris stromal thickening shows medium to highly reflectivity. The blood vessels show acoustic empty and cystic spaces on ultrasound. Water bath USG provides additional information regarding the extent of the tumour but is of limited resolution.

Fluorescein angiography can demonstrate vascular pattern of the tumour lesion.[5]

Differential diagnosis

- Iris nevi
- Iris cyst
- Leiomyoma
- Metastasis
- Juvenile xanthogranuloma[5]

Benign versus malignant iris tumours. Distinguishing features of benign versus malignant tumours are summarized in Table 13.1.

Treatment

Once the diagnosis of melanoma is established either clinically or with biopsy the management is limited to preserving maximum visual function.

1. *Sectoral iridectomy* is done for suspicious lesions. This involves removing the tumour and part of the normal iris. If the tumour is the near the iris root, then part of the ciliary body should also be considered. The complications include glare, hyphema, cataract, infection and IOP fluctuation.

2. *Iridocyclectomy or ophthalmic plaque radiation therapy* is employed for lesions extending to the ciliary body. Radiotherapy has a limited

Table 13.1 *Clinical distinguishing features between benign and malignant tumours*

Feature	Benign	Malignant
Elevation	Flat or slight elevation	Nodular
Number	One or more lesions	Solitary
Laterality	Unilateral/bilateral	Unilateral
Size	< 3 mm	> 3 mm
Growth	No	Yes
Vascularisation	No	Yes
Ectropion uvea	No	Yes
Iris infiltration	No	Yes
Pupillary distortion	No	Yes
Cataract	No	Yes
Sentinel vessels	No	Yes
Glaucoma	No	Yes

role in iris melanoma for the greater likelihood of impairing the visual function. In monocular or patients unwilling for enucleation, plaque therapy is considered.

3. *Enucleation* is done for diffuse tumours with intractable glaucoma and if the tumour involves more than 6 clock hours.[2, 5]

Prognosis

The prognosis of iris melanomas is generally good with spindle cell type histology with no metastasis. The rate of metastasis varies from 2.3 to 5% by 10 years.

IRIS METASTASIS

Iris metastasis accounts for 9% of the intraocular locations for metastatic tumours and the prognosis of survival with anterior uveal metastasis is usually poor.

Origin for metastasis

Common origin for metastasis is the breast in women and lungs in men. Other less common sites include gastrointestinal tract, kidney, thyroid, prostrate and testes.

Clinical presentation

• Metastasis is multifocal and bilateral which can be associated with concurrent brain and pulmonary metastasis.
• Metastasis typically presents as pink or yellow solitary or multifocal tumours.

• Metastasis can also present as hyphema, anterior uveitis or a psuedohypopyon.

Diagnosis

Ultrasonography. Diagnosis can be made by ultrasound/UBM which shows high internal reflectivity and irregular shapes.

Fine needle biopsy or incisional biopsy is done for confirming the diagnosis.

Treatment

• *Systemic chemotherapy and external beam radiation therapy* constitute the treatment for metastasis.
• *Enucleation and retrobulbar alcohol injection* are options for intractable painful blind eye.[5]

TUMOURS OF CILIARY BODY

Ciliary body tumours remain asymptomatic for a long period of time because of their peripheral location. Primary tumours of the ciliary epithelium are classified as congenital and acquired.

• *Congenital tumours* include: Glioneuroma and medulloepithelioma.
• *Acquired tumours* include Fuchs adenoma (psuedoepitheliomatous hyperplasia) and ciliary body non-pigmented, pigmented or mixed epithelial tumours: adenoma and adenocarcinoma.[5, 14]

TUMOURS OF CILIARY EPITHELIUM

CONGENITAL TUMOURS OF CILIARY BODY

Medulloepithelioma

Clinical features

It is an embryonal neoplasm arising from the primitive medullary epithelium or inner layer of optic cup and appears in the 1st deacde of life. Zimmerman classified it into teratoid and nonteratoid types. Both the types can be benign and malignant. There is no population based information on the incidence or prevalence of these tumours.[15]

Teratoid medulloepithelioma has hetroplastic appendages like cartilage, skeletal muscle and brain tissue.

Non-teratoid medulloepithelioma (diktyoma) is proliferation of cells of the medullary epithelium.

Symptoms. These tumours are slow growing tumours and are mostly overlooked due to the secondary complications and usually go undetected.[14]

Signs. Slit-lamp evaluation, they appear as irregular shaped, with smooth surface and grey to fleshy pink colour (Fig. 13.4). Visual loss may occur attributed to cataract formation (lens notch) and secondary glaucoma (neovascular glaucoma). It has a characteristic cyclitic membrane giving the apperance of PHPV.

Differential diagnosis is to be made from retinoblastoma and persistant hyperplastic primary vitreous. It can be distinguished, as it appears as a sheet of neoplastic membrane that migrated from the retina to the anterior vitreous.

Histopathology

Medulloepitheliomas are characterised by cords of primitive neuroepithelial cells that resemble the embryonic retina or neural tube surrounded by a loose mesenchymal tissue rich in hyaluronic acid. The teratoid medulloepithelioma is characterised by the presence of heteroplastic tissue, neuroblastic tissue.[16]

Diagnosis

Diagnosis is made from following features:

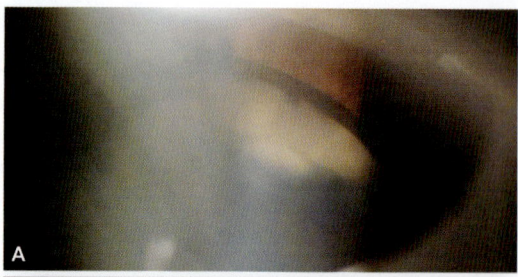
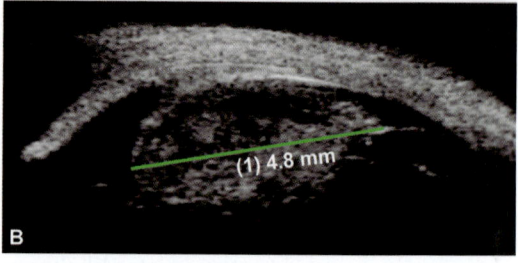

Fig. 13.4 *Medulloepithelioma: A 13-year-old girl presented with decreased vision and pain OS since 15 days. BCVA OS was 6/12. Examination revealed rubeosis iridis, ectropion uvea and cells in anterior vitreous cavity. IOP was 42 mm Hg. Gonioscopy revealed closed angles in all quadrants and greyish-yellow tumour originating from the ciliary body with a retrolental, cyclitic membrane (A). UBM confirmed a ciliary body tumour 4.8 × 3.6 × 2.4 mm with cystic spaces and retrolenticular membrane attached at the tumour apex (B). All the above features were suggestive of medulloepithelioma of ciliary body.*

- *Clinical evaluations.* MRI and ultrasound have limited role in diagnosis.[15] The diagnosis of medulloepithelioma can be made best by clinical recognition in the 1st decade of life.

- *Ultrasonography.* They may present with cysts inside the tumour, chalky white opacities with calcification on USG.

- *Fine needle aspiration* biopsy plays an important role in the diagnosis of medulloepithelioma.

Treatment

- *Local resection of tumour* is considered if tumour is small, well circumscribed (< 3 clock hours), as initial management but has high recurrence rate.

- *Iridocyclectomy* may be enough, if fortunately tumour is detected early.

- *Enucleation* is indicated, if the tumour has a friable apperance or there is adjacent free floating cyst.[15, 16]

ACQUIRED TUMOURS OF CILIARY BODY

Adenoma and adenocarcinoma of ciliary body

Acquired ciliary body tumours may arise from pigmented and non-pigmented ciliary epithelium. They are divided into benign (adenoma) and malignant (adenocarcinoma).

Clinical presentation

- *Clinical onset* occurs in adulthood (5th decde), with no sex predilection.
- *Patients remain either asymptomatic or present with* painless loss of vision, with a white to tan-coloured, irregular, multilobular mass. The patient can present with anterior chamber flare and cells, focal cataract, or subluxated lens.
- *Sentinel vessel* can occur in episceral tissue over the tumour.

Histopathology

Histopathologically, acquied tumours are categorised as: pseudoadenomatous, hyperplasia, adenoma, adenocarcinoma. The latter two are further classified as solid, papillary and pleomorphic.

Differential diagnosis

The tumour needs to be differentiated from melanoma of ciliary body, medulloepithelioma, adenoma/adenocarcinoma, leiomyoma, neurilemmoma, metastatic carcinoma and granuloma.

Tumour of non-pigmented epithelium of ciliary body occurrs internal to the pigment epithelium whereas a melanoma is located external to pigment epithelium and is pigmented with a smooth surface and mushroom-shaped appeerence.[17]

Medulloepithelioma is a congenital tumour and tends to be more cystic with associated lens notch, iris neovascularisation and persistent primary vitreous.

Diagnosis can be ascertained by transillumination as the tumour transmits light well, whereas melanoma blocks it. On ultrasound, the tumour shows abrupt elevation, acoustic solidity and high internal reflectivity.

Treatment includes local resection and enucleation.[16]

Leiomyoma occurs in younger patients and has a smooth surface and is less likely to cause cells in the vitreous.

Metastatic carcinoma will have a postive history of tumour elsewhere.

Granuloma of ciliary body is associated with severe uveal inflammation.

Note. Magnetic resonance imaging offers limited knowledge at diffrentiating adenoma from melanoma due to simlar imaging features.[5, 16, 17]

MELANOCYTIC TUMOURS OF CILIARY BODY

MELANOMA OF CILIARY BODY

Ciliary body melanomas are diagnosed at a later stage due to their location behind the iris. The age of presentation is in the 6th and 7th decade, with no sectoral preponderance.[5, 18]

Predictive factors of malignancy can be analyzed as direct and indirect signs (Table 13.2).

Histology

Ciliary body melanoma is divided in four histopathological subtypes by Modified Callender classification for uveal melanoma— Spindle A and B type melanoma, mixed cell melanoma, epithelioid cell melanoma and necrotic melanoma.

Type A spindle cells present small, fusiform nuclei with rare mitoses. The chromatin distribution follows the axis of the nuclei.

Type B spindle cells are a little bigger, more pleomorphic, with prominent nucleoli and mitotic activity.

The Spindle A and B type have the best prognosis and epitheloid and necrotic have unfavorable prognosis.

Epithelioid cell melanomas are the ones with the most unfavourable prognosis. Their cells present intense nuclear pleomorphism, with frequent mitoses and an anaplastic appearance.

Table 13.2 *Direct and indirect predictive signs of malignancy in ciliary body tumours*

Direct signs	Indirect signs
a. Unilateral solitary lesion	a. Dilation of episcleral vessels in the same quadrant as the tumour
b. Height greater than or equal to 3 mm, with or without pigment	b. Extrascleral extension
	c. Anterior uveitis
c. Pre-clinical presence of vascularisation	d. Presence of new vessels in the iris
d. Pigment dispersion	e. Infiltration of iris (with or without narrowing the angle)
e. Evidence of growth	f. Dyscoria
	g. Uveal ectropion
	h. Sectoral cataract
	i. Lens subluxation (lenticular astigmatism)
	j. Pigment dispersion and retinal detachment.

Immunohistochemically, ocular melanoma is reactive for S-100 protein, HMB-45, vimentin and different keratins with low molecular weight.

Genetic factors implicated in the triggering factors of melanoma are GNAQ, GNA11 in the 29 codon (the inactivation of INK4A, CDKN2a, CDKN1b, CCND1) of p53 gene. Other genetic changes are the monosomy 3-BAP gene (BRCA1 associated protein 1 or ubiquitin carboxyl-terminal hydrolase), frequently found in melanoma patients, as well as the duplication of long arm of 8th chromosome.[1]

Clinical evaluation

Clinical evaluation should include a detailed history of cancer, slit-lamp evaluation, indirect ophthalmoscopy, photodocumentation, transillumination, ultrasonography, CT/MRI, liver evaluation to rule out metastasis.

Treatment

The treatment protocol depends upon the tumour size, extent of intraocular involvement, status of the other eye, and general health of the patient.

1. *Plaque brachytherapy.* It is the widely accepted treatment for medium-sized tumours (thickness >3 to 5 mm, and greatest dimension >10–15 mm), using radioisotope I^{125} with an approximate dose of 40–45cGy/hr to the apex. The complications include radiation cataract, neovascular glaucoma, vitreous haemorrhage, retinal detachment and recurrence of tumour.[19]

2. *External beam radiation* is used for medium-sized tumours by irradiation with protons and helium ions. Radio-opaque tantalum rings are sutured to the sclera as a reference marker, the irradiation causes vascular damage and tumour necrosis. The complications include radiational cataract, dry eye, radiational retinopathy and neovascular glaucoma.

3. *Block excision or sclerouvectomy* is indicated when tumour is circumscribed, with no vitreous seeding and involvement is less than 5 o' clock hours of circumference. It involves full thickness excision, with in-block removal of ciliary body, cornea, iris, sclera with 2–3 mm margin of healthy tissue followed by grafting of banked sclera.[20, 21]

4. *Laser treatment* using laser photocoagulation and transpupillary thermotherapy is useful in small-sized tumours (size <3 mm) closer to macular area but are less valuable in ciliary body melanomas.

5. *Enucleation* is reserved for advanced cases (tumour size >18 mm in diameter and thickness >10 mm) or when other therapies have failed. Extreme caution is taken to minimise the amount of manipulation.

6. *Orbital exenteration* is done on rare occasions when the tumour has extrascleral spread into the orbit. This is done with an eyelid sparing technique which allows better healing and cosmetic appearance.

7. *Systemic therapy* is used to minimise the metastasis and includes intrahepatic artery delivery of chemotherapy, immunotherapy and intravenous chemotherapy.

8. *Future management techniques* will involve better and earlier tumour detection modalities and increased efficiency of focal ocular therapy and early cytogenetic evaluation specific for the tumour.[5, 18–22]

TUMOURS OF CHOROID

PRIMARY TUMOURS OF CHOROID

BENIGN PRIMARY TUMOURS

CHOROIDAL NEVI

These are the benign melanocytic lesions of posterior uvea (Fig. 13.5). The prevalence varies from 4.6–7.9% in Caucasians. The nevi are found in 6% of the white population with no specific sex predilection.[24] They are extremely rare in children.

Clinical features

They are usually asymptomatic, and are observed on routine dilated fundus evaluation. On clinical evaluation, choroidal nevi have clearly defined margins, flat or slightly elevated and remain stable in size and show a slow growth of about 0.5 mm over many years.

Accompanying features. These may be accompanied by other features such as overlying drusens, retinal pigment epithelial atrophy, hyperplasia or fibrous metaplasia.[23]

Risk of malignant transformation is rare, with an annual rate of 1 in 8,845. The rate of transformation increases with increasing age.

Management

The management of choroidal nevi requires close follow-up and routine evaluation. With lesions showing none of the risk factors, there is a 3% chance of growth at 5 years, if one of the risk factors is present, there is a 38% chance of growth and lesions having more than 3 risk factors have 50% chances of growth.

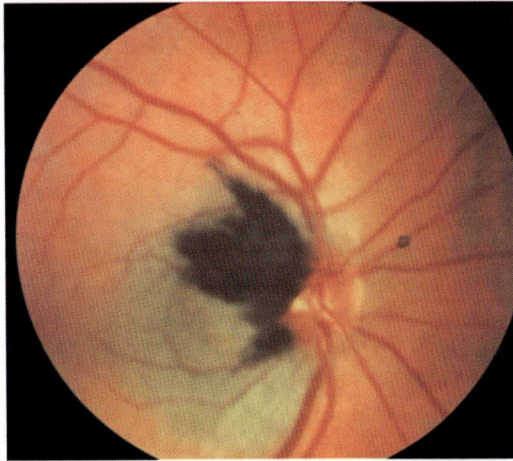

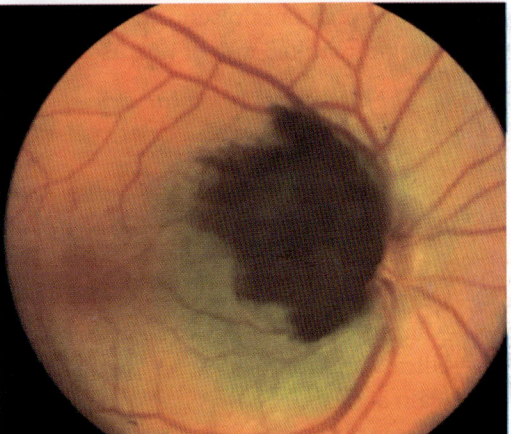

Fig. 13.5 *Melanocytoma of optic disc. Colour fundus photograph of right eye: A, showing a brown-black tumour over the optic disk; B, that had rapid growth suggestive of malignant transformation (right) (Courtesy: Jerry A Shields, MD)*

Lesions size <2 mm

Lesions size <2 mm, should be observed and followed regularly.

Lesions size >2 mm

In lesions > 2 mm, the management depends on the basis of associated risk factors.

During the 1st year, they should be followed twice year and after that annually.

Risk of ultraviolet exposure should be minimised with proper eyeglasses.

Dilated fundus evaluation and nevus photograph should be taken on subsequent visits.[24]

Distinguishing between a nevi and melanoma of the choroid is difficult and a thorough evaluation and keeping the risk factors in mind aids in early diagnosis and management of melanomas.

Mnemonic TFSOM (To find small ocular melanoma) for an early diagnosis was proposed by Shields et al in 1995 to analyze and detect the risk factors for malignant transformation of small melanocytic choroidal lesions on routine fundoscopic evaluation, the TFOSM stands for:

- T—Thickness greater than 2 mm
- F—Subretinal fluid
- S—Symptoms
- O—Orange pigment present
- M—Margin within 3 mm of the disc

Shields et al further modified the mnemonic to TFOSMHHD (To find small ocular melanoma using helpful hints daily)

- T— Thickness greater than 2 mm
- F—Subretinal fluid
- S—Symptoms
- O—Orange pigment present
- M—Margin within 3 mm of the disc
- H—Ultrasound hollowness
- H—Halo absent
- D—Drusen absent[25]

MELANOCYTOMA

Clinical features. Melanocytoma (magnocellular nevus) is a unilateral, benign tumour, most commonly affecting the optic disc and characterized by small, mildly elevated, pigmented lesion with peripapillary extension (Fig. 13.6).

These are visually asymptomatic but regular dilated fundus evaluation followed by disc photograph, ultrasound (tumour dimensions), and visual field evaluation should be done to rule out tumour growth.

Histological features. They are composed of intensely pigmented, round or oval nevus cells with benign features and copious quantity of cytoplasm.

Visual field defect is usually an enlarged blind spot which is visually asymptomatic in a large majority of patients.

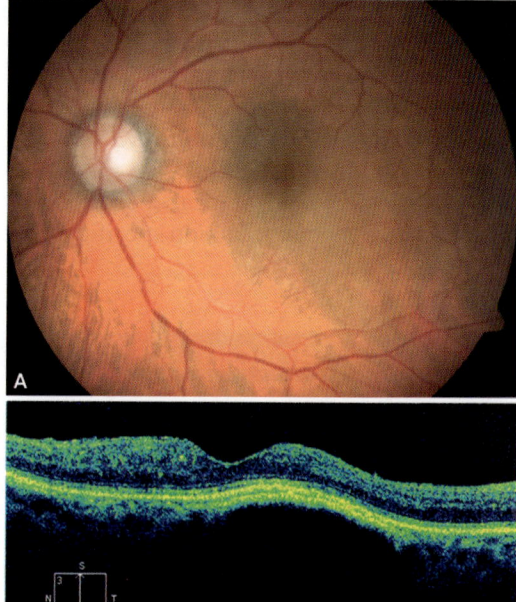

Fig. 13.6 *Choroidal naevus: A, Colour fundus photograph of left eye reveals a dark, minimally elevated subretinal lesion over the macula; B, Corresponding scan with EDI-OCT show slightly elevated mass in outer choroid, compressing choriocapillaris inward.*

Risk factor for vision loss is due to retinal extension of melanocytoma, subretinal fluid, retinal vascular occlusion, spontaneous tumour necrosis.

Risk of malignant transformations. There is a 1–2 risk of malignant transformation and should arouse suspicion, if the tumour size and thickness are increasing on subsequent follow-up.[2,5]

CHOROIDAL HAEMANGIOMA

Choroidal haemangioma occurs in two forms:
- Circumscribed
- Diffuse

Circumscribed choroidal haemangioma

Circumscribed choroidal haemangioma presents as a raised, dome-shaped, salmon pink swelling usually situated at the posterior pale of the eye. Overlying retina may show serous detachment cystoid degeneration and pigment epithelial moltering. The involvement of macula results in blurred vision and metamorphosis. Fluorescein angiography is usually diagnostic.

Diffuse choroidal haemangioma

Diffuse choroidal haemangioma usually occurs in association with Sturge-Weber syndrome. As presents diffuse red discolouration of the fundus (Tomato Ketchup fundus).

Complication. It may be complicated by secondary glaucoma and exudative retinal detachment.

Treatment consists of laser photocoagulation.

CHOROIDAL OSTEOMA

Choroidal osteoma is a rare benign tumour of the choroid. It typically affects young women suggesting the probable role of endocrinal or hormonal factors in its development.

Clinical features

Symptoms. It may be asymptomatic and detected on routine examination or may present with painless progressive loss of vision and/or micropsia and distortion of vision.

Signs. It may be unilateral (60–70% cases) or bilateral (20–30%) on fundus examination. It appears as an elevated, gellourish (justapofrillars) orange lesion located near cystic papillary or around the optic disc (circumpapillary) bilateral (20–30%) cases.

Margins of the lesion are typically well defined and smooth.

Associated features include:
- Progressive retinal degeneration overlying the lesion,
- Secondary macular choroidal degeneration, and
- Spontaneous decalcification in some cases.

Systemic associations include hyperparathyroidism with secondary alterations of serum calcium and phosphorus levels in few cases.

Pathologically, the choroidal osteoma is composed of mature bone that replaces the full thickness choroid in the involved area.

Diagnosis and investigations

Clinical diagnosis is suspected from the typical features described above.

Ultrasonography shows a bone density tumour characterised by highly reflective plate-like lesion that shadow the orbit.

Computed tomography reveals thickened posterior ocular wall which is isodense with rest of the skeletal bones.

Fluorescein angiography typically shows patchy early hyperfluorescence and late diffuse hyperfluorescence of choroidal lesion.

Indocyanine green angiography reveals generalised hyperfluorescence of the lesion with superimposed hyperfluorescence blood vessels in the early phase and diffuse hyperfluorescence in later phase.

Differential diagnosis

Differential diagnosis of choroidal osteoma includes:
- Circumscribed choroidal haemangioma
- Metastatic carcinoma of choroid
- Amelanotic choroidal melanoma
- Sclerochoroidal calcification
- Calcification in a phthisical eye

Treatment

Treatment to stop tumour growth consists of:
- Photodynamic therapy

Treatment options for choroidal neovascularisation associated with choroidal osteoma include:
- Laser photocoagulation
- Photodynamic therapy
- Intravitreal injection of anti-UEGF

MALIGNANT PRIMARY TUMOURS OF CHOROID

CHOROIDAL MELANOMA

Choroidal melanoma is the most common primary intraocular tumour of adults usually seen between 40 and 70 years of age. It can grow in diameter and height with further metastasis and cause death.

Incidence of choroidal melanomas is 6 in 1 million population in the United States and 7.5 cases/million in Denmark and Scandinavian countries.

Race. The melanoma most commonly affects Caucasians, followed by Hispanics and Asians, and least commonly, black population.

Age and sex. The median age of diagnosis is 56 years with a slight male preponderance.

Histology

The melanoma consists of four types of cells according to Callendar classification:

Epitheloid cells have abundant glassy cytoplasm, a well-defined border an abundant extracellular space, with large nucleoli and eosinophilic within the centre of nucleus.

Spindle cells are smaller, less pleomorphic, smaller nuclei which are stacked tightly in the extracellular space. Spindle cells are of two types:
- *Type A*—narrow nucleus with fine chromatin and indistinguishable nucleolus.
- *Type B* has rounder nucleus, thicker chromatin and prominent nucleoli.

Note. The most common form is the mixed epitheloid-spindle cell type (48%), spindle B cell type (32%), followed by necrotic (8%), spindle A (6%), and epitheloid (2%).[27]

Clinical features

Clinical presentation is usually symptomatic with complaints of decreased vision, photopsia and visual field defects. Symptoms of pain are suggestive of either inflammation or massive extraocular extension or neovascular glaucoma. Previous history of malignancy should be elicited. Choroidal melanomas are routinely classified as:
- *Small* (<10 mm in diameter and <3 mm in height)
- *Medium* (10 to 15 mm in diameter and 3 to 5 mm in height)
- *Large* (>15 mm in diameter and >5 mm in height)

Clinical appearance of the melanoma (Fig. 13.7) is a pigmented dome-shaped or collar button lesion with surrounding exudative retinal detachment. The melanoma may present as amelanotic lesion with lipofuscin pigmentation.

B-scan ultrasonography shows an acoustic silent zone within the melanoma, choroidal excavation and shadowing in the orbit (Fig. 13.7B). There is a 95% accuracy for tumours more than 3 mm in thickness on ultrasound.[7]

Fluorescein angiography is of limited value, but large melanomas show double circulation inside the tumour, extensive leakage with late staining of the lesion with multiple pinpoint leaks.

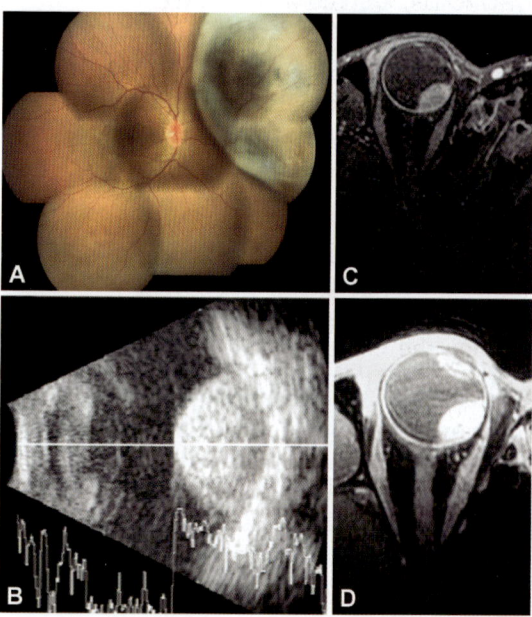

Fig. 13.7 *Choroidal melanoma: A 26-year-old male presented with metamorphopsia since 2 weeks: A, Fundus examination of right eye revealed a large, dome-shaped, partially pigmented subretinal mass lesion of size 18 × 12 × 10 mm in superonasal quadrant with shallow retinal detachment; B, Ultrasound revealed a dome-shaped retinochoroidal mass in superonasal quadrant with high surface reflectivity and decremental internal reflectivity along with choroidal excavation; C, MRI (brain + orbit) showed a decremental internal reflectivity along with choroidal excavation. MRI (brain + orbit) showed a well-circumscribed choroidal lesion (C), hyperintense on T1W1 and hypo-intense on T2W1. There was no extraocular extension; D, Post-contrast study revealed moderate contrast enhancement.*

Autofluorescence is also present due to the clumped orange pigments.

Indocyanine green angiography shows micro-circulation within the melanoma.[1,7]

Optical coherence tomography shows serous retinal detachment, retinal oedema, debris on the back of retina, with intact photoreceptor.[26, 28]

MRI brain and orbit shows decremental internal reflectivity along with choroidal excavation (Fig. 13.7C). Post-contrast study reveal moderate enhancement (Fig. 13.7D).

Differential diagnosis

The lesions mimicking melanoma are choroidal metastasis, choroidal haemangioma, benign lymphoid tumour, choroidal haemangioperi-cytoma, choroidal leiomyoma, extramacular disciform lesion, retinal pigment epithelial hypertrophy, haemorrhagic retinal detachment [from peripheral polypoidal choroidal vasculopathy (PCV) or peripheral exudative haemorrhagic chorioretinopathy (PEHCR)].[27]

Management

The management depends upon multiple factors, the visual acuity of the affected eye, visual acuity of the contralateral eye, tumour size, location, ocular structures involved and associated metastasis.

1. *Small tumours* can be treated with trans-pupillary thermotherapy, photodynamic therapy, plaque radiation therapy, external beam charged particle radiation therapy, and local tumour resection.

2. *Peripapillary tumours.* They are treated using notched radiation plaques that subtend the nerve head up to 180°. If it is more than 180°, then enucleation is better option.

3. *Medium-large-sized tumours.* The treatment options include I^{125} plaque brachytherapy, external beam charged particles radiation therapy and lamellar sclerouvectomy.

4. *Enucleation* is limited to advanced stage melanomas and eyes with intractable glaucoma with no visual prognosis.

5. *Metastasis* is treated with palliative systemic chemotherapy.

Prognosis and prognostic indicators in uveal melanoma

Prognosis

Even with the advancement in diagnosis and treatment, the prognosis and survival as determined in the collaborative ocular melanoma study (COMS) at 5, 10 and 15 years of study are 65%, 52% and 46%, respectively. The metastasis dissemination occurs by haemato-genous route and the common sites of metastasis are liver (90%), lung (24%), and bone (16%). Liver metastasis decreases the median survival time ranging from 2.2 to 12.5 months. [29-31]

Prognostic indicators

1. *Clinical features*
- Older age
- Male gender
- Large tumour basal diameter
- Thicker tumour
- Ciliary body tumour location
- Diffuse tumour configuration
- Associated with oculodermal melanocytosis
- Advanced stage as per AJCC (American Joint Committee on Cancer) grading

2. *Histopathologic features*
- Epitheloid cytology
- High mitotic activity
- High mean diameter of 10 largest nucleoli
- High microvacular density
- Microvascular loops
- Tumour infiltrating lymphocytes/macrophages
- High expression of insulin-like growth factor-I, HLA I and II

3. *Cytogenetic factors*
- Chromosome 3 loss
- Chromosome 8q gain or 8p loss
- Chromosome 1q loss
- Chromosome 6q loss

4. *Transcriptomic feature*
- Gene expression profile class 2[1]

RETICULUM CELL SARCOMA

Reticulum cell sarcoma, resembling histiocytes in histology, may arise within reticulo-endothelial system, central nervous system and rarely from the choroid.

Clinical features

Symptoms include:

- Decreased visual acuity,
- Floater, and
- Photopsia

Signs include:

- *Anterior segment* may show mild reaction without keratic precipitates.
- *Vitreous cell and floaters* refractory to steroid therapy constitute typical finding.
- *Fundus* examanitions may reveal lesions similar to subretinal infiltrates characterised by yellow-white fluffy outlines.

Differential diagnosis and diagnostic tests

Differential diagnosis needs to be made from the leukaemic infiltrate.

Vitreous biopsy is useful in tissue diagnosis. Tumour cells are large.

Treatment

Radiotherapy is quite effective and can lead to improvement in the visual acuity.

SECONDARY TUMOURS OF CHOROID

METASTATIC CARCINOMAS OF CHOROID

Carcinomas from elsewhere in the body may metastasise in uveal tissue—most commonly in choroid (90%) followed by iris and ciliary body (10%). The metastatic carcinomas constitute the most common intraocular malignant neoplasm. Uniocular involvement is seen in 80% and bilateral in 20% of cases.

Primary tumours to metastasise in the uveal tissue include:

Common primary tumours:

- Carcinoma breast, and
- Carcinoma of bronchus

Less common primary malignant tumours:

- Tumour of GIT
- Kidney tumour (renal cell carcinoma)
- Skin melanoma
- Follicular carcinoma of thyroid

Clinical features

Symptoms: The metastatic may be asymptomatic and defected on routine examination of fundus or patients may present with defective vision. Pain is very rare feature of advanced tumours presenting in glaucomatous stage.

Signs. Fundus examination reveals:

- *Golden yellow to creamy white oval lesion,* located at the posterior pole is a feature of metastatic carcinomas. Deposits are multifocal in about 30% and involves both eyes in about 20% cases.
- *Intensely melanotic* lesions are seen in metastatic skin melanoma.
- *Exudative retinal detachment,* that is out of proportion to the size of tumour, is after associated with metastatic carcinoma.

Investigation

1. *Fluorescein angiography (FA)* shows relative hypofluorescence in the early phase and diffuse hypofluorescence of the lesion in the late trauma. But, in contrast to choroidal melanoma, a dual circulation is not seen.

2. *Indocyanine green angiography (ICGA)* is useful in detecting subtle metastatic lesions seen on FA. ICGA shows hypofluorescence throughout the study.

3. *B-scan ultrasonography* is useful in the presence of exudative retinal detachment. Placoid tumour shows diffuse choroidal thickening. The dome-shaped metastatic lesions are sono-reflective (bright) as compared to choroidal melanomas which are sonolucent internally.

4. *Computed tomography (CT) and magnetic resonance imaging (MRI)* can demonstrate large metastatic tumours; these studies do not provide any reliable differential diagnostic information.

5. *Fine needle biopsy (FNB)* or biopsy using 25 gauge vitrectomy system is a reliable technique for establishing diagnosis in selected cases.

Systemic evaluation and investigations

Once metastatic carcinoma of choroid diagnosed, systemic evaluation and investigation should be carried out to detect unknown primary and other secondary tumours. These may include:

- Thorough history and physical examination including examination of breasts in females, palpation of abdomen and palpation of regional lymph nodes.
- Mammography in females to detect subtle primary tumour.
- Chest X-rays/CT scan and sputum analysis to delineate carcinoma of bronchi
- Whole body bone survey or scan PET/CT scan is very useful in detecting subtle primary and secondary tumours
- Faecal occult blood for GIT carcinoma
- Urine RBCs for renal cell carcinoma

Treatment

1. *Systemic chemotherapy or hormonal therapy* may be considered as first choice when other sites are detected to have secondaries; and the vision is not severely affected.

2. *Radiotherapy* with external beam or brachytherapy is very effective for choroidal metastasis and the vision is frequently stabilised. Mostly systemic therapy is also considered with radiotherapy. The treatment regime depends upon the type, extent, size and location of intraocular tumour.

3. *Transpupillary thermotherapy (TTT)* is useful for small tumour with minimal subretinal fluid.

INTRAOCULAR LYMPHOMAS

Intraocular lymphomas include:

Primary intraocular lymphomas (PIOL) are associated with following risk factors:

- Older age group,
- Female sex, and
- Immunosuppression (primary or acquired)

Metastatic tumour from visceral lymphomas.

- *Distant metasis* from carcinoma of breast or lung in late stage.
- *Local spread* from intraocular tumours such as retinoblastoma and uveal melanoma.

Note. For details see Chapter 8, page 359.

REFERENCES

1. Kaliki S, et al. Uveal melanoma: Estimating prognosis. Indian J Ophthalmol 2015;63:93–102.

2. Shields CL, et al. Review of cystic and solid tumors of iris. Oman J Ophthalmol 2013; 6:159–64.

3. Sheilds CL, et al. Clinical survey of 3680 iris tumor based on the patient age of presentation. Ophthalmology 2012; 119:407–14.

4. Biswas J, Krishnakumar S, Shanmugan S. Clinical and histopathological characteristics of uveal melanoma in Asian Indians. A study of 103 patients. Indian J Ophthalmol 2004;51(1):41–4.

5. Margio FA, et al. Anterior segment tumors current concept and innovations. Surv Ophthalmol 2003; 48:569–93

6. Henry HL, et al. Nevus of Ota: Clinical aspects and management. Sinmed, 2003;2920:89–98

7. Cronemberger S, et al. Nevus of Ota: Clinical-ophthalmological findings. Rev Bras Ofthalmol 2011;70(5):278–83.

8. Patidar OP, et al. Nevus of ota is a rare nevus and Q-switched laser is the best available option for successful treatment. Indian Journal of Clinical practice 2013; 24(4):338–7.

9. Lois N, et al. Primary cysts of the iris pigment epithelium. Clinical features and natural course in 234 patients. Ophthalmology 1998; 105(10):1879–85.

10. Shields JA. Primary cysts of the iris. Trans Am Ophthalmol Soc 1981; 79:771–809.

11. Grutzmacher R, et al. Congential cyst. Br J Ophthalmol 1987;71:227–34.

12. Conway MR, et al. Ultrasound biomicroscopy: role in diagnosis and management in 130 consecutive patients evaluated for anterior segment tumors. Br J Ophthalmol 2005; 89:950–55.

13. Myers TD, JR smith etal. Iris nodules with infectious uveitis. Br J Ophthalmol. 2002;86(9): 969–74.

14. Romanowska-Dixon B. et al. Adenoma of iris and ciliary body. Case report. Pol J Pathol 54,3, 187–190

15. Shields AJ, et al. Congenital neoplasms of non-pigmented ciliary epithelium (medulloepithelioma).1996,103(12),2007–16.

16. Saunders T, et al. Intraocular medulloepithelioma. Arch Pathol Lab Med. 2012;136.

17. Shields JA, et al. Acquired neoplasms of the non pigmented ciliary epithelium. Ophthalmology 1996;103:2007–16.

18. Costache M, et al. Ciliary body melanoma- a particularly rare type ocular tumor. Case report and general considerations. MAEDICA. 2013; 8(4):360–4.

19. Krema H, et al. Management of ciliary body melanoma with iodine-125 plaque brachytherapy. Can J Ophthalmol 2009;44:395–400.
20. Mclean IW, et al. Choroidal-ciliary body melanoma. Ophthalmology 1995;102:1060–4.
21. Garfield OH, et al. Block excision of tumors of the anterior uvea. Ophthalmology 1996; 103; 2017–28.
22. Lee CS, et al. Partial lamellar sclerouvectomy of ciliary body tumors in a kroean population. Am J Ophthalmol. 2013;156:36–42.
23. Shields CL, et al. Choroidal nevus transformation into melanoma. Arch Ophthalmol 2009;127(8): 981–7.
24. Singh AD, et al. Estimating the risk of malignant transformation of a choroidal nevus. Ophthalmology 2005;112:1784–9.
25. Rishi P, Koundanya W, Shields CL. Using risk factors for detection and prognosistication of uveal melanoma. Indian J Ophthalmol 2015; 63:110–6.
26. Singh P, et al. Choroidal melanoma. Oman Journal of Ophthalmology 2012;5(1):3–9.
27. Miyamoto C, et al. Uveal melanoma: Ocular and systemic disease. Saudi J Ophthalmol 2012: 26:145–9.
28. Say EA, Shah SU, Ferenczy S, Shields CL. Optical coherence tomography of retinal and choroidal tumors. J Ophthalmol 2012.
29. Shields JA, et al. Management of posterior uveal melanoma. Past, present and future. Ophthalmology 2015;122:414–28.
30. Robertson DM. Perspective changing concepts in management of choroidal melanoma. Am J Ophthalmol 2003;136:161–70.
31. Jovanovic P, et al. Ocular melanoma: an overview of current status. Int J clin Exp Pathol 2013;6:1230–44.

Part 2: | Disorders of Sclera

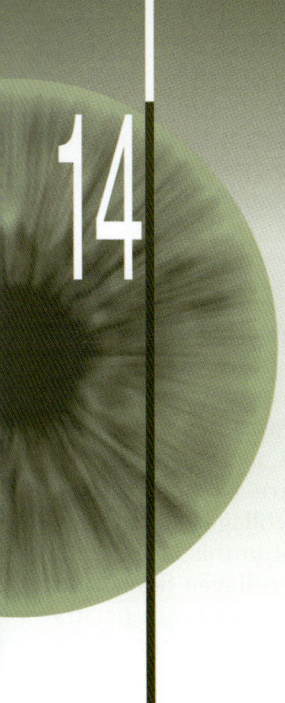

14

ANATOMY, DEVELOPMENT AND PHYSIOLOGY OF SCLERA

ANATOMY OF SCLERA
- Thickness of sclera
- Special regions of the sclera
- Scleral apertures
- Microscopic structure
- Nerve supply of the sclera

DEVELOPMENT OF SCLERA
- Changes in mesenchyme surrounding optic vesicle

- Formation of sclera

PHYSIOLOGICAL CONSIDERATIONS
- Biochemical composition
- Corneal lamellae versus scleral lamellae
- Swelling pressure, diffusion and bulk flow
- Tissue mechanics of sclera

ANATOMY OF SCLERA

The sclera forms the posterior opaque five-sixths part of the external fibrous tunic of the eyeball. Its whole outer surface is covered by Tenon's capsule and also by the bulbar conjunctiva in the anterior part. Its inner surface lies in contact with the choroid with a potential suprachoroidal space in between.

THICKNESS OF SCLERA

Thickness of the sclera varies considerably in different individuals and with age. The sclera is generally thinner in children than the adults and in females than the males.

Sclera is thickest posteriorly (1 mm) and gradually becomes thin when traced anteriorly. It is thinnest at the insertion of extraocular muscles (0.3 mm). Along with the muscle tendon, thickness becomes 0.6 mm. The thickness of the sclera at equator is about 0.4 to 0.6 mm and adjacent to the limbus it is about 0.8 mm.

SPECIAL REGIONS OF THE SCLERA

Scleral sulcus

It is an indentation (furrow) on the inner surface of the anterior most point of the sclera near the limbus. It houses the Schlemm's canal.

Scleral spur

It is a circular flang of the anterior most part of the sclera which lies deep to Schlemm's canal. It appears wedge-shaped in section and is known as "scleral spur". The corneoscleral part of trabecular meshwork extends from the scleral spur to Schwalbe's line. The meridional fibres of the ciliary muscle are attached to the scleral spur.

Lamina cribrosa

It is a sieve-like sclera from which the fibres of the optic nerve pass. When the intraocular pressure is increased for a prolonged period of time, such as in primary open-angle glaucoma, the lamina cribrosa gradually increases in posterior curvature.

SCLERAL APERTURES (EMISSARIA)

Sclera has three sets of apertures (Fig. 14.1).

1. Posterior apertures are situated around the optic nerve and transmit long and short ciliary nerves and vessels.

2. Middle apertures are situated 4–7 mm posterior to the equator. Through these pass four or more vortex veins (vena verticosae). The superior vortex veins are more posterior (7 mm) than the inferior veins (5–6 mm). The aperture which transmits the superior temporal veins lies close to the posterior edge of the insertion of superior oblique muscle.

3. Anterior apertures are situated 3–4 mm away from the limbus and transmit anterior ciliary vessels, perivascular lymphatics and the ciliary nerves.

MICROSCOPIC STRUCTURE

Histologically, sclera consists of following three layers (Fig. 14.2):

1. Episcleral tissue

It is a thin, dense vascularised layer of the connective tissue which covers the sclera proper.

Anteriorly, it becomes continuous with the Tenon's capsule. The capillary network present in the anterior part of the episclera becomes prominent during inflammation giving rise to ciliary flush.

2. Sclera proper

It is an avascular structure which consists of dense bundles of collagen fibres crossing each other in all directions. This arrangement makes the sclera opaque in contrast to cornea where the collagen bundles are arranged orderly. Mucopolysaccharides are present in the interfibrillar space of the collagen fibres. Few fibroblasts are also present in this layer. With advancing age, the scleral collagen fibres tend to become sclerosed and also there occurs deposition of lipids; consequently sclera becomes yellow.

3. Lamina fusca

It is the innermost part of sclera which blends with suprachoroidal and supraciliary lamina of the uveal tract. It is brownish in colour owing to the presence of pigment cells.

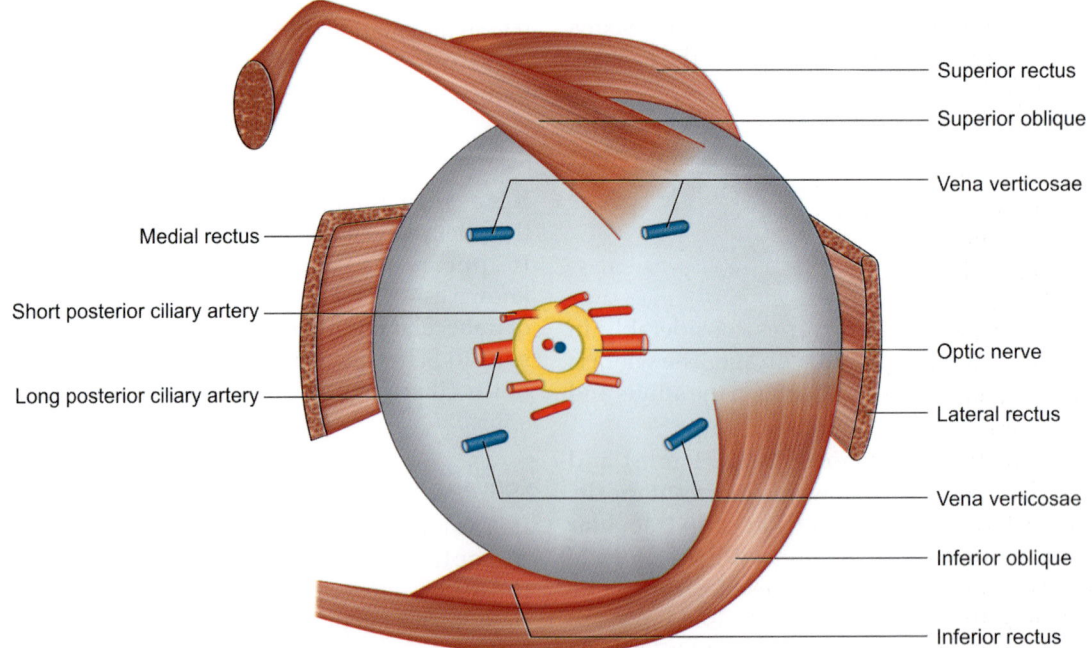

Fig. 14.1 *Posterior view of sclera showing apertures.*

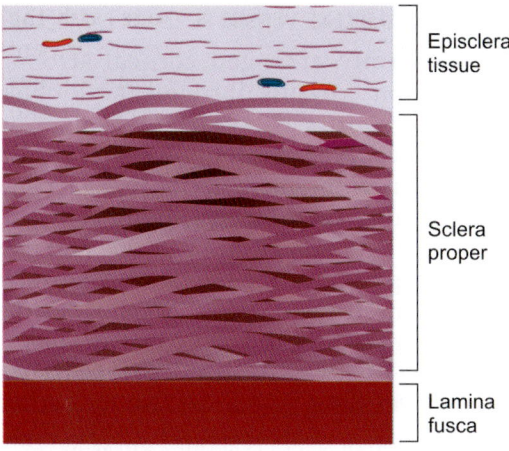

Episcleral tissue

Sclera proper

Lamina fusca

Fig. 14.2 *Microscopic structure of sclera.*

NERVE SUPPLY OF THE SCLERA

The sclera is supplied by branches from the long ciliary nerves anteriorly and short ciliary nerves behind the equator.

DEVELOPMENT OF SCLERA

CHANGES IN MESENCHYME SURROUNDING OPTIC VESICLE

The developing neural tube (from which central nervous system develops) is surrounded by mesenchyme. Mesenchyme is a loose tissue consisting of stellate, amoeboid mesenchymal cells embedded in a matrix rich in glycosamino-glycans.

Mesenchymal cells may be derived from serosal sources, namely mesoderm (dermatome or sclerotome component of the somite or lateral plate mesoderm) or neural crest. Thus this descriptive term mesenchyme does not imply an origin from any particular embryonic germ layer. The mesenchyme surrounding the neural tube subsequently condenses to form meninges. An extension of this mesenchyme also surrounds the optic vesicle, except at its apex, which is closely apposed to the surface ectoderm on the lateral side of the developing head. This mesenchyme may be derived from the cephalic neural crest and indeed from crest cells detaching from the outer surface of the optic vesicle itself. Later, this mesenchyme differentiates to form a superficial fibrous layer (corresponding to dura), which will form the sclera and cornea and a deeper vascular layer (corresponding to pia arachnoid) which will form stroma of uveal tissue (Fig. 14.3).

The fibrous layer of mesenchyme surrounding anterior part of optic cup forms the cornea.

In the posterior part of optic cup, the surrounding fibrous mesenchyme forms sclera and extraocular muscles, while the vascular layer forms the choroid and ciliary body.

FORMATION OF SCLERA

As mentioned above, sclera is developed from the mesenchymal cells surrounding the optic cup (corresponding to dura of CNS) (Figs 14.4 and 14.5). The mesenchymal cells are derived mainly from the neural crest. The process starts at the limbal-equatorial region (future site of extraocular muscle insertion) around 7th week of gestation and is completed by 5th month.

Formation of lamina cribrosa. By the third month of gestation, some undifferentiated mesenchymal cells have migrated between the nerve fibres in the optic nerve. These cells become oriented transversely and synthesize extracellular matrix materials to form the lamina cribrosa.

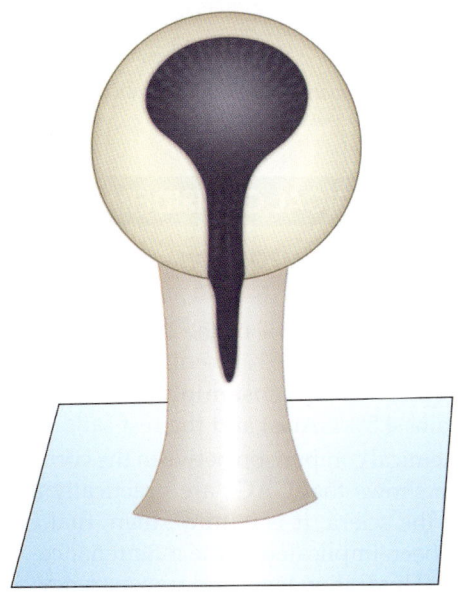

Fig. 14.3 *Optic cup and stalk seen from below to show the choroidal fissure.*

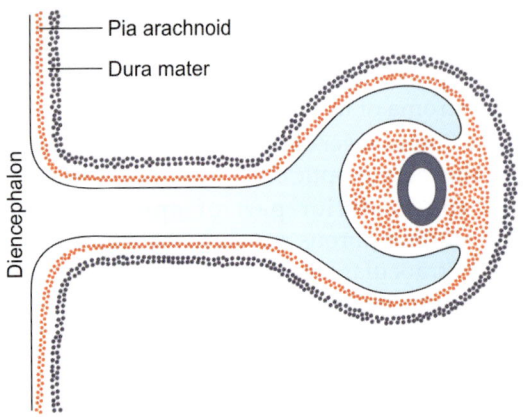

Fig. 14.4 *Developing optic cup surrounded by mesoderm.*

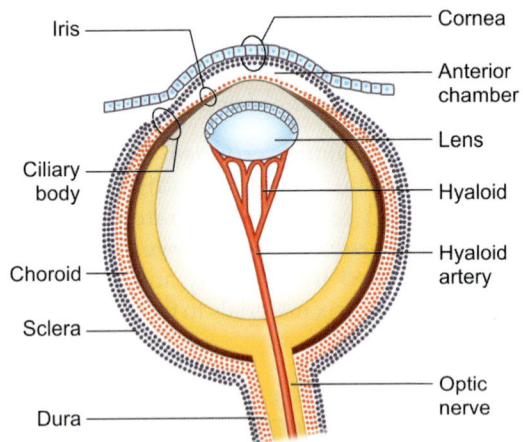

Fig. 14.5 *Derivation of various structures of the eyeball.*

PHYSIOLOGICAL CONSIDERATIONS

BIOCHEMICAL COMPOSITION

The water content of the sclera is about 70% compared to the 78% of the corneal stroma; of the solids about 75% is collagen, 10% other proteins, 10% glycosaminoglycans (cornea contains 4.5% GAGs) and the rest salts.

Chemical comparison between the cornea and sclera shows that GAGs are practically absent from the sclera. It is natural, then, that GAGs have been implicated in the maintenance of the corneal hydration level and transparency, since the sclera is not clear and reflects and scatters light under normal conditions.

CORNEAL LAMELLAE VERSUS SCLERAL LAMELLAE

The uniformly arranged corneal stromal lamellae, on crossing through the limbus, increasingly interweave (Fig. 14.6). The individual collagen fibrils of each lamella also change from their uniform 30 nm diameter and 60 nm centre to centre spacing in the cornea to wide variation in diameter (30 to 300 nm) and irregular spacing in the sclera. This peculiar arrangement of the lamellae accounts for the cornea being transparent and sclera opaque.

SWELLING PRESSURE, DIFFUSION AND BULK FLOW

The hydration of sclera is about 2 gm water/gm dry material near the limbus and corresponding swelling pressure is 10 to 17 mm Hg, while in the adjacent corneal stroma the hydration is 3.5 gm water/gm dry material and the swelling pressure is about 60 mm Hg. This difference is attributed to the lower GAG content of the sclera. The existence of difference in steady state swelling pressure in adjacent tissues indicates a constant flow of water from the sclera to the cornea.

Bulk fluid transport and the uveal effusion syndrome

Although most of the bulk transport of fluid out of the eye takes place through the anterior chamber drainage angle and/or uveoscleral meshwork, there is appreciable transretinal transport of fluid towards the choroids. Some of this is drained via the normal choroidal vessels but a proportion is drained directly transsclerally. The effect of this transscleral flow is to 'suction on' the retina to its adjoining RPE layer and maintain retinal apposition.

Fluid flowing across the sclera is absorbed by the matrix proteoglycans. Thus, the sclera is maintained in its normal state, by having proteoglycans with a low water binding capacity. In some conditions, such as the rare uveal effusion syndrome, and in non-ophthalmia, the sclera contains high levels of abnormal proteoglycans (PGs), especially dermatan sulphate containing PGs, which bind and trap large volumes of water. Thus the sclera thickens and may secondarily obstruct the choroidal venous drainage, causing further

Cornea   Sclera

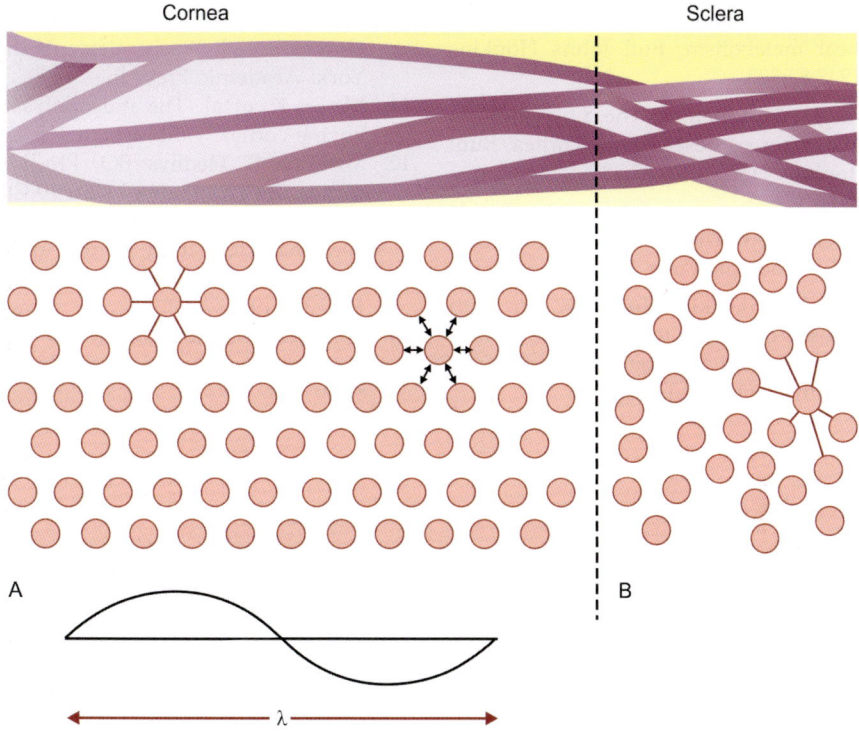

A   B

λ

Fig. 14.6 *Cross-section view showing regular arrangement of corneal fibrils as basis of corneal transparency (Maurice theory) (A) vis-à-vis irregular arrangement of sclera fibres (B).*

swelling and water retention. The disordered collagen/matrix structure in the uveal effusion syndrome has been demonstrated by the cuprolinic blue technique.

TISSUE MECHANICS OF SCLERA

The sclera is constantly under stress by the intraocular pressure. The pressure pushing outward is contained by the sclera, thereby providing a stable viscoelastic structure for the globe as a whole. Like most viscoelastic systems, the sclera will stretch proportionately more with initial elevations of intraocular pressure, and as the pressure increases, the resistance to further stretching also increases. Therefore, small increase in the intraocular volume at a low pressure causes a small increase of intraocular pressure, whereas similar small volume changes at high pressures will cause a much larger increase in intraocular pressure. This property of the sclera is known as *scleral rigidity*. This is an unfortunate term because most persons

associate the rigidity with resistance to bending rather than resistance to stretching. Therefore, the term *scleral distensibility* would be preferable to scleral rigidity.

BIBLIOGRAPHY

1. Allansmith MR, McClellan BH. Immunoglobulins in the human cornea. Am J Ophthalmol 1975; 80:124.

2. Collier E. The cornea. In: RA Moses, ed. Adler's Physiology of Eye: Clinical Application. St Louis: Mosby Co., 1975.

3. Davidson EA, Meyer K. Chondroitin, a new mucopolysaccharide. J Biol Chem 1954;211:605.

4. Dohlman CH. The function of the corneal epithelium in health and disease. Invest Ophthalmol 1971;10:375.

5. Freeman RD. Oxygen consumption by the component layers of the cornea. J Physiol (Lond) 1972;225:15-32.

6. Hermann H, Hickman F. Exploratory studies on corneal metabolism. Bull Johns Hopkins Hosp. 1948;82:225.

7. Hermann H, Hickman F. The utilization of ribose and other pentoses by the cornea. Bull. Johns Hopkins Hosp 1948;82:287.

8. Jakus M. The fine structure of the human cornea. In. Smelser G, ed. The Structure of the Eye, New York: Academic Press Inc. 1961,344.

9. Kwan M, NiimikoskiJ, Hunt TK. In vivo measurements of oxygen tension in the cornea, aqueous humor, and anterior lens of open eye. Invest Ophthalmol 1972;11:108–14.

10. Maurice DM, Riley MV. The cornea. In: CN Graymore, ed. Biochemistry of the Eye. New York: Academic Press Inc., 1970.

11. Meyer K, et al. The mucopolysaccharides of bovine cornea. J Biol Chem 1953;205:611.

12. Mishima S, Hedbys BO. Physiology of the cornea. Int Ophthalmol Clin 1968;8:527.

13. Piez KA, Weiss E, Lewis MS. The separation and characterization of the alpha and beta components of calf skin collagen. J Biol Chem 1960;235:1987.

14. Poise KA, Mandell RB. Critical oxygen tension at the corneal surface. Arch Ophthalmol 1970; 84:505–08.

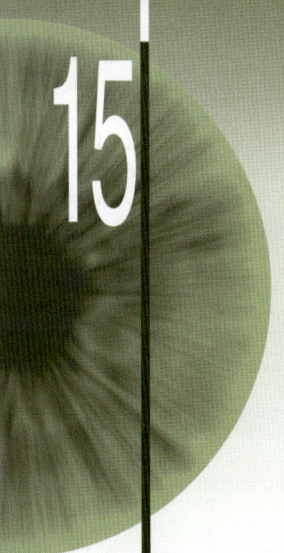

15

INFLAMMATIONS OF SCLERA

INTRODUCTION

Inflammation of episclera and sclera remain a diagnostic challenge to the ophthalmologists. Episcleritis and scleritis may represent the initial manifestation of an unsuspected systemic disease and can carry a prognostic message.

The classification system proposed by Watson and Hayreh is widely accepted. Broadly scleral inflammations can be divided into the episcleritis and scleritis. Both episcleritis and scleritis are recurrent inflammation. Though episcleritis is a benign, self-limiting disease, scleritis requires almost always systemic therapy. Scleritis can be divided into anterior and posterior scleritis. Anterior scleritis has been classified into four subgroups: diffuse, nodular, necrotising with inflammation, and necrotising

without inflammation. Necrotising scleritis without inflammation is also called sclero-malacia perforans (Fig. 15.1).

Since sclera is mainly dependent on episclera providing a response to an inflammatory stimulus, scleritis is almost always accompanied with overlying episcleritis. However, episcleritis is usually not associated with scleritis.

EPISCLERITIS

Episcleritis is benign, self-limiting but recurrent inflammation of the episclera, involving the overlying Tenon's capsule but not the underlying sclera.

Age and sex. It typically affects young adults, being twice as common in women than men.

449

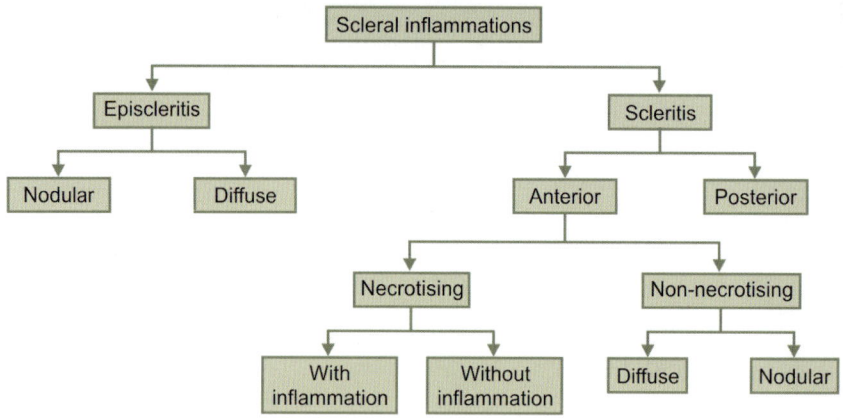

Fig. 15.1 *Watsen Hayrh's classification of inflammation of episcleral and scleral fissure.*

Laterality. More than one-third of patients have bilateral disease.

ETIOLOGY

1. *Idiopathic.* Exact etiology is not known in many cases.
2. *Systemic diseases* associated with episcleritis include gout, rosacea, psoriasis and connective tissue diseases such as rheumatoid arthritis, relapsing polychondritis, Cogan' syndrome, polyarteritis nodosa, etc.
3. *Hypersensitivity reaction* to endogenous tubercular or streptococcal toxins is also reported.
4. *Infectious episcleritis* may be caused by herpes zoster virus, syphilis, Lyme disease and tuberculosis.

PATHOLOGY

Histologically, there occurs localised lymphocytic infiltration of episcleral tissue associated with oedema and congestion of overlying Tenon's capsule and conjunctiva.

CLINICAL FEATURES

Symptoms

Episcleritis is characterised by redness, mild ocular discomfort described as gritty, burning or foreign body sensation. The redness typically persists for 24–72 hours and then resolves spontaneously. Very rarely, patients may experience more severe redness and mild pain.

Many a time it may not be accompanied by any discomfort at all. Rarely, mild photophobia and lacrimation may occur.

Signs

Episcleritis occurs most commonly in the exposed zone of the eye and is generally recurrent in nature. Careful examination with slit-lamp and meticulous history is usually sufficient for the diagnosis of episcleritis. *Episcleritis is diagnosed clinically* by the presence of inflamed episcleral vessels, which typically radiate from the limbus, have a salmon pink colour in natural sunlight, can be moved over the deeper sclera with a cotton-tipped applicator and will blanch with topical phenylephrine 10%. On examination, two clinical types of episcleritis, simple and nodular may be recognised.

Simple episcleritis is characterised by sectorial (occasionally diffuse) inflammation of episclera. The engorged episcleral vessels are large and run in radial direction beneath the conjunctiva (Fig. 15.2A).

Nodular episcleritis is characterised by a pink or purple flat nodule surrounded by injection, usually situated 2–3 mm away from the limbus (Fig. 15.2B). The nodule is firm, tender, can be moved separately from the sclera and the overlying conjunctiva also moves freely.

Clinical course

Episcleritis runs a limited course of 10 days to 3 weeks and resolves spontaneously. The majority

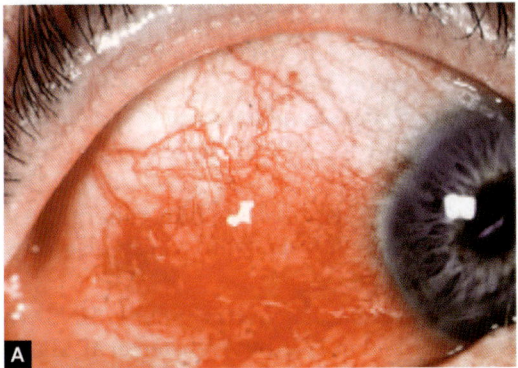
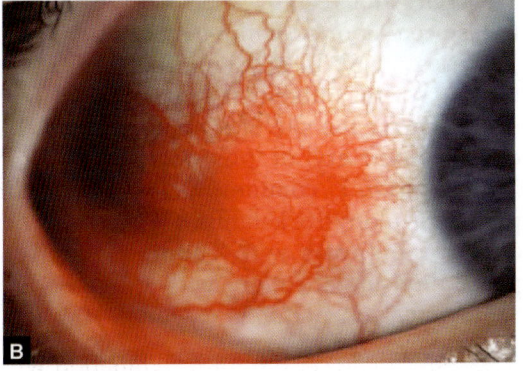

Fig. 15.2 *Episcleritis: A, Diffuse; B, Nodular.*

of patients with episcleritis recovers completely and has no residual changes. However, episcleritis can sometimes be associated with corneal involvement, uveitis, and glaucoma.

Recurrences are common and tend to occur in bouts. Rarely, a fleeting type of disease (*episcleritis periodica*) may occur.

DIFFERENTIAL DIAGNOSIS

Simple episcleritis may be confused rarely with conjunctivitis.

Nodular episcleritis may be confused with inflamed pinguecula, swelling and congestion due to foreign body lodged in bulbar conjunctiva and, very rarely with scleritis. The distinguishing features between episcleritis and scleritis are summarised in Table 15.1.

TREATMENT

Usually episcleritis is self-limiting, benign inflammation, whether treated or not, it will resolve in 10 to 21 days. Following medications are useful:

1. *Topical NSAIDs,* e.g. ketorolac 0.3% may be useful.

2. *Topical mild corticosteroid eyedrops,* e.g. fluorometholone or loteprednol instilled 2–3 hourly, render the eye more comfortable and resolve the episcleritis within a few days. However, prolonged use of topical corticosteroid should be avoided because of its potential side effects.

3. *Topical artificial tears,* e.g. 0.5% carboxymethylcellulose have soothing effect.

4. *Cold compresses* applied to the closed lids may offer symptomatic relief from ocular discomfort.

5. *Systemic nonsteroidal anti-inflammatory drugs.* Nodular episcleritis resolves slowly, responds slowly to topical therapy and often may require systemic medications. *NSAIDs,* such as flurbiprofen (300 mg OD), indomethacin (25 mg three times a day), or oxyphenbutazone, may be required in recurrent cases.

Table 15.1 *Distinguishing features between episcleritis and scleritis*

Episcleritis	Scleritis
Usually redness, irritations are the main presenting symptoms	Severe excruciating pain, which often wakes up the patient from sleep, is the main symptom
No or minimal tenderness	Moderate to severe tenderness
Congested vessels are bright red in colour and vessels can be moved easily with the help of cotton bud	Congested vessels are purple red in colour and vessels cannot be moved easily with cotton bud
Blanching of vessels occurrs with 10% phenylephrine	Blanching of vessels does not occur with 10% phenylephrine

SCLERITIS

GENERAL CONSIDERATIONS

Scleritis refers to a inflammation of the sclera proper. It is a comparatively serious disease which may cause visual impairment and even loss of the eye, if treated inadequately. Fortunately, its incidence is much less than that of episcleritis. It usually occurs in elderly patients (40–70 years) involving females more than the males.

ETIOLOGY

Overall about 50% cases of scleritis are associated with some systemic diseases, most common being connective tissue diseases.

Based on the etiology, scleritis may be labelled as below.

A. Idiopathic scleritis. Most of the time scleral inflammation starts with disturbances in equilibrium of scleral specific antigens towards collagen or glycosaminoglycans, the ground substances of sclera. This autoimmune reactions are usually idiopathic and mostly mediated by type IV delayed type of hypersensitivity reaction.

B. Scleritis associated with systemic rheumatic diseases or collagen vascular disorders. Rheumatoid arthritis is the most common systemic condition associated with scleritis. The incidence of rheumatoid arthritis in patients with scleritis ranges from 10 to 33%. Scleral inflammations in such systemic rheumatic disorders like Wegener's granulomatosis, polyarteritis nodosa, etc. are due to vasculitis which results from deposition of circulating immune complexes in superficial and deeper episcleral vessels.

C. Scleritis associated with other systemic disease. Metabolic disorders, like gout and thyrotoxicosis, have also been reported to be associated with scleritis.

Miscellaneous conditions. Vogt-Koyanagi-Harada syndrome, Behcet's disease and rosacea are also implicated in the etiology.

D. Infectious scleritis. Endogenous or exogenous spread of microorganism can give rise to scleral infections.

- *Neurotropic viruses,* like herpes viruses, can invade the scleral nerves and causes scleral inflammations.
- *Chronic staphylococcal and streptococcal infections* have also been known to cause infectious scleritis.
- *Granulomatous diseases,* like tuberculosis, syphilis, sarcoidosis, leprosy, can also cause scleritis.

E. Surgery-induced scleritis (SINS). SINS was first described in 1976 by Arensten et al. SINS is a rare but serious complication of ocular surgery. It has been reported with most types of ocular surgeries. SINS typically occurs after surgery as intense scleral inflammation associated with necrosis near the site of scleral incision. This dreaded variety of post-surgical scleral inflammation is commonly associated with peripheral ulcerative keratitis. The condition has a poor prognosis with chances of scleral perforation and, therefore, early diagnosis and rapid management is very essential.

Note. Common systemic associations of scleritis are depticted in Table 15.2.

PATHOLOGY

Histopathological changes are that of a chronic granulomatous disorder characterised by

Table 15.2 *Systemic associations of scleritis*
Scleritis may be associated with the following systemic diseases[3,4,7,10–13]:
• Rheumatoid arthritis
• Relapsing polychondritis
• Systemic lupus erythematosus and antiphospholipid syndrome
• Wegener's granulomatosis
• Polyarteritis nodosa
• Cogan syndrome
• Juvenile rheumatoid arthritis
• Ankylosing spondylitis
• Ulcerative colitis
• Polymyositis
• Sarcoidosis
• Syphilis
• Tuberculosis
• Herpes zoster ophthalmicus
• Acanthamoeba

fibrinoid necrosis, destruction of collagen together with infiltration by polymorphonuclear cells, lymphocytes, plasma cells and macrophages. The granuloma is surrounded by multinucleated epithelioid giant cells and old and new vessels, some of which may show evidence of vasculitis.

CLASSIFICATION

In general, scleritis can be classified as follows:

A. *Non-infectious scleritis*

I. *Anterior scleritis* (98%)

a. Non-necrotising scleritis (85%)

   1. Diffuse

   2. Nodular

b. Necrotising scleritis (13%)

   1. With inflammation

   2. Without inflammation (scleromalacia perforans)

II. *Posterior scleritis* (2%)

B. *Infectious scleritis*

NON-INFECTIOUS SCLERITIS

ANTERIOR SCLERITIS

CLINICAL FEATURES

Symptoms

- *Pain:* Patients with anterior scleritis presents with redness and pain. The onset is usually gradual, extending over several days. Patients typically complain of moderate to severe pain which is deep and boring in character and often wakes the patient early in the morning. Ocular pain radiates to the jaw and temple.
- *Redness* may be localized or diffuse.
- *Photophobia* and *lacrimation* may be mild to moderate.
- *Diminution of vision* may occur occasionally.

Signs

Scleral oedema and congestion of the deep episcleral plexus is the sine qua non of scleritis. Slit-lamp examination using red-free light is extremely helpful in determining the pattern and depth of episcleral vascular congestion and engorgement. In scleritis, the sclera assumes a violaceous hue in natural sunlight. It is very important to examine patients in daylight with the unaided eye to note the subtle colour differences of the vessels. Also inflamed scleral vessels have a crisscross pattern. They are adherent to the sclera and cannot be moved with a cotton-tipped applicator. Engorged scleral vessels cannot by blanched with 10% phenylephrine, whereas phenylephrine easily blanches engorged vessels in the superficial episcleral and conjunctival plexuses.

Tenderness of the globe is another important sign of sclera.

CLINICAL TYPES

Anterior scleritis is the most common form of scleral inflammation and can be broadly divided into non-necrotising scleritis and necrotising scleritis. Salient features of different clinical types of noninfectious anterior scleritis are described below.

I. Non-necrotising anterior scleritis

Non-necrotising scleritis is most common form of anterior scleritis, which can be further divided into nodular and diffuse varieties.

1. Non-necrotising anterior diffuse scleritis

It is the commonest variety, characterised by widespread inflammation involving a quadrant or more of the anterior sclera.

- Diffuse scleritis denotes diffuse involvement of scleral inflammation which is characterised by congestion of deeper episcleral plexuses and scleral oedema. Often it starts with sectoral congestion to involve the entire sclera. Involved area is raised and salmon pink to purple in colour (Fig. 15.3).
- Tenderness of globe of varying degree is almost always present.
- *Signs of uveal tract inflammation* in the form of anterior chamber reaction can be observed in some patients.
- *Corneal involvement*, e.g. corneal infiltrates, peripheral corneal ulcerations, thinning of peripheral cornea can also be seen in such patients.
- *Raised intraocular pressure* can occur from spread of the inflammation to the underlying trabecular meshwork.

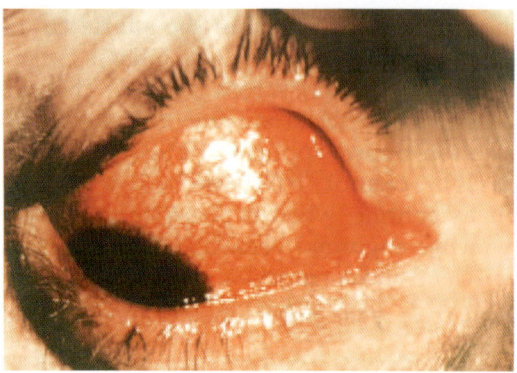

Fig. 15.3 *Non-necrotising anterior diffuse scleritis.*

2. Non-necrotising anterior nodular scleritis

Nodular anterior scleritis is characterised by a localised area of scleral oedema and congestion of the scleral vessels.

- *Scleral nodule* is deep red to purple in colour, immobile, tender to palpation and separated from the overlying episcleral tissue, which is elevated by the nodule.
- *Lack of necrosis within the nodule* and the localisation of inflammation within the borders of the nodule differentiate this form from necrotising anterior scleritis with inflammation.
- All of the vascular layers overlying the nodule are displaced forward.
- *Often there are one or two hard, purplish elevated immovable scleral nodules*, usually situated near the limbus (Fig. 15.4). Sometimes, multiple nodules may be present.[7–10] Rarely, the nodules are arranged in a ring around the limbus (*annular* scleritis).

II. Necrotising anterior scleritis

1. Anterior necrotising scleritis with inflammation

It is an acute severe form of scleritis characterised by intense localised inflammation associated with areas of infarction due to vasculitis (Fig. 15.5). It is the most severe of all the types and carries potential threat to visual loss. It is often seen in patients with rheumatoid arthritis. The condition is bilateral in 60% cases. The patient presents with severe pain and tenderness out of proportion to inflammatory signs. Examination reveals white, avascular areas of localised scleral oedema and congestion, edges of these lesions are more inflamed than the centre. The affected necrosed area is thinned out and sclera becomes transparent and ectatic with uveal tissue shining through it. It is usually associated with anterior uveitis. The condition has been found to be due to vasculitis secondary to immune complex depostion and results into shut down of the episcleral vascular bed. Because of the ectasia of the sclera, staphylomas are frequently seen. If not treated, the necrotising scleritis may spread to the equator and circumferentially and can involve the entire globe.

2. Anterior necrotising scleritis without inflammation

Van der Hoeve first used the term *scleromalacia perforans* in 1934 to describe this variety of scleritis. This specific entity typically occurs in elderly females usually suffering from long-standing rheumatoid arthritis. Though rare, the condition is vision-threatening. The condition is characterised by minimal signs of inflamma-

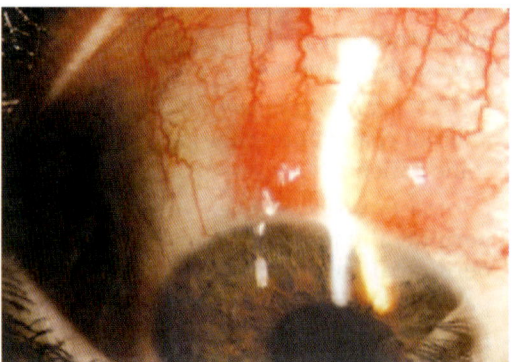

Fig. 15.4 *Non-necrotising anterior nodular scleritis.*

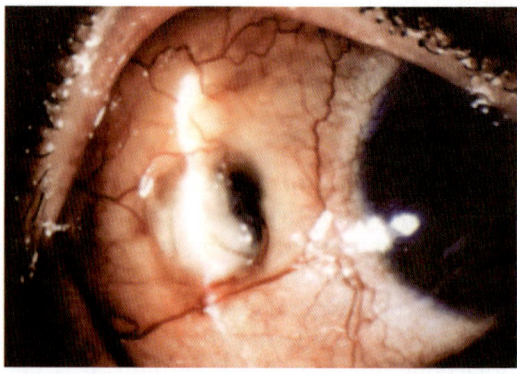

Fig. 15.5 *Anterior necrotising scleritis with inflammation.*

tion and absence of pain. In early phase of the disease, patient may present with blurred vision because of astigmatism due to thinning and distortion of the globe. It is characterised by development of yellowish patch of melting sclera (due to obliteration of arterial supply); which often together with the overlying episclera and conjunctiva completely separates from the surrounding normal sclera. This sequestrum of sclera becomes dead white in colour, which eventually absorbs leaving behind it a large punched out area of thin sclera through which the uveal tissue shines (Fig. 15.6). Staphylomas can develop during the course of scleral thinning. Peripheral corneal thinning is often seen, though direct corneal involvement is rare. Spontaneous perforation is rare but these eyes are prone to rupture with minimal trauma because of the extreme thinning of sclera.

Essential features of scleromalacia perforans are summarised below:

- Minimal or nil signs of inflammations
- No pain unlike other subtypes of scleritis.
- Most commonly associated with rheumatoid arthritis.

II. *POSTERIOR SCLERITIS*

CLINICAL PROFILE

Posterior scleritis is defined as an inflammation of the sclera, posterior to the ora serrata.

Posterior scleritis accounts for 2–12% of all scleritis cases. However, actual number of incidence of this clinical entity always underestimated

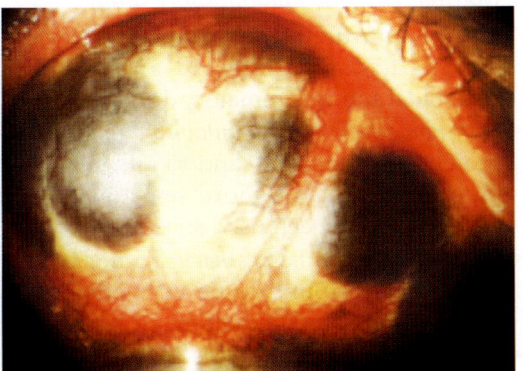

Fig. 15.6 *Anterior necrotising scleritis without inflammation (scleromalacia perforans).*

because of the lack of diagnosis and vivid presentation of posterior scleritis.

Patients with posterior scleritis present with pain, tenderness, proptosis, visual loss, and occasionally restricted motility, macular or paramacular oedema, choroidal folds, exudative retinal detachment, papilledema, and angle-closure glaucoma secondary to choroidal thickening.

Severe scleral inflammation of posterior segment can rarely manifest as proptosis or diplopia.

Posterior scleral thickening many a times may lead to altered refractive status—decrease in myopia or increase in hypermetropia and often mis-diagnosed as refractive errors.

Posterior scleritis may occur in association with anterior scleritis or may be isolated. Posterior scleritis, with anterior scleritis is relatively easy to diagnose.

ANCILLARY INVESTIGATIONS

1. *Fundus fluorescein angiogram.* Fundus fluorescein angiogram though aid in diagnosis of posterior scleritis, the findings of the angiogram are not specific for this clinical entity. Angiogram in a case of posterior scleritis with subretinal fluid shows pinhead leak in early phases and leakage of dyes in late phases of angiogram. Similar pattern of angiogram can also be encountered in Vogt-Koyanagi-Harada syndrome, sympathetic ophthalmia, punctate inner choroidopathy, choroidal malignant melanoma and various other conditions. However, it is helpful in cases with subretinal fluid in posterior pole, allowing one to differentiate multifocal leak central serous chorioretinopathy from posterior scleritis. The treatment of both of these conditions are paradoxical—while former need to avoid steroid, the later responds well to oral steroid. However, posterior scleritis presenting with choroidal folds, scleral mass does not show any leakage of dye and fundus fluorescein angiogram in such cases are of limited value.

2. *Ultrasonography.* Ultrasonography B scan of eye is considered as one of the most helpful ancillary investigation in diagnosis of posterior scleritis. Ultrasonography in a case of posterior scleritis shows thickening of the posterior coats of the eye and retrobulbar oedema. Widening of the subtenon spaces with T-sign often observed in cases with posterior scleritis (Fig. 15.7).

3. *Computed tomography and magnetic resonance imaging.* These modalities though rarely used for confirmation of the diagnosis, can aid to the diagnosis in difficult situations. An infiltration of extraocular muscles in the region of the posterior scleritis may lead to retraction of the lower lid in the upper gaze.[6,7,16,24]

DIFFERENTIAL DIAGNOSIS OF POSTERIOR SCLERITIS

The following conditions commonly mimick the posterior scleritis:

- Malignant melanoma
- Metastasis to choroid
- Choroidal haemangioma
- Uveal effusion syndrome
- Vogt-Koyanagi-Harada syndrome
- Central serous chorioretinopathy
- Cystoid macular oedema

The differential diagnosis of these clinical conditions is summarised in Table 15.3.

Complications

These are quite common with necrotising scleritis and include:

- Scleral thinning
- Stophylloma formation
- Scleral rupture/purforation
- Uveitis

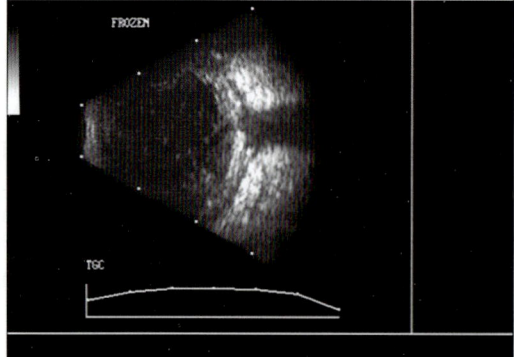

Fig. 15.7 *USG B-scan showing T-sign in a patient of posterior scleritis.*

- Sclerosing keratitis
- Keratolysis, complicated cataract
- Secondary glaucoma
- Phthisis bulbi

MANAGEMENT OF SCLERITIS

INVESTIGATIONS

Following laboratory studies may be helpful in identifying associated systemic diseases or in establishing the nature of immunologic reaction:

1. TLC, DLC and ESR.
2. Serum levels of complement (C3), immune complexes, rheumatoid factor, antinuclear antibodies and LE cells for an immunological survey.
3. FTA–ABS, VDRL for syphilis.
4. Serum uric acid for gout.
5. Urine analysis.
6. Mantoux test.
7. X-rays of chest, paranasal sinuses, sacroiliac joint and orbit (to rule out foreign body especially in patients with nodular scleritis).

TREATMENT

The primary aim of the treatment of scleral inflammation is to control the inflammatory process to relieve the symptoms and thereby reduce the damage to the eye. However, the effective management of a case of scleral inflammation involves timely diagnosis, prevention of complications and identification of underlying systemic or local cause, if any.

Medical treatment

1. Nonsteroidal anti-inflammatory drugs

Anterior non-necrotising scleritis readily responds to topical steroid and systemic nonsteroidal anti-inflammatory drugs (NSAIDs).

- *Both non-selective COX inhibitors* (e.g. flurbiprofen, indomethacin, and to a lesser extent ibuprofen) and the more selective COX-2 inhibitors have been used successfully.
- *Sustained-release indomethacin* 75 mg twice a day has been found to be very effective in controlling the inflammation.
- *However, prolonged use of NSAIDs* should be avoided in view of their significant side effect on long-term use.

Table 15.3 *Differential diagnosis of posterior scleritis*

Parameters of differentiation	Posterior scleritis	Malignant melanoma	Metastasis to choroid	Choroidal haemangioma
Age	Middle age, can occur in youngs	Old age group	Middle aged and older group	Middle aged and older group
Laterality	Unilateral	Unilateral	Unilateral	Unilateral
Pain	Moderate to severe	Rare	Rare	Rare
External appearance	Can present with anterior scleritis	Can present with dilated episcleral vessels.	Normal	Normal
Inflammation in anterior chamber and anterior vitreous	Seen	No	No	No
Posterior pole mass	Greyish-orange-coloured, associated with choroidal/retinal striae	Dark pigmented elevated ovoid mass lesion, can be amelanotic	Yellowish white mass, no choroidal/retinal striae seen	Well defined red orange, slightly elevated dome-shaped lesion usually located at the posterior pole. Sometimes associated with SRF
Fundus fluorescein angiogram	Multiple pinhead leak which gradually show pooling of dyes	Mottled hyper-fluorescence in the early phase with increased staining of the mass lesion in the late phase of the angiogram. Larger melanomas may show double circulation—simultaneous filling up of the normal retinal vessels and the tumour vessels.	Multiple small leaks	Early stippled hyperfluorescence with late leakage of the dye and staining of the tumour.
Ultrasonography	Thickening of the posterior sclera, retrobulbar oedema,	Choroidal mass with low internal activity and choroidal excavation	Moderately high reflectivity	High internal reflectivity
Age	Middle aged	20–50 years	30–50 years	Middle to older age
Laterality	Bilateral	Bilateral	Unilateral	Unilateral
Pain	Minimal	No	No	No
External appearance	Congestion	Ciliary congestion	Normal	Normal

(Contd.)

Table 15.3 *Differential diagnosis of posterior scleritis (Contd.)*

Parameters of differentiation	Posterior scleritis	Malignant melanoma	Metastasis to choroid	Choroidal haemangioma
Inflammation in anterior chamber and anterior vitreous Clinical findings in posterior pole	Can be seen	Present	No	No
Fundus fluorescein angiogram		Multiple pinhead leaks which gradually enlarges and show placoid pooling	Usually single leak which shows ink blot or smoke stock pattern.	Shows characteristic flower petal appearance.
Ultrasonography	Choroidal detachment with thickening	Shows choroidal thickening	Not contributory	Not contributory

2. Corticosteroids

Corticosteroids are helpful in patients not responding to COX-inhibitors or those with posterior or necrotising disease.

Oral corticosteroids. A starting dose of 1 mg/kg/day is standard with weekly reduction by 10 mg/week until a dose of 40 mg/day is reached. After this dose is reached, the rate of reduction is individualized, according to the clinical findings and patients' response but is in the order of 5 mg/week until cessation or an acceptable maintenance dose is reached.

Intravenous corticosteroids are sometimes needed in patients who need aggressive management of the scleral inflammation, for example, in cases with threatened scleral or corneal perforation in necrotising scleritis, which requires a rapid control of the inflammation. The most commonly used drug is methylprednisolone. The usual dosage is 500 mg to 1 gm intravenous infusion with 0.9% normal saline or sodium lactate solution over 30 to 60 minutes daily for 3 consecutive days, followed by high dose of oral corticosteroids. Caution should be taken as intravenous methylprednisolone can cause cardiac arrhythmias and cardiovascular collapse. Intravenous methylprednisolone is usually followed by high dose oral steroid or immunosuppressive agent.

Periocular application of steroid delivers the drug to the desired site and reduces the chances of side effects associated with systemically administered corticosteroid. It can be administered by subconjunctival or subtenon route. However, the role of periocular steroid in scleritis is controversial.

Note. Subconjunctival steroids are contraindicated because they may lead to scleral thinning and perforation.

3. Immunosuppressive drugs

Necrotizing scleritis, particularly associated with autoimmune diseases is difficult to treat and almost always requires systemic immunosuppressive therapy, not only for ocular involvement, also for life-threatening systemic complications. For example, prompt and effective immunosuppression is required to control the necrotising scleritis associated with systemic vasculitis like Wegener's granulomatosis because mortality is higher in this group of patients because of the systemic complications. This group of patients also requires a consultation with rheumatologist for their systemic ailments.

Indications for immunosuppressive therapy in scleral inflammation
- Anterior necrotizing scleritis
- Posterior scleritis
- Scleritis associated with a systemic disease

Various immunosuppressants have been tried for treatment of scleritis and these include anti-metabolites (methotrexate, azathioprine, and mycophenolate mofetil), alkylating agents (chlorambucil and cyclophosphamide), T cell inhibitors (cyclosporine and tacrolimus). Newer biological agents, like TNF-α inhibitors (infliximab or adalimumab), and rituximab, are reported to be used for the treatment of scleritis.

Methotrexate is commonly used to treat scleritis not responding to oral corticosteroid and less sever anterior necrotising scleritis with inflammation. Often the drug is used as a first-line treatment in patients in whom oral steroid cannot be started because of systemic ailments. Among steroid sparing immunosuppressives, methotrexate has gained the most widespread usage due to its relatively safe profile. Methotrexate, a folic acid analog, inhibits the enzyme dihydrofolate reductase and thus the production of thymidylate, which is essential for DNA replication. This results in the inhibition of rapidly dividing cells, including leucocytes. The drug is used with or without a short course of oral steroid in tapering dosage. Dosage of methotrexate is 0.1–0.5 mg/kg/week; low dose therapy is started at a dose of 7.5 mg/week and it can be increased up to 25 mg/week. Generally, it is given orally once a week. It has been observed that methotrexate immunosuppressive therapy is moderately effective. The drug takes months to achieve adequate tissue concentration for the therapeutic success. Severe side effects, such as hepatotoxicity, cytopenias, and interstitial pneumonia, are not uncommon.

Azathioprine is another antimetabolite, which is often used as steroid-sparing immuno-suppressives. Pasadhika et al have evaluated the use of this drug in scleritis patients. They used oral azathioprine in 27 eyes of 16 patients with scleritis and concluded that the azathioprine, as a steroid-sparing immunosuppressive mono-therapy, is moderately effective. In their study, sustained control of inflammation was observed in 29.9% of patients after tapering prednisone to less than 5 mg/day in one year.

Mycophenolate mofetil is an immuno-suppressive agent that selectively inhibits the proliferation of lymphocytes sparing other proliferating cells. Mycophenolate mofetil has been also used for the management of scleritis. However, the drug alone is not sufficient in control of acute scleritis cases and require additional immunosuppressants. The drug can be used as maintenance therapy in controlled scleral inflammations.

Treatment of scleritis associated with necrotising systemic vasculitis

In such cases, treatment should be prompt and effective. Treatment in such patients should be guided both by the ophthalmic response and control of the underlying disease. Most of the time, immunosuppressives are required in such cases.

Cyclophosphamide is an effective immuno-suppressive drug used in patients with necrotising scleritis associated with systemic vasculitis like Wegener's granulomatosis, relapsing polychondritis, polyarteritis nodosa, etc. Antineutrophil cytoplasmic antibody test is a useful laboratory parameter to monitor therapeutic response in patients with Wegener's granulomatosis. Cyclophosphamide in a dose of 100 mg per day (2 mg/kg/day) orally and tapered monthly, should be the first choice in treating patients with associated potentially lethal vasculitic diseases.

Oral steroids. Concomitant administration of prednisone at a dose of 1 mg/kg/day may be needed. Oral corticosteroids can usually be tapered and often discontinued over the first 6–12 weeks of cyclophosphamide therapy. The patient should be instructed to drink copious amounts of fluid to prevent haemorrhagic cystitis.

In severe and non-responsive cases, infusion of 500 mg of cyclophosphamide (given over 1 to 2 hours) is often required. Because of potential life-threatening complications, it should be administered under the supervision of a rheumatologist.

Other immunosuppressive agents, including methotrexate, azathioprine, cyclosporine, and newer agents, like biologicals, have been successfully used for the treatment of necrotising systemic vasculitis, but reports available are based on small case series.[6,18,20]

Biologicals, a group of drugs which are directed mainly against specific cytokines or their receptors, have been tried by various authors with promising results. However, most of these agents are not widely used in our country because of their high price and risks of life-threatening granulomatous infections.

Surgical treatment

Surgical treatment in the form of scleral patch graft may be required to preserve integrity of the globe in extensive scleral melt and thinning.

INFECTIOUS SCLERAL INFLAMMATION

Infectious scleritis accounts for 5–10% of all cases of scleritis.
- Scleritis with purulent exudates or infiltrates (Fig. 15.8) should raise the suspicion of an infectious etiology.
- Formations of granulomas or fistulas, painful nodules, conjunctival and scleral ulcers are often seen in infectious scleral inflammations.

ETIOLOGY

Infectious scleritis is a rare but devastating causes of scleral inflammation. Most of the literature reported *Pseudomonas aeruginosa* as the most common cause of infectious scleritis. Infectious scleritis can be endogenous or exogenous in origin.
- *Exogenous spread*. It can be secondary to corneal infection, accidental injury or surgical procedures. McCluskey et al in their series of 97 cases found that herpes zoster virus is the most common causes of infectious scleritis. Association of viruses in infectious scleritis has been reported by various authors, most commonly after pterygium excisions.
- *Endogenous spread* of *bacteria* (staphylococci, *H. influenzae, Treponema pallidum, M. tuber-culosis*); *fungi* (*Aspergillus*); *viruses* (Herpes simplex or H. zoster) or *parasites* (Toxocara, Toxoplasma, Onchocerca) is reported to cause infective scleritis.
- *Spreads of infection from adjacent structures*. In rare instances, infections of adjacent tissues, like the conjunctiva, cornea, may involve the sclera by contiguous spread.

- *In chronic cases*, foreign body must be ruled out.

Spread of infection of cornea: Keratoscleritis

Corneal infections can spread to the adjacent sclera and can cause keratoscleritis. Bacterial infections of cornea are most common to spread, but can be seen infections by virus, fungus and parasite too. Patients on long-term immuno-suppressant or patients with acquired immune deficiency syndrome are more prone to fulminent form of such keratoscleritis.

Reported causes of keratoscleritis or spread of corneal infection to sclera.
- *Pseudomonas aeruginosa*
- *Staphylococcus aureus*
- *Streptococcus pneumoniae*
- *Mycobacterium chelonei*
- Herpes simplex
- Herpes zoster
- Aspergillus
- Acremonium
- Acanthamoeba

Infectious scleritis after surgical intervention

1. *Post-scleral buckling surgery.* Scleral infections associated with scleral buckle are rare and the clinical presentations are varying. The patients complain of varying degree of pain and discomfort. Subconjunctival abscess, purulent discharge, conjunctival granulomas can be seen. Extruded buckle can be seen in cases of scleral infection. The most common organisms causing scleral buckle infection are coagulase-positive and coagulase-negative staphylococci species, which account for 70 to 90% of all such infections.

Various organisms have been reported to cause such infections and include *Staphylococcus, Pseudomonas, Proteus*, atypical *Mycobacterium, Corynebacteria* and fungi.

2. *Post-pterygium excision.* Scleral infections after pterygium excision are usually associated with the application of mitomycin-C or β-irradiation. However, infective scleritis were reported following bare sclera technique without these adjunctive therapies also. *Pseudomonas aeruginosa* is the most common organism found in such cases.

CLINICAL PROFILE

One must be careful while treating the infectious scleritis, as diagnosis of such cases is difficult and presentations are same as immune-mediated scleritis.While the oral steroid and immunosuppressives are known to cause rapid resolution of the immune-mediated scleritis, it worsens or deteriorates infectious scleritis.

Clinical profile of some forms of infectious scleritis is described briefly.

Pyogenic bacterial scleritis

Most common cause of acute bacterior infectious scleritis is *Pseudomonas aeruginosa*.

- *Infectious scleritis accounts for 5–10% of all cases.*
- *In the early stage,* diagnosis becomes difficult as presentation is similar to as non-infectious scleritis.
- *Scleritis with purulent exudates* (Fig. 15.8) or infiltrates should raise the suspicion of an infectious etiology.
- *Formation of fistulae, painful nodules, conjunctival and scleral ulcers* are usually the signs of infectious scleritis.

Herpetic scleritis

Herpes zoster. Scleral inflammations related to herpes zoster are caused by infections or reactivation of latent varicella zoster viruses.

Though rare, sclera can be involved in primary varicella zoster and in herpes zoster ophthalmicus and usually associated with some form of corneal involvement. Involvement of the vessels with ischaemia is common.

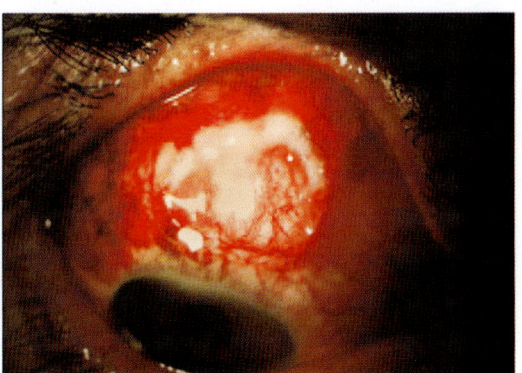

Fig. 15.8 *Infectious scleritis.*

Scleral infection in herpes simplex is rare and most of the times associated with milder inflammation of the perilimbal sclera. Scleritis and episcleritis occur in 8% of the cases with herpes zoster ophthalmicus.

Syphilitic scleritis

Syphilitic scleritis is rare and most of the time inflammation is restricted to episclera in such patients. Often they are associated with inter-stitial keratitis. Though the exact pathogenesis of syphilitic scleritis is not clear, the positive serological tests in patients, response to anti-microbial therapy, absence of collagen vascular diseases indicates direct role of spirochete.

Mycobacterium tuberculosis scleritis

Mycobacterium tuberculosis-related scleritis are thought to be due to hypersensitivity reaction to mycobacterial protein rather than direct role of the microorganism. Most of the time the scleritis is anterior nodular subtypes. Often multiple scleral nodules are seen.

DIAGNOSIS

Clinical diagnosis of infectious scleritis is made from following features:

- Scleritis with purulent exudates or infiltrates
- Scleritis associated with scleral or conjunctival ulcers
- Scleritis associated with visible pus points or scleral abscesses
- Scleritis associated with hypopyon

Obtaining a specimen for diagnosis. Usually specimens from scleritis with ulcerative lesions are collected by scrapping with the help of a surgical blade (no 15 blade attached to Bard Parker handle). This procedure can be carried out in out-patient department under topical anaesthesia. However, in scleritis with scleral abscesses, nodular scleral nodules with visible pus points the specimens are collected from base of the lesions after dissecting conjunctiva and deroofing of the lesions. Such procedures are better to be carried under peribulbar anaesthesia in operating room and surgeon must be ready to tackle the accidental inadvertent perforation while collecting the sample.

Scleral biopsy. Fungal causes of infectious scleritis are most difficult to diagnose because of their varied clinical picture and often scleral biopsy is required to confirm the diagnosis in such cases.

TREATMENT

Treatment of the infectious scleritis is frustrating and cumbersome. Microbial invasion of the sclera is difficult to treat and eradicate becuase of the poor penetration of various antimicrobial agents into avascular sclera.

- Most of the time, diagnosis is delayed and patients are put on topical and oral steroids which worsen the infective scleritis.
- *Antimicrobial therapy*, both with topical and oral agents, is required in an aggressive manner.
- *Surgical debridement* is found useful by debulking the infected scleral tissue and also facilitating the effect of antibiotics.

BIBLIOGRAPHY

1. Agrawal R, Lavric A, Restori M, Pavesio C, Sagoo MS. Nodular posterior scleritis: Clinico-Sonographic Characteristics and Proposed Diagnostic Criteria Retina, 2015.
2. Axmann S, Ebneter A, Zinkernagel MS. Imaging of the sclera in patients with scleritis and episcleritis using anterior segment optical coherence tomography. Ocul Immunol Inflamm 2015;1–6.
3. Goldstein DA, Patel SS, Tessler HH. Episcleritis and scleritis. In: Yanoff M, Duker JS, eds. Ophthalmology, 4th ed. St. Louis, MO: Mosby Elsevier; 2013:chap 4.11
4. González-López JJ, Lavric A, Dutta Majumder P, Bansal N, Biswas J, Pavesio C, et al. Bilateral Posterior Scleritis: Analysis of 18 Cases from a Large Cohort of Posterior Scleritis. Ocul Immunol Inflamm 2015;1–8.
5. Jabs, Douglas A, Mudun, Abdulbaki, Dunn, J.P, Marsh, Marta J. "Episcleritis and scleritis: clinical features and treatment results". Am J Ophthalmol 2000;130(4):469–476.
6. McGavin DD, Williamson J, Forrester JV, Foulds WS, Buchanan WW, Dick WC, Lee P, MacSween RN, Whaley K. "Episcleritis and scleritis. A study of their clinical manifestations and association with rheumatoid arthritis". Br J Ophthalmol 1976;60(3):192–226.
7. Sainz de la Maza M, Foster CS, Jabbur NS. Scleritis associated with systemic vasculitic diseases. Ophthalmology 1995;102(4):687–92.
8. Sainz de la Maza M, Tauber J, Foster CS. Scleral grafting for necrotizing scleritis. Ophthalmology 1989;96(3):306–10.
9. Sainz de la Maza, M; Jabbur, NS; Foster, CS. "Severity of scleritis and episcleritis." Ophthalmology 1994;101(2):389–96.
10. Watson P. Diseases of the sclera and episclera. In: Tasman W, Jaeger EA, eds. Duane's Ophthalmology 15th ed. Philadelphia, Lippincott Williams & Wilkins; 2009:chap 23.
11. Watson PG, Hayreh SS. Scleritis and episcleritis. Br J Ophthalmol 1976;60:163–192.
12. Watson PG. Episcleritis. Current Ocular Therapy. 5th ed. 809.
13. Yadav S, Rawal G. Tubercular Nodular Episcleritis: A Case Report. J Clin Diagn Res 2015;9(8):ND01-2.

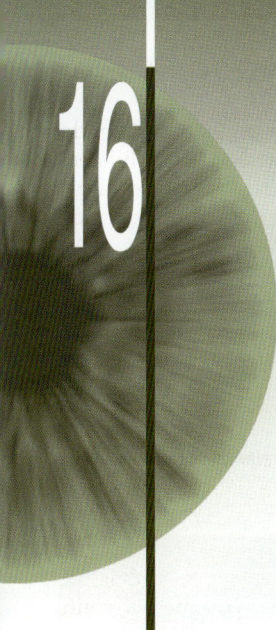

STAPHYLOMAS AND MISCELLANEOUS SCLERAL CONDITIONS

STAPHYLOMAS

- Anterior staphyloma
- Intercalary staphyloma
- Ciliary staphyloma
- Equatorial staphyloma
- Posterior staphyloma

MISCELLANEOUS SCLERA CONDITIONS

- Blue sclera
- Metabolic deposits in sclera
- Scleral pigmentations
- Scleral tumours
  - Secondary tumours

STAPHYLOMAS

Staphyloma refers to a localised bulging of weak and thin outer tunic of the eyeball (cornea or sclera), lined by uveal tissue which shines through the thinned out fibrous coat.

Types

Anatomically, it can be divided into anterior, intercalary, ciliary, equatorial and posterior staphyloma (Fig. 16.1).

1. *Anterior staphyloma.* An ectasia of pseudo-cornea (the scar formed from organised exudates and fibrous tissue covered with epithelium) which results after total sloughing of cornea, with iris plastered behind it is called *anterior staphyloma* (Figs 16.2A and B).

2. *Intercalary staphyloma.* It is the name given to the localised bulge in limbal area lined by root of iris (Figs 16.1A and 16.3).

- It results due to ectasia of weak scar tissue formed at the limbus, following healing of a perforating injury or a peripheral corneal ulcer.
- *Secondary angle closure glaucoma,* may cause progression of bulge if not treated.

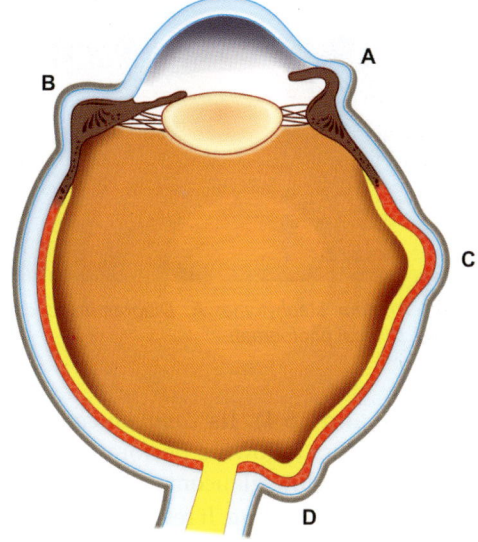

Fig. 16.1 *Staphylomas (diagrammatic depiction): A, Intercalary; B, Ciliary; C, Equatorial; D, Posterior.*

- *Defective vision* occurs due to marked corneal astigmatism.

  Treatment consists of localised staphylectomy under heavy doses of oral steroids.

3. *Ciliary staphyloma.* As the name implies, it is the bulge of weak sclera lined by ciliary body. It occurs about 2–3 mm away from the limbus

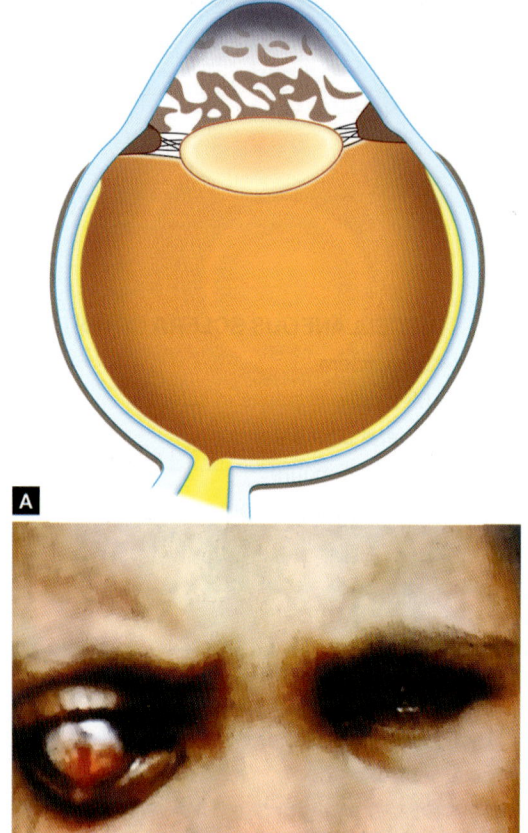

A

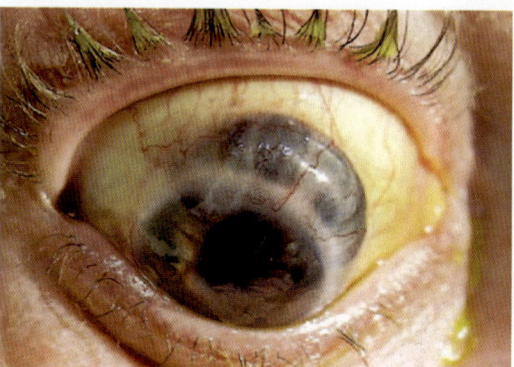

Fig. 16.3 *Intercalary staphyloma.*

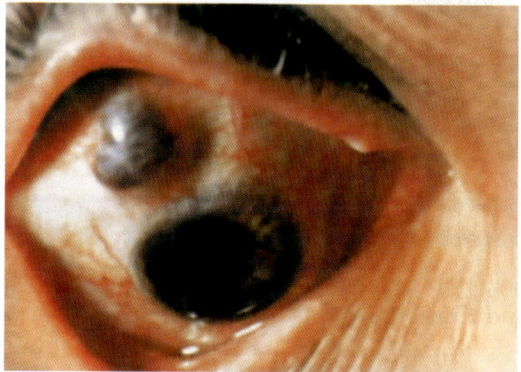

Fig. 16.4 *Ciliary staphyloma.*

B

Fig. 16.2 *Anterior staphyloma: A, Diagrammatic cross-section; B, Clinical photograph.*

(Figs 16.1B and 16.4). Its *common causes* are thinning of sclera following perforating injury, scleritis and absolute glaucoma.

4. *Equatorial staphyloma*. It results due to bulge of sclera lined by the choroid in the equatorial region (Fig. 16.1C). Its causes are scleritis and degeneration of sclera in pathological myopia. It occurs more commonly at the regions of sclera which are perforated by vortex veins.

5. *Posterior staphyloma*. It refers to bulge of weak sclera lined by the choroid behind the equator (Fig. 16.1D). Here again the *common causes* are pathological myopia, posterior scleritis and perforating injuries. It is diagnosed on ophthalmoscopy. The area is excavated with

retinal vessels dipping in it (just like marked cupping of optic disc in glaucoma) (Fig. 16.5). Its floor is focussed with minus lenses in ophthalmoscope as compared to its margins.

MISCELLANEOUS SCLERAL CONDITIONS

BLUE SCLERA

It is an asymptomatic condition characterised by marked, generalised blue discolouration of sclera due to thinning (Fig. 16.6).

Causes

Blue ling occur due to of underlying ciliary bud and choroid through the transparant sclera. Blue sclera is typically associated with osteogenesis imperfecta (Paget's disease). Its other causes are Marfan's syndrome, Ehlers-Danlos syndrome,

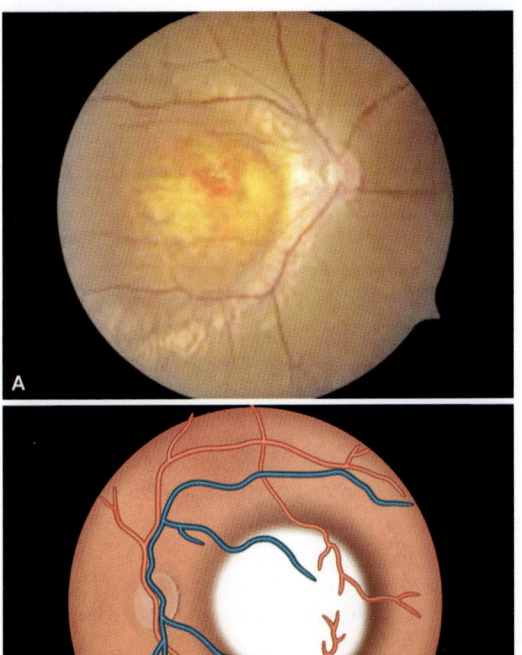

Fig. 16.5 *Fundus photograph (A) and diagrammatic depiction (B) of excavation of retinal tissue and blood vessels in posterior staphyloma.*

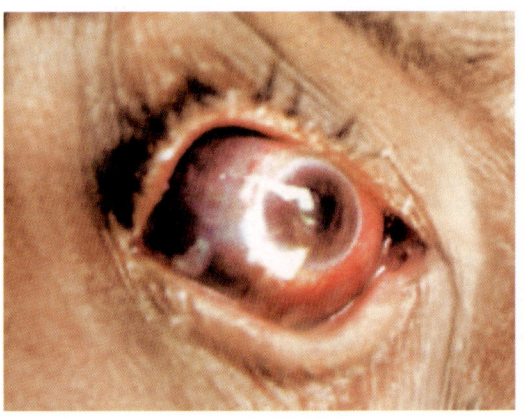

Fig. 16.6 *Blue sclera.*

pseudoxanthoma elasticum alkaptonuria, acid phosphatase deficiency, Al Gazali Sabrinathan Nair syndrome, Diagmond-Blackfan anaemia, buphthalmos, high myopia and healed scleritis.

METABOLIC DEPOSITS IN SCLERA

Following metabolic deposits may occur in the sclera:

- *Uric acid* deposits may occur in gaut.
- *Cystine crystals* may be deposited in the sclera in patients with cystinosis.
- *Alkaptonuria*, a condition associated with altered metabolism of homogenetic acid, can lead to pigmentary deposits in sclera.
- *Calcium deposits*, causing whitish plaques, may occur in conditions with high levels of circulating calcium.
- *Lipid deposits* may occur in disorders of fat metabolism, giving the sclera a yellowish appearance.
- *Bilirubin deposits* in patients with jaundice, is the commonest known scleral deposits.
- *Amyloid deposition* may occur following severe inflammations of sclera.

SCLERAL PIGMENTATIONS

Pigmented abnormalities of sclera include:

Blue sclera, described above, is the commonest pigmented abnormality of sclera, occurring due to shining of underlying uveal tissue through the thinned sclera.

Melanotic pigmentation can be seen as below:

- Normally in pigmented races. This usually appears after birth and so is not a congenital condition. Often small cuffs of pigmentation are seen surrounding the entry point of vessels.
- The pigmentation occurring along the neural, vascular bundle is known as *Axenfeld's loop*.
- *Pigmentation due to malignant melanoma* of uveal tissue is not uncommon.

SCLERAL TUMOURS

Primary tumours of sclera are not known.

Secondary tumours may occur due to:

- *Distant metastasis* from carcinoma of breast or lung in late stage.
- *Local spread* from intraocular tumour sush as retinoblastoma and uveal melanoma.

BIBLIOGRAPHY

1. Caldwell JB, Sears ML, Gilman M. Bilateral peri-papillarystaphyloma with normal vision. Am J Ophthalmol 1971;71(1 Pt 2):423–5.
2. Curtin BJ, Karlin DB. Axial length measurements and fundus changes of the myopic eye. I. The posterior fundus. Trans Am Ophthalmol Soc 1970;68:312–34.
3. Giunta C, Randolph A, Steinmann B. Mutation analysis of the PLOD1 gene: an efficient multistep approach to the molecular diagnosis of the kyphoscoliotic type of Ehlers-Danlos syndrome (EDS VIA). Mol Genet Metab 2005; 86(1–2):269–76.
4. Goldstein D, Tessler H. Episcleritis, scleritis, and other scleral disorders. In: Yarnoff M, Duiker J editor. Ophthalmology 2nd ed St Louis: Mosby; 2007; p. 511–9.
5. Haaga JR, Boll D. CT and MRI of the whole body. Mosby. (2009) ISBN:0323053750.
6. Karlin DB, Curtin BJ. Peripheral chorioretinal lesions and axial length of the myopic eye. Am J Ophthalmol 1976;81(5):625–35.
7. Kral K, Svarc D. Contractile peripapillary staphyloma. Am J Ophthalmol 1971;71(5):1090-2.
8. Kuhn F, Halda T, Witherspoon D. Sclera. In: Roy F editors. Ocular Differential Diagnosis, 6th ed. Baltimore: Williams & Wilkins; 1997; p.265–75.
9. Mafee MF, Valvassori GE, Becker M. Imaging of the head and neck. George Thieme Verlag. (2004) ISBN:1588900096.
10. Osborne DR, Foulks GN. Computed tomographic analysis of deformity and dimensional changes in the eyeball. Radiology 1984; 153(3):669–74
11. Paller A, Mancini A. Hurwitz Clinical Pediatric Dermatology, 3rd ed. Philadelphia: Elsevier Saunders; 2006;133–4.
12. Pemberton JW, Freeman HM, Schepens CL. Familial retinal detachment and the Ehlers-Danlos syndrome. Arch Ophthalmol 1966; 76(6):817–24.
13. Phillips CI, Dobbie JG. Posterior staphyloma and retnal detachment. Am J Ophthalmol 1963 55:332-5.
14. Riise D. Visual field defects in optic disc malformation with ectasia of the fundus. Acta Ophthalmol (Copenh) 1966;44(6):906–18.
15. Siam A. Macular hole with central retinal detachment in high myopia with posterior staphyloma. Br J Ophthalmol. 1969;53(1):62–63.
16. Sillence D, Butler B, Latham M, Barlow K. Natural history of blue sclerae in osteogenesis imperfecta. Am J Med Genet 1993;45(2):183–6.
17. Steiner R, Pepin M, Byers P. (2005). Osteogenesis imperfecta. Retrieved February 20, 2008, from http://www.ncbi.nlm.nih.gov/books/bv.fcgi?highlight = presentation, osteogenesis imperfect
18. Streeten BW. Development of the human retinal pigment epithelium and the posterior segment. Arch Ophthalmol 1969;81(3):383–94.
19. Sugar HS, Beckman H. Peripapillarystaphyloma with respiratory pulsation. Am J Ophthalmol 1969;68(5):895–7.
20. Ts'o MO, Friedman E. The retinal pigment epithelium, Growth and development. Arch Ophthalmol 1968;80(2):214–6.
21. Wenstrup RJ, Murad S, Pinnell SR. Ehlers-Danlos syndrome type VI: clinical manifestations of collagen lysyl hydroxylase deficiency. J Pediatr. 1989;115(3):405–9.
22. Wise JB, MacLean AL, Gass JD. Contractile peri-papillary staphyloma. Arch Ophthalmol 1966; 75(5):626–30.

Index